INNOVATIONS IN CLINICAL PRACTICE: A SOURCE BOOK

Volume 5

Edited by
PETER A. KELLER, PhD
LAWRENCE G. RITT, PhD

PROFESSIONAL RESOURCE EXCHANGE, INC.
P.O. Box 15560
Sarasota, Florida 34277-1560

Looseleaf Edition ISBN: 0-943158-17-6
Hardbound Edition ISBN: 0-943158-16-8
Set (Vols. 1, 2, 3, 4, & 5) Looseleaf Edition ISBN: 0-943158-04-4
Set (Vols. 1, 2, 3, 4, & 5) Hardbound Edition ISBN: 0-943158-05-2
ISSN 0737-125x

Printed in the United States of America

by

McNaughton & Gunn Lithographers

PREFACE

This volume marks half a decade in our *Innovations in Clinical Practice: A Source Book* series. Over the 5 years nearly 200 authors have contributed to make the *Innovations* series a unique resource for practicing mental health clinicians. Although each volume follows the same basic format, no single volume in the series is comprehensive or designed around a particular theme. We continue to view this as a wide ranging clinician resource series. If there exists a single theme, it is one of sharing information among clinicians. We are proud of the role that we have played in disseminating so much information.

Over the years many of our readers have told us about the value of the *Innovations* series in their practice. They note that *Innovations* has become a ready resource to which they can turn for a wide range of materials. One of our criteria for including contributions in the series is that they be practical. Many readers have told us they rely heavily on the series for up-to-date clinical information.

We believe that our series has been successful and now look forward to another half decade of sharing resources among practicing clinicians. To help us in this task, we invite our readers to call or write and let us know about your comments, criticisms, and suggestions. What can we do to make the *Innovations* series even better? What ideas do you have for a contribution?

We would like to thank the many individuals who have contributed their efforts toward the quality of this volume. Various reviewers and colleagues have made valuable suggestions which contributed directly to the quality of the fifth volume, and we are very appreciative of their efforts. However, we as editors must assume ultimate responsibility for the contents.

Finally, it is important to acknowledge the essential efforts of many people in the production of the fifth *Innovations* volume. These include Debbie Worthington, Eva Green, Judy Warinner, and Janet Nunez for their many hours of work on the manuscripts. Without their diligence, this volume would not be a reality. Again, we would also like to thank our spouses, Rhonda Keller and Judy Ritt, for their valued suggestions and support. Making *Innovations in Clinical Practice* an annual reality is a task which requires considerable support from our families, and we are grateful for their willingness to tolerate our efforts.

CONTINUING EDUCATION

The Professional Resource Exchange is approved by the American Psychological Association as a continuing education sponsor, and credits can be obtained by readers required to participate in such programs, as well as those who wish to validate their learning. Interested readers are referred to the material at the back of this volume to learn how to obtain home study continuing education credits through the *Innovations in Clinical Practice* series. This service provides an economical means of obtaining continuing education credits while acquiring relevant clinical knowledge. Readers have been consistently positive about the experience of obtaining CE credits through the series.

AN INVITATION TO SUBMIT A CONTRIBUTION

We are currently soliciting contributions for future volumes in the *Innovations* series as well as seeking ideas for other publications or ways to share information among practitioners. If you are doing something innovative in your work, let us hear from you. Specific guidelines for contributors are included at the end of this volume. Please contact us if you would like more detailed information.

COPYRIGHT POLICY

Most of the material in this volume may be duplicated. You may photocopy materials (such as office forms and instruments) or reproduce them for use in your practice or share contributions with your students in the classroom. For materials on which the Professional Resource Exchange holds the copyright, no further permission is required for noncommercial professional or educational use. However, unauthorized duplication or publication for resale or large scale distribution of any material in this volume is expressly prohibited.

Any material which you duplicate from this volume (with the exception mentioned below) must be acknowledged as having been reprinted from this volume and must note that copyright is held by the Professional Resource Exchange, Inc. The format and exact wording required in the acknowledgment are shown on the copyright page of this volume. The only exception to this policy is that clinical and office forms (not instruments) for use with clients may be reprinted without including the acknowledgment mentioned above.

There are exceptions to our liberal copyright policy. We do not hold copyright on some of the materials included in this volume and, therefore, cannot grant permission to freely duplicate those materials. When copyright is held by another publisher or author, such copyright is noted on the appropriate page of the contribution. Unless otherwise noted in the credit and copyright citation, any reproduction or duplication of these materials is strictly and expressly forbidden without the consent of the copyright holder.

Peter A. Keller
Lawrence G. Ritt

Professional Resource Exchange, Inc.
Post Office Box 15560
Sarasota, FL 34277-1560

TABLE OF CONTENTS

PREFACE — iii

INTRODUCTION TO THE VOLUME — 1

SECTION I: CLINICAL ISSUES AND APPLICATIONS

INTRODUCTION TO SECTION I — 3

THE CLINICAL ASSESSMENT OF ANOREXIA NERVOSA
AND BULIMIA NERVOSA
David M. Garner and Ron Davis — 5

THE FUNDAMENTALS OF PSYCHOTHERAPY FOR
ANOREXIA NERVOSA AND BULIMIA NERVOSA
David M. Garner and Paul Isaacs — 29

ERICKSONIAN APPROACHES TO STRATEGIC HYPNOTHERAPY
Andrew P. Musetto — 45

THE STEPS AND METHODS IN EXPERIENTIAL
PSYCHOTHERAPY SESSIONS
Alvin R. Mahrer and Patricia A. Gervaize — 59

PRACTICAL ISSUES FOR THE CLINICIAN
TREATING SUBSTANCE ABUSE
*William Grady Ryan, Nancy J. Ryan,
Andrew Rosen, and Antonio R. Virsida* — 71

COLLABORATING WITH SELF-HELP GROUPS
FOR SUBSTANCE ABUSERS
*William Grady Ryan, Nancy J. Ryan,
Andrew Rosen, and Antonio R. Virsida* — 83

NEW DEVELOPMENTS IN PSYCHIATRIC DIAGNOSTIC TECHNOLOGY
Earl L. Loschen — 91

BORDERLINE PERSONALITY DISORDER: DEFINITION,
DIAGNOSIS, AND ASSESSMENT
William S. Pollack — 103

BORDERLINE PERSONALITY DISORDER:
TREATMENT CONSIDERATIONS
William S. Pollack — 113

COGNITIVE-BEHAVIORAL TECHNIQUES IN MARITAL THERAPY
Stephen E. Schlesinger and Norman B. Epstein — 137

THE EFFECTIVE USE OF HUMOR IN PSYCHOTHERAPY
Waleed A. Salameh
157

THE THERAPLAY TECHNIQUE FOR CHILDREN
Ann M. Jernberg
177

BEHAVIORAL ASSESSMENT AND TREATMENT OF FACIAL PAIN
Robert M. Malow and Ronald E. Olson
189

CONSTRUCTING AND INTERPRETING GENOGRAMS:
THE EXAMPLE OF SIGMUND FREUD'S FAMILY
Randy Gerson and Monica McGoldrick
203

TREATING CLIENTS WHO HAVE AIDS
John C. Gonsiorek
221

SECTION II: PRACTICE MANAGEMENT AND PROFESSIONAL DEVELOPMENT

INTRODUCTION TO SECTION II
231

THE PRIVATE PRACTICE OF PSYCHOLOGY: FOUR VARIATIONS
Herbert J. Freudenberger, Mark H. Lewin,
Carroll L. Meek, and Lawrence G. Ritt
233

HOW TO USE SMALL CLAIMS COURT FOR COLLECTIONS
William R. Hussey
245

CLIENT SNATCHING: A DEFENSE
Carroll L. Meek
257

CHANGES IN HEALTH CARE DELIVERY:
A GUIDE FOR THE INDEPENDENT PRACTITIONER
A. Steven Frankel
261

GUIDELINES FOR USING AN ANSWERING MACHINE IN YOUR PRACTICE
Carroll L. Meek
271

SECTION III: INSTRUMENTS AND OFFICE FORMS

INTRODUCTION TO SECTION III
277

THE MENTAL STATUS EXAMINATION - REVISED
Christopher M. Faiver
279

THE COPING STRATEGIES SCALES FOR DEPRESSED PATIENTS
E. Edward Beckham
287

THE SOCIAL ADJUSTMENT SELF-REPORT QUESTIONNAIRE
Myrna M. Weissman
299

THE STRAIN QUESTIONNAIRE
R. Craig Lefebvre and Sandra L. Sandford
309

SECTION IV: COMMUNITY INTERVENTIONS

INTRODUCTION TO SECTION IV   315

PSYCHOLOGICAL SCREENING OF LAW ENFORCEMENT CANDIDATES
Forrest Scogin and Larry E. Beutler   317

AN INTRODUCTION TO OCCUPATIONAL HEALTH PSYCHOLOGY
George S. Everly, Jr.   331

A CLINICIAN'S GUIDE TO SELECTING PARENT TRAINING PROGRAMS
Richard F. Dangel and W. Ted Blevins   339

SECTION V: SELECTED TOPICS

INTRODUCTION TO SECTION V   349

A PRIMER ON PSYCHOLOGICAL PRACTICE IN MEDICAL SETTINGS
James M. Raczynski   351

PSYCHOLOGICAL ASSESSMENT AND INTERVENTION
IN THE EMERGENCY ROOM
Keith A. Wood   365

THE DUTY TO PROTECT: LEGAL PRINCIPLES
AND THERAPEUTIC GUIDELINES
Samuel Knapp, Leon VandeCreek, and Cindy Herzog   383

TECHNIQUES FOR ENGAGING "DIFFICULT"
CHILDREN IN THE PLAYROOM
Stanley Kissel   391

AN INTRODUCTION TO DIVORCE MEDIATION
Stanley N. Cohen   405

RECENT DEVELOPMENTS IN ASSESSMENT OF THE MENTALLY
DISABLED FOR SOCIAL SECURITY AND SSI BENEFITS
Jack R. Anderson   417

INTRODUCTION TO CLIENT HANDOUTS   425

   STRESS MANAGEMENT: TEN SELF-CARE TECHNIQUES
   Kent. T. Yamauchi   427

   COMMUNICATING MORE EFFECTIVELY
   Waleed A. Salameh   431

INFORMATION FOR CONTRIBUTORS   435

INDEX TO THE INNOVATIONS SERIES   437

CONTINUING EDUCATION   465

INTRODUCTION TO THE VOLUME

The fifth volume in the *Innovations in Clinical Practice* series is organized in the same manner as previous volumes. Materials are grouped into five sections which reflect the diversity of contributions within the volume. In addition to the table of contents, a cumulative subject index facilitates rapid access to materials in this as well as the previous four volumes.

The first section, ISSUES AND APPLICATIONS, deals primarily with therapeutic concerns. The various contributions, however, go beyond the traditional therapeutic issues and also address important questions of assessment as well as treatment. Issues that relate to a number of different types of clients and situations are all covered.

The second section addresses PRACTICE MANAGEMENT and related professional development issues. This section is included because of the number of clinicians who work independently and require a source of current information on practice management and related professional issues. Practice management concerns are undergoing rapid transition, and almost from month to month there are developments which are important for the practitioner to follow. Some of our discussions in this section will also be of interest to students and those who practice in organizations or agencies.

The third section includes ASSESSMENT INSTRUMENTS AND OFFICE FORMS. The assessment instruments are primarily informal and designed to assist the clinician in collecting information about clients. Our intention is to publish screening instruments and forms that assist in the organization of data rather than the making of formal inferences. There are some exceptions to this rule, but we believe that they all fall well within the bounds of professional ethics in the format in which they are presented. We believe that the materials contained here should be of use to psychologists and other professionals, with minimal potential for misuse. Readers are advised to carefully review the introductory material which accompanies contributions to this section.

The fourth section on COMMUNITY INTERVENTIONS reflects our view that mental health practitioners have much to offer in the community beyond traditional clinical services. Although preventive interventions with appeal to clinicians have developed slowly, the community orientation continues to have an important impact on the mental health field. We trust that the material in this section will be of assistance to those who are interested in consultation and education efforts.

The fifth section on SELECTED TOPICS includes a variety of contributions that do not fit neatly into one of the other sections. Topics range from the "Duty to Protect" to "Divorce Mediation." In addition, this section introduces roles which may be relatively new to some clinicians. Also included here are two useful client handouts.

INTRODUCTION
TO THE VOLUME

INTRODUCTION TO SECTION I: CLINICAL ISSUES AND APPLICATIONS

The ISSUES AND APPLICATIONS section includes contributions that primarily relate to assessment and treatment. There is no other unifying theme intended, and the range of topics is quite broad. This section provides a means for experienced practitioners to stay up to date with newer techniques that might be incorporated into their practices, or to learn of new developments in specialized areas.

Garner and his colleagues have contributed two articles that address, first, the clinical assessment of anorexia nervosa and bulimia nervosa and, second, the fundamentals of psychotherapy for these two disorders. Eating disorders are of growing concern in our culture, and these authors have provided readers with a helpful perspective on dealing with these problems.

Next, Musetto provides an introduction to Ericksonian approaches to strategic hypnotherapy. Following that, Mahrer and Gervaize describe the steps and methods in a session of experiential psychotherapy. Both of these articles provide practical illustrations of therapeutic interventions.

Two articles in this section address treatment of substance abuse. William G. Ryan and his colleagues provide a practical background on identifying and intervening with the substance abuser and then discuss basic treatment strategies. In their view, it is essential for the therapist to collaborate comfortably with self-help groups. They provide a framework for this perspective.

Recent years have seen a number of new developments in psychiatric diagnostic technology. Loschen provides a practical perspective on several of the most important developments with which the clinician should be familiar.

Also in recent years there has been a growing discussion about the topic of borderline personality disorder. In two related contributions, Pollack provides an overview of the definition, diagnosis, assessment, and treatment of borderline personality disorder.

Schlesinger and Epstein address cognitive-behavioral techniques in marital therapy. After outlining a framework for cognitive-behavioral interventions, they illustrate practical techniques for helping couples.

Salameh describes the effective use of humor in psychotherapy. He distinguishes between humor that can be destructive and humor that can free the client and allow him or her to act more constructively. Salameh skillfully involves the reader in examining the use of humor.

Other contributions in this section cover a diversity of techniques and issues. Jernberg illustrates her theraplay technique for children; Malow and Olson describe the behavioral assessment and treatment of facial pain which is a common problem for many individuals; Gerson and McGoldrick introduce and illustrate the use of genograms, citing the example of Freud's family; and, finally, Gonsiorek provides an up-to-date look at treating the client who has AIDS.

THE CLINICAL ASSESSMENT OF ANOREXIA NERVOSA AND BULIMIA NERVOSA

David M. Garner and Ron Davis

In writing this contribution we have attempted to fulfill three objectives. Our first objective is to present a framework for assessing eating disorder patients that nonmedical clinicians, primarily psychologists, would find appropriate for their practice in the applied setting. In our experience, most eating disorder patients are best managed as outpatients unless there are specific medical or psychological issues which warrant inpatient attention. Our second objective is to highlight key clinical issues in assessment rather than present a more theoretical coverage of the range of controversies regarding the etiology of eating disorders. In doing so, we assume the reader already has some basic familiarity with the theoretical, experimental, and clinical literature (see Garfinkel & Garner, 1982, for a review). Our third objective is to present an assessment framework that will allow clinicians to formulate an appropriate diagnosis and a course of treatment. The companion contribution on treatment (p. 29) was written as an extension of the assessment framework presented here. Although assessment and treatment are covered separately, they are not necessarily distinct processes; assessment influences the course of treatment and reassessment is an ongoing process during therapy.

This contribution is comprised of four major sections. In the first section the terms anorexia nervosa and bulimia nervosa are defined. In the second section an assessment framework is offered as a guide to the clinician's line of inquiry when conducting the assessment. It is intended to provide a means by which the clinician may comprehend the overall clinical picture when patients present with seemingly disparate psychological symptoms and physical complaints. The third section covers the important issues of diagnostic criteria and differential diagnosis. Some of the major problems with the *DSM-III* criteria are discussed. The final section is devoted to a presentation of the assessment techniques that will enable the clinician to reach a diagnosis and plan a course of treatment for the eating disorder patient.

DEFINITION OF TERMS

BULIMIA NERVOSA (BULIMIA)

The individual conforms to the diagnostic criteria for the syndrome of bulimia nervosa (Russell, 1979) or bulimia (*DSM-III*; American Psychiatric Association, 1980) which are outlined in Table 2 (p. 12). The use of the term bulimia to describe both a symptom and a syndrome has led to considerable confusion in the eating disorder literature. As a symptom it is relatively common, but as a syndrome it appears in a small minority of women (Pyle et al., 1983). In the current chapter we will follow the convention suggested by Russell (1979) by referring to the symptom of uncontrollable eating as "bulimia" and the syndrome as "bulimia nervosa." Although individuals meeting the diagnostic criteria for bulimia nervosa or bulimia are not emaciated in appearance, many have lost as much weight as those with anorexia nervosa, but they have begun their descent from a higher absolute level (Garner, 1986). Some have argued that bulimia nervosa patients may be differentiated on the basis of a history of anorexia nervosa, but initial studies have shown that patients referred to specialized eating disorder treatment centers present similar clinical and psychometric features regardless of their history of emaciation (Fairburn & Cooper, 1984; Garner, Garfinkel, & O'Shaughnessy, 1985; Garner, Olmsted, & Garfinkel, 1985).

ANOREXIA NERVOSA

The individual conforms to weight loss and other conventional criteria for anorexia nervosa as outlined in Table 2. Those with the "bulimic" subtype of anorexia nervosa experience bouts of uncontrollable eating or binge eating, while those with the "restricting" subtype do not. In some cases the distinction between these subtypes is unclear because the patient may primarily display the restricting patterns and rarely experience episodes of bulimia.

THE ASSESSMENT FRAMEWORK

Figure 1 illustrates the formulation of both anorexia nervosa and bulimia nervosa as multidetermined disorders which present with specific clinical features and which persist over time because of the self-perpetuating nature of certain sequelae of the disturbed eating patterns. An incomplete evaluation of one or more of these factors can lead to a misdiagnosis and inappropriate course of treatment. Thus it is absolutely essential for the clinician to have a firm understanding of specific predisposing, initiating, and perpetuating factors.

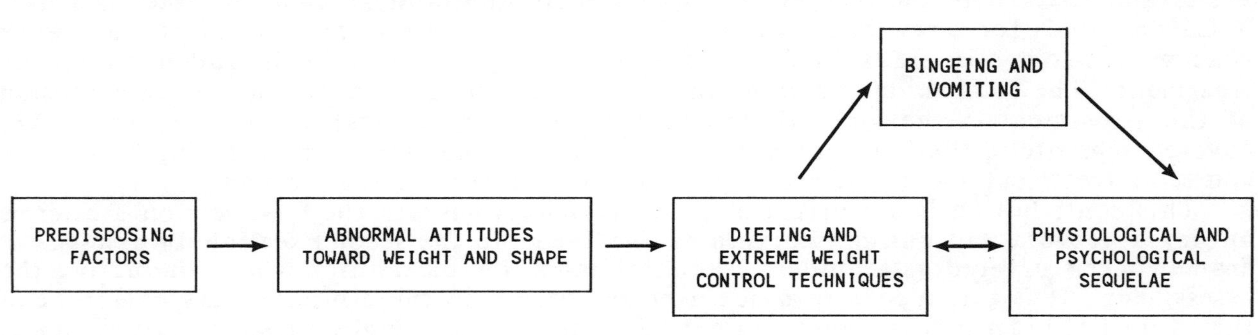

Figure 1. Anorexia Nervosa and Bulimia Nervosa as Multidetermined and Self-Perpetuating Disorders. The schematic illustrates that anorexia nervosa and bulimia nervosa are linked together in terms of common predisposing, initiating, and perpetuating factors which are outlined in Table 1. The categorical distinction between these disorders is blurred by the facts that (a) approximately 50% of anorexia nervosa patients have the symptom of bulimia, and (b) extreme weight loss from moderately obese levels is common in bulimia nervosa. Their distinction is made on terms of absolute weight, with anorexia nervosa defining those who are emaciated. Both disorders are "final common pathways" which are multidetermined in the sense that various combinations of predisposing factors lead to the expression of similar symptom patterns.

PREDISPOSING FACTORS

The eating disorders discussed here primarily affect women. Hence the feminine pronoun is used throughout this contribution. Factors that have been proposed to play a predisposing role within the individual are summarized in Table 1 (p. 7). A major predisposition to anorexia nervosa and bulimia nervosa concerns the difficulties these individuals may have in autonomous functioning and in experiencing a sense of personal identity which leaves them unable to function separately from their family or other external "guideposts." Bruch (1973) has related the core predisposition of the eating disorders to fundamental ego deficits in autonomy and mastery over one's body which she described as the overall sense of "personal ineffectiveness." According to Bruch, feelings of ineffectiveness are characterized by patients' experiences of "not being in control of their behavior, needs and impulses, as not owning their own bodies, as not having a center of gravity within themselves. Instead, they feel under the influence and direction of external forces" (p. 55). This feeling of ineffectiveness and subsequent lack of personal identity may often result in major difficulties when the individual is removed from the concrete guidelines of her parents or is placed in situations in which there are new expectations (Igoin-Apfelbaum, 1985). For the individual vulnerable to eating disorders, these times set the stage for the body to become the overvalued symbol and source of autonomy, control, and identity through the misinterpretation of thinness as a sign of specialness and starvation as an indication of self-control.

TABLE 1:   CLINICAL MANIFESTATIONS OF THE CORE FEATURES OF ANOREXIA NERVOSA AND BULIMIA NERVOSA

<u>Predisposing Factors</u>

Deficits in autonomous functioning.
Overall sense of personal ineffectiveness.
Self-esteem deficits.
Personality traits of perfectionism, compliance, obsessionality.
Characterologic depression.
Fears of psychological maturity.
Family conflicts.

<u>Abnormal Attitudes toward Weight and Shape</u>

Preoccupation with proportion and size of one's own body.
Hypervigilance over, and extreme sensitivity to, cues about weight and shape.
Dissatisfaction with weight and shape.
Morbid fear of weight gain and strong drive for thinness.
Reasoning errors related to food, weight, and shape (dichotomous thinking, personalization, superstitious
    thinking, magnification, selective abstraction, overgeneralization).

<u>Dieting and Extreme Weight Control</u>

Sustained caloric restriction in both quantity and type of food intake.
Evacuative techniques (self-induced vomiting, laxative and diuretic abuse).
Frequent bouts of strenuous exercise.

<u>Bingeing and Vomiting</u>

Consumption of prodigious amounts of food which is experienced as excessive and beyond voluntary control.
Induced vomiting which instills a false sense of security that the fattening effects of the binge have been
    avoided.
Tremendous fluctuation in mood over the binge-purge sequence.

<u>Physiological and Psychological Sequelae</u>

Starvation produces emotional symptoms and a hypometabolic state (hypotension, hypothermia, bradycardia).
Self-induced vomiting, starvation, and laxative or diuretic abuse cause electrolyte disturbance leading to
    muscle cramping, paresthesias, edema, and cardiac arrhythmias.
Preoccupation with food.
Social maladjustment in leisure activities and interpersonal relationships.

There has been a diversity of opinion regarding pre-morbid personality and the eating disorders. Some believe that there is no characteristic pre-morbid personality structure in these disorders (Morgan & Russell, 1975; Russell, 1979). Others have described the compliant, perfectionistic, and dependent characteristics of many patients (Bruch, 1973; Crisp, 1965). Many patients do show comparable levels of obsessional personality traits to those seen in obsessive-compulsive patients (Solyom et al., 1983). Depressive personality or "characterologic depression" (Akiskal, 1983) has also been documented (Hatsukami, Mitchell, & Eckert, 1984). However, these findings are of questionable value in determining the nature of predisposing psychopathology since it is very difficult to separate characteristics that are possible precursors of the eating disorder from those that are by-products of a serious illness or are secondary to starvation. Yet, it is clear that there is some variability in personality features among patients, with several characteristics being particularly prominent. These include an extraordinary need for approval from others, conformity, conscientiousness, perfectionism, depression, and a lack of responsiveness to inner needs. These qualities suggest a group of individuals with extremely high personal expectations and a need to please others in order to maintain a sense of self-worth.

ABNORMAL ATTITUDES TOWARD WEIGHT AND SHAPE

Abnormal attitudes toward weight and shape are pathognomonic for both anorexia nervosa and bulimia nervosa. Much of the patient's stream of consciousness is filled with concerns related to the proportion and size of her body parts and the distribution of lean versus adipose tissue, with the overriding desire to lose or control body weight. The patient may become hypervigilant of the bodies of women around her and those depicted in the media. Comparing body parts and "shopping" around for the perfect figure in her immediate environment usually results in emotional upset, because she can always find someone who is thinner and more shapely. One emaciated patient we treated was jealous of a greyhound dog she had seen in a park because she felt more of the dog's ribs were sticking out than her own. This preoccupation in the extreme indicates the degree of concern many patients have about body shape.

The preoccupation can manifest itself in many ways. Most patients are generally dissatisfied with their shape and weight *regardless* of their actual weight. An emaciated patient of 90 lbs is just as likely to be dissatisfied with her body as a normal weight patient of 125 lbs. The dissatisfaction varies in intensity from a dislike of specific body parts, like thighs and abdomen, to a revulsion of the entire body. While most patients focus upon the parts of the body which change conspicuously during puberty (i.e., breasts, hips, thighs, waist, and buttocks), some develop revulsion for their face, arms, or even fingers. Many patients will lament the fact that the "fat" they grab could not be surgically removed, and some have seriously considered or undergone cosmetic surgery. Previously emaciated bulimia nervosa patients frequently talk about their former bodies as one would talk about a deceased loved one; they find it difficult to accept the loss of a thinner body which they once possessed. As will be discussed later, a thorough weight history usually reveals that most bulimic patients who present at a normal weight once achieved a significantly lower weight following a period of severely restrictive dieting, and this usually coincided with the onset of bulimic symptoms (Abraham & Beumont, 1982; Davis, 1985; Fairburn & Cooper, 1984; Johnson et al., 1982; Pyle, Mitchell, & Eckert, 1981; Russell, 1979). Patients idealize this previous weight, and it is therefore not surprising to find that they view their current weight and shape as both foreign and loathsome in contrast to their previously attained lighter weight. Emaciated anorexic patients also regard their bodies with contempt. However, in addition to dissatisfaction they may actually experience their bodies in a distorted way, pointing to areas where they are quite convinced there is too much fat when objective evidence indicates mere skin and bone.

Eating disorder patients have a phobic-like avoidance of fatness which results in a preoccupation with their shape and weight; this may be expressed as a belief that current weight is unacceptable or a fear of what it could become if they were to relax their vigilance over food intake for even a single day (Garner & Bemis, 1982). A "drive for thinness" (Bruch, 1973) or an extreme fear of weight gain or a "morbid fear of fatness" (Russell, 1979) are essential diagnostic features for patients with anorexia nervosa and bulimia nervosa. This fear of fatness or drive for thinness stems from the inexorable conviction that strict control over body weight or thinness is necessary for happiness and well-being. The fear of fatness also stems from the fact that most eating disorder patients once weighed substantially more than their current weight. Virtually all anorexia nervosa patients arrive at the diagnosis through extreme weight loss of between 20% and 25% of former body weight, depending upon the formal criteria employed (American Psychiatric Association, 1980; Feighner et al., 1972; Garfinkel & Garner, 1982). However, some early adolescent patients become emaciated by dieting and fail to gain weight as they become taller (American Psychiatric Association, 1980). A substantial number of bulimic patients, while currently of normal weight, were "overweight" or greater than 110% of matched population mean weight at some point (Abraham & Beumont, 1982; Fairburn & Cooper, 1984; Garner, 1986; Johnson et al., 1982; Mitchell et al., 1985).

Most patients have a specific maximum weight which they are unwilling to exceed for fear this will lead to further uncontrolled weight gain. For the emaciated anorexic, the weight of 99 lbs often has been given almost "magical" significance because, as the highest two-digit figure, it represents a special performance threshold; the patient believes that if she goes above 99 lbs there will be nothing stopping her from uncontrolled weight gain. This weight may also have special significance because it is just below the menstrual weight threshold for many patients and is associated with an entirely different hormonal profile. Other nonemaciated bulimics may have a buffer zone or narrow range of weight above their current one which they will not allow themselves to exceed. In all cases this tolerable maximum is substantially below their healthy pre-morbid weight (Russell, 1979), and exceeding this maximum weight can be quite distressing for the patient. For many patients, self-esteem is tied directly to those cues which signal changes in weight and shape (e.g., mirrors, bathroom scales, clothing, rings, and bracelets). Patients are extremely vigilant of these cues and sensitive to the messages they convey. Complete social withdrawal, profound dysphoria, and feelings of inadequacy often follow the discovery that weight has crept above the "safe zone." Patients often remark that a weight change of 1 or 2 lbs can "make or break" their entire day or week.

These abnormal attitudes toward weight and shape become crystallized into a fairly specific set of reasoning errors which characterize the faulty thinking patterns of eating disorder patients. The following recurring errors have been identified by Beck and his colleagues in various psychological disorders (Beck, 1976; Beck & Emery, 1985; Beck et al., 1979), and we have described their idiosyncratic content with eating disorders (Garner & Bemis, 1982, 1985; Garner, Garfinkel & Bemis, 1982).

1. *Dichotomous Thinking.* This involves thinking in extreme, absolute, or all-or-none terms and is typically applied to food, eating, and weight, although it extends to the pursuit of sports, careers, and school. For example, breaking a rigid eating routine produces panic because it means complete loss of control to the individual. A 1 lb weight gain may be equated with incipient obesity.
2. *Personalization and Self-Reference.* This involves the egocentric interpretations of impersonal events or the overinterpretation of events related to the self. The eating disorder patient frequently displays the conviction that strangers or casual friends would notice if she gained a pound.
3. *Superstitious Thinking.* This error in reasoning reflects the belief in cause-effect relationships between noncontingent events. It often involves magical thinking which is applied to the maintenance of eating or exercise rituals. Eating a small amount of a "forbidden" food may precipitate taking laxatives despite the knowledge that they do not result in malabsorption of calories. Extreme anxiety is often experienced following a minute deviation from exercise rituals because of the belief that weight gain will result.
4. *Magnification.* This involves overestimation of the significance of undesirable events. For the eating disorder patient, the significance of small increases in weight is reliably overinterpreted.
5. *Selective Abstraction.* This error in thinking is characterized by focusing on isolated details while ignoring contradictory or more salient evidence. This style of thinking is illustrated by the belief that thinness is the sole frame of reference for inferring self-worth. It is also represented by the reciprocal belief that fatness is a clear indication of incompetence. These beliefs persist in defiance of examples to the contrary.
6. *Overgeneralization.* This involves extracting a rule on the basis of one event and applying it to dissimilar situations. Overgeneralization is evident in the inferences drawn about thinness. For example, a patient may conclude that weight loss would be the secret to competence because someone she knows who is competent is also thin. She may assume that because she was unhappy at a normal weight, weight gain will produce unhappiness.

DIETING AND EXTREME WEIGHT CONTROL

Dieting and extreme weight control are the second hallmark of the eating disorders. They distinguish the individual who is dissatisfied with her weight and shape from the anorexic or bulimic patient whose extreme drive for thinness translates into behaviors which are aimed at producing weight loss or preventing weight gain. One recent magazine survey showed that while most women feel "too fat," few go to such extremes to control weight as self-induced vomiting, laxative and diuretic abuse, or fasting ("Feeling Fat," 1984). These methods of weight control are the rule rather than the exception in eating disorder patients.

Severe dieting or sustained caloric restriction in both quantity and type of food is the most common method of weight control practiced by eating disorder patients. The U.S. Recommended Dietary Allowance (RDA; Food and Nutrition Board Committee on Dietary Allowances, 1980) for young adult women is 1,700 to 2,500 calories per day, yet the intake for anorexic patients typically does not exceed 600 to 900 calories (Huse & Lucas, 1984; Marshall, 1978). Most normal weight bulimic patients consume nutritionally inadequate diets of not more than 1400 calories (Dalvit-McPhillips, 1984; Kirkley, Agras, & Weiss, 1985). Infrequent consumption of meals has been noted in bulimic patients compared to normal women (Davis, Freeman, & Solyom, 1985).

In addition to dieting, most patients engage in one or more evacuative techniques to control weight. A recent survey of 275 bulimic patients seeking treatment revealed that 84% induced vomiting, 47% took laxatives, and 25% took diuretics one or more times per week (Mitchell et al., 1985). Estimates of the percentage of anorexic patients who induce vomiting or abuse laxatives are 33-43% and 32-58%, respectively (Casper et al., 1980; Crisp et al., 1980; Garner, Garfinkel, et al., 1985; Halmi, 1974). Patients also resort to frequent bouts of strenuous exercise in an effort to "burn off" the day's accumulation of calories.

BINGEING AND VOMITING

Self-induced vomiting or laxative abuse frequently follows a binge, which is defined in *DSM-III* as the "rapid consumption of a large amount of food in a discrete period of time, usually less than two hours" (American Psychiatric Association, 1980, p. 70). This definition is problematic because it defines a binge according to such topographical aspects as speed of eating and quantity of food rather than how the episode is experienced by the individual. Patients invariably comment on the ego-dystonic nature of their binges, in which both rate of consumption and quantity of food are experienced as outside their voluntary control (Fairburn, 1982). It is this phenomenological experience which the clinician must attend to during the assessment, because it distinguishes the eating disorder patient from most healthy adults who occasionally engage in binge eating (i.e., 65% of college students according to Halmi, Falk, & Schwartz, 1981).

Most bulimic patients present themselves for treatment because they are perplexed and guilt-ridden about their bingeing behavior. They typically conceptualize their binges as lapses in rigid self-control over food intake and completely fail to recognize that bingeing is a consequence of dieting for a number of psychological and biological reasons (Garfinkel & Kaplan, 1985; Garner, Rockert, et al., 1985; Polivy & Herman, 1985). At the psychological level, many binges are precipitated by the consumption of forbidden foods which the patient fears will metabolize instantly into an equivalent amount of fat. Ironically, it is precisely those foods the patient fears (i.e., calorie dense carbohydrates) which she constantly craves prior to the binge (Abraham & Beumont, 1982; Mitchell et al., 1985; Pyle et al., 1981). Having sampled the food, she feels she has "blown the diet" and can now satisfy her craving with the false sense of security that vomiting will undo any fattening effects of food.

Binges are usually of prodigious amounts, often exceeding 1,200 calories; about 2.5 times greater than the caloric value of meals consumed by both bulimic and nonbulimic women (Davis, 1985). At the biological level, insulin-induced hypoglycemia following ingestion of the carbohydrate dense forbidden foods may specifically increase appetite for more carbohydrates, especially sugar (Geiselman & Novin, 1982). It is therefore important for the clinician to assess the patient's bingeing behavior within the context of her daily dieting practices. Protracted periods of abstention from carbohydrates increase the patient's risk for bingeing, which typically occurs at home and alone in the latter part of the day (Crowther, Lingswiler, & Stephens, 1984; Davis et al., 1985). Assessing the patient's bingeing and vomiting behaviors from a functional analytic perspective will be discussed in the final section of this contribution.

PHYSIOLOGICAL AND PSYCHOLOGICAL SEQUELAE

Dieting, bingeing, vomiting, and laxative abuse all have important physiological and psychological sequelae of which the clinician must be aware when conducting an assessment of the anorexic or bulimic patient. In some cases these need to be attended to immediately by a physician because of the grave medical dangers they pose for the patient. Other sequelae are important for understanding the patient's current psychological state. Starvation, for example, produces such depressive symptoms as mental confusion, lability of mood, lethargy, social and sexual anhedonia, and sleep disturbance (Altshuler & Weiner, 1985; Keys et al., 1950). It is important for the clinician to construe these symptoms as consequences of the patient's semistarvation state rather than as an underlying affective disorder, because the symptoms reliably improve with refeeding and weight gain (Eckert et al., 1982; Keys et al., 1950). If they persist after weight has been restored, the depression should be re-examined for other causal factors.

Depressive symptoms are also frequently observed in the normal weight bulimic patients where starvation effects may not be as evident (Gwirtsman et al., 1983; Hatsukami, Eckert, et al., 1984; Herzog, 1984; Mitchell et al., 1984; Piran et al., 1985). However, they too may often be attributed to the patient's disturbed eating pathology. Cooper and Fairburn (in press) found that bulimic patients were as severely depressed as women with an affective disorder, yet many of the symptoms were specifically related to eating pathology (e.g., tiredness due to vomiting; obsessional ideas specific to food, weight, and shape; pathological guilt regarding the consumption of forbidden foods and binges). These symptoms usually abate after the patient relinquishes her core eating pathology during psychotherapy (Fairburn et al., 1985). Social maladjustment is also common (Johnson & Berndt, 1983; Norman & Herzog, 1984), especially in those patients who spend much of the day bingeing and vomiting in secrecy, or avoiding people and places that they fear will encourage them to break rigid dietary restraint.

Starvation, self-induced vomiting, and laxative abuse have pernicious consequences for the patient's physical health. The most serious clinical situation is the emaciated anorexic patient who induces vomiting, abuses laxatives on a daily basis, and engages in a rigorous exercise program. This combination of weight control techniques works in a synergistic manner to increase the patient's risk for cardiac failure (Garfinkel & Garner, 1982). In one study, grossly aberrant electrocardiographic changes were detected in 74% of anorexic patients (Silverman, 1983). Electrolyte disturbance in the form of shifts in total body potassium is a consequence of semistarvation and may contribute to cardiac arrhythmias (Dempsey et al., 1984; Welle et al., 1984). Vomiting and laxative abuse also produce electrolyte disturbance by depleting potassium, chloride, and sodium levels (Mitchell et al., 1983; Richardson, Forbath, & Karanicolas, 1983). This depletion can cause weakness, constipation, edema, muscle cramping, paresthesias, and cardiac arrhythmias (Garfinkel & Garner, 1982; Webb & Gehi, 1981).

Clinicians must be alerted to these sequelae and have the patient's cardiac functioning and serum/urine electrolytes monitored by a physician if the combination of starvation and frequent vomiting or laxative abuse is present (Isner et al., 1985). In some cases, psychotherapy cannot proceed until these conditions are stabilized through medical intervention, not only because of the grave medical danger to the patient, but also because her clouded sensorium stemming from a toxic state negates any psychotherapeutic progress.

A final sequelae of starvation we wish to mention is that of a hypometabolic state (e.g., reduced basal metabolic rate, hypotension, hypothermia, bradycardia). This is important for understanding why some patients exist on as few as 600 calories per day and that weight gain can result from even minor increments in caloric intake.

ISSUES IN DIAGNOSIS

In this section we focus on two issues related to the diagnosis of anorexia nervosa and bulimia nervosa. First, we present a number of criticisms of the *DSM-III* (American Psychiatric Association, 1980) diagnostic criteria for bulimia, along with recommendations for dealing with these criteria. Next, we highlight those symptoms that are critical to assess when making a differential diagnosis between the eating disorders and other psychiatric syndromes that they superficially resemble.

DIAGNOSTIC CRITERIA

The *DSM-III* criteria for anorexia nervosa and bulimia nervosa* are presented in Table 2. Reviewing the formal diagnostic criteria may lead to the impression that the disorders are distinct with no overlapping symptoms. While some authors view bulimia as a syndrome entirely distinct from anorexia nervosa (e.g., Hamilton, Gelwick, & Meade, 1984; Schlesier-Stropp, 1984), we feel this is unwarranted and misleading for a number of

---

TABLE 2: *DSM-III* **DIAGNOSTIC CRITERIA FOR ANOREXIA NERVOSA AND BULIMIA NERVOSA****

<u>Anorexia Nervosa</u>

A. Intense fear of becoming obese, which does not diminish as weight loss progresses.

B. Disturbance of body image (e.g., claiming to feel fat even when emaciated).

C. Weight loss of at least 25% of original body weight or, if under 18 years of age, weight loss from original body weight plus projected weight gain expected from growth charts may be combined to make the 25%.

D. Refusal to maintain body weight over a minimal normal weight for age and height.

E. No known physical illness that would account for the weight loss.

<u>Bulimia</u>

A. Recurrent episodes of binge eating (rapid consumption of a large amount of food in a discrete period of time, usually less than 2 hours).

B. At least three of the following:

    1. consumption of high-caloric, easily ingested food during a binge
    2. inconspicuous eating during a binge
    3. termination of such eating episodes by abdominal pain, sleep, social interruption, or self-induced vomiting
    4. repeated attempts to lose weight by severely restrictive diets, self-induced vomiting, or use of cathartics or diuretics
    5. frequent weight fluctuations greater than 10 pounds due to alternating binges and fasts

C. Awareness that the eating pattern is abnormal and fear of not being able to stop eating voluntarily.

D. Depressed mood and self-deprecating thoughts following eating binges.

E. The bulimic episodes are not due to anorexia nervosa or any known physical disorder.

**From <u>Diagnostic and Statistical Manual of Mental Disorders</u> (3rd ed., pp. 67-71) by American Psychiatric Association, 1980, Washington, DC: Author.

---

reasons. First, approximately 50% of anorexia nervosa patients engage in binge eating, despite the fact that in the *DSM-III* it is presented as a symptom for bulimia only (Casper et al., 1980; Garfinkel, Moldofsky, & Garner, 1980). Second, it is well-established that some patients move between bulimia and anorexia nervosa at different points in time (Holmgren et al., 1983). Third, these disorders have many common clinical features, and patient profiles are similar on virtually all clinical and psychometric dimensions that have been measured (Garner, Garfinkel, et al., 1985; Garner, Olmsted, et al., 1985).

---

*Although <u>DSM-III</u> refers to the syndrome as "bulimia," we prefer to follow the less ambiguous convention of Russell (1979) by referring to it as bulimia nervosa.

Because anorexia nervosa and bulimia nervosa share so many clinical features, the validity of the diagnostic distinction is questionable. However, it may be premature to conclude that these are simply different manifestations of the same fundamental disorder, because there is almost no information regarding prognosis for the two diagnostic groups. Moreover, the generally accepted treatment for anorexia nervosa differs from that of bulimia nervosa in that weight restoration is an essential initial stage in the management of the anorexic patient but not the bulimic patient, who typically has a weight within the statistically normal range. However, as mentioned earlier, many nonemaciated bulimic patients have been considerably overweight prior to the onset of their disorder, and most have had lifetime weight fluctuations which are equivalent to those in anorexia nervosa (Garner, 1986). Interpreted in light of "set point" theory (Keesey, 1980; Nisbett, 1972), these patients may present at a statistically normal weight but may be considerably below their optimal weight, and may not experience permanent relief from their urges to binge unless they return to a higher "healthy weight" (Russell, 1979).

Nevertheless, at present it seems appropriate to retain the distinction between anorexia nervosa and bulimia nervosa by ruling that bulimia nervosa not be diagnosed if the *DSM-III* criteria for anorexia nervosa are met, *even though the patient may in addition meet all criteria for bulimia nervosa.* In effect, this means that the diagnosis of bulimia nervosa should not be given if the patient's weight control behavior results in her weight falling substantially below either her previous weight or the matched population mean weight.

The *DSM-III* criteria for anorexia nervosa revolve around the two core clinical features of abnormal attitudes toward weight and shape (see criteria A, B, and D in Table 2), and the use of extreme weight control techniques (criterion C). In contrast, abnormal attitudes toward weight and shape are not mentioned at all in the *DSM-III* criteria for bulimia nervosa, and weight control techniques are relegated to an optional status (see criterion B-4). These omissions mean that the *DSM-III* criteria, as they now stand, are overinclusive and do not only define individuals with a clinically significant condition who typically present for treatment. By focusing primarily on binge eating, they define a group of individuals who have the symptom of bulimia (i.e., gross overeating) rather than the specific syndrome which involves the core clinical features of (a) abnormal attitudes toward weight and shape, (b) dieting and extreme weight control, and (c) bulimic episodes. Fairburn and Garner (1986) have proposed that these three features are necessary criteria for a diagnosis of bulimia nervosa. However, a diagnosis of anorexia nervosa, bulimic subtype, must be given if the patient additionally experiences a weight loss of at least 25% of original body weight. The diagnosis of anorexia nervosa, restricting subtype, is given to the patient who meets the attitudinal, weight control, and weight loss criteria *but* does not engage in bulimic episodes. The revised *DSM-III R* criteria which have been proposed for the "bulimic disorder" are also presented in Table 2a (p. 14), and it is evident that some, but not all, of the criticisms raised earlier have been addressed (see Fairburn and Garner, 1986 for a more complete discussion).

DIFFERENTIAL DIAGNOSIS

In the diagnosis of a disorder, the clinician is vitally dependent upon the patient's genuine self-report. In anorexia nervosa, the ego-syntonic nature of many of the symptoms may lead to denial of the disorder or a less-than-accurate description of the motivation behind weight loss. Although failure to identify cases of anorexia nervosa and bulimia nervosa despite obvious signs was a major problem in the past, the recent interest in these disorders may result in a different form of misclassification. Because many of the symptoms of anorexia nervosa and bulimia nervosa can present in patients with other functional disorders, there is some risk of erroneously classifying patients with schizophrenia, affective disorder, obsessive-compulsive disorder, conversion disorder, and even nonclinical weight preoccupation as primary eating disorders (Garfinkel, Garner, et al., 1983). Issues related to differential diagnosis of these disorders from primary eating disorders will be briefly reviewed.

TABLE 2A: PROPOSED DIAGNOSTIC CRITERIA FOR INCLUSION IN *DSM-III R**

Bulimic Disorder

A. Recurrent episodes of binge-eating (rapid consumption of a large amount of food in a discrete period of time, usually less than 2 hours).

B. During the eating binges there is a feeling of lack of control over the eating behavior.

C. The individual regularly engages in either self-induced vomiting, use of laxatives, or rigorous dieting or fasting in order to counteract the effects of the binge-eating.

D. A minimum average of two binge-eating episodes per week for at least 3 months.

Anorexia Nervosa

A. Intense fear of becoming obese, even when underweight.

B. Disturbance in the way in which one's body weight, size, or shape is experienced, for example, claiming to "feel fat" even when emaciated; belief that one area of the body is "too fat" even when obviously underweight.

C. Refusal to maintain body weight over a minimal normal weight for age and height, for example, weight loss leading to maintenance of body weight 15% below expected; failure to make expected weight gain during period of growth, leading to body weight 15% below expected.

D. In females, absence of at least three consecutive menstrual cycles when otherwise expected to occur (primary or secondary amenorrhea).

Eating Disorders NOS

This is a residual category for disorders of eating that does not meet the criteria for a special Eating Disorder.

Examples include:

1. An individual of average weight who does not have binge-eating episodes, but frequently engages in self-induced vomiting for fear of gaining weight.
2. All of the features of Anorexia Nervosa in a female except for absence of menses.
3. All of the features of Bulimic Disorder except for the frequency or duration of binge-eating episodes.

---

*From <u>DSM-III R in Development (10/5/85)</u> by American Psychiatry Association, 1985, Washington, DC: Author.

Affective Disorder. Most eating disorder patients exhibit symptoms of depression, and some researchers have suggested that eating disorders are a marked form of depression (Cantwell et al., 1977; Hudson, Pope, Jonas, Laffer, et al., 1983). In addition, weight loss is a common symptom of depression. Because of the significant overlap between the symptoms of these disorders, they may be difficult to distinguish in some cases (Altshuler & Weiner, 1985). Although many patients with a primary affective disorder lose weight and complain of true "anorexia," they may be differentiated from the eating disorder patient who consciously loses weight despite the experience of hunger because of a drive to be thinner or a morbid fear of becoming fat. For the eating disorder patient, loss of self-esteem is directly related to failure to control eating and weight. In the patient with primary depression, loss of self-esteem is more general or is linked to issues other than weight control. Activity level is reduced with primary depression and may be increased with eating disorders with the expressed purpose of "burning up" calories.

Although the distinction between primary depression and anorexia nervosa is relatively clear in most instances, the differences between a mood disorder and bulimia nervosa may be less clear in many cases. Bulimia nervosa patients have a higher than expected incidence of mood disorder in first degree relations (Hudson, Pope, Jonas, & Yurgelun-Todd, 1983) and some may respond to antidepressant therapy (Pope et al., 1983; Walsh et al., 1984). The primary distinguishing feature between the mood disorders and eating disorders relates to attitudes toward weight and shape as well as what we have referred to as "weight-losing" behaviors.

Schizophrenia. Cases of schizophrenia presenting with weight loss and self-induced vomiting have been described recently (Garfinkel, Garner, et al., 1983). The self-induced vomiting and refusal to eat may be closely related to the delusion that the food is possessed or contaminated, or the belief that food cannot be accepted into the stomach for some other reason. There is no drive for thinness in schizophrenia, and there is an absence of hallucinations, delusions (other than those related to eating and weight), and other psychotic ideational aberrations in eating disorder patients.

Conversion Disorder. Recently a group of patients initially resembling those with anorexia nervosa have been described, but upon closer examination they appear to lack many of the core clinical features. These individuals have been previously described as having "atypical" anorexia nervosa (Bruch, 1973) and also have been referred to as having conversion disorder because their symptoms may primarily function to control others or sustain fundamental conflicts at a conversion level (Garfinkel, Kaplan, et al., 1983). In these cases the eating symptoms may be linked to an identifiable traumatic event, and there is an absence of the drive for thinness which is seen in the typical eating disorder patient.

Nonclinical Weight Preoccupation. Recent attempts have been made to distinguish between women who display the same aberrant attitudes toward weight and shape seen in true eating disorders but who lack the characteristic severe ego deficits of the clinical syndromes (Garner, Olmsted, & Garfinkel, 1983; Garner et al., 1984). These women are highly weight conscious and engage in rigid dieting, but they do not seem to be motivated by the level of unhappiness typical of the eating disorder patients, and they do not exhibit the profound behavioral symptoms designed to bring about weight loss.

Other Disorders. Occasionally, weight loss will present in patients due to other primary symptoms. For example, we recently consulted on a case in which the woman's weight loss resulted directly from a morbid fear of dental procedures. She was terrified of visiting the dentist, and this had first led to the avoidance of sweets which might cause tooth decay and second to the avoidance of foods which required chewing because they might result in a tooth breaking. There was no drive for thinness, and she sincerely wished to gain weight since she viewed herself as far too thin.

ASSESSMENT TECHNIQUES

Psychological assessment is the process of making hypotheses about the patient's disorder and testing their conceptual validity through the collection of relevant data (Maloney & Ward, 1976). In a sense the process is like a funnel, beginning broad band and extensive, and becoming increasingly narrow and intensive (Cone & Hawkins, 1977). We advocate beginning the assessment with a clinical interview which covers the five core features outlined in Figure 1. From this conceptual framework, tentative hypotheses are made about the patient's diagnosis, and converging evidence from the interview, psychometric tests, and self-monitoring procedures will either confirm or refute the diagnosis.

THE INTERVIEW

When interviewing potential eating disorder patients, we advocate what Spitzer and Williams (1984) have termed the "canine approach." In this approach, the clinician has in mind a specific clinical feature or "bone" he or she would like to assess; questions are asked until this is achieved, at which time the clinician moves on to search for another core issue. Our interview focuses on a search for the five core features depicted in Figure 1 and elaborated further in Table 1.

The clinician might begin the interview with the following question: "I would like you to spend a minute or two and say what brought you here today." As nebulous as this question may seem, it serves three very important functions. First, it allows the patient to verbalize what really troubles her about her relationship to food, after perhaps having gone to numerous professionals who might never have given her the chance to discuss this issue (Garner, 1985). Second, the way in which the patient responds verbally, emotionally, and posturally to the question will indicate how structured and direct succeeding questions will have to be. Finally, this question allows the patient to reveal her own agenda or purpose in consulting you, which has relevance for determining how quickly a therapeutic alliance may be formed. Many anorexic patients present themselves at the behest, and under the duress, of relatives who view them as "sick," while they view their own symptoms as ego-syntonic. Launching a barrage of questions at the patient about her symptoms under these circumstances without first determining her own agenda bodes poorly for both the attainment of accurate information and the establishment of a therapeutic alliance.

The next major question we ask may be paraphrased as follows: "I am interested to find out about your weight history. Let us begin at the age when you reached your current adult height and proceed from there. (This is typically around 12 to 14 years and it is important for the patient to have this clearly in mind.) I want you to give me a 'guided tour' of both your weight and your relationship to food beginning at this age and working up to the present. Tell me everything you think would be important for me to know. I am particularly interested in when your weight changed significantly, both up and down, according to your own perceptions of it."

We never cease to be amazed about how open patients are in relating their weight history in a detailed and factual manner. Usually without further questioning, patients reveal in the first few minutes of the interview both the history and current breadth and severity of the core feature of dieting and weight control. Specific probes may be necessary to clarify the following: (a) highest and lowest past weight; (b) rates of weight change; (c) a description of all diets previously embarked upon and their effects on weight and menstruation; (d) if and when they began to binge, induce vomiting, or abuse laxatives, diuretics, or diet pills; (d) periods when dieting and weight control were exacerbated and attenuated; and (e) the circumstances surrounding these changes in dieting and weight control including familial, interpersonal, and work or school issues.

During this weight history the patient usually reveals information which will allow the clinician to formulate hypotheses about the four remaining core features. These should then be pursued with more direct probing:

Predisposing Factors. As we stated earlier, it is very difficult to examine pre-morbid personality in isolation from the patient's focal eating disorder because what we very likely perceive in the patient is the interaction between the two (Zubin, 1979). This is why no two eating disorder patients are exactly alike. Their core features may be the same, but the way in which the patient manifests them is variable because of differences in pre-morbid personality. The patient begins to allude to the latter when she discusses her weight history during adolescence. Patients invariably recall feeling fat at this age and this typically coincides with one or more significant events: (a) friends or relatives commented on her development of breasts and thighs, (b) she moved or changed schools, (c) the family broke up. The patient's inability to function autonomously and her overall sense of ineffectiveness during these times may predispose her to embark on a diet with the view of restoring control and autonomy in her otherwise chaotic life. In the interview, the clinician might examine the circumstances surrounding the onset of the disturbed eating pathology, not so much because this will lead to a developmental understanding of her disorder, but because it will help to understand how she is dealing with autonomy and control issues in the present. It may also be important to assess for history of depressive episodes in conjunction with important shifts in weight, eating pathology, and interpersonal functioning.

Abnormal Attitudes toward Weight and Shape. In contrast to the relative ease with which dieting and weight control information can be obtained, assessing abnormal attitudes toward weight and shape is a much more difficult and delicate task. This is because the patient arrives at the assessment session operating from a basic assumption that her self-worth is fundamentally dependent upon achieving and maintaining a low weight. Direct confrontation of this set of beliefs may be construed as a personal attack and provoke a defensive retreat. It is therefore crucial that the patient's attitudes and beliefs about her shape and weight be accepted as genuine (Garner & Bemis, 1982). All of the clinical manifestations listed in Table 1 under "Abnormal Attitudes toward Weight and Shape" must be assessed with tact and questions framed appropriately because of the very emotionally laden nature of the subject. For example, when assessing the patient's degree of dissatisfaction with her weight and shape, it would be inappropriate to ask "Which parts of your body are you dissatisfied with most?" without first asking "How do you feel about your current shape and weight?" The reverse direction of questioning is consistent with the "funnel" line of inquiry which we endorse.

To assess fear of weight gain and drive for thinness, the following probes would be appropriate: (a) "If you could magically change your weight, how much would you really like to weigh right now?"; (b) "How important is it for you to weigh this?"; (c) "How would it affect your life if you achieved it?"; (d) "If you were to gain weight, what would be the maximum that you could tolerate without panicking?"; (e) "How likely do you feel it is that you will achieve this higher weight?"; (f) "What would have to happen in order for you to get there?"; (g) "What do you think would happen if you do get there?" This line of inquiry is based on the working hypothesis that, according to the patient, thinness is happiness and fatness is misery; these questions are designed to test out the conceptual validity of this reasoning.

Bingeing and Vomiting. If the patient alludes to bingeing and vomiting during the weight history, the clinician needs to probe for current patterns within a functional analytic framework, looking for proximal antecedents and consequences of the bingeing and vomiting behavior. Emotional antecedents are important because many bulimic patients experience a negatively decelerating mood state in the hours leading up to a binge (Davis et al., 1985; Johnson & Larson, 1982). Determining the qualitative nature of the mood is also important because it is often the case that the patient's dysphoric mood stems from having eaten a small amount of forbidden food; having broken her dietary restraint, she feels guilty and ineffective for lapses in her otherwise rigid self-control over food (Fremouw & Heyneman, 1984). Other antecedent factors related to location, time of day, and social circumstance need to be assessed through direct probing. Above all, one needs to examine the degree to which the patient restricts her food intake in the hours preceding a binge. Mounting hunger and food preoccupation in the absence of food intake greatly increases the patient's risk for bingeing if the circumstances permit. Frequency of bingeing and vomiting, method of inducing vomiting, and quantity and types of food consumed during the binge also require assessment. Mood states following self-induced vomiting typically worsen even further (Davis et al., 1985), and it is important to ask the patient how she feels after a bulimic episode. Fatigue, guilt, and social interruption are frequently experienced.

Physiological and Psychological Sequelae. The patient may allude to these during her weight history, but more often than not they require direct questioning. Many sequelae cannot be directly examined by the nonmedical clinician (e.g., cardiac functioning, electrolyte balance, metabolic state). However, if the patient is in a state of semistarvation or is abusing laxatives and vomiting on a daily or greater basis, one can ask if associated physical symptoms are present (edema, paresthesias, muscle cramping, clouded sensorium). If there is reason to suspect physical abnormalities, the patient should be referred to a physician for a thorough examination. Complications of anorexia nervosa and bulimia nervosa have been discussed in detail elsewhere (Garfinkel & Garner, 1982; Garner, Rockert, et al., 1985; Mitchell et al., 1983). Depressive symptoms can and should be routinely evaluated; in particular, suicidal ideation is not uncommon and should be assessed (Hatsukami, Mitchell, et al., 1984).

Social Functioning. Social impairment in family and peer relationships is commonly observed in eating disorder patients (Johnson & Berndt, 1983; Mitchell et al., 1985). The patient's ability to function autonomously should be evaluated, particularly if she is still living with her family. In some cases, a parent's critical attitude toward the patient is predictive of whether she will drop out of treatment (Szmukler et al., 1985). Most patients complain that they lack meaningful peer or intimate relationships, and it is important to determine the degree to which this is a consequence of their focal eating pathology. For example, social anhedonia is a symptom of starvation (Keys et al., 1950) and this typically abates with renourishment; intimacy issues, interpersonal anxieties, and deficiencies in social skills do not, and these need to be addressed in psychotherapy. Assessing living arrangements is particularly important for the patient who binges because she is most vulnerable when at home alone. Job and school functioning should also be assessed. In some cases patients excel in their job or academic performance, but for others the focal eating pathology is so pernicious as to render gainful employment or scholastic achievement impossible.

Personality Features. Although a review of personality features associated with anorexia nervosa and bulimia nervosa is beyond the scope of this contribution, there are two specific comments that we believe are relevant regarding assessment. First, there is a consensus among most clinical theorists that no one personality structure is characteristic of either eating disorder. Based upon clinical observation, some have described subgroups which differ in terms of personality (Dally, 1969; Sours, 1980; Swift & Stern, 1982); others have proposed empirically derived typologies (Garner et al., 1984; Strober, 1983). Several authors have suggested that these disorders can develop within the context of "normal" personality development (Garner, Rockert, et al., 1985; Morgan & Russell, 1975). Second, regardless of whether personality is being assessed using interview or psychometric methods, it must be emphasized that presenting features can be significantly affected by starvation. Attempts should be made to gather information on pre-morbid functioning, and assessments on patients who have experienced significant weight loss must be tentative. Patients with poor pre-morbid functioning, borderline personality features, or severe characterological deficits may require more intensive treatment and may have a relatively poor prognosis.

Body Image Disturbances. The clinical relevance of body image disturbances to eating disorders often has been observed; however, there are many conceptual and methodological concerns related to assessment (Garner & Garfinkel, 1981). Different methods have been proposed to measure body size distortion; some are aimed at assessing overestimation of specific regions of the body (i.e. face, hips, waist) and others focus on estimation of body size using the subject's actual image distorted along the horizontal axis. At this time, the clinical utility of size overestimation is not clear, and therefore, it is probably of limited importance in clinical practice. There is, however, a logical connection between body dissatisfaction and eating disorders which makes assessment of this dimension of body image intuitively appealing. This construct has been assessed in anorexia nervosa and bulimia nervosa using the Body Dissatisfaction subscale of the Eating Disorder Inventory (Garner, Olmsted, & Polivy, 1983) and the Offer Self-Image Questionnaire (Casper, Offer, & Ostrov, 1981).

Impulse Related Behaviors. A number of empirical reports have documented that a significant number of eating disorder patients, particularly those with the symptom of bulimia, indicate more general problems with impulse control. Although this pattern may reflect characterological disturbance, it must be emphasized that these behaviors may be secondary to the eating disorder. For example, stealing may only involve food or laxatives, drug or alcohol abuse may be aimed at curbing appetite, mood fluctuations may be secondary to starvation, and suicide attempts may be directly related to despair associated with unremitting symptoms of the eating disorder. If careful assessment reveals more general problems in the area of impulse control, therapy may be more turbulent and a close liaison with an inpatient setting may be desirable.

Autonomy and Dependence. Although anorexia nervosa has been conceptualized from many points of view, most authors have presumed that issues related to separation, individuation, or heightened demands at adolescence are fundamental in the development of many cases of the disorder (cf. Crisp, 1980; Goodsitt, 1985). The failure to cope with maturational expectations may primarily reflect the patient's own psychopathology or it may be more related to separation fears communicated by the parents and the resulting interactional patterns within the family system. Assessment should be directed toward slowly uncovering salient maturational themes, with the recognition that the patient and her family may not have a clear awareness of these issues and that their precipitous exploration may be overwhelming. It is our clinical impression that these themes are most common among the classical anorexia nervosa patient; they also may be relevant in some cases of bulimia nervosa.

Family Functioning. The role of the family in the development of anorexia nervosa has received considerable attention in the clinical literature. The stereotypic family has been described as displaying high performance expectations, overprotectiveness, enmeshment, overconcern about weight or food, a façade of harmony, and various ambiguous communicational patterns (Bruch, 1973; Kalucy, Crisp, & Harding, 1977; Leibman, Minuchin, & Baker, 1974; Selvini-Palazzoli, 1974; Yager, 1982). Although a complete assessment must include an evaluation of family functioning, it is extremely difficult to separate pre-morbid contributing factors from disturbances which could be expected from having a serious illness within the family. Nevertheless, the identified patient and other family members may benefit from an assessment which avoids blame but conveys the message that everyone can play a meaningful role in the process of recovery.

Motivation for Change. Most patients approach treatment with considerable ambivalence because many of their symptoms are ego-syntonic. Therefore, the clinician must assess the motivation for change and implement specific strategies designed to enhance commitment to recovery (Garner, 1986). These involve providing the patient with detailed educational material regarding her disorder, reviewing certain ego-dystonic symptoms, and slowly developing a trusting therapeutic relationship. The issue of motivation must be repeatedly addressed throughout treatment since it is perhaps the single most important variable affecting outcome.

PSYCHOMETRIC EVALUATION

Self-report instruments provide the advantages of economy, actuarial scoring, lack of interviewer bias, and access to certain types of information which may not be as forthcoming in a personal interview. Recently, a number of psychometric instruments have been developed for the purpose of assessing symptoms characteristic of anorexia nervosa and bulimia nervosa (see Garner, Olmsted, & Polivy, 1983, for a review).

The psychometric evaluation of the eating disorder patient may be divided into two broad areas: (a) attitudes or behaviors related to food, eating, and body shape; and (b) psychological symptoms and personality features which may not be specific to eating disorders, but which may be fundamental in assessing the individual's psychological and social functioning.

The Eating Attitudes Test (EAT) was originally proposed to measure the symptoms of anorexia nervosa (Garner & Garfinkel, 1979) and abbreviated based upon a factor analysis (Garner, Olmsted, et al., 1982). The 26-item version of the EAT has been included on page 22 along with item scoring and notation of factors. The EAT has been used as a measure of symptomatology in clinical samples and as a screening instrument in nonclinical populations (Button & Whitehouse, 1981; Garner & Garfinkel, 1980). More recent investigations have revealed that individuals with bulimia nervosa score in a similar range on the EAT to those with anorexia nervosa (Fairburn & Cooper, 1982; Garner, Olmsted, et al., 1985). Table 3 on page 20 indicates that patients with bulimia nervosa, regardless of whether or not they have a history of anorexia nervosa, have similar scores to patients with the bulimic subtype of anorexia nervosa.

The Eating Disorder Inventory (EDI) was developed to go beyond the EAT in measuring various psychological traits found in eating disorders, as well as assessing disturbed attitudes related to eating and shape (Garner & Olmsted, 1984; Garner, Olmsted, & Polivy, 1983). Table 4 on page 20 illustrates mean scores for anorexia nervosa and bulimia nervosa patients on the eight subscales of the EDI. The first three subscales are aimed at weight and shape concerns that are present in anorexia nervosa and bulimia nervosa but are also evident in nonclinical groups of dieters (Garner & Olmsted, 1984). The remaining five subscales of the EDI measure traits that have been identified by clinical therapists as core elements in the psychology of eating disorders.

It must be remembered that the EAT, EDI, or any other self-report instrument should not be used as the sole means of diagnosing an eating disorder. First, considering the

TABLE 3: COMPARISON OF THE BULIMIC PATIENT GROUPS ON THE EATING ATTITUDES TEST

	Anorexia Nervosa: Bulimic Subtype < 80% (n = 32)	Bulimia Nervosa Hx AN < 80% (n = 34)	Bulimia > 25% weight loss (n = 28)	Bulimia < 25% weight loss (n = 36)
EAT-26 Total	44.3 (12.8)*	39.2 (13.1)	36.0 (12.5)	38.4 (10.5)
Dieting	24.6 (8.2)	22.2 (8.8)	20.6 (8.3)	23.4 (6.7)
Bulimia	11.3 (4.8)	11.9 (4.1)	12.0 (3.9)	11.7 (3.8)
Oral Control	8.4 (5.4)**	5.1 (4.9)	3.4 (3.4)	3.3 (2.8)

* Mean (Standard Deviation)
** Indicates this group significantly different ($p < .05$) from all groups to the right.

Adapted from "Similarities among Bulimic Groups Selected by Weight and Weight History" by D. M. Garner, M. P. Olmsted, and P. E. Garfinkel, 1985, Journal of Psychiatric Research, 19, p. 131.

TABLE 4: SCORES ON THE EATING DISORDER INVENTORY FOR WOMEN WITH BULIMIA NERVOSA, THE BULIMIC SUBTYPE OF ANOREXIA NERVOSA, AND THE RESTRICTING SUBTYPE OF ANOREXIA NERVOSA

Item	Bulimia Nervosa (n = 49)		Anorexia Nervosa: Bulimia Subtype (n = 45)		Anorexia Nervosa: Restricter Subtype (n = 40)	
	M	SD	M	SD	M	SD
Eating Disorder Inventory Subscales						
Drive for thinness	16.6	4.2	14.6[b]	5.8	11.2[c]	7.2
Bulimia	11.6	5.6	10.7[c]	5.4	2.1[c]	2.5
Body dissatisfaction	17.9	7.5	16.8	8.8	13.9[a]	7.5
Ineffectiveness	11.7	7.1	12.8	8.6	10.0	8.6
Perfectionism	8.7	5.1	8.4	5.4	8.2	5.1
Interpersonal distrust	4.4[a]	4.3	6.5	5.1	6.3	5.1
Interoceptive awareness	12.3	6.7	12.2[a]	7.0	9.3[a]	6.4
Maturity fears	4.7	4.8	6.5	7.1	6.0	6.0

[a] $p < 0.05$, for a family of 8 comparisons, the family-wise error rate = .34
[b] $p < 0.01$, for a family of 8 comparisons, the family-wise error rate = .08
[c] $p < 0.001$, for a family of 8 comparisons, the family-wise error rate = .008

Adapted from "The Validity of the Distinction Between Bulimia With and Without Anorexia Nervosa" by D. M. Garner, P. E. Garfinkel, and M. O'Shaughnessy, 1985, American Journal of Psychiatry, 142, pp. 581-587.

relatively low base rates for these syndromes, it would be impossible to devise an instrument that would have acceptable sensitivity, specificity, and positive predictive value. Second, the diagnosis of these disorders is relatively straightforward in a clinical interview. As a general rule, psychological tests should be used as an adjunct, not a replacement for clinical judgments. Nevertheless, self-report instruments provide a reliable, valid, and qualifiable measurement of important symptom dimensions.

The complete psychiatric assessment of the eating disorder patient should include standard measures of personality functioning and symptom areas such as anxiety, depression, and impulse related features (Strober, 1980). Ideally, convergent information from various sources will lead to the identification of distinct psychological typologies which may be meaningfully related to treatment and predictors of outcome.

SELF-MONITORING PROCEDURES

Self-monitoring refers to the systematic self-recording of one's own behavior as it occurs in the natural environment (Nelson, 1981). There are two principal advantages to using self-monitoring procedures in the clinical assessment of anorexia nervosa and bulimia nervosa. First, the information allows the clinician to fine tune the functional analysis of the patient's disturbed eating pathology which was tentatively formulated during the interview. For example, if the patient says in the interview that she binges in the evenings, the clinician could ascertain whether dietary restriction throughout the day is an antecedent by reviewing the frequency and quantity of food intake according to the patient's self-monitoring records. The second advantage to the procedure is that it allows the clinician to monitor the patient's progress over the course of treatment in areas which have been specifically targeted for therapeutic intervention. This, of course, necessitates continuous self-monitoring on the part of the patient. We have patients monitor the following on a daily basis over the course of assessment and treatment: (a) quantity and type of food and liquid consumed; (b) the time and date of the intake; (c) episodes of bingeing and vomiting; (d) urges to binge or vomit; and (e) thoughts and feelings associated with eating (see the Daily Eating Record on page 23). Most patients readily adopt the procedure, but some require more extensive instruction and encouragement. Following the guidelines set forth by Nelson (1981) usually results in satisfactory compliance and accuracy in self-monitoring. These include instruction in ongoing recording rather than recall, explicit definition of the facets to be monitored, modeling the appropriate use of the self-monitoring records, and emphasizing the integral value of the procedure to the therapeutic approach.

SUMMARY

A detailed clinical assessment is vital to the understanding of any psychological problem; however, it is particularly important for eating disorders since many of the focal symptoms may be masked by symptoms such as depression, anxiety, or disturbed social functioning. The foregoing contribution provides basic information regarding the definition of anorexia nervosa and bulimia nervosa. The similarities between these disorders is emphasized and they are distinguished from other disorders resulting in weight loss or dieting symptoms. Because many of the symptoms associated with eating disorders are the consequence of starvation, assessment must continue throughout the process of renourishment in the case of anorexia nervosa. Because the metabolic disturbances associated with bingeing and vomiting also produce a range of psychological symptoms, the bulimia nervosa patient must be reassessed once eating patterns are normalized. Clinical and psychometric techniques are described which enable the clinician to arrive at a diagnosis and to plan treatment which will focus initially on altering disturbed eating patterns and modifying distorted attitudes toward weight or shape. Once some symptomatic improvement has been achieved, it is recommended that assessment of personality, family, and social functioning be conducted using traditional methods. These areas become the focus of later stages of treatment.

EATING ATTITUDES TEST (EAT-26)

Name:_________________________________ Date:_____________________ Age:_______________

Present Weight:________________(lbs) Height:_____________________ Sex:_______________

Highest Past Weight:________________ How Long Ago?___________________

Lowest Past Adult Weight:____________ How Long Ago?___________________

<u>INSTRUCTIONS</u>

Please place an (X) under the column which applies best to each of the numbered statements. All of the results will be <u>strictly</u> confidential. Most of the questions directly relate to food or eating, although other types of questions have been included. Please answer each question carefully. Thank you.

ALWAYS USUALLY OFTEN SOMETIMES RARELY NEVER

1. Am terrified about being overweight.

2. Avoid eating when I am hungry.

3. Find myself preoccupied with food.

4. Have gone on eating binges where I feel that I may not be able to stop.

5. Cut my food into small pieces.

6. Aware of the calorie content of foods that I eat.

7. Particularly avoid foods with a high carbohydrate content (e.g., bread, rice, potatoes, etc.).

8. Feel that others would prefer if I ate more.

9. Vomit after I have eaten.

10. Feel extremely guilty after eating.

11. Am preoccupied with a desire to be thinner.

12. Think about burning up calories when I exercise.

13. Other people think that I am too thin.

14. Am preoccupied with the thought of having fat on my body.

15. Take longer than others to eat my meals.

16. Avoid foods with sugar in them.

17. Eat diet foods.

18. Feel that food controls my life.

19. Display self-control around food.

20. Feel that others pressure me to eat.

21. Give too much time and thought to food.

22. Feel uncomfortable after eating sweets.

23. Engage in dieting behavior.

24. Like my stomach to be empty.

25. Enjoy trying new rich foods.

26. Have the impulse to vomit after meals.

EAT - D. M. Garner and P. E. Garfinkel (1979), Toronto General Hospital, Toronto, Canada.

<u>Scoring Instructions</u>: Sum the responses to each item to arrive at a total score. "Always" = 3; "Usually" = 2; "Often" = 1; "Sometimes," "Rarely," and "Never" = 0 except for item 25 where the scoring is reversed. Items loading on Factor I (Dieting) are 1, 6, 7, 10, 11, 12, 14, 16, 17, 22, 23, 24, and 25. Items loading on Factor II (Bulimia and Food Preoccupation) are 3, 4, 9, 18, 21, and 26. Items loading on Factor III (Oral Control) are 2, 5, 8, 13, 15, 19, and 20.

DAILY EATING RECORD

DATE	FOOD AND LIQUID CONSUMED	EPISODES OF BINGEING AND VOMITING	URGES TO BINGE OR VOMIT	COMMENTS

<u>INSTRUCTIONS</u>: The information you provide on this record will help us to plan a course of treatment for you and monitor your progress. It is therefore very important that you follow these instructions. As soon as you consume any food or liquid, write a complete description of it including quantity in the second column. In the first column indicate the time and date of the intake. In the third column indicate which of these intakes was a binge and whether you induced vomiting or took laxatives. In the fourth column rate your urges to binge or vomit according to a 10 point rating scale where 0 means no urge and 9 means a very strong urge. In the last column make note of any thoughts and feelings you had while eating. Keep this record with you at all times and bring it to your next appointment.

David M. Garner, PhD, is currently an Ontario Mental Health Foundation Research Associate. He is also Professor of Psychiatry at the University of Toronto and the Director of Research in Psychiatry at the Toronto General Hospital. He received his degree in clinical psychology at York University in 1975 and has been active in research and clinical practice since that time. His current research involves the efficacy of two different therapies for eating disorders in a psychotherapy outcome study. Dr. Garner may be contacted at Toronto General Hospital, Bell Wing 4-639, 200 Elizabeth Street, Toronto, Ontario, M5G 2C4.

Ron Davis, PhD, is presently an Ontario Mental Health Foundation Post-Doctoral Fellow, and a Lecturer in Psychiatry at the University of Toronto. He received his clinical psychology degree in 1985 from Simon Fraser University, Burnaby, British Columbia. He is currently investigating the role of cognitive factors in eating disorders. Other interests include basic issues in therapeutic process and outcome. Dr. Davis can be contacted at Toronto General Hospital, Bell Wing 4-636, 200 Elizabeth Street, Toronto, Ontario, M5G 2C4.

RESOURCES

Abraham, S. F., & Beumont, P. J. V. (1982). How patients describe bulimia or binge eating. *Psychological Medicine, 12,* 625-635.

Akiskal, H. S. (1983). Dysthymic disorder: Psychopathology of proposed chronic depressive subtypes. *American Journal of Psychiatry, 140,* 11-21.

Altshuler, K. Z., & Weiner, M. F. (1985). Anorexia nervosa and depression: A dissenting view. *American Journal of Psychiatry, 142,* 328-332.

American Psychiatric Association. (1980). *Diagnostic and Statistical Manual of Mental Disorders* (3rd ed.). Washington, DC: Author.

Beck, A. T. (1976). *Cognitive Therapy and the Emotional Disorders.* New York: International Universities Press.

Beck, A. T., & Emery, G. (1985). *Anxiety Disorders and Phobias: A Cognitive Perspective.* New York: Basic Books.

Beck, A. T., Rush, A. J., Shaw, B. F., & Emery, G. (1979). *Cognitive Therapy for Depression.* New York: Guilford Press.

Bruch, H. (1973). *Eating Disorders.* New York: Basic Books.

Button, E. J., & Whitehouse, A. (1981). Subclinical anorexia nervosa. *Psychological Medicine, 11,* 509-516.

Cantwell, D. P., Sturzenberger, S., Burroughs, J., Salkin, B., & Green, J. K. (1977). Anorexia nervosa; an affective disorder? *Archives of General Psychiatry, 34,* 1087-1093.

Casper, R. C., Offer, D., & Ostrov, E. (1981). The self-image of adolescents with acute anorexia nervosa. *Journal of Pediatrics, 98,* 656-661.

Casper, R. C., Eckert, E. D., Halmi, K. A., Goldberg, S. C., & Davis, J. M. (1980). Bulimia: Its incidence and clinical importance in patients with anorexia nervosa. *Archives of General Psychiatry, 37,* 1030-1035.

Cone, J. D., & Hawkins, R. P. (Eds.). (1977). *Behavioral Assessment: New Directions in Clinical Psychology.* New York: Brunner/Mazel.

Cooper, P. J., & Fairburn, C. G. (in press). The depressive symptoms of bulimia nervosa. *British Journal of Psychiatry.*

Crisp, A. H. (1965). Some aspects of the evolution, presentation and follow-up of anorexia nervosa. *Proceedings of the Royal Society of Medicine, 58,* 814-820.

Crisp, A. H. (1980). *Anorexia Nervosa: Let Me Be.* New York: Grune and Stratton.

Crisp, A. H., Hsu, K. G., Harding, B., & Hartshorn, J. (1980). Clinical features of anorexia nervosa: A study of 102 female patients. *Journal of Psychosomatic Research, 24,* 179-191.

Crowther, J. H., Lingswiler, V. M., & Stephens, M. A. P. (1984). The topography of binge eating. *Addictive Behaviors, 9,* 299-303.

Dally, P. J. (1969). *Anorexia Nervosa.* New York: Grune and Stratton.

Dalvit-McPhillips, S. (1984). A dietary approach to bulimia treatment. *Physiology & Behavior, 33,* 769-775.

Davis, R. (1985). *The Functional Analysis and Treatment of Bulimia.* Unpublished doctoral dissertation, Simon Fraser University, Burnaby, British Columbia.

Davis, R., Freeman, R., & Solyom, L. (1985). Mood and Food: An analysis of bulimic episodes. *Journal of Psychiatric Research, 19,* 331-335.

Dempsey, D. T., Crosby, L. O., Lusk, E., Oberlander, J. L., Pertschuk, M. A., & Mullen, J. L. (1984). Total body water and total body potassium in anorexia nervosa. *The American Journal of Clinical Nutrition, 40,* 260-269.

Eckert, E. D., Goldberg, S. C., Halmi, K. A., Casper, R. C., & Davis, J. M. (1982). Depression in anorexia nervosa. *Psychological Medicine, 12,* 115-122.

Fairburn, C. G. (1982). *Binge-Eating and Bulimia Nervosa.* London: Smith, Kline & French Publications.

Fairburn, C. G., & Cooper, P. J. (1982). Self-induced vomiting and bulimia nervosa: An undetected problem. *British Medical Journal, 284,* 1153-1155.

Fairburn, C. G., & Cooper, P. J. (1984). The clinical features of bulimia nervosa. *British Journal of Psychiatry, 144,* 238-246.

Fairburn, C. G., Cooper, P. J., Kirk, J., & O'Connor, M. (1985). The significance of the neurotic symptoms of bulimia nervosa. *Journal of Psychiatric Research, 19,* 135-140.

Fairburn, C. G., & Garner, D. M. (1986). The diagnosis of bulimia nervosa. *International Journal of Eating Disorders, 5,* 403-419.

Feeling fat in a thin society. (1984, February). *Glamour Magazine,* pp. 198-201, 251-252.

Feighner, J. P., Robins, E., Guze, S. B., Woodruff, R. A., Winokur, G., & Munoz, R. (1972). Diagnostic criteria for use in psychiatric research. *Archives of General Psychiatry, 26,* 57-63.

Food and Nutrition Board Committee on Dietary Allowances. (1980). *Recommended Dietary Allowances* (9th ed.). Washington, DC: National Academy of Sciences.

Fremouw, W. J., & Heyneman, N. E. (1984). A functional analysis of binge episodes. In R. C. Hawkins, W. J. Fremouw, & P. F. Clement (Eds.), *The Binge-Purge Syndrome: Diagnosis, Treatment and Research* (pp. 254-263). New York: Springer.

Garfinkel, P. E., & Garner, D. M. (1982). *Anorexia Nervosa: A Multidimensional Perspective.* New York: Brunner/Mazel.

Garfinkel, P. E., Garner, D. M., Kaplan, A. S., Rodin, G., & Kennedy, S. (1983). Differential diagnosis of emotional disorders that cause weight loss. *Canadian Medical Association Journal, 129,* 939-945.

Garfinkel, P. E., & Kaplan, A. S. (1985). Perpetuating starvation based mechanisms in anorexia nervosa and bulimia. *International Journal of Eating Disorders, 4,* 651-665.

Garfinkel, P. E., Kaplan, A. S., Garner, D. M., & Darby, P. L. (1983). The differentiation of vomiting/weight loss as a conversion disorder from anorexia nervosa. *American Journal of Psychiatry, 140,* 1019-1022.

Garfinkel, P. E., Moldofsky, H., & Garner, D. M. (1980). The heterogeneity of anorexia nervosa: Bulimia as a distinct subgroup. *Archives of General Psychiatry, 37,* 1036-1040.

Garner, D. M. (1985). Iatrogenesis in anorexia nervosa and bulimia nervosa. *International Journal of Eating Disorders, 5,* 701-726.

Garner, D. M. (1986). Cognitive therapy for bulimia nervosa. *The Annals of Adolescent Psychiatry, 13.*

Garner, D. M., & Bemis, K. M. (1982). A cognitive-behavioral approach to anorexia nervosa. *Cognitive Therapy and Research, 6,* 123-150.

Garner, D. M., & Bemis, K. M. (1985). Cognitive therapy for anorexia nervosa. In D. M. Garner & P. E. Garfinkel (Eds.), *Handbook of Psychotherapy for Anorexia Nervosa and Bulimia* (pp. 107-146). New York: Guilford Press.

Garner, D. M., & Garfinkel, P. E. (1979). The eating attitudes test: An index of the symptoms of anorexia nervosa. *Psychological Medicine, 9,* 273-279.

Garner, D. M., & Garfinkel, P. E. (1980). Socio-cultural factors in the development of anorexia nervosa. *Psychological Medicine, 10,* 649-656.

Garner, D. M., & Garfinkel, P. E. (1981). Body image in anorexia nervosa: Measurement, theory and clinical implications. *International Journal of Psychiatry in Medicine, 11,* 263-284.

Garner, D. M., Garfinkel, P. E., & Bemis, K. M. (1982). A multidimensional psychotherapy for anorexia nervosa. *International Journal of Eating Disorders, 1,* 3-46.

Garner, D. M., Garfinkel, P. E., & O'Shaughnessy, M. (1985). The validity of the distinction between bulimia with and without anorexia nervosa. *American Journal of Psychiatry, 142,* 581-587.

Garner, D. M., & Olmsted, M. P. (1984). *Eating Disorder Inventory Manual.* Odessa, FL: Psychological Assessment Resources.

Garner, D. M., Olmsted, M. P., Bohr, Y., & Garfinkel, P. E. (1982). The eating attitudes test: Psychometric features and clinical correlates. *Psychological Medicine, 12,* 871-878.

Garner, D. M., Olmsted, M. P., & Garfinkel, P. E. (1983). Does anorexia nervosa occur on a continuum? Subgroups of weight-preoccupied women and their relationship to anorexia nervosa. *International Journal of Eating Disorders, 2,* 11-20.

Garner, D. M., Olmsted, M. P., & Garfinkel, P. E. (1985). Similarities among bulimic groups selected by weight and weight history. *Journal of Psychiatric Research, 19,* 129-134.

Garner, D. M., Olmsted, M. P., & Polivy, J. (1983). Development and validation of a multidimensional eating disorder inventory for anorexia nervosa and bulimia. *International Journal of Eating Disorders, 2,* 15-34.

Garner, D. M., Olmsted, M. P., Polivy, J., & Garfinkel, P. E. (1984). Comparison between weight-preoccupied women and anorexia nervosa. *Psychosomatic Medicine, 46,* 255-266.

Garner, D. M., Rockert, W., Olmsted, M. P., Johnson, C., & Coscina, D. V. (1985). Psychoeducational principles in the treatment of bulimia and anorexia nervosa. In D. M. Garner & P. E. Garfinkel (Eds.), *Handbook of Psychotherapy for Anorexia Nervosa and Bulimia* (pp. 513-572). New York: Guilford.

Geiselman, P. J., & Novin, D. (1982). The role of carbohydrates in appetite, hunger and obesity. *Appetite: Journal for Intake Research, 3,* 203-223.

Goodsitt, A. (1985). Self psychology and the treatment of anorexia nervosa. In D. M. Garner & P. E. Garfinkel (Eds.), *Handbook of Psychotherapy for Anorexia Nervosa and Bulimia* (pp. 55-82). New York: Guilford.

Gwirtsman, H. E., Roy-Burne, P., Yager, J., & Gerner, R. H. (1983). Neuroendocrine abnormalities in bulimia. *American Journal of Psychiatry, 140,* 559-563.

Halmi, K. A. (1974). Anorexia nervosa: Demographic and clinical features in 94 cases. *Psychosomatic Medicine, 36,* 18-26.

Halmi, K. A., Falk, J. R., & Schwartz, E. (1981). Binge-eating and vomiting: A survey of a college population. *Psychological Medicine, 11,* 697-706.

Hamilton, M. K., Gelwick, B. P., & Meade, C. J. (1984). The definition and prevalence of bulimia. In R. C. Hawkins, W. J. Fremouw, & P. F. Clement (Eds.), *The Binge-Purge Syndrome: Diagnosis, Treatment, and Research* (pp. 3-26). New York: Springer.

Hatsukami, D., Eckert, E., Mitchell, J. E., & Pyle, R. (1984). Affective disorder and substance abuse in women with bulimia. *Psychological Medicine, 14,* 701-704.

Hatsukami, D. K., Mitchell, J. E., & Eckert, E. D. (1984). Eating disorders: A variant of mood disorder? *Psychiatric Clinics of North America, 7,* 349-365.

Herzog, D. B. (1984). Are anorexic and bulimic patients depressed? *American Journal of Psychiatry, 141,* 1594-1597.

Holmgren, S., Humble, K., Norring, C., Roos, B. E., Rosemark, B., & Sohlberg, S. (1983). The anorectic bulimic conflict: An alternative diagnostic approach to anorexia nervosa and bulimia. *International Journal of Eating Disorders, 2,* 3-14.

Hudson, J. I., Pope, H. G., Jonas, J. M., Laffer, P. S., Hudson, M. S., & Melby, J. C. (1983). Hypothalamic-pituitary-adrenal-axis hyperactivity in bulimia. *Psychiatry Research, 8,* 111-117.

Hudson, J. I., Pope, H. G., Jonas, J. M., & Yurgelun-Todd, D. (1983). Family history study of anorexia nervosa and bulimia. *British Journal of Psychiatry, 142,* 133-138.

Huse, D. M., & Lucas, A. R. (1984). Dietary patterns in anorexia nervosa. *American Journal of Clinical Nutrition, 40,* 251-254.

Igoin-Apfelbaum, L. (1985). Characteristics of family background in bulimia. *Psychotherapy and Psychosomatics, 43,* 161-167.

Isner, J. M., Roberts, W. C., Heymsfield, S. B., & Yager, J. (1985). Anorexia nervosa and sudden death. *Annals of Internal Medicine, 102,* 49-52.

Johnson, C. L., & Berndt, D. J. (1983). Preliminary investigation of bulimia and life adjustment. *American Journal of Psychiatry, 140,* 774-777.

Johnson, C. L., & Larson, R. (1982). Bulimia: An analysis of moods and behavior. *Psychosomatic Medicine, 44,* 341-351.

Johnson, C. L., Stuckey, M. K., Lewis, L. D., & Schwartz, D. M. (1982). Bulimia: A descriptive survey of 316 cases. *International Journal of Eating Disorders, 2,* 3-16.

Kalucy, R. S., Crisp, A. H., & Harding, B. (1977). A study of 56 families with anorexia nervosa. *British Journal of Medical Psychology, 50,* 381-395.

Keesey, R. E. (1980). A set point analysis of the regulation of body weight. In A. J. Stunkard (Ed.), *Obesity* (pp. 144-165). Philadelphia: W. B. Saunders.

Keys, A., Brozek, J., Henschel, A., Mickelsen, O., & Taylor, H. L. (1950). *The Biology of Human Starvation.* Minneapolis: University of Minnesota Press.

Kirkley, B. G., Agras, W. S., & Weiss, J. J. (1985). Nutritional inadequacy in the diets of treated bulimics. *Behavior Therapy, 16,* 287-291.

Leibman, R., Minuchin, S., & Baker, L. (1974). An integrated treatment program for anorexia nervosa. *American Journal of Psychiatry, 131,* 432-436.

Maloney, N., & Ward, M. (1976). *Psychological Assessment: A Conceptual Approach.* New York: Oxford University Press.

Marshall, M. H. (1978). Anorexia nervosa: Dietary treatment and re-establishment by body weight in 20 cases studied on a metabolic unit. *Journal of Human Nutrition, 32,* 349-357.

Mitchell, J. E., Hatsukami, D., Eckert, E. D., & Pyle, R. L. (1985). Characteristics of 275 patients with bulimia. *American Journal of Psychiatry, 142,* 482-485.

Mitchell, J. E., Pyle, R. L., Eckert, E. D., Hatsukami, D., & Lentz, R. (1983). Electrolyte and other physiological abnormalities in patients with bulimia. *Psychological Medicine, 13,* 273-278.

Mitchell, J. E., Pyle, R. L., Hatsukami, D., & Boutacoff, L. I. (1984). The dexamethasone suppression test in patients with bulimia. *Journal of Clinical Psychiatry, 45,* 508-511.

Morgan, H. G., & Russell, G. F. M. (1975). Value of family background and clinical features as predictors of long-term outcome in anorexia nervosa: Four year follow-up study of 41 patients. *Psychological Medicine, 5,* 355-371.

Nelson, R. O. (1981). Realistic dependent measures for clinical use. *Journal of Consulting and Clinical Psychology, 49,* 168-182.

Nisbett, R. E. (1972). Eating behavior and obesity in men and animals. *Advances in Psychosomatic Medicine, 7,* 173-193.

Norman, D. K., & Herzog, D. B. (1984). Persistent social maladjustment in bulimia: A 1-year follow-up. *American Journal of Psychiatry, 141,* 444-446.

Piran, N., Kennedy, S., Garfinkel, P. E., & Owens, M. (1985). Affective disturbance in eating disorders. *The Journal of Nervous and Mental Disease, 173,* 395-400.

Polivy, J., & Herman, C. P. (1985). Dieting and bingeing: A causal analysis. *American Psychologist, 40,* 193-201.

Pope, H. G., Hudson, J. I., Jonas, J. M., & Yurgelun-Todd, D. (1983). Bulimia treated with Imipramine: A placebo-controlled, double-blind study. *American Journal of Psychiatry, 140,* 554-558.

Pyle, R. L., Mitchell, J. E., & Eckert, E. D. (1981). Bulimia: A report of 34 cases. *Journal of Clinical Psychiatry, 42,* 60-64.

Pyle, R. L., Mitchell, J. E., Eckert, E. D., Halvorson, P. A., Newman, P. A., & Goff, G. M. (1983). The incidence of bulimia in freshman college students. *International Journal of Eating Disorders, 2,* 75-85.

Richardson, R. M. A., Forbath, N., & Karanicolas, S. (1983). Hypokalemic metabolic alkalosis caused by surreptitious vomiting: Report of four cases. *Canadian Medical Association Journal, 129,* 142-146.

Russell, G. F. M. (1979). Bulimia nervosa: An ominous variant of anorexia nervosa. *Psychological Medicine, 9,* 429-448.

Schlesier-Stropp, B. (1984). Bulimia: A review of the literature. *Psychological Bulletin, 95,* 247-257.

Selvini-Palazzoli, M. (1974). *Anorexia Nervosa.* London: Chaucer.

Silverman, J. A. (1983). Medical consequences of starvation; the malnutrition of anorexia nervosa. In P. L. Darby, P. E. Garfinkel, D. M. Garner, & D. V. Coscina (Eds.), *Anorexia Nervosa: Recent Developments* (pp. 293-299). New York: Alan R. Liss.

Solyom, L., Freeman, R. J., Thomas, C. D., & Miles, J. E. (1983). The comparative psychopathology of anorexia nervosa: Obsessive-compulsive disorder or phobia? *International Journal of Eating Disorders, 3,* 3-14.

Sours, J. A. (1980). *Starving to Death in a Sea of Objects: The Anorexia Nervosa Syndrome.* New York: Jason Aronson.

Spitzer, R. L., & Williams, J. B. W. (1984). *The Initial Interview: Evaluation Strategies for DSM-III Diagnosis; Interviewer's Manual.* New York: BMA Audio Cassette Publications.

Strober, M. (1980). Personality and symptomatological features in young, nonchronic anorexia nervosa patients. *Journal of Psychosomatic Research, 24,* 353-359.

Strober, M. (1983). An empirically derived typology of anorexia nervosa. In P. L. Darby, P. E. Garfinkel, D. M. Garner, & D. V. Coscina (Eds.), *Anorexia Nervosa: Recent Developments.* New York: Alan R. Liss.

Swift, W. J., & Stern, S. (1982). The psychodynamic diversity of anorexia nervosa. *International Journal of Eating Disorders, 2,* 17-35.

Szmukler, G. I., Eisler, I., Russell, G. F. M., & Dare, C. (1985). Anorexia nervosa, parental "expressed emotion" and dropping out of treatment. *British Journal of Psychiatry, 147,* 265-271.

Walsh, B. T., Stewart, J. W., Roose, S. P., Gladis, M., & Glassman, A. H. (1984). Treatment of bulimia with Phenelzine: A double-blind, placebo-controlled study. *Archives of General Psychiatry, 41,* 1105-1109.

Webb, W. L., & Gehi, M. (1981). Electrolyte and fluid imbalance: Neuropsychiatric manifestations. *Psychosomatics, 22,* 199-202.

Welle, S. L., Amatruda, J. M., Forbes, G. B., & Lockwood, D. H. (1984). Resting metabolic rates of obese women after rapid weight loss. *Journal of Clinical Endocrinology and Metabolism, 59,* 41-44.

Yager, J. (1982). Family in the pathogenesis of anorexia nervosa. *Psychosomatic Medicine, 44,* 43-60.

Zubin, J. (1979). Research in clinical diagnosis. In B. B. Wolman (Ed.), *Clinical Diagnosis of Mental Disorders: A Handbook* (pp. 3-14). New York: Plenum Press.

THE FUNDAMENTALS OF PSYCHOTHERAPY FOR ANOREXIA NERVOSA AND BULIMIA NERVOSA

David M. Garner and Paul Isaacs

Psychotherapy with eating disordered patients is different in important ways from psychotherapy with any other group of patients. We believe that recognition of the intimate interplay between physiology and psychology in eating disorders is a prerequisite to successful treatment of the majority of such patients. In the material which follows, we will introduce concepts and techniques that will aid the clinician in adapting his or her treatment approach to take this interplay into account. The primary goal of this contribution is to present a practical set of principles for management of anorexia nervosa and bulimia nervosa on an outpatient basis. This framework is also appropriate for inpatient treatment of these disorders; however, other recent contributions have been specifically tailored to the multidisciplinary inpatient regimen (Andersen, Morse, & Santmyer, 1985; Garner & Garfinkel, 1985). In keeping with the practical focus, the current contribution will not include exhaustive citations for each section because much of the material has been presented by our group elsewhere (Garfinkel & Garner, 1982; Garner, 1986, in press; Garner & Bemis, 1982, 1985; Garner & Isaacs, 1985; Garner, Garfinkel, & Bemis, 1982; Garner et al., 1985). The more academically oriented reader is advised to consult the sources cited above for further clarification.

Much has been written regarding the etiology of anorexia nervosa and, to a lesser extent, bulimia nervosa.* Many plausible theories have been proposed to account for the development of anorexia nervosa from a wide variety of conceptual vantage points. These vantage points include Freudian drive theory, object relations theory, self-psychology, family interactional concepts, and cognitive theory. Despite this diversity among theoretical formulations, many clinicians who specialize in the treatment of patients with eating disorders have evolved certain common strategies. Our own view is that a search for a single common developmental pattern for all patients with anorexia nervosa is unlikely to yield meaningful results. We regard eating disorders as common final pathways arrived at from different developmental histories that are at least as diverse as the various etiological theories (Garfinkel & Garner, 1982).

As discussed in the preceding contribution on assessment of eating disorders, anorexia nervosa and bulimia nervosa share certain essential features; primary among these is an extreme preoccupation with weight and shape. The central theme which unites the diverse symptomatology of these disorders is the patient's conviction that "it is absolutely essential that I be thin(ner)." Secondary to this conviction is behavior intended either to produce weight loss or to prevent weight gain. In any given patient's history this belief will have become crystallized during a period of stress, often one which carries demands for autonomous functioning. The patient embraces the idea that losing weight will somehow alleviate her distress, and weight loss becomes a vehicle for achieving a kind of salvation without having to directly tackle difficult interpersonal issues (since the eating disorders discussed here primarily affect women, the feminine pronoun is used throughout this contribution).

---

*The use of the term bulimia to describe both a symptom and a syndrome has led to considerable confusion in the eating disorder literature; we will follow the convention suggested by Russell (1979) by referring to the symptom of uncontrollable overeating as bulimia and the syndrome as bulimia nervosa.

PREDISPOSING FACTORS

Many factors have been found to predispose individuals to develop anorexia nervosa. The primary psychological factor within the individual is a deficit in autonomous functioning. Bruch (1962, 1978) has identified this as a sense of personal ineffectiveness. This may be related to general difficulties in the area of identity formation or separation from parents, or to particular stressors such as early pubertal development, difficulties in autonomy due to being a twin, or other fears associated with maturation. Higher than average weight is a predisposing factor in some cases, especially among bulimia nervosa patients. Higher weight could act as a predisposing factor via several different mechanisms. The most obvious is the creation of a negative social stigma within the peer group. A less obvious mechanism may be the association during adolescence of higher weight with early pubertal development and hence an earlier confrontation with the demands of adolescence and emergent sexuality. Last, some investigators believe that the disturbed body image, which is characteristic of the eating disorders, may come about as a result of a perceptual deficit that is predisposing to the illness (cf. Garner & Garfinkel, 1981). Research has yet to establish, however, whether this deficit is a predisposing factor or sequel to the disorders.

PERPETUATING FACTORS

Once a patient has embarked on a diet, there are many factors which act to perpetuate the pursuit of thinness. Most patients are relieved and exhilarated by the early success of their weight-reduction campaign. Having struggled for much of their lives with a pervasive sense of inadequacy and impotence, they are delighted by the discovery that their figures and appetites are among the few things over which they can exercise some control. They derive a gratifying sense of power from their self-restraint (Garner & Bemis, 1982). Initially they are also likely to receive strong environmental support in the form of compliments from friends and family on their thinner appearance and on their self-control. The compliments may eventually turn to expressions of concern if extreme thinness or emaciation is achieved, but the behaviors and beliefs surrounding the value of thinness become functionally autonomous over time, so that even punishment from the environment will have little impact. Contributing to this isolation of the symptom from environmental influences is the increasing role of avoidance behavior. The initial pleasure at weight loss is transformed into a fear of weight gain, and much of the patient's behavior is directed at avoiding eating. Both anorexic patients and many nonemaciated bulimia nervosa patients starve themselves for many hours during the day, eat large quantities of food, and subsequently vomit. Most eating disorder patients are very much preoccupied with avoiding normal eating, which they perceive to be a threat to their weight goals. Since environmental cues for eating are so widespread, and so prominent to hungry individuals, a great many stimuli become occasions for avoidance.

GENERAL ISSUES PERTAINING TO TREATMENT

We have found that the features shared between anorexia nervosa and bulimia nervosa permit similar treatment strategies to be formulated for the two disorders. There are differences that revolve around specific strategies for achieving weight gain in the emaciated population and for dealing with the symptom of bulimia with either the bulimia nervosa or the anorexia nervosa patient. These strategies will be described in separate sections of this contribution.

THE TWO-TRACK APPROACH

We advocate a two-track approach to treatment (Garner & Isaacs, 1985). The first track pertains to achieving behavioral change in the patient's current eating pattern. This track distinguishes therapy with eating disorder patients from other forms of psychotherapy. It involves what may seem to be the mundane tasks of specifically addressing the patient's eating and weight control patterns; however, it is an essential element in bringing about meaningful changes. The second track pertains to examining psychological issues which underlie the disorder. There are two broad categories into which these issues may be grouped. The first category subsumes those issues which are most obviously connected to the symptomatology, namely concerns with weight or shape and the multiple meanings which have come to be associated with feeling "fat" or feeling "thin." The second category is comprised of other psychological issues such as low self-esteem, separation anxiety or guilt, difficulty with autonomous functioning, impulse control, affective disturbances, and interpersonal relationships in general. This second category has much in common with issues that are salient in other noneating disordered populations.

MEDICAL CONSULTATION AND HOSPITALIZATION

Both anorexia nervosa and bulimia nervosa are serious disorders with significant risks of mortality or morbidity. Awareness of the complications of these disorders is a prerequisite for conducting outpatient psychotherapy. Patients who are at a low weight, who lose weight precipitously, induce vomiting, or abuse purgatives or other medications, should be monitored frequently by a physician. Hospitalization may be required for renourishment, to control bingeing and vomiting, to assess or treat various physical complications, or to disengage the patient from an interpersonal system which is maintaining the disorder. Although there are no established guidelines regarding the amount of weight loss or the frequency of vomiting which necessitate hospitalization, it is our impression that a conservative approach based upon common sense and an understanding of potential complications leads to a clear decision in most cases. Particularly with patients who are at risk for cardiac abnormalities due to emaciation, frequent vomiting, or both, aerobic exercise should be discouraged.

We feel that, whether or not hospitalization is required, it is both ethically necessary and therapeutically useful to inform patients of the potential complications arising from severe weight loss, vomiting, and laxative abuse. This illustrates to the patient, often for the first time, the risks involved by persisting in these self-destructive behaviors. We have found that many patients can benefit from reading an educational manual (Garner et al., 1985) which describes many of the complications of disordered eating. However, many patients persist in disturbed eating patterns despite an awareness that their behavior is dangerous because the prospect of a higher body weight is completely unacceptable. In these cases the patient's physical status must be monitored frequently, and hospitalization should be considered if weight decreases or eating patterns become chaotic.

SOURCES OF RESISTANCE TO TREATMENT

For many eating disorder patients, some of the most insidious symptoms are ego-syntonic. The sense of control over their weight may be one of the few sources of positive feeling. This is in marked contrast to patients who present with subjectively distressing symptoms, as is the case in depression or anxiety based disorders. While it might seem that the bulimic patient's motivation to receive treatment would be greater than that of the anorexic because of the distress that is associated with bingeing and vomiting, this motivation may quickly fade with the recognition that the goals of treatment go beyond mere control of these symptoms. Both groups of patients tend to be resolved in their commitment to dieting and the maintenance of a "suboptimal" weight. Although it is not articulated as such, a minority of bulimic patients essentially want therapy to convert them to restricting anorexics. If initially asked what their goal for therapy is, they will state that it is to "stop bingeing and vomiting and to be thin." In instances in which they wish to maintain a more statistically normal weight, the goal may be no less realistic if they have a personal history of obesity. In our setting, many of the so-called "normal weight bulimic" patients have lost as much weight as patients with anorexia nervosa - the only difference is that the bulimia nervosa patients began their weight loss from much higher levels (Garner, 1986). When it is explained that the bingeing and vomiting cycle is partially a consequence of extreme dieting, many patients become quite distressed, preferring instead to see these symptoms as manifestations of poor self-control. Unfortunately, this view is unwittingly shared by some treatment approaches to bulimia which emphasize self-control procedures without an apparent understanding of the biological factors that may precipitate or maintain binge-eating (cf. Garner et al., 1985).

Another source of resistance to treatment is wariness as a result of previous treatment failures. There are a variety of treatment approaches that represent direct attacks on the patient's sense of personal autonomy or ignore food and weight issues in the course of psychotherapy. These treatments may leave patients feeling either violated or not understood. The potentially harmful effects of treatment and their role in resistance have been discussed elsewhere (Brotman, Stern, & Herzog, 1984; Garner, 1985).

Finally, a significant number of patients are coerced by family or friends into seeking therapy. The primary symptoms of these patients are more distressing to those around them than they are to themselves. Even though they may desperately require therapy due to the physical and emotional effects of their illness, they may be difficult to engage in the therapeutic endeavor. For younger patients these issues are probably best resolved within the context of family therapy (Minuchin, Rosman, & Baker, 1978). Clinical experience and preliminary research evidence indicate that patients from about 16 years of age or older may benefit from an individual therapy that initially highlights goals that are separate from those expressed by family members who have pressured the patient to seek help.

THE IMPORTANCE OF THE THERAPEUTIC RELATIONSHIP

One of the key ingredients in helping a patient to exchange the positive feelings engendered by dietary and weight "control" for the promise of ultimate improvement is a trusting therapeutic relationship. Almost all writers in this field agree that it is particularly important to achieve a strong therapeutic alliance with eating disorder patients. Our view on the significance of the therapeutic relationship has been presented elsewhere (Garner & Bemis, 1985; Garner et al., 1982); however, there are several fundamental points worthy of emphasis. Receiving help is itself conflictual for many of these patients, and great sensitivity is needed because the therapy may require the therapist to assume some degree of control or guidance of the patient's eating. A caring attitude and a genuine concern for the patient are necessary, and the patient must understand that this concern extends beyond issues of food and weight. Nevertheless, excessive or inappropriate warmth will also cause difficulties. Eating disorder patients are prone to feeling worthless and undeserving, and too much warmth may be perceived as an attempt at manipulation or may evoke feelings of guilt. Most patients have difficulty with closeness in relationships, and are guarding against feelings of dependence associated with relationships in which they have felt insignificant and subject to influence. Fears of abandonment or of engulfment may lead to overtly disruptive behavior designed to provoke rejection and thereby assert mastery over the situation. The therapist must be tolerant while still maintaining appropriate limits. Occasionally, genuine but dramatic expressions of concern, such as scheduling an emergency appointment, will have positive impact on the patient and provide early signs of the therapist's trustworthiness. Talking to the patient about her fears and expectations surrounding the therapeutic relationship is also beneficial. The relationship provides a conduit for examining the expectations that the patient applies to her interpersonal world.

THE INITIAL INTERVIEWS

The goals for the few initial interviews are to establish a therapeutic alliance, to conduct an assessment, and to begin the process of therapy. These are discussed below.

The anorexic patient usually comes to therapy with the conviction that her experiences are idiosyncratic and that no one (especially someone without the disorder) could possibly appreciate life from her perspective. The bulimic patient often presents with feelings of shame regarding her behavior. In both cases the therapist must demonstrate an understanding of the range of unusual behaviors associated with the disorder and its phenomenology. Along with communicating warmth, concern, and empathy, demonstrating familiarity with the patient's problem helps to establish the trusting therapeutic alliance which is a prerequisite to therapy. Thus, the assessment component of the initial interviews may itself be used to foster the therapeutic alliance.

The assessment aspects are presented in detail in the preceding contribution. Of particular concern in the initial sessions is the set of circumstances surrounding the initiation of treatment. Some patients will have sought therapy on their own, and others will have reluctantly acquiesced to the demands of parents after months of bitter struggle. Regardless of the antecedent events, the therapist should clarify that the purpose of therapy is to address the patient's underlying unhappiness, which has been responsible for the symptom development. If "unhappiness" is denied, the point should not be pressed, and greater attention should be focused on the psychological and physiological effects of starvation and bulimia. Information regarding weight history, current eating patterns, and behaviors employed to lose weight should always be collected.

The therapist should also obtain information regarding family context, personal history, and living circumstances. This information should be gathered slowly and with particular sensitivity to the way in which the patient sees herself, her goals, her family relationships, and the meaning she attributes to potentially frightening issues associated with adolescence and separation from parents.

As described earlier, the therapy itself may be introduced to the patient as a two-track process. In emphasizing the initial importance of track one issues (normalization of eating and weight), much information can be imparted to the patient. The gentle questioning and sensitive imparting of information provide an important opportunity to establish rapport in early meetings. In particular, we find it very useful to outline the effects of starvation and to differentiate these symptoms from other primary psychological symptoms.

THE CONSEQUENCES OF STARVATION

An essential informational base that a therapist must first acquire when treating eating disordered patients is a familiarity with the physical and psychological consequences of starvation (see Garfinkel & Garner, 1982; Garner et al., 1985). Many of the symptoms that have been ascribed to the syndrome of anorexia nervosa are actually a direct result of the starvation process. Experimental research on starvation, conducted with normal volunteers over 35 years ago, has shed light on the extent of the psychological disturbances associated with starvation (Keys et al., 1950). One of the most salient consequences of starvation is the preoccupation with food. Most anorexic patients, while steadfastly avoiding eating, collect recipes, read books about food, and are often enthusiastic cooks. Unusual ritualistic behavior associated with eating and increasingly lengthy periods of time spent eating are also characteristic of semistarvation. Other starvation effects include depression, anxiety, irritability, lability of mood, sleep disturbance, loss of sexual interest, and social withdrawal.

NORMALIZATION OF EATING AND WEIGHT

The effects of abnormal eating patterns, vomiting, and strict dieting are both psychological and physical. Patients who have lived with abnormal eating patterns for months or years will not typically be aware of the extent to which the gradual shift in their psychological well-being has been influenced by their eating behavior.

The patient's motivation for normalizing her eating behavior prior to changing her basic attitude toward weight and dieting is derived primarily from distress based upon physical symptoms that become attributed to starvation or vomiting, and faith in the therapist's judgment which grows from the therapeutic alliance. It is only when patients begin to experience the psychological benefits of normalized eating that they recognize the extent to which their whole experience has been colored by their abnormal behavior. As one patient indicated after 2 weeks of eating normally for the first time in many years: "It is as though a veil were lifted. I never realized the difference between anxiety and hunger and was always on edge. Now I feel calm. For the first time in years, my thoughts aren't racing inside my head."

The therapist is confronted with a host of practical issues in helping a patient give up entrenched, perhaps ritualistic behavior in favor of normal eating patterns. Most patients have literally lost the concept of what constitutes a "normal" meal. Our therapeutic strategy provides considerable structure initially; this is decreased as the patient becomes less fearful of weight gain. Most patients have very unrealistic notions of what will happen to their weight if they eat normally. Monitoring weight and discussing the way in which their bodies are using the food that they eat will help patients relinquish their fears and develop a more realistic appraisal of the effects of eating on weight gain. Because the relationship between the number of calories consumed and change in body weight is not a simple linear function, it is necessary to provide specific information on the metabolic effects of eating on weight gain. One reason that clinical experience is so important with these patients is that it provides the therapist with confidence that initial rapid weight gain with large quantities of food is followed by a much more gradual rate of gain, and eventually a plateau which may require a further increase in calories. For patients who, at least on a theoretical level, can accept a somewhat more realistic body shape, knowledge of the metabolic adaptation to increased caloric intake provides some reassurance that their body weight is not destined to skyrocket out of control.

We have found that providing patients with a manual which describes the metabolic and psychological consequences of starvation, as well as other information about weight regulation, is a useful adjunct to psychotherapy. By explaining to the patient that many of her distressing symptoms are consequences of her abnormal eating behavior and reinforcing this with educational material, it becomes more apparent that it is only by achieving a normal pattern of eating and maintaining this pattern for awhile that both patient and therapist will be able to determine which problems are due to starvation and which problems require resolution through psychotherapy.

The therapist may then begin to gently promote the view that it would be both misleading and futile to try to deal psychologically with problems that are in fact being maintained by her eating behavior. This concept presents a major stumbling block to many psychotherapists and patients alike. While intellectually we all acknowledge that mind and body are not separate domains, most clinicians tend to discount the degree to which chronic hunger, vomiting, or general physiological disruption affects psychological state. If a patient does not appear to be in grave physical danger, there is a tendency among therapists who have been psychologically trained to rapidly dismiss this half of the mind-body interaction in favor of concentrating on the psychological underpinnings of the disorder. The experience of seeing a rapid transformation in psychological characteristics (e.g., increased frustration tolerance, improved mood, and enhanced ego strength) in just a few patients is enough to convince most therapists that it is indeed worth emphasizing track one early in the treatment process.

MEAL PLANNING

Most bulimic and anorexic patients are or have been chronic dieters. Even if they are not currently dieting, bulimic patients typically experience extreme guilt eating foods that they consider to be "fattening." Exposing and clarifying many of the myths and overgeneralizations that have been promoted by the dieting industry are the first steps in easing these patients out of their current pattern. Ideally, the therapist should be aware of the basics of nutrition which may be used to counter these extreme ideas about food, eating, and weight. The long-term goal is for the patient to be able to eat enough to maintain a healthy physiology (including menstruation) without feeling abnormally hungry or feeling strong urges to binge eat. Unfortunately, a history of disturbed eating patterns leads to confusion around feelings of satiety and hunger. Until these signals normalize, it is necessary to essentially "imitate" a normal eating plan despite feelings of psychological and occasionally physical discomfort.

We find a reasonable starting point is three regularly spaced meals a day with one or two snacks, totaling about 2000 calories. Patients often fear that if they eat this much food their weight will increase dramatically. Their fears in this regard must be explored and met with two lines of reassurance. First, their weight will be monitored and the diet adjusted if they are gaining weight too rapidly (this is true for emaciated patients who require controlled weight gain, as well as for nonemaciated patients who are below their "natural" body weight). Second, as mentioned earlier, patients who have lowered their basal metabolic rate through dieting must understand that their basic requirements for calories can increase dramatically with the consistent consumption of greater amounts of food. Most patients are aware of isolated nutritional axioms, such as "3500 excess calories creates a 1 pound weight gain," without understanding that changes in basal metabolic rate will allow them to ultimately accommodate a considerable number of calories without further weight gain. While their weight may have to be higher than they prefer, they may be reassured that there is little danger that their worst fear (i.e., uncontrollable weight gain) will be realized. Any statements regarding predicted weight changes should be qualified by explaining that individual differences in metabolism and shifts within their own metabolism or activity level mean that the same amount of calories may have slightly different effects at different times as they begin to normalize the physiological and psychological response to food. Patients should also be prepared for an initial weight gain due to rehydration; this weight gain does not consist of body fat, and weight gain will not continue at this same rate.

Eliciting a patient's agreement that normal eating is a reasonable goal is often not a difficult therapeutic task. However, if the patient leaves the office having agreed to this plan without having thought through in vivid detail what is required, no significant behavioral change can be expected. The reason for this is that the patient's starting point for thinking about meal planning is a diet designed to achieve weight loss. If left to her own devices, she will modify her intake slightly and still fear that she is eating too much.

The aim of meal planning is to help a patient who becomes anxious at the thought of eating normally or who is very confused about what constitutes normal eating. The degree of structure and the specific components that are included should be determined by assessing these two facets of the patient's response to eating. At the least structured end, suitable for patients who are highly motivated, who have a good understanding of the concept of "nondieting," and who have overcome most of their fears of weight gain, regularly discussing what they are eating, providing information, and exploring their residual anxieties may be enough to sustain them. This, however, is not sufficient for most patients who experience guilt at the mere prospect of eating. For these patients it is often essential to begin by planning individual meals in advance. This process can be time-consuming and probably stands in sharp contrast to the kinds of sessions with which most therapists are familiar; however, this is not wasted time, because it conveys to the patient that the therapist understands the extent to which her anxieties about eating are incapacitating.

The planning process involves presenting the patient with some choices and having her make decisions from among these choices based on her own preferences. Diet foods and any foods which evoke associations of dieting are avoided. This process may be extremely anxiety arousing for a patient who lacks a concept of eating that is not bound to dieting. Also, it pre-supposes a trusting therapeutic relationship through which agreement has been established regarding the goal of ultimate recovery from the eating disorder.

For some patients it is desirable to monitor food intake, as well as incidents of bulimia or vomiting, on self-monitoring sheets. Although the details of different strategies for meal planning and self-monitoring vary, all provide structure which can facilitate the gradual development of more appropriate eating patterns (Fairburn, 1983; Garner et al., 1985; Long & Cordle, 1982; Loro, 1984; Mitchell et al., 1985; Russell, 1979). The decision to use self-monitoring should be based on whether or not this strategy will provide the patient a desired sense of security and control.

In cases where self-monitoring is viewed as a threat to autonomy or is otherwise unpalatable, these reservations can often be overcome by discussing the purpose of recording food intake. However, sometimes the patient needs to try normalizing her eating on her own and may discover that, despite agreeing in principle, she is unable to achieve the desired normalization. She may then be ready to accept the therapist's offer of a more structured approach. As the patient becomes more confident, structured eating and monitoring of food intake may be gradually replaced by more natural eating behavior. A sustained resistance to self-monitoring usually indicates the patient's lack of acceptance of eating and weight goals; the contradiction between this stance and her goal of recovery should be explored in detail.

INTRODUCTION OF AVOIDED FOODS

Rigid avoidance of certain foods or food groups is characteristic of anorexia nervosa and bulimia nervosa. The avoidance follows directly from fears that these foods will cause weight gain or loss of control. Because self-induced vomiting may be at least partially maintained by the belief that it is the only means by which the patient can consume highly palatable foods, it is imperative that these "forbidden foods" be gradually introduced into the regular diet. Qualitative restriction usually creates a greater desire for these foods and intensifies the fear of being out of control when they are available.

The therapist should gradually challenge the patient's beliefs that certain foods are intrinsically harmful, even in moderate quantities, and help her to understand that the real threat to her well-being is her eating disorder. The avoided foods may be gradually introduced in normal quantities into the patient's meal plan at times specified in advance. She is encouraged to mechanically eat these foods as "medication" or as a "therapeutic inoculation" against binge eating in the future. The powerful urge to overeat on certain foods usually subsides once they become a regular part of the meal plan and after weight has stabilized at an appropriate level.

DETERMINING AN APPROPRIATE BODY WEIGHT

Throughout history and even today for most of mankind, conscious decisions regarding how to determine an appropriate body weight have been largely irrelevant. Although there are factors that appear to exert some influence on set point (e.g., exercise, food palatability, climate), significant changes in weight result in physiological compensations designed to return the individual to a state of equilibrium in terms of body weight. There appear to be individual differences in the degree of plasticity in the mechanisms that determine the set point for body weight, but, in general, short-term fluctuations in food intake and exercise are met by metabolic adaptations aimed at body weight stability. Although there is some scientific controversy surrounding the construct of "set point," it is a useful concept clinically and has sound empirical support. For further discussion of the set point concept, see Keesey (1980) and Mrosovsky and Powley (1977); we have discussed its relationship to anorexia nervosa and bulimia nervosa elsewhere (Garner et al., 1985).

Determining the target weight for a patient for whom the equilibrium between intake, activity level, and metabolism has been disturbed requires an estimate based upon ideographic factors. It is most definitely in contrast with the view of weight as something which should be determined on the basis of esthetic considerations; it is also contrary to the view that target weights should be set on the basis of tables of population norms based on aggregate statistics. Our view is that "healthy" body weights, like other physical attributes, are distributed normally in the population (Garner et al., 1985). According to this view, originally expressed by Nisbett (1972), many people who are heavier than average or even "obese" may not be suffering from a weight disorder, but may be naturally over the mean weight for their height, sex, and age. This viewpoint is consistent with the growing evidence that the health risks associated with moderate obesity have been exaggerated (cf. Fitzgerald, 1981). The weight histories of bulimic patients indicate that many have been obese, and that many have lost as much body weight as typical patients diagnosed as having anorexia nervosa, even though they have never appeared emaciated (Garner, 1986). Bulimia nervosa or anorexia nervosa patients with a history of obesity may need to maintain a higher weight than they would prefer in order to reduce the biological pressure toward binge eating.

There are several possible practical approaches for arriving at a target weight. For emaciated anorexic patients the immediate goal is to help the patient out of physical danger. An effective starting point in this case is usually a goal of 90% of the mean matched population weight. However, this must be modified to take into consideration the patient's own weight history. Some patients are able to describe a stable body weight, which pre-dated their eating disorder and which they maintained without dieting. In many instances this was followed by a period of precipitous weight gain and the intensification of feeling "fat." Most college age women who are not intensely concerned about their body weight seem to maintain a body weight that is less than 10% below their highest weight (Garner et al., 1984). Most bulimic patients report that their highest stable body weight prior to the onset of their disorder was approximately 10% below their highest weight (Abraham & Beumont, 1982). This may be terrifying for patients with pre-morbid obesity and distressing for others who consider their ideal weight to be much lower than their highest pre-morbid stable weight. Moreover, this guideline may have to be modified based upon the patient's capacity for change.

Bulimic patients should be advised that once they refrain from vomiting or purgative abuse, they may gain a considerable amount of weight due to "rebound" water retention. They should be reassured that this is not body fat and that it will "normalize" naturally if they avoid vomiting and purgatives.

Sometimes the target weight must be arrived at very gradually or in several stages. Patients who fear that their "set point is extraordinarily high" can be given some reassurance that it is very unlikely that their set point is higher than their previous highest stable weight. Moreover, not all patients are destined to remain at a weight that they find unacceptable. Many bulimic patients actually maintain or lose weight when they cease dieting and vomiting with the resolve that they are no longer willing to sacrifice personal health or comfort in the struggle to achieve a lower weight than their physiology will easily permit.

MONITORING WEIGHT

Monitoring of weight on a regular basis serves several functions. It allows the therapist and patient to separate feelings of "fatness" and "thinness" from the reality represented by the scale. Monitoring of weight also provides a source of reassurance that weight gain is gradual and will not be permitted to proceed in an uncontrolled fashion; this allows the patient to focus on other salient psychological issues.

As with the determination of a target weight, there are several alternative strategies for deciding on the frequency and manner of weighing. Fairburn (1983, 1985) has recommended that patients weigh themselves on one particular morning each week. With patients who are extremely sensitive about weight changes, we recommend that they discontinue weighing themselves at home and that they be weighed on a weekly basis by their therapist (Garner et al., 1985). Some patients prefer to be informed of their weight so that potential distress may be addressed in therapy; others who tend to become preoccupied with minute shifts in weight prefer to be "blind" to the weighings. These latter patients step on the scale facing backwards and are only informed if there is a consistent trend up or down over several weeks.

ADDITIONAL ISSUES IN THE
TREATMENT OF BULIMIA NERVOSA

THE SELF-PERPETUATING CYCLE OF BULIMIA AND VOMITING

Russell (1979) originally conceptualized bulimia nervosa as a self-perpetuating cycle involving an interaction between psychological and physiological mechanisms. Shape dissatisfaction that is usually, but not necessarily, accompanied by low self-esteem and, in some cases, by more severe personality disturbance, leads to an organized system of beliefs aimed at strict dieting and weight loss. Weight loss and a sustained "suboptimal" weight produce physiological responses reflected by increased hunger, food preoccupations, and bouts of overeating, all of which are designed to return the organism to a "healthy weight" or a constitutionally determined "set point" for body weight. Cognitive and emotional factors determine whether binge eating will be triggered or prevented. The reliance on self-induced vomiting perpetuates the disorder by keeping weight at a reduced level and by diminishing anxiety associated with consuming foods perceived as fattening. Occasionally, self-induced vomiting may be maintained by positive contingencies such as attention from family members or pleasurable sensations (Stoller, 1982).

PSYCHOLOGICAL AND PHYSIOLOGICAL DETERMINANTS OF BINGE EATING

It is widely recognized that binge eating may be triggered by certain stressful circumstances, relationship conflicts, or negative feeling states. Bulimia is, however, an unlikely response among stressed or emotionally disturbed individuals who are not dieting. Because binge eating is more ego-alien than dieting, patients are often extremely distressed by the question "Why do I binge?" They expect from psychotherapy a psychological answer to this question, and will usually have some hypotheses of their own about interpersonal conflict or feelings of frustration and anger as explanations for their binge eating. Frequently, however, the patient neglects to report that the binge was preceded by 8 to 12 hours or more of virtual starvation. In these cases, it is important that the dieting and weight suppression be confronted in the therapy and that the therapist not collude with the patient's proffering of interesting material which ignores the physiological component of her binge. We find that once the patient understands the role of dieting in triggering binge eating and is willing to normalize her eating, therapy takes on a somewhat different focus. Discussion of what triggers the occasional "emotional" binge becomes meaningful and constitutes a vehicle for dealing with important psychological issues.

SPECIFIC INTERVENTIONS TO REDUCE BINGEING AND VOMITING

There are two fundamental reasons for dealing with the vomiting as the highest priority: (a) vomiting acts to legitimize overeating by reducing anxiety and guilt, and (b) vomiting is also more directly associated with medical complications. The essential strategy for reducing bingeing is to convince the patient to inhibit the urge to vomit while beginning to eat normal meals. While strongly suggesting that dieting and vomiting are inconsistent with the goal of recovery, we recognize that total abstinence from these practices may take some time for certain patients to achieve. Dealing with the patient's post-binge feelings of failure and the belief that they have "blown everything" can be a useful therapeutic task.

Bulimia evolves as a response to complex biological, social, and psychological forces and there will inevitably be periodic relapses. While bingeing and vomiting should not be taken casually, patients should be discouraged from overinterpreting the significance of either success or failure early in the course of treatment. These are not always reliable indices of one's psychological status. Instead, the task is to recover immediately from each relapse by reinstituting their plans for control - not just the urge to binge but the desire to diet as well.

One of the most common reactions to an episode of bingeing and vomiting is to skip the next meal or to abandon eating for the entire day. Such self-punitive measures merely reintroduce the vicious cycle. Relapse must be followed by the commitment to begin at the first step of prevention by consuming the entire next meal without avoiding any of the foods outlined in the meal plan.

We have emphasized that prevention of vomiting and normalization of eating are the two key ingredients in the treatment of bulimia. A secondary or adjunct set of strategies involves teaching the patient to find ways of identifying cues which are typically associated with bingeing and then either avoiding or coping with them more adaptively. Such stimulus control techniques as distraction, delay, planned imagery, and thought stopping can be of benefit. These are all control techniques which can be applied when the urge to binge is present. The primary techniques, described earlier, are aimed at removing the biological bases for the urge to binge, and their full effect may not be realized for many weeks or months. Patients may be somewhat reassured by reading about the experiences of normal victims of semistarvation whose urge to "binge eat" subsided only after many months of renutrition and having returned to the pre-experiment weight (see Garner et al., 1985).

COGNITIVE BEHAVIORAL METHODS

The cognitive behavioral approach to anorexia nervosa and bulimia nervosa emphasizes the logical connection between beliefs or assumptions held by the patient and the symptom patterns which are characteristic of her disorder. The apparently bizarre symptoms of self-starvation, bingeing followed by purging, and extreme weight control are more understandable within the context of the assumption that "thinness is absolutely vital to happiness and well-being."

Modifications of conventional cognitive-behavioral methods have been suggested recently to deal with the special problems posed by the eating disorder patient (Fairburn, 1981, 1985; Garner, 1986, in press; Garner & Bemis, 1982, 1985; Garner et al., 1982). Although the context and style of cognitive-behavioral therapy with eating disorders may differ somewhat from that described for other disorders (e.g., Beck, 1976), the fundamental goals of the therapy are the same and may be summarized as follows:

1. The patient is taught to monitor her own thinking or to heighten awareness of her own thinking. This involves extracting the essential or core aspects of particular dysfunctional beliefs. Beliefs must be articulated, clarified, and operationalized in order to determine their consequences.
2. The patient is helped to recognize the connection between certain dysfunctional thoughts and maladaptive behaviors and emotions.
3. Together, the patient and therapist examine the evidence for the validity of particular beliefs. The implications of certain attitudes or assumptions should be followed to their logical conclusion.
4. The patient is taught to gradually substitute more realistic and appropriate interpretations based upon the evidence.
5. The ultimate goal is the modification of underlying assumptions which are fundamental determinants of specific dysfunctional beliefs.

One of the advantages of the cognitive-behavioral model is that it is not necessarily incompatible with other approaches to treatment. While the cognitive-behavioral model may be distinguished by its explicit concern with values and beliefs, to varying degrees most psychotherapeutic models emphasize the surplus or distorted meanings held by the patient, and many interventions are aimed at providing the reality-oriented feedback designed to alter these misperceptions. Other advantages of the cognitive-behavioral approach with eating disorders have been described elsewhere (Fairburn, 1985; Garner & Bemis, 1982, 1985; Guidano & Liotti, 1983).

Specific cognitive interventions such as "decentering," "decatastrophizing," "prospective hypothesis testing," "reattribution," and "palliative techniques" have been described in detail elsewhere (Garner & Bemis, 1985). The mere articulation of beliefs may be helpful for many patients who are struggling to determine how their values may differ from those of their parents. Finally, encouraging patients to engage in certain behavioral exercises such as normal eating, inhibition of symptoms such as vomiting and laxative abuse, and exercise rituals invariably exposes a plethora of assumptions which may become the focal point of meetings. The success of these exercises depends upon a trusting therapeutic alliance and a realistic expectation for progress.

PSYCHOLOGICAL ISSUES IN THE TREATMENT OF ANOREXIA NERVOSA AND BULIMIA NERVOSA

To achieve a lasting cure of an eating disorder, more is required than control of the maladaptive eating behaviors. The second therapeutic track deals with the proximal underpinnings of the eating pathology, namely the patient's distorted attitudes towards weight and shape, and the more distal underpinnings, namely underlying psychological issues that may have contributed to the development of an eating disorder. In presenting the material that follows, we will focus more on delineating the various themes that are likely to emerge in therapy with eating disorder patients than on specific techniques of intervention. Salient themes will vary from patient to patient. While the initial focus on track one creates a certain consistency to the therapy across patients, the diversity in track two issues causes the long-term therapy to be shaped by each patient's unique circumstances and developmental history.

ATTITUDES TOWARD WEIGHT AND SHAPE

The preoccupation with thinness which is seen in its most extreme form in the eating disorders is not just an individual preoccupation but a societal one. One of the major obstacles in the treatment of anorexia nervosa and bulimia nervosa is the fact that many of the therapeutic objectives are contrary to the emphasis on dieting and slimness which are currently pervasive in Western society. Challenging the patient's association between slenderness and feelings of self-worth becomes onerous in light of the consistent bombardment with messages such as those embodied in the lyrics of a recent commercial for a diet soft drink: "I believe in being the best I can be. I believe in counting every calorie."

We believe that this sociocultural pressure on women is enormously influential and cannot be overlooked in treatment (see Garner & Garfinkel, 1980; Garner et al., 1980). Considerable emphasis in therapy is devoted to questioning the unrealistic and potentially destructive definition of feminine attractiveness in terms of a pre-pubertal shape. This must be done while scrupulously avoiding a direct assault on the patient for adhering to this aesthetic standard. The notion that slimness is the road to beauty, happiness, security, and approval may be gradually disputed by carefully determining its implications and sources of validity.

It is important for the therapist to understand and possibly to re-examine his or her own attitudes towards weight when treating these patients. We believe that it is helpful for the therapist to be a counterbalancing force, someone who can take a stand that opposes the prevailing cultural norms when they are clearly destructive. This stance serves the dual functions of modeling a well integrated capacity for autonomy and attacking the specific attitudes which hamper the patient's progress.

SELF-ESTEEM

Deep-seated feelings of worthlessness are characteristic of both anorexic and bulimic patients. These patients typically try to view their performances through the eyes of others, hoping to see some measure of approval reflected there, while being quite convinced that they are unlikely to find it. Anorexic patients, in particular, tend to feel incompetent at what they do and are very much preoccupied with evaluating themselves, only finding satisfaction from "flawless" performances. To quote one patient: "Each day is a hurdle to be overcome, each action a performance which must be rehearsed before being executed perfectly." Spontaneous access to her own feelings was impossible. The only happiness she experienced was the momentary joy of hearing applause, knowing that one hurdle had been overcome successfully.

Therapy is, in part, directed at helping the patient to find other ways of feeling good about herself. This is achieved by validating any hints of self-expression or risk taking and by encouraging efforts at mastery in areas that are feared. It is also done by providing a relationship in which she is nurtured in developing and applying her own standards based on trusting her own subjective feeling states. Other specific methods for encouraging self-esteem have been articulated elsewhere (Garner & Bemis, 1985; Garner et al., 1982).

SELF-TRUST OR SELF-AWARENESS

A number of authors have suggested that anorexia nervosa patients exhibit a remarkable lack of confidence or trust in the validity of their own thoughts, feelings, and perceptions (Bruch, 1962, 1973; Frazier, 1965; Goodsitt, 1977; Selvini-Palazzoli, 1978; and others). Similar observations have been made more recently about those with bulimia nervosa (Johnson & Larson, 1982; Orleans & Barnett, 1984; White & Boskind-White, 1984). The inner confusion may relate to distorted beliefs about the legitimacy of experiencing certain emotions such as anger, or it may reflect a conflict between the experience of sensations such as those associated with hunger, sexual excitement, or fatigue, and beliefs about the moral acceptability of these experiences. A detailed presentation of therapeutic strategies aimed at the gradual development of self-awareness is beyond the scope of this contribution and has been recently presented by several writers (cf. Garner & Garfinkel, 1985).

DEVELOPMENTAL ISSUES

One of the features of normal development is a gradual transition in which the child learns to trust his or her own perceptions, partly by finding a reasonable match between these and parents' perceptions. According to a number of theorists who have speculated about the etiology of anorexia nervosa, when this match does not exist, a developmental roadblock is created, and the child is left constantly in need of external direction and is vulnerable to the development of conflicts in the areas of separation and autonomy (Bruch, 1962, 1973; Selvini-Palazzoli, 1978).

Bruch (1962, 1973) has attributed the anorexic patient's low self-esteem and confusion about internal state to early disturbances in parenting. She postulates that the mother's failure to accurately respond to the child's inner needs by superimposing her own inaccurate perception of those needs, leads to the child developing confusion surrounding inner experiences. Being deprived of these "inner guideposts" leaves the child dependent upon others and vulnerable to feelings of helplessness or loss of control. Similar views have been expressed by others to account for the development of anorexia nervosa (Goodsitt, 1985; Masterson, 1977; Selvini-Palazzoli, 1978; Sours, 1980).

Crisp (1965, 1980) has advanced a somewhat different developmental explanation for anorexia nervosa. According to his model, the anorexic patient's dieting and starvation become mechanisms by which she regresses to a pre-pubertal appearance, hormonal status, and experiential posture. She is thus able to avoid various elements of adolescent turmoil and family conflicts for which she feels unprepared.

Various therapeutic strategies have been proposed to address the developmental fears and uncertainties observed in many anorexia nervosa and bulimia nervosa patients. Individual therapy may help the patient face the feared state of physical maturity and the resulting developmental expectations that it implies. Either individual or family therapy may facilitate the development of autonomy by repeatedly differentiating between parental expectations and those of the patient. Both parents and the anorexic child may experience anxiety or even guilt surrounding the entire process of separation.

Recently a distinction has been drawn between the kind of separation anxiety just discussed and a related aspect of separation, namely, guilt (Friedman, 1985). In some families the message is conveyed that the separation or maturity of the patient will cause harm to a parent or sibling. Where this is the case, one often gets a clear sense that the patient is protecting someone by holding herself in check. This "protection of the parent" theme, and the associated sense of guilt at autonomous functioning, should be addressed in its own right and distinguished from the patient's concerns about her own performance, or separation anxiety. Whereas family therapy affords an opportunity to directly challenge dysfunctional thought patterns that imply difficulties in separation, individual therapy may provide the support to enable the patient to break away from an enmeshed and overprotective environment.

MULTIDIMENSIONAL PSYCHOTHERAPY

From a review of the diverse theoretical accounts of anorexia nervosa and bulimia nervosa, it is apparent that many are describing the same type of patient using a different language or perspective. Others seem to focus upon a subgroup of patients for whom particular themes are salient. For example, Masterson (1977) illustrates the impulse control and separation themes which are readily apparent in some patients but not in others. Minuchin et al. (1978) describes themes which are dominant with most younger patients but may be less important or even irrelevant for some older patients. Our view of these disorders as multidetermined has led to the development of multifaceted treatment strategies which incorporate principles from different orientations (Garfinkel & Garner, 1982; Garner & Bemis, 1982, 1985; Garner et al., 1982).

Many themes commonly found to pervade the psychology of the eating disorder patient are not directly tied to food or weight. Therapeutic strategies for dealing with these themes need not differ from those applied to other patient populations. However, it is our impression that the orthodox practice of traditional methods without attention to issues which are specific to the eating disorder patient (e.g., management of eating and body weight) may alienate the patient, frustrate the therapist, and result in unnecessary treatment failure. By contrast, traditional methods may be adapted to accommodate those special needs (Bruch, 1982; Goodsitt, 1985; Rosen & Leitenberg, 1985; Schwartz, Barrett, & Saba, 1985).

SUMMARY

The aim of this contribution has been to review a range of clinical strategies which we have found useful in the treatment of anorexia nervosa and bulimia nervosa. A two track approach to psychotherapy was described: The first track applies to issues related to symptom management and the second track addresses psychological themes which may lead to the development or maintenance of these disorders. The current contribution has emphasized the track one aspects of management, because these are most often overlooked by clinicians who have had limited experience with eating disorder patients. In actual practice, the majority of time in therapy is spent on track two; however, this pre-supposes that consistent progress is being made in the areas of eating and weight.

In our experience, the content of therapy is altered remarkably when patients actually begin to normalize eating and weight. If fears related to eating and shape are not addressed directly, the patient generally does not have the capacity to progress to the point of exploring other meaningful psychological topics. Educational materials can be extremely useful in motivating the patient in therapy; they may be employed to challenge erroneous assumptions and self-defeating behaviors which perpetuate the disorders.

Several psychological themes which are common to eating disorders were briefly presented. It was emphasized that there is no one psychology of anorexia nervosa or bulimia nervosa - both are final common pathways that derive from a range of individual, familial, and sociocultural predisposing factors.

David M. Garner, PhD, is currently an Ontario Mental Health Foundation Research Associate. He is also Professor of Psychiatry at the University of Toronto and the Director of Research in Psychiatry at the Toronto General Hospital. He received his degree in clinical psychology at York University in 1975 and has been active in research and clinical practice since that time. His current research involves the efficacy of two different therapies for eating disorders in a psychotherapy outcome study. Dr. Garner may be contacted at Toronto General Hospital, Bell Wing 4-639, 200 Elizabeth Street, Toronto, Ontario, M5G 2C4.

Paul Isaacs, PhD, is presently a Research Associate in the Department of Psychiatry at Toronto General Hospital in Toronto, Canada. His training is in clinical psychology and his other areas of interest include individual differences in mental imagery and cerebral laterality. Dr. Isaacs can be contacted at Toronto General Hospital, Bell Wing 4-636, 200 Elizabeth Street, Toronto, Ontario, M5G 2C4.

RESOURCES

Abraham, S. F., & Beumont, P. J. V. (1982). How patients describe bulimia or binge eating. *Psychological Medicine, 12,* 628-635.

Andersen, A. E., Morse, C., & Santmyer, K. (1985). Inpatient treatment for anorexia nervosa. In D. M. Garner & P. E. Garfinkel (Eds.), *Handbook of Psychotherapy for Anorexia Nervosa and Bulimia* (pp. 311-343). New York: Guilford Press.

Beck, A. T. (1976). *Cognitive Therapy and the Emotional Disorders.* New York: International Universities Press.

Brotman, A. W., Stern, T. A., & Herzog, D. B. (1984). Emotional reactions of house officers to patients with anorexia nervosa, diabetes and obesity. *International Journal of Eating Disorders, 3,* 71-77.

Bruch, H. (1962). Perceptual and conceptual disturbances in anorexia nervosa. *Psychosomatic Medicine, 24,* 187-194.

Bruch, H. (1973). *Eating Disorders: Obesity, Anorexia Nervosa and the Person Within.* New York: Basic Books.

Bruch, H. (1978). *The Golden Cage: The Enigma of Anorexia Nervosa.* Cambridge: Harvard University Press.

Bruch, H. (1982). Anorexia nervosa: Therapy and theory. *American Journal of Psychiatry, 139,* 1531-1538.

Crisp, A. H. (1965). Clinical and therapeutic aspects of anorexia nervosa: A study of 30 cases. *Journal of Psychosomatic Research, 9,* 67-78.

Crisp, A. H. (1980). *Anorexia Nervosa: Let Me Be.* London: Academic Press.

Fairburn, C. G. (1981). A cognitive-behavioral approach to the management of bulimia. *Psychological Medicine, 141,* 631-633.

Fairburn, C. G. (1983). The place of a cognitive-behavioral approach in the management of bulimia. In P. L. Darby, P. E. Garfinkel, D. M. Garner, & D. V. Coscina (Eds.), *Anorexia Nervosa: Recent Developments* (pp. 393-402). New York: Alan R. Liss.

Fairburn, C. G. (1985). Cognitive-behavioral treatment for bulimia. In D. M. Garner & P. E. Garfinkel (Eds.), *Handbook of Psychotherapy for Anorexia Nervosa and Bulimia* (pp. 160-192). New York: Guilford Press.

Fitzgerald, F. T. (1981). The problem of obesity. *Annual Review of Medicine, 32,* 221-231.

Frazier, S. H. (1965). Anorexia nervosa. *Diseases of the Nervous System, 26,* 155-159.

Friedman, M. (1985). Survivor guilt in the pathogenesis of anorexia nervosa. *Psychiatry, 48,* 25-39.

Garfinkel, P. E., & Garner, D. M. (1982). *Anorexia Nervosa: A Multidimensional Perspective.* New York: Brunner/Mazel.

Garner, D. M. (1985). Iatrogenesis in anorexia nervosa and bulimia nervosa. *International Journal of Eating Disorders, 5,* 701-726.

Garner, D. M. (1986). Cognitive therapy for bulimia nervosa. *The Annals of Adolescent Psychiatry, 13.*

Garner, D. M. (in press). Cognitive therapy for anorexia nervosa. In K. D. Brownell & J. P. Foreyt (Eds.), *Physiology, Psychology and Treatment of Eating Disorders.* New York: Basic Books.

Garner, D. M., & Bemis, K. M. (1982). A cognitive-behavioral approach to anorexia nervosa. *Cognitive Therapy and Research, 6,* 123-150.

Garner, D. M., & Bemis, K. M. (1985). Cognitive therapy for anorexia nervosa. In D. M. Garner & P. E. Garfinkel (Eds.), *Handbook of Psychotherapy for Anorexia Nervosa and Bulimia* (pp. 107-146). New York: Guilford Press.

Garner, D. M., & Garfinkel, P. E. (1980). Sociocultural factors in the development of anorexia nervosa. *Psychological Medicine, 10,* 649-656.

Garner, D. M., & Garfinkel, P. E. (1981). Body image in anorexia nervosa: Measurement, theory and clinical implications. *International Journal of Psychiatry in Medicine, 11,* 263-284.

Garner, D. M., & Garfinkel, P. E. (Eds.). (1985). *Handbook of Psychotherapy for Anorexia Nervosa and Bulimia.* New York: Guilford Press.

Garner, D. M., Garfinkel, P. E., & Bemis, K. M. (1982). A multidimensional psychotherapy for anorexia nervosa. *International Journal of Eating Disorders, 1,* 3-46.

Garner, D. M., Garfinkel, P. E., Schwartz, D., & Thompson, M. (1980). Cultural expectations of thinness in women. *Psychological Reports, 47,* 483-491.

Garner, D. M., & Isaacs, P. (1985). Psychological issues in the diagnosis and treatment of anorexia nervosa and bulimia. In R. E. Hales & A. J. Francis (Eds.), *Psychiatry Update* (Vol. 4, pp. 503-515). Washington, DC: American Psychiatric Association.

Garner, D. M., Olmsted, M. P., Polivy, J., & Garfinkel, P. E. (1984). Comparison between weight-preoccupied women and anorexia nervosa. *Psychosomatic Medicine, 46,* 255-266.

Garner, D. M., Rockert, W., Olmsted, M. P., Johnson, C. L., & Coscina, D. V. (1985). Psychoeducational principles in the treatment of bulimia and anorexia nervosa. In D. M. Garner & P. E. Garfinkel (Eds.), *Handbook of Psychotherapy for Anorexia Nervosa and Bulimia* (pp. 513-572). New York: Guilford Press.

Goodsitt, A. (1977). Narcissistic disturbances in anorexia nervosa. In S. C. Feinstein & P. L. Giovacchini (Eds.), *Adolescent Psychiatry* (Vol. 5, pp. 304-312). New York: Jason Aronson.

Goodsitt, A. (1985). Self-psychology in the treatment of anorexia nervosa. In D. M. Garner & P. E. Garfinkel (Eds.), *Handbook of Psychotherapy for Anorexia Nervosa and Bulimia* (pp. 55-82). New York: Guilford Press.

Guidano, V. F., & Liotti, G. (1983). *Cognitive Processes and Emotional Disorders: A Structural Approach to Psychotherapy*. New York: Guilford Press.

Johnson, C. L., & Larson, R. (1982). Bulimia: An analysis of moods and behavior. *Psychosomatic Medicine, 44,* 333-345.

Keesey, R. E. (1980). A set point analysis of the regulation of body weight. In A. J. Stunkard (Ed.), *Obesity* (pp. 144-165). Philadelphia: W. B. Saunders.

Keys, A., Brozek, J., Henschel, A., Mickelsen, O., & Taylor, H. L. (1950). *The Biology of Human Starvation*. Minneapolis: University of Minnesota Press.

Long, G. C., & Cordle, C. J. (1982). Psychological treatment of binge eating and self-induced vomiting. *British Journal of Medical Psychology, 55,* 139-145.

Loro, A. D. (1984). Binge-eating: A cognitive-behavioral treatment approach. In R. C. Hawkins, W. J. Fremouw, & P. F. Clement (Eds.), *The Binge/Purge Syndrome: Diagnosis, Treatment and Research* (pp. 183-210). New York: Springer.

Masterson, J. F. (1977). Primary anorexia nervosa in the borderline adolescent: A object-relations view. In P. Hartocollis (Ed.), *Borderline Personality Disorders* (pp. 475-494). New York: International Universities Press.

Minuchin, S., Rosman, B. L., & Baker, J. (1978). *Psychosomatic Families: Anorexia Nervosa in Context*. Cambridge: Harvard University Press.

Mitchell, J. E., Hatsukami, D., Goff, G., Pyle, R. L., Eckert, E. D., & Davis, J. M. (1985). Intensive outpatient group treatment for bulimia. In D. M. Garner & P. E. Garfinkel (Eds.), *Handbook of Psychotherapy for Anorexia Nervosa and Bulimia* (pp. 240-253). New York: Guilford Press.

Mrosovsky, N., & Powley, T. L. (1977). Set points for body weight and fat. *Behavioral Biology, 20,* 205-223.

Nisbett, R. E. (1972). Eating behavior and obesity in men and animals. *Advances in Psychosomatic Medicine, 7,* 173-193.

Orleans, C. T., & Barnett, L. R. (1984). Bulimarexia: Guidelines for behavioral assessment and treatment. In R. C. Hawkins, W. J. Fremouw, & P. F. Clement (Eds.), *The Binge/Purge Syndrome: Diagnosis, Treatment and Research* (pp. 144-182). New York: Springer.

Rosen, J., & Leitenberg, H. (1985). Exposure plus response prevention treatment of bulimia. In D. M. Garner & P. E. Garfinkel (Eds.), *Handbook of Psychotherapy for Anorexia Nervosa and Bulimia* (pp. 193-209). New York: Guilford Press.

Russell, G. F. M. (1979). Bulimia nervosa: An ominous variant of anorexia nervosa. *Psychological Medicine, 9,* 429-448.

Schwartz, R. C., Barrett, M. J., & Saba, G. (1985). Family therapy for bulimia. In D. M. Garner & P. E. Garfinkel (Eds.), *Handbook of Psychotherapy for Anorexia Nervosa and Bulimia* (pp. 280-307). New York: Guilford Press.

Selvini-Palazzoli, M. (1978). *Self-Starvation: From Individual to Family Therapy in the Treatment of Anorexia Nervosa*. New York: Jason Aronson.

Sours, J. A. (1980). *Starving to Death in a Sea of Objects: The Anorexia Nervosa Syndrome*. New York: Jason Aronson.

Stoller, J. (1982). Erotic vomiting. *Archives of Sexual Behavior, 11,* 361-365.

White, W. C., & Boskind-White, M. (1984). An experimental behavioral treatment program for bulimarexic women. In R. C. Hawkins, W. Fremouw, & P. F. Clement (Eds.), *The Binge/Purge Syndrome: Diagnosis, Treatment and Research* (pp. 77-103). New York: Springer.

ERICKSONIAN APPROACHES TO STRATEGIC HYPNOTHERAPY

Andrew P. Musetto

Words convey meaning. As they mediate to us realms beyond our immediate perception and personal experience, they reveal the common, everyday worlds in which people of similar and diverse cultures live out their lives. Through the pages of literature and the records of historians, they put us in touch with the drama of human decisions by which men and women more or less successfully manage their lives and influence the course of civilization. For some, they give access to worlds of science, religion, and philosophy. Through words, written and spoken, we come to know a much larger world than we could realize immediately through direct experience.

Not only do words convey the meaning of different worlds, more specifically they also evoke feelings, challenge attitudes, and teach behavior. The drama of great literature or even the dime store romance can provoke sadness, joy, contempt, and a full range of human feelings. The gospel parables and ancient fables, for example, question and mold our attitudes about ourselves and others. Words can also teach, whether it is how to repair a faucet or raise children.

It is through the power and range of words, especially in the context of stories and the meaning to which they refer, that hypnosis accomplishes its purposes. Through the subtlety of human communication, by putting us in touch with alternative ways of thinking, feeling, and behaving and by drawing upon the vast experience of other people, their high points and their downfalls, hypnosis is able to elicit, alter, and reorganize human experience and human thinking. Consequently, if psychotherapy attempts to change and heal human experience, break old patterns of feeling, perceiving, thinking, and reacting and establish new ones, hypnosis and its multiple trance phenomena can be an excellent vehicle to accomplish these goals.

It is my contention in this contribution that hypnosis can be a vital part of psychotherapy. In general, I will be discussing hypnotherapy, or the strategic use of a trance state and trance phenomena, and not simply hypnosis, a distinction which I will explain later. More specifically, I will be referring to the strategic use of hypnotherapy as exemplified in the genius of Milton Erickson. My reflections on Erickson are influenced heavily by the emerging artistry of Stephen and Carol Lankton (1983), as well as by Erickson's own works (1980a, 1980b, 1980c, 1980d; Erickson, E. L. Rossi, & S. Rossi, 1976; Erickson & E. L. Rossi, 1979). It is, however, my perception of Erickson and of the Lanktons' view of him that is being offered. I am not proposing an original or completely faithful portrait of Erickson, but because he valued creativity, uniqueness, and finding the answers from within oneself, I believe I am not far off the mark. It should also be noted that a thorough, nuanced, and comprehensive understanding of Erickson or the Lanktons would exhaust many volumes and the minds and talents of many individuals.

Erickson believed that cure results from a reassociation of a client's experiential life - the association of therapeutic responses and latent resources to problem areas (Erickson et al., 1976; Erickson & E. L. Rossi, 1979). In simple terms, if something that previously elicited anxiety now evokes joy or satisfaction, a reorganization of the person's experiential life has occurred. In broader terms, when a couple can look at each other and notice the caring each has for the other, whereas previously all they could see was animosity, there is a reorganization of each person's experiential life; a change in their thinking, perceiving, and feeling in relation to the other.

The trance state offers an excellent framework to reorganize experiences. It does this by creating or retrieving subtle mental processes (e.g., thinking, remembering, imagining) and trance phenomena (e.g., dissociation, positive and negative hallucination, amnesia, age regression, and others) that can be used as resources and applied to problem areas. Much of this mental activity is stimulated indirectly, through the use of metaphors (dramatic stories that capture and hold attention and offer an altered framework through which uncustomary or latent therapeutic experiences can be entertained) and anecdotes (shorter stories that elaborate a point) (S. Lankton & C. Lankton, 1983), paradox, indirect and direct suggestions and binds.

The effectiveness of the trance state has to do in part with the management of resistance - the limiting conscious attitudes and expectations that individuals hold. Problems often result from people's conscious attitudes that restrict the use of their abilities and prohibit certain feelings, or which drive them to repeat faulty solutions to their problems. To suggest to a person that criticism from a significant other need not evoke anger or anxiety is to suggest the seemingly impossible. But to speak to a client in trance by means of a metaphor about how a person has learned to not notice criticism, just as there are many things people do not notice, or to hold on to a pleasant experience when criticized, starts a reorganization of that person's experiential life, outside the doubts and limits of the conscious mind.

But the artistry of Erickson is not just a grab bag of clever gambits. It is thoroughly strategic, systematic, planned, and purposeful. To make such interventions work requires a thorough assessment of the individual and the system of relationships in which that individual operates. Strategic hypnotherapy is not, therefore, just hypnosis - the use of trance phenomena, especially by direct suggestion, to remove isolated symptoms. It is, rather, the planned use of the trance state and trance phenomena that takes into account individual, family, social, and developmental levels so that the symptom becomes unnecessary.

Strategic is a key word here. It refers to interventions that are supposed to achieve well-defined goals which may go beyond those stated by the client or clients. Formulating such goals means understanding not only the history of the symptom, but its current purpose and function, its current reinforcers, what it may be expressing about a client or a family's developmental challenges, and what it implies about the missing skills needed to obviate the symptom and advance along the developmental path that individuals and families must navigate throughout their lives.

It needs to be stressed that since symptoms do refer to factors beyond themselves - to individual, developmental, family, and social conflicts - hypnotherapy should generally not be used just to eliminate isolated symptoms. It is best used, rather, as one of several strategic interventions in a comprehensive treatment plan. Erickson was quite fond of paradox, symptom prescription, social interfacing, and many other interventions. In this contribution, however, I will focus on how hypnosis can be hypnotherapy, and how trance phenomena and the trance state can be effectively utilized as a part of therapy.

HYPNOSIS DEFINED

Hypnosis can be defined simply as a heightened state of inner concentration. As a state of focused awareness, it contrasts with the usual waking state in which individual attention bends to the multiple distractions and stimuli present in the environment. It also makes more available ideas and mental processes usually outside of awareness and not readily accessible, or those that conflict with conscious beliefs. In the trance state, new ideas - an altered frame of reference - can be communicated, retrieved, and developed. Erickson defined hypnosis, then, as a way of communicating potentially therapeutic ideas.

Implied here is that conscious attitudes and the conscious state are limited and limiting. First of all, much learning - walking, talking, driving a car, for example - takes place unconsciously or becomes unconscious. Second, conscious attitudes can be restrictive and are a major reason why people have problems, as when individuals believe that emotions are inferior and should be suppressed. The implication to people like this that emotions are indispensable and provide an extremely valuable if incomplete access to human and social realities would be readily rejected. But to communicate such a concept in the trance state, making use of metaphors, anecdotes, and indirect suggestions, offers an altered framework in which this new idea can be considered. And, if relevant, it can be incorporated into the person's belief system, but not necessarily with conscious awareness. The trance state of inner concentration, therefore, gives access to the much larger world of human experience that words mediate and metaphors dramatize; a world of meaning and experience that lies outside the boundaries of a person's current psychological horizon.

The split between conscious and unconscious processes is crucial to the Ericksonian approach. *Unconscious* in this sense refers to subtle mental processes - such as imagining things that are not there (positive hallucination), not noticing those that are (negative hallucination), and seeing oneself in detail from a distance or feeling apart from one's body (dissociation) - and not to the content of aggressive and sexual impulses referred to by psychoanalytic authors. In Ericksonian terms, the unconscious refers primarily to mental processes, not so much to specific content.

ERICKSONIAN VERSUS TRADITIONAL APPROACHES

Ericksonian hypnotherapy, or strategic hypnotherapy, is characterized by possibility and creativity. It embodies possibility because a client is free to respond in a variety of ways (including noncompliance) to the therapist, to accept or reject suggestions, and to develop personal answers to the presenting problem. The range of possible responses is virtually unlimited. It is creative inasmuch as no single method, approach, induction, or therapy is used with everyone. There is no stereotyping of clients or therapy. Erickson has remarked that he invented a different therapy for each client. He loved finding new ways to solve problems.

Traditional hypnosis (e.g., H. Spiegel & D. Spiegel, 1978) tends to be symptom focused, relies largely on progressive relaxation and guided imagery, uses standardized induction methods for most clients, aims at symptom removal, and is directed and controlled mostly by the therapist. Strategic hypnotherapy, in contrast, is personal and symptom centered. It understands symptoms as partially relational events (Haley, 1973). It diagnoses a symptom as a function of a client's biological, experiential, interpersonal, and developmental worlds. Departing from guided imagery, it takes advantage of indirect suggestions, therapeutic binds, metaphors, and anecdotes to create or access the mental processes that help make the symptom unnecessary. Its target for change is a reorganization of a client's experiential or inner world. Rather than trying to eliminate or oppose symptoms directly, it utilizes the presenting complaint as the gateway to change. Finally, since it allows maximum freedom for clients to respond relevantly, it is permissive and indirect. These distinctions will become clearer as this contribution develops.

INDIRECTION

Two key words are *indirection* and *utilization*, important concepts that differentiate Ericksonian approaches from others (S. Lankton & C. Lankton, 1983).

Whereas direct suggestions ("Sit down") appeal to the conscious mind and initiate voluntary and readily available behavior, indirect suggestions ("Can you be comfortable as you begin to sit down?") initiate an unconscious *search* for an appropriate response. It is the client's own search for relevant mental processes (e.g., imagining, remembering, comparing, distinguishing) and the resulting response potentials that are engaged (e.g., relaxation, dissociation, age regression, amnesia, and many others) that typify strategic hypnotherapy. Since these processes and responses are outside conscious awareness, they tend to bypass conscious criticism and allow for the consideration of an altered framework that is essential to therapy.

Direct suggestions tend to be stereotyped statements ("You will go deeper and deeper in a trance") that draw upon a narrow range of response (compliance or rejection). Indirect suggestions and binds, because they are vaguer and more ambiguous, allow for the clients' own interpretation and unique response: "There are a variety of ways to go into trance." Stimulated to think about the meaning and possible relevance of the therapist's suggestions, the client's attention is focused inward and the trance state begun or enhanced. Indirect suggestions and binds, therefore, engage clients in hypnosis more creatively and more actively than do direct suggestions.

Indirect suggestions and binds also encourage self-reliance. Clients are not just complying with the therapist's directives; they are utilizing their own latent mental processes that can resolve their problem. The therapist is not doing something to them, nor imposing values on them. Rather, it is the client's own thinking and experiences that bring about the therapeutic change. If dissociation of a painful limb occurs in compliance with direct suggestions, clients are more likely to rely upon further directives from the therapist to recreate the dissociation. But if dissociation is stimulated by therapeutic suggestions and created by clients' own potentials, it becomes more easily available and more under clients' control.

Indirect Suggestions and Binds. S. Lankton and C. Lankton (1983), in summarizing Erickson's work, describe several indirect suggestions and therapeutic binds that Erickson commonly used.

1. *Open-ended suggestions*: These are vague statements subject to a wide range of interpretations (e.g., "People respond in various ways to trance"). They are at the next highest level of abstraction, one step from the specific response desired (in this case, relaxation).
2. *Implications*: The trance state or trance phenomena are pre-supposed by such words as before, when, as, after, and one. "One way to go into trance is to think about what interests you."
3. *Questions or statements that focus or reinforce awareness*: "How does a person think about trance?" The question itself focuses attention on the desired response while not directly demanding it.
4. *Truisms*: These are statements about human living that are virtually universal. "Everyone has had the experience of imagining something." They are often used to introduce a concept, such as imagining, which is going to be developed.
5. *Suggestions covering all possible alternatives*: These are statements that cover all the existing alternatives, so that there is no way for the client to fail to cooperate. "You may go into trance at your own speed, quickly, gradually, suddenly, slowly, sooner or later, or in a different way, with your eyes open or closed."
6. *Apposition of opposites*: These involve the juxtaposition of two behaviors which are changing in opposite directions. "Just as difficult as it was for you to start therapy, that's how easily you can find yourself going into trance."

The following indirect suggestions are also called therapeutic binds: No matter which alternative the client selects to respond to, the response is therapeutic.

7. *Binds of comparable alternatives*: "Would you like to go into trance with your eyes opened or closed, listening to me or not paying attention consciously at all?" No matter which part of the statement the client responds to, going into trance is pre-supposed.
8. *Conscious/unconscious double binds*: Comparable alternatives are offered in terms of a conscious/unconscious split. "Your conscious mind may not be aware of just how deeply your unconscious can go into trance."
9. *Double dissociative conscious/unconscious double binds*: This is a variety of #8, except that both parts of the comparable alternative are attributed to the conscious and unconscious minds. "Your conscious mind may not be aware of just how deeply your unconscious can go into trance, or perhaps your conscious may go into a level of trance that your unconscious doesn't notice."
10. *Non sequitur double binds*: Each part of the suggestion contains the desired response but at a different level of abstraction. "Can you go into trance or just turn your attention to your own thoughts?"

Metaphors and Anecdotes. In addition to indirect suggestions and binds, the other major vehicles for indirection are *metaphor*, stories that capture attention through drama and offer an altered framework which allows clients to entertain novel or uncustomary therapeutic experiences and ideas, and *anecdotes*, shorter tangents that elaborate certain points (S. Lankton & C. Lankton, 1983). By means of the details of a story about how a woman was repeatedly instructed to "say goodbye" to a beloved farm that she was selling, to leave something that she cherished, Erickson intended her to experience sadness and a grief reaction, which would be augmented by indirect suggestions and binds. In another story about how a woman from a privileged, sophisticated background goes to work among the poor and needy and discovers that she herself is needy in a different way, while her clients have a hidden beauty and strength of their own, attitudes about what it really means to be well-off and needy can be questioned.

Metaphors can be used in any of the goals listed above, as the Lanktons (1983) have delineated. Attitude metaphors contrast, teach, or challenge attitudes and expectations. Affective metaphors bring out emotional responses, as protagonists move to and from positive or negative objects. Metaphors about behavioral responses describe and teach how to do something, how it looks from the outside, and how it is thought about from within. Self-image metaphors detail scenarios in which protagonists rehearse new behavior and exercise new skills in different contexts, especially those that are troublesome. Family structure metaphors show how new roles or ways of relating in families can be rewarding. And discipline/enjoyment metaphors offer advice that clients can apply to their own lives. The Lanktons' valuable writing and teaching have given us a way to understand and reproduce these metaphors in clinical work.

It is not the cleverness of the story, its outcome, or the story line, however, that is effective, but the experience and resources (e.g., sadness and grief; the message that having a lot does not preclude being needy) that are evoked and reassociated in the process of listening to the story. For Erickson, it will be remembered, cure comes from the reassociation of a client's experiential life. If during a metaphor describing compassion a client experiences compassion which is then associated with a loved one towards whom the client is feeling antagonistic, a therapeutic reassociation is taking place. If the memory and experience of determination can be evoked and linked to a recalcitrant habit, reassociation is taking place here, too. Metaphor is an effective way to reassociate experiences; while the client is consciously paying attention to the story line, the unconscious responds to the indirect suggestions and therapeutic binds, to the myriad associations and various meanings that can be derived from the story.

UTILIZATION

Erickson is also recognized for his utilization of the presenting problem and personality orientation of the client. Haley (1973), for one, has detailed Erickson's creativity in this regard. Erickson and E. L. Rossi also speak about it. "We view hypnotherapy as a process whereby we help people utilize their own mental associations, memories and life potentials to achieve their own therapeutic goals" (1979, p. 1). "The initial step in the utilization approach, as in most other forms of psychotherapy, is to accept the patients' manifest behavior and to acknowledge their personal frames of reference. This openness and acceptance of the patients' worlds facilitate a corresponding openness and acceptance of the therapist by the patients" (Erickson & E. L. Rossi, 1979, p. 53). Resistance, therefore, is not considered a function of clients' inability or unwillingness to respond to therapy, but the therapist's difficulty appreciating and utilizing what clients present and can do, so that clients can be helped to do what they need to do. It is difficult to read Erickson without being impressed by his ability to deal with almost any type of behavior or presenting problem. If he was challenged, he responded with a challenge of his own; insulted, he described himself with a better insult. Cooperative clients received compassionate replies. Doubt met doubt, and caution greeted hesitation.

Utilization applies as a therapeutic intervention and as a way of facilitating trance. An agoraphobic client, panicked over the anticipated loss of control she expects in trance, opens and closes her eyes during the induction. She is advised to continue to do this as a way of reassuring herself that she controls the process and that she herself will find the appropriate level of trance. The authoritarian husband of a woman client, a prosecuting attorney, is asked to come to therapy in order to advise the therapist as to how the therapist can best help his wife. A compulsively compliant client is told that the most responsible way to go into a trance, the way that she can cooperate the most, is by having her own unique trance, one that reflects her personal values. A highly intelligent, critical, obsessive-compulsive client is asked to be on the alert (consciously) to criticize and analyze the therapist's suggestions, keeping track of any mistakes so that the therapist can be even more helpful the next time, while at the same time criticizing his own reactions, thus leaving his unconscious free to respond spontaneously. The application of utilization is bounded only by the inventiveness of the therapist.

Utilization is often accomplished through paradox. S. Lankton and C. Lankton (1983) cite Bateson (1979, p. 23), who defines paradox as a contradiction in conclusions that were correctly argued from consistent premises. The Lanktons have detailed Erickson's frequent utilization through paradox. As an example of paradox, I told a jealous wife that her jealousy reflected her loyalty and desire to hold onto what she prized, her husband, and evidenced the respect she had for him. Since she was grateful for what she had, she should congratulate herself for her good sense. I then advised her to continue to show loyalty and good sense, but stated that she did not have to feel bad about it or check up on her husband to accomplish it. Paradox takes what the client presents (jealousy) and provides a positive interpretation (a sign of loyalty and good sense). It also includes a prescription to continue the symptom after a split has been offered between the intention (prizing) and the specific behavior (checking up) and in the way the symptom is experienced ("You don't have to feel bad about it"). It falls to the process of therapy to help her find alternative ways to show her loyalty.

The paradox should begin, the Lanktons tell us, with verbal empathy and nonverbal matching, not be given in a one-up manner, and come either first or last in the therapeutic sequence or session. It often starts a formal induction, as when clients are told to continue doing what they would normally do (e.g., doubting, criticizing, complying, listening carefully) while their unconscious is free to respond differently and creatively.

HYPNOTHERAPY OR THE STRATEGIC USE OF HYPNOSIS IN PSYCHOTHERAPY

To understand how hypnosis can be a part of psychotherapy, we might recall that, for Erickson, hypnosis is a way of communicating ideas. Not that the ideas could not be communicated in other ways, but in the trance state conscious resistance is lowered, receptivity is higher, learning is facilitated by relaxation, what can be considered possible is expanded, and underutilized resources are more available. But for hypnosis to effectively communicate potentially therapeutic ideas, it is first necessary to have some idea of what might be therapeutic; it is necessary to have an adequate diagnosis and treatment plan.

Strategic hypnotherapy treats the whole person without singling out one dimension as intrinsically more important than another. It does not esteem the private self to the exclusion of the public self, the social more than the personal, or the interpersonal network and family to the devaluation of the biological, for all are interrelated. Strategic hypnotherapy goes beyond biological influences, beyond psychoanalytic and dynamic processes, beyond behavioral learning and habit patterns, beyond interpersonal transactions, beyond the social network, to an assessment of all as they interface together. It treats particular symptoms as partly interpersonal events, as veiled means of influencing and communicating between people.

Not only is Erickson's approach systemic, it is also practical. To be practical in this sense means to understand the symptom and the system sufficiently so as to intervene in whatever level or levels the therapist assesses to be most receptive to therapeutic change. It is to use the therapist's energy, time, and resources purposefully and strategically, in accord with personal preference, clients' needs, and therapeutic acumen. Erickson might have treated a bedwetting problem by seeing only the child, or just the parents, or both one after the other. He could prescribe the symptom as easily as put the child or his parents in trance, or give each a homework assignment, or tell the parents to leave the child to him.

SYSTEMIC CONSIDERATIONS

Strategic hypnotherapy is systemic but not stereotyped. It does not use a generalized, standardized format to undo any smoking habit, for example, but it undertakes a thorough investigation of the individual and those surrounding attitudes and variables that condition and are conditioned by the smoking behavior. For instance, is it a social activity with the person's spouse, a way to relax, a form of rebellion, a perceived mark of adulthood, a diversion from conflicts, or a stable companion? No matter what the presenting problem is, from smoking to depression, from obsessive-compulsive behavior to sexual dysfunction, it begins with a systematic assessment.

The Lanktons (1983, p. 36) have identified six major parameters that Erickson seems to have considered most often in his treatment planning. These are (a) the structures of the family system and social network, that is, the boundaries and communication styles as examined by structural family therapists such as Minuchin (1974); (b) the stage of family development, such as the courtship or birth of a first child, as studied by Haley; (c) the developmental age or task of the individual; (d) the availability of resources, whether directly or indirectly retrievable, such as confidence, tenderness, or determination; (e) the flexibility and sensitivity of each member in areas of perception, cognition, meaning, behavior role, and emotions; and (f) the verifiable function or purpose of the symptom in the current life of the client or family, that is, what it does to and for these people.

The following questions represent *some* of the relevant issues to be explored:

- What is the history of the presenting problem, especially in terms of specific learning experiences or traumas associated with it (such as in simple phobias)?
- Who or what currently reinforces the behavior of the symptom?
- What is the current developmental level of the individual (e.g., identity formation) and family (e.g., birth of the first child), and what is the next stage of development?
- What skill or skills do the individual and family need to negotiate the present stage of development, move on to the next, and obviate the presenting complaint?
- What are the relevant demographic variables: age, living arrangements, occupation, social strata, religious affiliation?
- What does the client think is needed to solve the problem?
- What are the client's goals?
- What are the clinician's goals, which may go beyond the explicit, conscious goals of the client? (These are based upon the clinician's expertise in assessing the individual and the presenting problem.)
- When and where does the symptom occur or not occur?
- What and who are most affected by it and who would be most threatened by its absence?
- What would the client be like without it?
- What is the client's family of origin like; are there similarities to the presenting complaint?
- What are the repetitive patterns of individual behavior and interpersonal transactions that express the problem?
- How has the client already tried to solve the problem?
- Has there been any previous therapy, or hypnotherapy?
- What are the client's attitudes towards therapy and hypnosis?
- What are the client's interests and activities, since these can be helpful in formulating appropriate metaphors?

Other therapists will, no doubt, extend the list depending upon their specific theoretical backgrounds.

STRATEGIC CONSIDERATIONS

Erickson's approach, like others, is strategic: specific interventions designed to reach specific goals. These goals are not only those stated explicitly by the client, but also those the clinician sees as necessary to eliminate the symptom and provide the necessary growth experiences for the client to advance developmentally. It is the clinician's responsibility to think beyond the presenting complaint and stated goals and to devise effective and economical interventions. At the same time, these goals and interventions are always subject to revision based upon feedback from clients, so that there is a continual interplay between what the therapist hypothesizes as worthwhile goals and effective interventions and how clients respond to them. A depressed client, for example, may or may not need to consciously identify her difficulty in moving gracefully into old age and accepting retirement to improve her moods. A woman with headaches may not realize that not speaking her mind and compulsively taking care of people lies at the heart of her problem.

If the goals must be specific, so must the interventions. Again the Lanktons have delineated six categories of goals, identical with the six types of metaphors listed previously, which they believe Erickson most often considered. These are behavioral or task (e.g., how to be assertive), affective (e.g., the feeling of tenderness), attitudinal (e.g., that it is healthy to be aware of one's anger), self-image (i.e., seeing oneself interacting with those positive traits and resources learned or accessed in therapy), discipline and enjoyment, a catchall for giving advice (e.g., that mistakes can be appreciated because of the learning that results), and family structure (e.g., seeing oneself enjoyably spending more time with one's children).

PROCESS OF HYPNOTHERAPY

Erickson and E. L. Rossi (1979) break down their approach into three distinct stages: (a) preparation; (b) therapeutic trance; and (c) recognition, evaluation, and ratification of therapeutic trance. The preparation stage is an opportunity to study and evaluate clients, as well as to allow them to become comfortable with the hypnotist. Sound rapport or the feeling of mutual understanding and respect marks the interaction as potentially helpful. Once their attention is engaged, clients are said to be response-ready or ready to respond to the subtleties of therapeutic communication. The clinician, to be effective, must understand clients' habitual conscious framework that limits creative responses to current problems. People, Erickson assumed, get into difficulty because they get caught in responses that worsen instead of resolve their problems, and in mind sets that block access to their underutilized potential. As clients become receptive to therapeutic communication, the possibility of new responses and an expectancy of hope are fostered.

Therapeutic trance is the second phase. It is "...a period during which patients are able to break out of their limited frameworks and belief systems so they can experience other patterns of functioning within themselves" (Erickson & E. L. Rossi, 1979, p. 2). Trance moves from a fixation of the client's attention to distracting, interrupting, or depotentiating habitual mind sets, so that an unconscious search can take place; relevant unconscious processes are then activated and unrealized potentials can be automatically applied to the problem areas. Throughout the process, indirect suggestions and binds, metaphors, and anecdotes are employed to evoke resources, relevant experience, and subtle mental processes. By utilizing clients' presenting problems and preferred interpersonal styles, therapy proceeds from where clients are, towards where they are capable of being, with alternative ways of functioning derived from personally generated creative solutions.

Not only must clients be properly prepared and disposed to hypnosis, and relevant therapeutic responses be elicited, but so also must those responses be recognized and ratified by the hypnotist. Recognizing a therapeutic response in place of a previous untoward one helps to negate unhealthy patterns while allowing for the emergence of new, salutary ones. Recognition and ratification imply that the therapist is able to read the signs of a therapeutic response. Since individuals go into trance and respond uniquely, this requires perceptive (but always fallible) recognition of clients' ideomotor signals that indicate therapeutic response. These signals are multiple. Classically, they include such responses as catalepsy, relaxation, dissociation, loss or retardation of reflexes, slowed pulse, and deepened breathing. Guided by these, clinicians can discern the impact of therapeutic communication. A flushed face accompanied by tears probably indicates sadness; a slight smile and sigh, possibly relief or amusement.

STEPS OF INDUCTION

While Erickson found that he could bring about trance in many ways, and anything that captures and heightens attention and directs it inward might be considered trance-inducing, perhaps he is best known for the conscious/unconscious dissociation method, which is widely used by clinicians. The Lanktons (1983) have described seven overlapping steps in a conscious/unconscious induction protocol:

1) Orient to trance (including physical, attitudinal and psychological orientation).
2) Fixate attention and rapport.
3) Create conscious/unconscious dissociation.
4) Ratify and deepen the trance state.
5) Establish a learning frame or learning set.
6) Utilize trance state and hypnotic phenomena for clinical goals.
7) Reorient to normal waking state. (p. 142)

Preparing clients for the trance includes a physical orientation, usually sitting comfortably in a chair; an attitudinal orientation involving discussion of the clients' beliefs and misconceptions about trance; and a psychological orientation which deals with previous trance experiences and present expectations. In our culture, misconceptions about trance prevail. Not only is there a popularized notion that trance equals oblivion or loss of control, but there are also exaggerated claims made by hypnotists. That trance is a state of heightened inner concentration, of increased awareness, in which clients control the process, respond relevantly, and accept only those suggestions that make sense to them, is presented implicitly and perhaps explicitly. I may give clients an article that describes hypnosis and how it can be helpful and addresses some of their questions and objections. I suggest to some clients that they allow me to tape the session so they can listen again at their leisure (but not while driving their cars).

The orientation or preparatory phase depends on clients' attitudes and previous trance experiences. Doubtful or distrusting clients are advised to continue their skepticism, which only indicates their good sense in not being willing to just hand over their experience to a process they don't adequately understand. Clients who are afraid of losing control are reassured that they are in charge of the induction and the depth of trance they reach. For those clients who refuse formal induction, therapeutic ideas still can be communicated in everyday language, interspersed with indirect suggestions, binds, and metaphors.

Next, Erickson would establish rapport and fixate the client's attention. Clients are told that people often start going into trance by staring at a spot, but anything that captures their attention, even their own distracting thoughts or tension, suffices. At some point in the trance process, Erickson was fond of reminding clients that they know more about themselves than he does and that their unconscious knows even more; that they hypnotize themselves, hopefully stimulated by his suggestions which they are free to change; and that they decide what to concentrate on. Rapport is the subtle communication of mutual understanding and respect between clients and therapists (Erickson & E. L. Rossi, 1979). By using words that fit clients' cultural backgrounds and metaphors that appeal to their life experiences, by matching clients' facial expressions, bodily postures, vocal and tonal patterns, and breathing, the clinician helps to engage their unconscious mind. Just fixating attention inward begins to disrupt the usual conscious thought patterns and prepares for the therapeutic reorganization of experience that Erickson prized as the benchmark of therapy.

Erickson next used conscious/unconscious dissociation to help reorganize the client's inner experiences. As part of the induction and dissociation, clients are educated about the different workings of the conscious and unconscious minds: that the conscious mind, for example, is oriented to the moment, thinks linearly, is easily distracted, may doubt the validity of trance, and might be curious, skeptical, or analytical; the unconscious pulls on past learnings and resources, thinks globally, perceives latent possibilities, and acts in a client's best interests. The therapist encourages clients to continue doing what their conscious minds do normally (being critical, for example), while engaging the unconscious by indirect suggestions, binds, metaphors, and anecdotes. As the conscious mind is distracted, it is depotentiated as a source of resistance and as an obstacle to change. The learning and reassociation of experience can then take place unconsciously, outside the hegemony of conscious beliefs, as clients learn (without necessarily realizing it) that criticism can elicit humor instead of anxiety.

Next, the trance state would be ratified and deepened. By commenting on those experiential and sensory alterations (e.g., deepened breathing or slowed reflexes) that occur as a result of fixation, relaxation, and conscious/unconscious dissociation, the therapist ratifies trance. Deepening can be accomplished in many ways: by anecdotes about deeply relaxing experiences, by indirect suggestions and binds, by confusion, by counting backwards from 20 to 1, or by whatever more fully distracts the conscious mind and engages the unconscious.

During the hypnotic trance a learning set is established. Learning, for Erickson, was associational: Experiences which happen to be associated tend to get linked together. Cure results from a reassociation of experiences, by pairing a resource (such as confidence) with a problem area (such as public speaking). Obviously, the complexity of this can be substantial. That clients are learning things in trance, even if they are unaware of what they are learning, is implied in many ways and expressed explicitly.

The stage is now set for effecting change. As helpful experiences are elicited and associated to problem areas, trance becomes an excellent vehicle for change. Trance allows the elicitation of unconscious processes that either can be resources or can retrieve such resources. Metaphors, indirect suggestions, and binds provide the altered framework in which new options can be entertained and resources retrieved, created, intensified, and finally reassociated, according to the previously established goals. Usually, this is the most lengthy and difficult part of therapy and often requires a series of metaphors and sessions, perhaps over many months, to be accomplished.

Actually, several metaphors can be embedded within each other, as Erickson himself did and the Lanktons (1983) now do. In brief, a series of metaphors are told to a client in trance, each metaphor designed to address one of the six areas listed previously. When three metaphors are used, the first is begun and suspended, the second is also started but not completed, and the third is told completely, followed by the completion of the second, and then the first. For example, if the goal were to help a client deal with criticism, the first metaphor might be an attitudinal one in which two attitudes towards criticism - one in which it is utilized as constructive feedback and the other in which it is defensively resisted - are contrasted. The second metaphor might detail the feeling of comfort which will later be applied to situations in which the client feels criticized. The third or middle metaphor, which Erickson called the direct work phase, may teach alternative ways to deal with criticism (e.g., by humor, or by ignoring it). The second is completed as the client imagines anxiety situations while maintaining the feeling of comfort. Finally, the attitudinal metaphor is completed, showing the merits of using criticism constructively.

This multiple embedded metaphor format enriches an already powerful therapeutic device. Suspending metaphors increases the drama and hopefully, therefore, the clients' involvement. The embedding and complexity of several metaphors with the interspersal of advice and suggestions more effectively bypasses conscious resistance, thus permitting a greater unconscious receptivity and creating a variety of subtle therapeutic mental processes. Because the stories are about other people, clients are free to respond or not respond according to their own needs, as they search for the meaning and relevance of what is being said.

Finally, the client must be reoriented to normal waking state. Reorientation takes place in a variety of ways, either rapidly, gradually, or in whatever way is suitable for a given client. This is the time to complete the trance experience, to tie together or summarize some of the main points, to develop or initiate amnesia, to provide post-hypnotic suggestions, or to present or complete a paradoxical prescription which may have been developed throughout the trance itself.

A CASE STUDY

The following case study illustrates the strategic use of hypnosis with the presenting problem of public speaking anxiety.

BACKGROUND INFORMATION

The client is a young executive, successful by his own standards. He has a law degree but is pursuing a business career, and claims his only problem is public speaking anxiety. In the first few minutes of a talk in front of any audience, he feels extremely anxious and fears losing control so that he will not be able to continue. His anxiety is expressed as a stammer, stomach spasms, shaking, cold and clammy hands, and a rash which develops on his neck. The problem arose some time during college, although he cannot identify what started it or exactly when it began. Interestingly, he was a good debater in high school.

Although he is relatively happy with himself, he is able to identify several destructive attitudes that he thinks might underlie the problem. At times, for example, he feels inadequate and socially awkward. He thinks of himself as tending to be perfectionistic, and when he is anxious about giving a talk he tends to imagine the worst, that he will become utterly humiliated because he is unable to speak at all. Working about 50-55 hours per week, success-oriented, hard-driving, and not able to relax easily, he might be described as a Type A personality. At one time he had high blood pressure, which is now controlled. He enjoys jogging and other sports.

Married, with two children, he describes the marriage as happy yet "fiery" at times. His only prior treatment occurred a few years ago when he had 4-5 sessions of psychotherapy for generalized anxiety. He has taken a course in self-hypnosis, which he enjoyed and thinks would be a worthwhile approach for this problem. His goal is simply to be able to speak publicly without so much anxiety that he feels out of control and shakes visibly.

Relevant family background revealed that the client has always felt unable to please his successful, critical father, who also has public speaking anxiety, as does the client's younger and only brother.

His nonverbal presentation does not contradict his verbal one. Well-dressed, articulate, somewhat friendly, he appears comfortable speaking about himself. The Adjective Checklist, developed by Leary (1957) and used extensively by the Lanktons, describes him as a friendly dominant personality, prone to self-criticism, capable of being competitive and hostile, but lacking in the ability to offer help or be affectionate, supportive, and sympathetic towards others. If he cannot dominate a situation and be in charge, his next response is to blame himself, and if that fails, he tries to allay anxiety by being competitive or assertive.

TREATMENT GOALS

Using the six types of goals mentioned previously, the following specific goals were formulated. They are designed not only to eliminate the public speaking anxiety, but also to help with individual and family developmental goals: to consolidate and enhance his career and to increase his intimacy and cooperation with his wife and children. These goals go beyond those stated explicitly by the client, but are seen to underlie and be associated with the public speaking anxiety and the client's current developmental concerns.

Attitudinal Goals:

1. One failure or mistake is not equivalent to total failure and can be helpful as constructive feedback; therefore, mistakes can be appreciated.
2. Offering help and being able to cooperate with others are positive traits; this is introduced by the attitude that the person with the most response possibilities, including cooperation and offering help, controls the situation (to appeal to his dominance).
3. Each person is different and unique and, therefore, adequacy does not have to be based upon comparison with or pleasing other people, but upon one's own uniqueness which is a given.

Through a variety of metaphors, his current attitudes will be challenged while these new ones are offered.

Affective Goals:

1. Feeling good about cooperation with others.
2. Enjoying offering help and support to others, and being tender with people.
3. Joy.
4. Confidence.

The first two emotional goals will be utilized in self-image scenarios, where the client will envision himself interacting with other people with these new skills. The second two will be paired with his public speaking anxiety as a form of reciprocal inhibition (S. Lankton & C. Lankton, 1983).

Behavioral Goals:

1. Disrupt the sequence of experience that leads to public speaking anxiety. This will be done by means of Erickson's scramble technique as described by the Lanktons (1983, pp. 334-336): breaking down the symptom into five stages, from its minimal occurrence to its completion, and then having the client scramble the sequence.
2. Reciprocally inhibit the public speaking anxiety by associating it with relaxation arising from trance, and with joy and confidence, developed in the affect metaphors.

Discipline/Enjoyment:

Punchlines will be provided that are designed to offer advice about how the client can perceive himself and his problem differently. Metaphors will be told about other clients and will contain such statements as: "Imagine the worst until you can appreciate the absurdity of it"; "Why not learn to laugh at yourself and improve upon your ability to criticize yourself"; "Be sure to make enough mistakes so you can appreciate your ability to continue to learn"; "Worry enough before the speech so you won't have to be anxious when it's time to give it."

Self-Image Thinking:

In metaphors about other clients, the client will be guided to imagine himself in various situations giving speeches without anxiety, with the experiences of confidence and joy during these times, worrying beforehand and not at the time of the speech, and learning from any mistakes he might make.

Family Role:

Again through metaphor, the client will be helped to picture himself with his wife and children, while feeling and acting tenderly, offering help, and being cooperative.

THERAPEUTIC INTERVENTION

The multiple embedded metaphor was used. As an example of the metaphors used, the attitude metaphor about the value of mistakes is as follows: A story was told about two collegians trying out for a place on the college basketball team. The story is introduced by the comment about how surprised people were to find that the better, more talented player was cut, while the less talented one made the team. The first player, the more skilled, becomes discouraged and self-blaming whenever he makes a mistake in a game or practice period. He is not receptive to feedback from his coach about his mistakes. The second player, less talented, learns from his mistakes, accepts feedback, and improves steadily. The first player, we find out, is cut, while the second makes the team.

The hypnotherapy is introduced by means of paradox as the therapist observes that the client is on the verge of full adulthood and more success. So eager is he to grow and improve that he wants to do everything just right, and so he becomes anxious as a result. The anxiety, in turn, blocks him from doing what he really wants (rapport building). Actually, his anxiety is just a sign of how much he wants to succeed (positive interpretation of the symptom). He is advised to continue to work hard to succeed, but is told that he does not have to be anxious about it (splitting the intention from the behavior). Parenthetically, therapy will have to help him find other ways to succeed without undue anxiety. It is suggested that he might even worry and be anxious before a talk (just to remind him how much he wants to do well) so that he won't have to be anxious at the time of the speech (symptom prescription plus an alteration in the time of its occurrence).

During the induction he is asked to help the therapist and direct the trance. "You help me the most by realizing that you control the trance and that you do most of the work yourself." He is told that he might be anxious at first, but that this is only a sign of how important hypnosis and treatment is to him and how much he wants to overcome his problem. "Be sure to criticize yourself and your responses as a way of really relaxing and deepening trance." "The most perfect way to go into trance is your own way, your own unique way."

The client was seen for six sessions: an initial evaluation, four for hypnotherapy, and one wrap-up session. After the second session of hypnotherapy he reported a decrease in public speaking anxiety, and by the end of the fourth hypnotherapy session, the anxiety was very manageable. He indicated no other specific changes; his home life continued to be satisfactory. At the wrap-up session he reported that he was very happy about receiving a major promotion. His anxiety, he said, was no longer bothersome. Treatment was terminated at this point; but it was expected and hoped that more subtle developmental and personal changes would come about slowly, since salutary ideas and burgeoning resources were seeded in the client's unconscious.

CONCLUSION

There is something particularly rewarding about reaching up to the mind of a great thinker, a man of genius. Not only is there the advance in clinical skills, and the stimulation that comes from his clever interventions and amusing and poignant stories; there is also the personal transformation and inspiration that comes from stretching the boundaries of one's own mind and awareness, as one is stopped short by Erickson's love of living and regard for the human person. For me, Erickson stands as a clarion call to live life fully: to trust one's instincts, to continue the joy of learning in every situation, to look forward to the future, to not be afraid to break the boundaries of present limitations, to see beyond insults, to be free to express the childlike wonder that lives within us all, to take care of ourselves and nurture our talents, to discern the positive in every negative, and to realize that death in all its disguises can be embraced by life. Perhaps in the following quote, cited by Rosen (1982), we can also hear Erickson speaking to each of us: "And I want you to choose some time in the past when you were a very, very little girl. My voice will go with you. My voice will change into that of your parents, your neighbors, your friends, your schoolmates, your playmates, your teachers. And I want you to find yourself sitting in the schoolroom, a little girl feeling happy about something, something that happened a long time ago, that you forgot a long time ago" (p. 23).

Andrew P. Musetto, PhD, is a partner in private practice with Psychological Service Associates, Haddonfield, New Jersey. He has been a clinical psychologist since 1973. Among his areas of interest and publication are child custody problems, agoraphobia, and marital and family therapy. He has taken hypnotherapy training with Stephen and Carol Lankton and hopes to continue learning more about the uses of hypnosis in therapy. Dr. Musetto may be contacted c/o Psychological Service Associates, Suite C, Haddonfield, NJ 08033.

RESOURCES

Bateson, G. (1979). *Mind and Nature.* New York: Dutton.

Erickson, M. H. (1980). The nature of hypnosis and suggestion, edited by E. L. Rossi. *The Collected Papers of Milton H. Erickson on Hypnosis* (Vol. I). New York: Irvington. (a)

Erickson, M. H. (1980). Hypnotic alteration of sensory, perceptual and psychophysiological processes, edited by E. L. Rossi. *The Collected Papers of Milton H. Erickson on Hypnosis* (Vol. II). New York: Irvington. (b)

Erickson, M. H. (1980). The hypnotic investigation of psychodynamic processes, edited by E. L. Rossi. *The Collected Papers of Milton H. Erickson on Hypnosis* (Vol. III). New York: Irvington. (c)

Erickson, M. H. (1980). Innovative hypnotherapy, edited by E. L. Rossi. *The Collected Papers of Milton H. Erickson on Hypnosis* (Vol. IV). New York: Irvington. (d)

Erickson, M. H., & Rossi, E. L. (1979). *Hypnotherapy: An Explanatory Casebook.* New York: Irvington.

Erickson, M., Rossi, E. L., & Rossi, S. (1976). *Hypnotic Realities.* New York: Irvington.

Haley, J. (1973). *Uncommon Therapy: The Psychiatric Techniques of Milton H. Erickson, M.D.* New York: Norton.

Lankton, S., & Lankton, C. (1983). *The Answer Within: A Clinical Framework of Ericksonian Hypnotherapy.* New York: Brunner/Mazel.

Leary, T. (1957). *Interpersonal Diagnosis of Personality: A Functional Theory and Methodology for Personality Evaluation.* New York: John Wiley & Sons.

Minuchin, S. (1974). *Families & Family Therapy.* Cambridge, MA: Harvard University Press.

Rosen, S. (1982). *My Voice Will Go with You.* New York: Norton.

Spiegel, H., & Spiegel, D. (1978). *Trance and Treatment: Clinical Use of Hypnosis.* New York: Basic Books.

THE STEPS AND METHODS IN EXPERIENTIAL PSYCHOTHERAPY SESSIONS

Alvin R. Mahrer and Patricia A. Gervaize

Experiential psychotherapy is derived from an existential-humanistic conception of human beings (Binswanger, 1967/1978; Mahrer, 1978a; May, Angel, & Ellenberger, 1958). It is based on the belief that change is a matter of therapeutic experiencing rather than insight or understanding, a special relationship, modifications in whatever the patient's behavior is supposed to be contingent upon, or other techniques espoused by various therapies. Our larger family includes provocative, feeling-expressive, Gestalt, client-centered, logotherapy, existential, Daseinsanalytic, encounter, intense feeling, psychoimagination, crisis mobilization, focusing, phenomenological, humanistic, and other therapies.

Every session of experiential psychotherapy begins with the patient reclining in a large comfortable chair, feet on a hassock, and eyes closed. The therapist is likewise reclining in a chair a few feet away, also with eyes closed. The session continues until therapeutic work finishes the steps, which generally runs about 2 hours.

Each session proceeds through the same steps (Figure 1 on the next page) whether it is the initial session, a middle session, or the final one. We go through the same steps whether the patient has one session a week or five sessions a week, or whether the patient has a total of just one session or hundreds of sessions. We also follow the same steps whether the patient is old or young, is reasonably satisfied personally or abysmally unhappy, whether attention is on the exciting new life event or the virulent cancer, or whether others consider the patient a model human being or a deranged lunatic.

Our goal in this contribution is to outline the steps and methods which the experiential psychotherapist uses in each session. Therapists who are already familiar with the theory and methods of some of the therapies in the larger experiential family may be inclined to adopt some of the steps and methods outlined here. However, the goal is not to describe the underlying conceptualization of this particular approach; the important underlying theory is given in other sources (Mahrer, 1978a, 1983a, 1985a, 1985b). Nor is the goal to encourage therapists to rush into the wholesale use of these steps and methods. Given a skilled and competent experiential therapist, and given a patient who is ready and willing to enter into experiencing, the history of these methods stamps them as potentially rather powerful. Accordingly, it is the professional responsibility of the therapist to insure that he or she has solid basic training to provide competent expertise in the supervised use of these methods. Given these disclaimers, the goal of the balance of this contribution is to provide an introductory outline of the steps and methods of experiential psychotherapy.

STEP 1: GETTING INTO THE EXPERIENTIAL STATE

The first step is getting into an experiential state. This involves several elements:

1. The patient's attention is predominantly focused on some "center." This may be any center at all, inside or outside the patient, vivid or vague, recent or remote, real or fanciful.

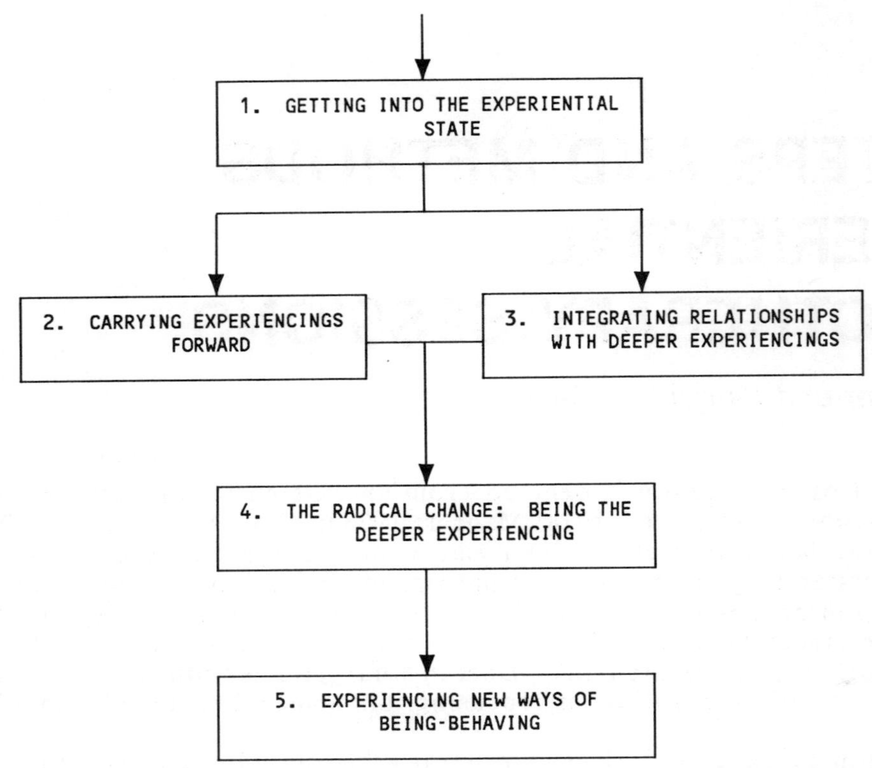

Figure 1. The sequence of steps in each experiential session.

2. Symmetrically, very little of the patient's attention is on the therapist; the patient is focused on the cancer, or mother's face, or the words spoken by the spouse, and not on talking to the therapist (Mahrer, 1978c, 1980b, 1983a).
3. At least moderate sensations are experienced in the patient's body, for example, butterflies in the stomach, tension in the chest, or lightness in the head.
4. The patient is in a state of at least moderate "experiencing" such as feeling loving, experiencing a sense of aloneness, feeling defiant, or any other experiencing which comes forth.

CLOSING EYES AND ALLOWING THE BODY TO SETTLE

The therapist instructs the patient to keep his or her eyes closed throughout the session, and to start by allowing the body to get settled. Rather than a state of relaxation, it is a state in which whatever is occurring at the moment is allowed to occur a little more.

SHARING THE PATIENT'S IMMEDIATE BODILY SENSATIONS

The therapist invites the patient to locate and identify the major ongoing bodily sensations so that the therapist can approximate similar bodily sensations in his or her own body. It may feel good or it may feel bad, but the therapist is to share the major bodily sensations occurring "right now" in the patient's body, whatever their nature and wherever they are located, as long as they are being experienced.

FOCUSING ATTENTION AND ENTERING AN EXPERIENTIAL STATE

The therapist shows the patient how to let attention go to whatever is so personal and meaningful that the more attention is focused onto and into it, the more the patient drifts into an experiential state. Instead of talking to the therapist, the patient focuses attention on a recent incident, an old scene, the cancer, a grandfather's face, a chance remark - anything which is meaningfully present and yoked to feelings. The patient allows more and more attention to pour into the meaningful center until a state of experiencing is entered which is rather strong and enveloping; it occurs instead of an interaction with the therapist.

Experiential Listening. Once the patient enters a state of experiencing, what the patient says and does seems to come from and through the therapist. It is as if the therapist is saying and doing it. It is as if the therapist is inside the patient, or the patient is inside the therapist. The content of what is said and done and the way it is being said and done, are as if they are coming in, to, through, and from the therapist.

When the therapist "listens" in this way, he or she exists in a world of images, scenes, and situations. The patient's momentary words and doings invoke experiencings and imagery. Some are real and some are fanciful, some current and some remote, some gripping and some mundane. The therapist also has experiencings accompanied with bodily sensations and feelings. Some of these experiencings are superficial but some are deeper.

When patient and therapist have entered into the experiential state, when the therapist is experientially listening, the first step is attained.

STEP 2: CARRYING EXPERIENCINGS FORWARD

As the patient's words flow through the therapist, the therapist is attending to some focal center, and the therapist is having some experiencing. For example, the therapist is attending to the cancer, and the experiencing is a sense of helpless vulnerability (Mahrer, 1980a). Or the therapist is attending to mother's face, the way she is when she reads a novel in her favorite chair after supper, and the experiencing is warm and loving closeness. This second step is achieved when the experiencing deepens and intensifies, becomes more saturated, and attains a higher plateau, or in other words, *carries forward.* Whatever the nature and content of the immediate experiencing, the process is that of carrying it forward so that the patient experiences it much more deeply and fully (Bugental, 1978; Mahrer, 1978b, 1983a, 1985b).

The therapist carries forward the experiencing by means of any or all of the following methods.

CLARIFYING THE SITUATIONAL CONTEXT

When the therapist's attention is drawn by the image, scene, or situational context, he or she describes what is seen. It is a matter of simple description of whatever is witnessed, seen, or attended to. The therapist says, "The cancer is white, milky, and it is eating the flesh around it" or "Mother seems so peaceful and happy; she is putting her finger in her hair and playing with the feel of the hair." The therapist lives in this imagined scene. Clarifying the situational context means that the patient also lives in this imagined scene, and then the experiencing carries forward so that the patient has a greater sense of warm and loving closeness.

EXPRESSING THE VOICE OF THE EXPERIENCING

As the patient talks, what may be induced or invoked in the therapist is the experiencing rather than attending to the situational context. It is as if the patient's words invite the therapist to be the active voice of the experiencing - to say it and do it. The therapist accommodates, and serves as the patient's agent, or expressive self. For example, when this occurs as patient and therapist are here with the cancer, the therapist is the helpless dependency, and this is expressed: "What am I going to do? It's going to kill me! There's nothing I can do, nothing, nothing." Within the context of mother, the warm and loving closeness induces the therapist to express this: "I love you, Mom. I feel so good with you. I love touching your face and being with you." The experiencing then carries forward.

WELCOMING DESCRIPTION OF THE EXPERIENTIAL STATE

The experiencing is inside the therapist, but instead of pulling for direct and open expression, it is merely "here," inside, glowing. Accordingly, the therapist welcomes the experiencing and describes what it is like. When there is a helpless vulnerability, the therapist welcomes and describes its felt nature. The therapist says, "I'm shaking and trembling! My insides feel like mush, all weak and vulnerable. No strength! Dirty, garbage, helpless!" When the experiencing is a warm and loving closeness, the therapist welcomes and describes what this is: "All tender and warm, and soft, just soft and gentle, and close. Like being with, like being so close, so close and soft." Welcomed and careful description carries forward the experiencing.

DISCOVERING EARLY EXPERIENCES

These methods open up the experiencing, allow it to carry forward, to become fuller and deeper, and to fill the patient more. When this occurs, the patient may, for example, feel a sense of passivity, giving in, being reached and invaded, as the cancer is virulent, unreachable, and coldly devouring. Or the patient's whole body radiates a sense of safety, protection, comfort as he or she is cuddled into mother, becoming a part of mother, fondled and touched by mother.

Earlier experiences are discovered through the vehicle of the ongoing, carried forward experiencing and through the alive and real situational context. The patient sinks into earlier life events as the therapist describes the experiencing: "Passive, just giving in, being reached and invaded, done to...," and the patient, for example a woman, becomes a child, having her arm twisted by the older boys, and she is giving into the fainting, the heavy dizziness. Alternatively, the therapist describes the context: "Something or someone who is cold and unreachable, devouring, eating...," and she freezes up with an image of her father making strange animal sounds, poking mother's limp body with his thrusting, bobbing torso. By describing the nature of the experiencing and of the situational context, earlier events and experiences are brought forth. Now the patient is in these very special early life experiences, and the process of carrying forward continues as the therapist is invoked and induced to clarify the early situational context, to give voice to the experiencing, or to welcome and describe the nature of the experiencing.

Once the patient enters into a state of experiencing (Step 1), what the patient says and does may invite the further carrying forward of the experiencing (Step 2), and that is what the therapist does. On the other hand, what the patient says and does may activate something deeper; then the therapist deals with this relationship between the patient and the deeper experiencing in Step 3.

STEP 3: INTEGRATING THE RELATIONSHIPS
WITH DEEPER EXPERIENCINGS

As the patient's words seem to come through and from the therapist, there are moments when a relationship is constructed between the patient and a deeper, inner experiencing. It is a charged relationship, as if the patient is recoiling, defending, and struggling against the alive and present deeper experiencing. The interactive arena is now the patient and the deeper experiencing, and the relationship is tense and antagonistic. When this occurs, what ensues is an enlivened confrontational encounter between the patient and the patient's own deeper experiencing, which is given identity and voice through the therapist. At first this interaction is charged and tense. As it continues, it reaches a clashing peak, a full-feelinged, internal encounter wherein the patient and the deeper experiencing have it out with one another, grappling, twisting and fighting; it is a final confrontation between the patient and the deeper experiencing which the patient has always avoided and defended against.

The consequence is a radical change into a relationship of mutual welcoming, acceptance, and assimilation (Mahrer, 1982, 1983b). The patient attains a new found sense of oneness, harmony, peacefulness, soundness, and wholeness. It is a qualitative change wherein relationships with the deeper experiencing are integrated. Along with this is a symmetrical change in the nature of the deeper experiencing. What had been monstrous and grotesque, twisted into its bad form, is now allowed to occur in its wholesome, friendly, playful, benign, good form. This is the additional consequence and meaning of integrating the relationships with deeper experiencings.

There are several methods that guide what the therapist does as the identity and voice of the deeper experiencing.

EXPRESSING THE DEEPER EXPERIENCING'S TRUTH ABOUT THE PATIENT

The deeper experiencing knows the patient all too well, has uncannily accurate "insight" into the patient, and an unerringly penetrating understanding of the devastating truth about the patient. From within the bowels of the deeper experiencing, the therapist says, "Well, you can fool a lot of people, but I know you're scared silly of your mother, frightened to death of disobeying her...Oooo, you dirty old man, what nasty sexy thoughts you got! Wicked!...Better watch out, Jack, that's a tell-tale sign of your craziness; your lunacy is starting to show!"

The deeper experiencing is the sense of superiority, and that is all it knows. It accuses the patient of being that way ("You really think you're better than everyone"), playfully describes the patient as being that way ("You old dog; they're finally seeing your greatness!"), pushes the patient into being that way ("Tell them that you know better because you're a genius"), and understands everything about the patient that way ("All superior people have occasional periods of uncertainty"). The patient is pushed, goaded, nagged, chided, and generally blasted with the truth of the deeper experiencing.

FEEDING THE AVOIDANCES BACK INTO THE ENCOUNTER

As the internal encounter starts to heat up, patients will use all sorts of maneuvers to cool the relationship. They will construct safe distancing moats, slide into avoidant states, or do anything to prevent the encounter from getting more intense. The therapist feeds these avoidances back into the internal encounter: "Here's where you get nauseous and feel like vomiting. Go ahead, see if it works!...Ah, the old 'I'm going crazy' ploy. Mind if I join you?...Good show! The crying is neat. 'Course all little boys who are scared to death of their mothers are great criers." Everything the patient does to seal off or get away from the encounter is used as grist for the encountering mill.

THE THERAPIST AS THE REAL "I"

By speaking as the voice of the deeper experiencing, the therapist naturally refers to himself or herself as "I" and "me," and this makes for a strange encountering dialogue. It is as if the therapist is the authentic "I," and the patient is consequently forced to speak on behalf of the balance of the personality, that is, the more superficial, conscious portion. It is a dialogue between two selves, between the patient and his or her other, deeper self. It is an encounter over who is the most genuine, most real of the "I"s.

The therapist says, "You can find excuses for Dad all you want, but I think he's a tyrant and I don't like him...Just who do you think you are? I like Tom, and I want to have lunch with Tom. Just get out of the way and stop interfering in my life!...Will you listen to that jerk whining! I think he's nothing but a little Mama's boy. What do you think about him, huh? Agree with me?"

EXPRESSING INTEGRATIVE FONDNESS FOR THE PATIENT

While the patient is threatened by, distrusts, and avoids the deeper experiencing, it encounters the patient with unswerving fondness, loving playfulness, assimilative intimacy, deep warmth, and affection. The therapist expresses this directly and openly: "I like you! You're a wonderful person...You're great! What a delightful person you are!...What are you saying to me? That's terrible! You shouldn't talk that way to me!" Whether directly expressed or lacing whatever the therapist-as-deeper-experiencing says to the patient, there is an ever-present fondness.

A RELENTLESS COMMITMENT TO THE ENCOUNTER

Once the internal encounter locks into place, the therapist plays out the whole string. There is a ruthlessly single-minded commitment to the total encounter. Nothing the patient can do is capable of dislodging or disengaging the therapist from seeking the encounter through its crescendoing clash, its emotional peak, and out onto the inevitable plateau of internal integration (cf. Schutz, 1973).

By combining all or most of these components, the therapist insures that there is a dramatic change in the relationships between the patient and the deeper experiencings, for they are now integrative.

STEP 4: THE RADICAL CHANGE:
BEING THE DEEPER EXPERIENCING

Steps 2 and 3 open the way for the patient to disengage from his or her very identity, the continuing, substantive, ordinary boundaries of who and what he or she is. In this step, the patient is to be the deeper experiencing (Boss, 1963). This is a rare, profound, wholesale, and radical personality change. When it occurs, the very core of the patient is now existing as the deeper experiencing, the inner personality process. Here is a qualitative wholesale shift into being an entirely new person. The patient is free of the constraints and problems of who and what he or she has always been; all of this is left behind. Now there is a new person with new experiencings.

There are several methods for negotiating Step 4.

SELF ENCOUNTERING

The very center of the sense of self or "I-ness" must see a distinctly clear image. It is as if one sees a film or videotape of oneself. Then, as the center of the self or I-ness interacts with that image, relating more and more intimately with that image, the process draws the center of I-ness further into the deeper experiencing. It is as if you back into the deeper experiencing by having an emotional interaction with the exceedingly alive image of your ordinary, continuing identity.

The patient literally sees a clear, vivid self-image. For instance, a woman clearly sees an 11-year-old girl, scrunched up in the chair, devastated because her younger brother got to go skiing with her beloved Daddy. The image is so real that the patient can have an alive encounter with that hurt little girl, and as the interaction occurs, her very center backs into being the deeper experiencing of loving compassion: "Oh you wonderful person you! Just let me hold you. There, there. I know it hurts. God, I love you. You really feel hurt, don't you? Just come with me. I'm a great skier, and we can ski, and when they get back, let's have some fun bawling Dad out for not even thinking of you. I love you. I just love you!" By seeing, describing, interacting with, and encountering the self, the very heart of the patient undergoes the radical change of being the deeper experiencing.

DOING TO THEM WHAT THEY DO TO YOU

There are moments when the deeper experiencing comes alive in the form of the important figures who do "it" to you, where you are the passive receiver, the victim, the helpless pawn. For instance, a man's own deeper experiencing of dominating power comes alive in the form of his grandfather who disdainfully looks upon him as the unwanted, disgusting, repulsive little nobody. In the Copernican switch, he reverses the interaction and becomes the deeper experiencing by doing to the grandfather what the grandfather does to him (Loevinger, 1966; Perls, 1976). The patient says, "That is just about enough from you! Now you apologize, you worthless old man! If you are going to remain in my Mommy and Daddy's home, you are going to start to behave! From now on you are going to start helping out around here! You are going to clean your room! And you look at me when I'm talking to you!!" The radical change into the deeper experiencing is achieved when the patient does to another what the other does to the patient.

SUCCUMBING TO THE DEEPER EXPERIENCING

The patient fully succumbs to that which he or she had avoided, denied, hid from, or fought against. It is a total surrender into being the secret, hidden, menacing, awful, monstrous, and grotesque. Now the patient is into the deeper experiencing of the horrible inner coldness and uncaring metallic hardness. The patient says, "I give the impression of being concerned. Lies! A lifelong act! I'm skilled! I really don't give a damn about anyone! It's me, me, me first and only! I'm tough and hard, and nothing can ever reach me! I manipulate everyone, and I am damned good at it!" By giving in completely, the radical change is achieved and the patient *is* the deeper experiencing.

ALTERNATIVE EXPERIENCING IN OLD CRITICAL MOMENTS

There were old critical moments which were fraught with feelings. Those were the special moments when the deeper experiencing might have occurred, but it was blocked. Almost always the patient felt miserable, torn apart, and frozen. Those old critical moments stand as the awful highlights in one's life, the traumatic early incidents which hurt and pain. As the therapeutic process discloses the deeper potential, there is a new opportunity to go back into the old critical moments and, this time, rewrite history by living through the moment as the deeper experiencing.

For instance, the patient is a 7 year old whose divorced father has visited him on Sunday morning, sadly kissed him goodbye, and walked toward his car. Frustrated and hurt, his insides churned as he froze, watching his father walk dejectedly away. Therapeutic work has uncovered a deeper scurrilous toughness which, in the alternative experiencing of the old critical moment, explodes in wholesome expression: "No! Come back! I'm going to catch you and throw all my toys at you and grab onto you! I love you! I'm going to slug you and Mommy until the two of you make up! Wake up and love me!"

In the beginning of the session, methods were used to enable the patient to enter an experiential state. Thereafter, therapeutic work takes place. Depending upon how the patient is experiencing, methods are used to carry forward experiencing (Step 2), and the patient is filled a little more with experiencing which is both on the surface and deeper. Alternately, methods are used to soften, open up, and integrate the relationships between the patient and the deeper experiencing (Step 3). As the deeper experiencing is carried forward, and as relationships with the deeper experiencing become integrated, the way is clear for the patient to undergo the radical change of disengaging from the ordinary, continuing identity and entering into being the deeper experiencing (Step 4).

These are genuine changes, whether they occur for only a few seconds or much longer. They are profound changes; each step has provided the patient with a sample of what it is like to be a different person. We are now at the threshold of the final step in each session.

STEP 5: EXPERIENCING NEW WAYS OF BEING AND BEHAVING

The purpose of the final step is to enable the patient to gain a sense of being a substantially new and different person in a substantially new and different world. For some moments in the session, the patient was a changed person whose experiencings carried forward, whose relationships with deeper experiencings were integrative, who was being the deeper experiencing. Suppose this substantially changing person were to live and behave in the extratherapy world. Suppose the context now turns to the real world of today and tomorrow. If the person who was substantially different in the session were to step out into the extratherapy world, what would that new world feel like; how would this new person live and behave in this world? Given the changes which occurred, even momentarily, in the session, how would that person change even further to become the kind of optimal person which the individual in this session is capable of becoming? What are the directions of change open to this person in the extratherapy world? What can this person's world be like, and how can this person be and behave? The possibilities may be slight, restricted to specific little behaviors for a person who essentially lives in the same world as before. Or the possibilities may be dramatic, comprised of wholesale changes in the entire world, and in who the person is and how he or she behaves.

The purpose of this final step is to enable the patient to gain an experiential tasting of the possible new ways of being and behaving in the extratherapy world (Mahrer, 1985a). What follows is a summary of the methods for accomplishing this purpose.

INVITE THE NEW POTENTIAL TO BE AND BEHAVE IN ITS OWN WAY AND IN ITS OWN WORLD

For some moments in the session, the patient is a whole new and different person, qualitatively different from the ordinary, continuing person. It might occur when the potentials are carrying forward, or when the internal encounter attains a state of integration. It certainly occurs when the sense of I-ness disengages from the operating domain and enters into being the deeper experiencing.

The therapist brings this new person forward by addressing him or her and by carefully differentiating this new and different personality from the old, continuing, ordinary operating personality. Then the therapist invites the patient to define the kind of world he or she chooses to live in, to be and behave in his or her own distinctive ways. The therapist says, for example, "You are quite a woman! Sixty-four years old and full of all sorts of sexy thoughts. Leave old Louise alone, with her aches and pains and problems living with her daughter, and all depressed. What is *your* life like? How do *you* live? I know you don't want to get stuck in old Louise's life, so what's yours like?" The new and different personality will frame out its own world and its own ways of being and behaving in this new world.

INVITE THE NEW POTENTIAL TO COMMUNICATE WITH THE OLD SELF ABOUT HOW TO BE AND BEHAVE IN THE EXTRATHERAPY WORLD

The therapist also talks to the new person, the new potential. In differentiating the new person from the old self, the therapist invites this new person to communicate with the old self about how to be and behave in the extratherapy world. Talk to the old self. Say what you think about the way that person is, about the way he or she operates in life. The new person says, "You poor old sucker! You don't have to spend your life trying to please your mother. Wake up! You're young. You're vital and alive. Let Mommy ruin her own life. Go get an apartment and live with Christine. She's waiting for you to grow up! It's time, little fellow. Say goodbye to Mommy!"

INVITE THE PATIENT TO SEE THE PICTURE OF THE DIRECTIONS OF POTENTIAL CHANGE

The therapist carefully differentiates the ordinary, continuing patient from the picture of the directions of potential change. Safety is provided by emphasizing the picture as quite distinct from the patient, as a picture of the merely possible, a picture of a twin or clone or ideal possibility. Then the therapist paints the picture in a hypnagogically slow manner, with careful, detailed concretizing of how this new person can be and behave in his or her extratherapy world (Erickson, 1980). By means of a richly vivid picture, the patient is provided with an experiential feel of these new ways of being and behaving within the context of a new external world.

ACT AS THE IDENTITY WHO CARRIES OUT THE NEW WAY OF BEING AND BEHAVING

The therapist speaks as the voice and identity of the new experiencing who exists and behaves in the extratherapy world. Leaving the patient as the old identity, the therapist speaks as the (deeper) I, and the old patient is distinguished as "you." The therapist says to the patient, "I'm going to move to Vancouver and accept that job, and see what it's like to have a real executive position...Tonight I am going to call Nancy, give her flowers, and tell her I am really sorry...I have decided I'm going to ask Bill to move in. It's about time!" Through the identity of the integrated and actualized deeper potential, the therapist has carried out the new behavior in the context of the extratherapy world, quite separate and apart from the "you," the continuing, ordinary self. It is the therapist who risks the new way of being and behaving: "I'll do it; you stay here...You keep on sulking; I'm going to call her tonight...You don't have to do it; I will."

ACT AS THE VOICE OF THE OLD SELF, INTEGRATIVELY OBJECTING TO THE NEW PERSON

There are occasions where the patient dares to be the new potential and, even more audaciously, takes steps toward new ways of being and behaving in the extratherapy world. When this occurs, the therapist speaks as the voice of the old self who objects to the new possibilities, but who does so integratively. The therapist objects playfully, resists wholesomely, brings up an endless cascade of problems as he or she catastrophizes, yelps and yowls, scolds and berates, flusters and frets.

As the integratively objecting old self, the therapist says, "What are you trying to do - be different?...But if you are that way with Francis, what about me? I got to feel like a failure! What about me...What is this? You can't get rid of Homer! He's your son, and he has a responsibility to take care of you! He's only 29! Plenty of time for him to get married when he grows up!...You sound normal, and uh happy! I hate that! Stop that, you'll ruin everything!...But what happens to your whole life of being scared of going crazy? Tell me that, huh! You're not even the same person any more! What have you done?"

USE THE NEW BEHAVIOR IN THE EXTRATHERAPY WORLD

Each therapeutic step is designed to invite new behaviors. Yet none of these occurs within the context of the imminent new extratherapy world. The final method consists of using these various new behaviors in the extratherapy world. Several techniques may be used.

1. *The therapist may fabricate extratherapy situations in which to use the behavioral achievement from the session.* Patients will demonstrate "behavioral achievements" in the course of the session. They will behave in new ways and with good feelings. For the first time, patients will cry hard, bellow and scream, be confused and bewildered, tell a significant figure to shut up, and defiantly refuse to do what others want. The therapist's task is to fabricate extratherapy situations in which the new behavior is to occur, and to provide for the experiential tasting and sampling of these behavioral achievements within the context of the extratherapy situations.

   The therapist applies the new behavior to the patient's favorite "problem" situation, to situations where the patient ordinarily avoids and blocks being this new way, to situations mentioned by the patient earlier in the session, to current and future versions of remote situations where the patient as child used to behave that way magnificently, or to new situations which the patient actively constructs and fashions in new ways in the future extratherapy life.

   When the patient finally bellows out in anger, the therapist searches for appropriate life situations where being this way starts to happen and then is shunted off, or the therapist inserts this way of behaving into the patient's problem situations with superior and dominating others. The therapist invents ridiculous situations which demand such explosive reactions, and then the therapist either enacts the angry bellowing or describes it in minute detail. The therapist concocts absurd situations which are to be constructed by the patient, and in which the angry bellowing is most appropriate.

2. *The therapist recycles old effective behaviors as substitutes for the current problematic behaviors in the situation.* Therapy will discover magnificently useful and

effective behaviors within the context of early situations. Here are effective behaviors in situations where today the patient behaves in ways which are accompanied with bad feelings. It is refreshing to go back to childhood precursors of current problematic situations, and to discover the generally forgotten package of effective behaviors accompanied with delightful feelings. With a little technical refurbishing, they are inserted into today's situations and offer exciting experiencings of new ways of being and behaving.

3. *The therapist fabricates situations in which to use the acquired "therapy process skills."* Patients in experiential therapy learn a set of skills as part of the therapy process itself. They acquire the behavioral skills of stepping aside from the way they are, and playfully reacting to themselves; they learn how to be aware of and to describe bodily sensations and spontaneous images; they learn how to allow experiencings and bodily sensations to become fuller and stronger, how to concentrate attention upon a meaningful center, how to use ongoing bodily sensations to monitor and guide behavior, how to enter into deeper experiencings, how to engage in integrative encounters, how to express openly and directly, how to do to others what others do to them, and other "therapy process skills."

All of these new behaviors are available for use in the extratherapy world. Again, the therapist selects or invents situations in which these new behaviors may be used. For example, the process skill of allowing ongoing bodily sensations to monitor behavior means that patients learn to be aware of sudden bodily sensations such as being numb and frozen, for these are particular indications of threat, or of something wrong. They learn to use these bodily sensations in threatening situations, such as when visiting in-laws. They also learn how to act upon the warning signals by stopping what they are doing and exiting from the scene: "Sorry, all this is too much for me. I am stopping. I must leave. Bye bye." Each therapy process skill may be individually fitted to the particular patient and used in the particular patient's own life situations.

SUMMARY

Each session starts with the patient entering an experiential state, proceeding through the carrying forward of that experiencing and/or the internal encountering relationship between the patient and the deeper experiencing, and the radical change into being the deeper potential. Each session ends with the tasting and sampling of new ways of being and behaving. These are the steps of experiential psychotherapy. Each of these steps calls for its own methods. By competent use of the methods, each session proceeds through the same steps in the actualizing and integrating of new ways of being and behaving, whether the initial, the middle, or final session, or whether there is only one session or many.

There are sources for those who wish to go beyond this distilled introduction to experiential psychotherapy. The theoretical and philosophical foundations are given in Binswanger's (1967/1978) pioneering work, in the bible of clinical existentialism (May et al., 1958), and in the existential-humanistic theory of human beings (Mahrer, 1978a). The theory and methods of practice of this experiential psychotherapy are contained in two books. One (Mahrer, 1983a) concentrates on a general overview and on the basic practices for the initial step of getting into the experiential state. The second (Mahrer, 1985b) presents the theory and methods for the subsequent steps in the session. Finally, for those interested in psychotherapy research, an additional source (Mahrer, 1985a) introduces an alternative paradigm for studying psychotherapeutic change, one which is cordial to the existential-experiential therapist.

Alvin R. Mahrer, PhD, is currently Professor of Psychology, School of Psychology, University of Ottawa, in Ottawa, Canada. He is also in private practice. He has published in the areas of existential-humanistic theory of psychology and psychiatry, experiential psychotherapy, and psychotherapeutic research. Dr. Mahrer may be contacted at the School of Psychology, University of Ottawa, Ottawa, Ontario, Canada K1N 6N5.

Patricia A. Gervaize, PhD, is currently in the private practice of psychotherapy, and is also a Clinical Professor of Psychology at the School of Psychology, University of Ottawa, in Ottawa, Canada. Her publications are in the areas of psychotherapy and women's health. Dr. Gervaize can be contacted at the School of Psychology, University of Ottawa, Ottawa, Ontario, Canada K1N 6N5.

RESOURCES

Binswanger, L. (1978). *Being-in-the-World: Selected Papers of Ludwig Binswanger.* (J. Needleman, Trans.). New York: Harper. (Original work published in 1967)

Boss, M. (1963). *Psychoanalysis and Daseinsanalysis.* New York: Basic Books.

Bugental, J. F. T. (1978). *Psychotherapy and Process: The Fundamentals of an Existential-Humanistic Approach.* Reading, MA: Addison-Wesley.

Erickson, M. H. (1980). *The Collected Papers of Milton H. Erickson on Hypnosis.* New York: Irvington.

Gendlin, E. T. (1968). Client-centered: The experiential response. In E. F. Hammer (Ed.), *Use of Interpretation in Treatment* (pp. 208-227). New York: Grune & Stratton.

Gendlin, E. T. (1969). Focusing. *Psychotherapy: Theory, Research and Practice, 6,* 4-15.

Gendlin, E. T. (1978). *Focusing.* New York: Everest House.

Loevinger, J. (1966). Three principles for psychoanalytic psychology. *Journal of Abnormal Psychology, 5,* 432-443.

Mahrer, A. R. (1978). *Experiencing: A Humanistic Theory of Psychology and Psychiatry.* New York: Brunner/Mazel. (a)

Mahrer, A. R. (1978). Sequence and consequence in experiential psychotherapies. In C. L. Cooper & C. P. Alderfer (Eds.), *Advances in Experiential Social Processes* (pp. 39-65). New York: John Wiley. (b)

Mahrer, A. R. (1978). The therapist-patient relationship: Conceptual analysis and a proposal for a paradigm-shift. *Psychotherapy: Theory, Research and Practice, 15,* 201-215. (c)

Mahrer, A. R. (1980). The treatment of cancer through experiential psychotherapy. *Psychotherapy: Theory, Research and Practice, 17,* 335-342. (a)

Mahrer, A. R. (1980). Research on theoretical concepts of psychotherapy. In W. DeMoor & H. R. Wijngaarden (Eds.), *Psychotherapy: Research and Training* (pp. 33-46). Amsterdam: Elsevier/North Holland Biomedical Press. (b)

Mahrer, A. R. (1982). Humanistic approaches to intimacy. In M. Fischer & G. Stricker (Eds.), *Intimacy* (pp. 141-158). New York: Plenum.

Mahrer, A. R. (1983). *Experiential Psychotherapy: Basic Practices.* New York: Brunner/Mazel. (a)

Mahrer, A. R. (1983). An existential-experiential view and operational perspective on passive aggressiveness. In R. D. Parsons & R. J. Wicks (Eds), *Passive-Aggressiveness: Theory and Practice* (pp. 98-133). New York: Brunner/Mazel. (b)

Mahrer, A. R. (1985). *Psychotherapeutic Change: An Alternative Approach to Meaning and Measurement.* New York: Norton. (a)

Mahrer, A. R. (1985). *Therapeutic Experiencing: The Process of Change.* New York: Norton. (b)

May, R., Angel, E., & Ellenberger, H. F. (1958). *Existence: A New Dimension in Psychiatry and Psychology.* New York: Basic Books.

Perls, F. (1976). *The Gestalt Approach and Eyewitness to Therapy.* New York: Bantam.

Schutz, W. C. (1973). Encounter. In R. Corsini (Ed.), *Current Psychotherapies* (pp. 401-443). Itasca, IL: F. E. Peacock.

PRACTICAL ISSUES FOR THE CLINICIAN TREATING SUBSTANCE ABUSE*

William Grady Ryan, Nancy J. Ryan, Andrew Rosen, and Antonio R. Virsida

Horrendous examples of unintentioned malpractice occur daily in the area of substance abuse treatment. Prior to this epidemic era, the clinician could take refuge in the thought: "I wasn't trained to deal with those people." Today's patients, however, are driving us out of our ignorance. Whether or not we choose to acknowledge it, almost every mental health practitioner is dealing with substance abuse.

Ignorance and bias all too frequently are the lens that accounts for (a) addiction being diagnosed as depression and anxiety; (b) therapists having the illusion of trying to help a patient make thought-feeling connections when the patient's brain is altered with either illegal or prescribed legal drugs; (c) clinicians sometimes compartmentalizing their diagnoses, consciously or preconsciously, to systematically bury the substance abuse process working behind the cardiovascular, gastrointestinal, or other somatic disorder; (d) clinicians offering addicts truly ludicrous statements like "Just cut back," "Get off the hard stuff," "Try this Xanax"; or (e) clinicians denying that a significant percentage of the patients in a routine psychotherapy practice have been touched by substance abuse, either directly or indirectly.

The purpose of this contribution is to convey to the clinician a mind set and a sense for how to grapple more effectively with the addiction that is frequently overlooked. We will briefly review models of addition and attempt to provide reference points for the treating clinician. We will also address treatment planning, with special emphasis on dealing with initial denial.

Contained within the above, the reader will see reflected our treatment biases. First, addiction is a physiological-psychological state of being that must be accepted through the elimination of denial. Semantically, "alcoholic," "addict," and "substance abuser," are interchangeable. Second, we believe that the *most* efficacious method of recovery combines treatment (psychotherapy) and self-help groups such as Alcoholics Anonymous (AA). Treatment taken in conjunction with the "12 Steps of AA" provides an effective behavior modification program with a values-clarification component that is compatible with various perspectives. We will attempt to strike a balance between explaining and changing behavior throughout our discussion.

WHAT IS ADDICTION?

The issue of just what constitutes addiction will not be settled definitively in this paper. However, in passing, it is interesting to note the range and diversity of thinking, from an illness or medical-model concept, emphasizing, at times, a genetic propensity or physiological substrate; to more psychologically oriented models such as "family" systems or maladaptive Transactional Analysis scripts; and finally, to some remnant of outmoded societal or religious notions of a lack of willpower.

We believe a balanced view appropriately incorporates elements of the first two concepts. While no one has specified exactly what comprises the illness of addiction,

---

*This contribution and the one which follows are expansions of the article entitled "Practically Everything Practical the Clinician Wants to Know about Substance Abuse" by William Grady Ryan, Spring, 1984, <u>Voices: The Art and Science of Psychotherapy</u>, <u>20</u>(1) and is included here by permission. Copyright © 1984.

there is a general agreement that addiction is multidetermined. Interestingly, without either the aid or burden of professional training, self-help groups such as AA have globally described addiction as a threefold debilitative process interfering with loving and working. It is described as a physical, emotional, and spiritual (i.e., values clarification) problem. Although lacking any specificity or precision concerning the etiology or dynamics of addiction, this is a surprisingly well-balanced and sophisticated experiential description of addiction, consistent with research findings to date.

Those interested in an excellent overview of addiction from the viewpoint of a biochemical-genetic approach may wish to consult the work of Talbott (Talbott, 1983; Talbott & Cooney, 1982). Schuckit (1972) has also done research on alcoholism that supports Talbott's view of genetic involvement. Schuckit found that the students sired by alcoholic parents metabolized alcohol differently and had a higher tolerance for alcohol, reporting less dizziness and so on, than their counterparts. Interestingly, this meshes with what alcoholics usually report in their case histories: "Doctor, I had a high tolerance - after the party, I drove the others home."

Perhaps encompassing both issues of genetic predisposition and ongoing changes of biochemistry, Ohlms, 1983, reviewed in *The Disease Concept of Alcoholism* the production and storage of Tetrahydroisoquinoline (THIQ) in the brains of alcoholics. THIQ is a morphine-like substance which is a residue of acetaldehyde by-products which are left in the brains of alcoholics - in contrast with nonalcoholics - partially as a result of faulty biochemical elimination. This substance is more powerful and addicting than morphine (based on animal studies); and, serves as a potential basis for explaining the progressive danger of the illness, once either activated or reactivated (as in a slip); and, finally serves as a conclusive foundation for the necessity of an abstinence treatment model for alcoholics.

This research illustrates some of the interesting research on alcoholism and offers an antidote to any moralistic biases lurking in the clinician. Hard evidence that certain groups are at higher risk is accumulating (e.g., Valliant & Milofsky, 1982). Within Talbott's model, abuse must precede addiction and obviously, drawing on Schuckit's work, the higher the tolerance for abuse, the greater the probability that one will cross the "barrier" into addiction.

Despite some of the moving experiential descriptions by adult children of alcoholics and of substance abusers in the self-help groups, no common personality character structure exists for the alcoholic or drug addict. Addiction does not discriminate between personality and diagnostic groups nor, to a lesser extent, socio-economic groups. *What addicts and alcoholics have in common is an obsessive-compulsive trait that should never be thought of in isolation from an underlying genetic-biochemical substrate.* Such a trait need not stem from an obsessive-compulsive character structure. We have worked with addicts who ranged from inadequate personalities to the now defunct *DSM-II* garden variety of not-so-happy neurotics, to manic-depressives and paranoid-schizophrenics, where all of the above processes were diagnosed, after a sufficient (at least 3 months) period of sobriety, and were interactive with the prior addiction process.

For purposes of this contribution, hereafter dealing only with psychological variables, addiction may be considered an obsessive-compulsive trait involving a profound, primarily unconscious fantasy or belief that if I "take something from the outside and put it on the inside, I will feel better." The "something," to distinguish addiction from other forms of psychopathology, involves a mood- and mind-altering drug. This "something" is free and unconditional, which meshes with the orality of the addict, an important component if one wishes to expand addiction to include other forms of irrational behavior such as gambling. Finally, the locus of control is perceived as an initially external "something."

MIND SETS FOR THE CLINICIAN

PSYCHOLOGICAL TESTING - A DISTORTED LENS?

We believe that clinicians should never rely heavily on personality testing to diagnose character structure during the first 6 months of intervention with a substance abuser.

Neuropsychological testing is a general exception to this admonition in that it may be attempted after the patient is detoxified and stable. To illustrate this problem, the MMPI asks the patient to endorse or deny some pathological experiences (e.g., "I have had very peculiar and strange experiences"). Indeed, any serious alcoholic has had more than a few strange experiences and does not have sufficient experience in early sobriety to mentally decide "mostly false"; he or she is caught between Scylla and Charybdis, leading to the likelihood of artifactually high "F," "Sc," "MA," and "D" scales. We recommend that test-retest procedures be performed 6 months apart. The second testing should instruct patients to respond on the basis of their experiences during the period of sobriety.

Projective tests such as the Rorschach yield similar problems in early sobriety. Such tests are analogous to the classic "upside-down lens" perception experiments that demonstrated how the brain adapts to pathological conditions by seeing the world right-side up even through upside-down lenses. Metaphorically, removing the lenses of addiction at first leaves the the patient seeing the world upside down. The period might be likened to early sobriety when it is important, as the AA people say, to deal with the "thinking that went behind the drinking." Thinking or perception measured by the Rorschach during early sobriety yields misleading information regarding anything but a tentative diagnosis. This may be due either to microsubstance by-products of the final phases of detoxification or to the "thinking behind the drinking," as distinguished from relatively enduring personality characteristics. Of course, from a case management point of view, early testing is not misleading if it is taken merely as a base line or as a functional assessment of the patient at that point in time.

ADDICTION AS A SYMPTOM?

In the spirit of Allport's (cited in Rappaport, 1960) concept of "functionally autonomous" processes (p. 56), it is helpful, from a treatment point of view, to understand substance abuse as a relatively independent syndrome rather than as a symptom of underlying conflict that, once analyzed and worked through, will remit. It is analogous to a prolonged, functionally autonomous, post-traumatic stress syndrome with both organic and functional factors.

Professionals have been slow to move toward this position, long ago inherently postulated in the self-help groups' approach. Fortunately, rehabilitation centers around the country share the former position, which recognizes that certain drugs (alcohol merely being one of the oldest in use) are inherently powerful reinforcers. For example, few people would question the primary reinforcing effect of heroin, yet many underestimate the same effect with alcohol or Valium. The various psychosexual issues or self-esteem deficits existing at the inception of the problem can only be viewed as catalysts or one part of an ongoing, multidetermined, self-destructive self-system that increasingly comes under the tyranny of the primary reinforcers themselves.

SHOULD ADDICTS EVER HAVE DRUGS?

A brief clarification of terminology is first in order. There is no one satisfactory term for the process of substance abuse in this age of polydrug usage: "Addict" connotatively seems to exclude the alcoholic; "chemically dependent" sounds too diluted. "Cross-addiction" may well be denotatively inaccurate given the prevailing preference of most clinicians and researchers to talk about "drug of preference" as the figure contrasted against the shifting ground of all other mood- and mind-altering substances. Pursch (1978) talks about "sedativism" as the illness; however, this is not comprehensive enough to encompass such categories as hallucinogens and mood elevators.

The basic point is that all drugs are relatively interchangeable for the sensitized substance abuser. The implication is that a mood- and mind-altering drug of lesser preference physiologically or psychologically triggers a chain reaction that increases the probability - as in a habit hierarchy - that there will be a progression toward or immediate reinstatement of the drug of preference.

Clinicians accordingly must be attuned to the delicate issue, long a controversy between AA and psychiatry, of the appropriate use of prescription drugs. Neither physicians nor clinical psychologists necessarily receive much formal training in substance abuse and, in their attempt to help addicts, abuse often preconsciously becomes transformed into issues of depression or anxiety, problems with which the clinician is trained to work. The psychiatrist typically prescribes, while the psychologist provides psychotherapy or various behavioral interventions. In our view, both miss the central role of addiction; both gloss over the reality that addicts have good reason to experience anxiety and depression as a result of cortical depressants or stimulants and a chaotic personal and occupational life. The lives of addicts are a crashing mess - an important reference point for the clinician who desires to maintain his or her own reality testing.

At the Family Institute of Broward and Palm Beach, we resolve the dilemma by making a distinction between drugs that "take you to reality" and drugs that "take you from reality." As a general rule, chemotherapy is provided to manic-depressives and other patients who have an overt or underlying thought disorder, usually with paranoid features. These psychotic or psychotic-like processes (e.g., even Kohut's [1982] "borderline" personalities experiencing wild regressive swings without the palliative self-medicating effects of substance abuse), diagnosed with a clinical interview, Rorschach, and MMPI, seem to respond well to such varied substances as Lithium, the phenothiazines, or MAO inhibitors (with Kohut's "borderline-borderline" personalities where there are also pronounced depressive features). Rarely are the newer antidepressants used because some patients have reported a "racing" effect that triggers thoughts of an antidote to one form or another of downers. Hence, the degree and type of depression must be carefully assessed in order to prescribe the appropriate medication.

We have found numerous patients who, on the one hand, felt misunderstood in self-help groups and frustrated in "working their AA steps" and, on the other hand, were misdiagnosed by the professional community which ignored the role of addiction. We have not found that issuing appropriate medications to such patients produced a reversion to the "drug of preference." A typical patient taking prescribed medication reported, "I feel like I imagine normal people feel." An important caution to add, however, is that the use of medication is buttressed by the other components of our outpatient program. Clinicians who have developed their own internal norms regarding these matters with the adjunctive observations of enlightened AA sponsors carefully monitor these patients.

On an anecdotal basis, we cite the case of an alcoholic who was dry for 5 years but would break into gales of laughter at inappropriate moments in a speaker's AA talk, triggering laughter in other members. While the speaker told his story of how he lost his job, killed two pedestrians in a blackout, and lost his wife to cancer, this patient incessantly laughed, and eventually was asked to leave the meeting room, which in itself triggered assaultive behavior. The patient was actually suffering from a paranoid-schizophrenic process with fixed delusions. The appropriate prescription of Haldol in the right dosage controlled the process, and fellow AA members were amazed at how this patient now "worked his steps." This eclectic approach of chemotherapy, psychotherapy, and the self-help groups quickly gained the acceptance of many AA members. This was facilitated by also involving the AA sponsor in the program, providing information, and encouraging him to be supportive of the patient.

When there are the pathognomonic Rorschach signs of contamination, confabulation, F-minus responses, frequent reversal of figure-ground, morbid content, and signs of poor individuation, the clinician should begin to think of the possibility that chemotherapy, in conjunction with AA and psychotherapy, may be appropriate. It is also important to note that, unless there is a clear-cut pattern of thought encroachment, medication should be given most cautiously, especially for affective problems. If there is a blatant manic-depressive process (with documented family history), the physician may begin Lithium after the first 28 days but more preferably only after 3 months. Affective disorders very frequently are merely the residue of substance abuse. However, with the above Rorschach signs and 3 months of consistent clinical behavior, the clinician may proceed cautiously with medication.

When there is resistance to such recommendations from self-help groups, we frequently note two facts: (a) The founders of AA, Dr. Bob and Bill Wilson, apparently took some form of antidepressants; and (b) In Chapter V of *Big Book of Alcoholics Anonymous* (1976), referred to by members as "the Big Book," it clearly states, "There are those too who suffer from grave emotional and mental disorders, but many of them do recover if they have the capacity to be honest" (p. 58). "Honest" certainly connotes good reality testing and looking at things objectively. It is not unreasonable to assume that a separate but interacting psychiatric process must also be taken into consideration in a sound treatment plan. After all, alcoholics and addicts are susceptible to various physical problems that should be treated. The ultimate question, however, in the area of prescribed drugs for psychiatric processes in conjunction with addiction is whether the drugs take someone "to reality" or "away from reality." Such evaluation must not be limited to the subjective report of the addict but must be carefully considered by a clinician experienced in treating substance abuse.

Special problems arise with pain medications because patients quickly build a tolerance to medication that no longer eliminates pain, but to which they have become emotionally habituated. This issue would require a separate paper, but the treating clinician should speak with the physician or dentist who recommended such medication. Both common sense and clinical experience dictate that all such medications be taken only when absolutely necessary and for the shortest duration possible.

As a final note, it is imperative that no minor tranquilizer (Librium, Valium, Tranxene, Xanax) be prescribed to any addict. It is our opinion that such medications, along with sleeping compounds, lead back to the drug of preference. People rarely die of anxiety and almost never from lack of sleep - but they inevitably die from addiction. One can speculate that the latter grouping is destructive because (a) it has a sedative-like effect which is all too similar to alcohol, and (b) it reinforces the central unconscious fantasy in addiction: "If I take something from the outside and put it on the inside, I will feel *better* (in contrast to *normal*)."

WHAT ABOUT CONTROLLED INGESTION?

Theoretically, the issue of drug preference might be likened to the old controversy of symptom substitution debated by the behavioral and psychoanalytic camps. The heart of that issue involved differences in semantics, theoretical models, and identification of the problem. Additionally, it was a quasi-philosophical issue. In our view, the behavioral researchers missed a central aspect of addiction. Addiction is a narcissistic regression, acting in conjunction with a genetic-biochemical substrate that drives the addicting need. Controlled drinking in this context, therefore, can only be seen as prolonged self-tortuous foreplay which ultimately leads to self-destruction.

Another dimension to the issue is a purely philosophical matter. Most personality theories and abnormal psychology paradigms key in on "adapting to reality." Yet what constitutes reality is an issue of intuition and judgment outside the realm of applied science that can only describe patterns but cannot evaluate them. The latter task is philosophical, and we have no difficulty making the judgment that the pattern of controlled ingestion of mood- and mind-altering substances for the addict is an exercise in masochism and hence a poor form of adapting to reality.

We have almost never seen a heavy user control his or her substance ingestion. To deal with resistance and clarify diagnosis, we have new patients chart their drug intake, after mutual agreement regarding the level of intake. (For example, with alcohol consumption, no more than 2 ounces per day is allowed. If a day or days of intake are skipped, no combining of missed quantities is permitted. Charting is done. No other drugs are allowed.) Rarely has any heavy drinker been able to adhere to this. The same results have been obtained with other abusers using only minute quantities of their drug of preference. Few bother to lie; more frequently there is initial resistance to charting (an excellent tool to destroy denial). In sum, we seriously doubt that individuals who present with a drinking problem and later learn to control their problem with moderate use were even true addicts.

GRAPPLING WITH DENIAL AND RATIONALIZATIONS

Diagnostic criteria for addiction, as implied above, involve a philosophical judgment of behavioral patterns. Although a thorough discussion of this point is beyond the scope of this contribution, it should be noted that differing chemicals produce differing patterns of psychophysical deterioration.

For all practical purposes, it is important for the therapist not to enter the complicated system of rationalizations regarding addiction. Two key notions can serve the clinician well in the initial interview. First, the ingestion, whatever the sequencing, patterning, or contingencies, is experienced by the patient as an ego-alien, obsessive-compulsive process. Second, in line with Freud's value judgment that the purpose of living is loving and working, does the patient's ingestion of the substance interfere with either? If it does, why can't he or she stop? It is important to remember that denial is a primary defense in protecting the obsessive-compulsive process; therefore, the self-evaluation of work-love interference must be taken in conjunction with clinical judgment.

But clinical judgment is just that - clinical. Like a butterfly net that fails to capture the essence of a living, suffering patient, a clinical abstraction can fail to communicate a feeling for what to do when confronted with denial and rationalizations. We believe that as a clinician you must let your mind's eye see the murky, imprecise canvas of evasion, self-deceit, self-destruction, and desperate manipulation. If you let yourself, you will intuitively identify addiction when you see it.

Later, we will discuss some more theoretical issues while outlining a comprehensive practical treatment program. First, consider some typical clinical data occurring in the early interventive sessions.

A SCENARIO

1. The Set: Doctor, I'm here because my wife (interchangeable with boss, court, physician, clergyman) thinks I have a little problem - you know how wives are - well, she thinks I drink too much. I don't think so - but you are the doctor. What is an alcoholic?

   Inner Translation:

   My wife has a problem because she thinks I have a problem. Preconsciously I, too, know I have a problem - otherwise I wouldn't have to minimize it. I'd rather project my irritability, instability, and so on, onto my wife, because if I admitted I had a problem, I'd have to give up something my body craves, booze. I might have to solve my chemical problem and the emotional issues related to it. Out of my grandiosity, I will flatter you by reassuring you that you are indeed the doctor even if you can't define alcoholism. I'd rather go up into my head and intellectualize my feelings while I seductively trap you.

2. Director's Suggestions:

   a. Never, never discuss definitional issues of alcoholism. At the Family Institute, we will provide the substance abuser and his or her family with literature from varying sources. However, great pains are taken early on to not discuss varying formulations of "how much and how often is enough" to qualify as an alcoholic. This is an intellectual trap for both patient and therapist. Invariably, the more sophisticated patient will even refer to some of the methodologically questionable controlled drinking studies.
   b. Urge the patient to talk about his or her feelings about substance use and abuse. We might say, "I help individual people, not experimental and control groups," or "Tell me why it concerns you." Statements such as the latter act through the externalization, denial, or projection and help patients to focus on their inner world, which they probably sense is in a shambles.
   c. Almost invariably, if the therapist asks "Do you have a problem?" the patient will say "No." Don't paint yourself in a corner. More helpful statements would be "I don't know whether or not you have a problem; by working together, perhaps we (assuming the patient is not in need of impending withdrawal and institutionalization) can make a determination about whether you want to change your lifestyle. Your wife's perceptions are your wife's." Remarks of this sort help disentangle the therapist from the net of family and third-party judgments that the substance user or abuser will throw out in an effort to associate them with significant judgmental others (some probably appropriately judgmental) and in order to disqualify them.

THE SCALLOP TEST: A CASE STUDY

Recently, an extremely demanding, defensive, 49-year-old patient brought his harping wife, his medical records, and his abrasive demeanor to the Family Institute to settle once and for all the ridiculous controversy he claimed his wife had created over his consumption of what was his drug of preference, alcohol. Decade-long use of Librium provided the background music while brief experimentation with cocaine provided relief from depression. In his mind the latter was an obvious by-product of what he perceived as an overcontrolling wife. Regardless of etiology, he was depressed; his professional respectability was wavering and considerable legal accomplishments as an attorney were discussed by colleagues in the past tense. Finances were not yet a problem, enabling the maintenance of denial; somewhat surprisingly, child and teen management problems were still only impending.

"Here are the medical records; just give me a complete psychological test battery...without the Halstead-Reitan. I'll tell you in advance...you'll find an allergic reaction to Florida is the only positive medical finding. You may find depression and I can't tell you there is a marriage problem...not much difference between what you and I do, Doc."

Ironically, the patient got his demand for a full battery. An MMPI revealed a tentative picture of a narcissistic personality with a strong possibility of borderline and depressive features. Further projective testing and in-depth substance abuse clinical interviews, however, strongly suggested that the personalized thinking on the MMPI was primarily the biochemical and psychological sequelae of not-so-simple addiction, rather than character structure.

In working with substance abusers, it is often best to forget, at least while confronting denial, traditionally taught non-directive techniques. The clinician must maintain a developmental dimension and realize that, no matter how sophisticated the orally conflicted addict may appear, he is orally-conflicted. The nature of the conflicts often calls for intervention techniques that a child would understand, wrapped in the language and thinking of the patient.

"Mr. X, having thoroughly reviewed your records with our medical consultant, there indeed is an allergy. It is an idiosyncratic reaction to seafood and specifically to scallops." Seizing upon this already known piece of information, the patient leapt off the sofa as if to make closing argument to his wife that indeed the secret of his universe had been discovered: There was probably a network of allergies responsible for his emotional difficulties (progress from making the marriage the Maginot Line) - a network waiting to be affirmed by a local allergist with more tests! "I'm swearing off scallops; I'm going to get into nutrition. As much as I love seafood, I need to be in good shape...red meat...probably no good either."

We continued: "The allergy we had in mind, Mr. X, is to booze, pills, and coke." Caught off guard, this sophisticated trial lawyer got a brief glimmer of what his impulsivity had wrought. For a brief moment, he realized the ludicrous, desperate need to seize upon anything else as the problem to maintain the umbilical connection with "chemical love." With the speed of an aged fighter in the ring, he regained his footing somewhat: "Well, you're not the first...I don't need help, I can do it myself." Then, with his wife in tears, Mr. X. interrupted himself and asked, sarcastically but weakly, "Any final pronouncement before you give me your bill?" Reflecting the sadness of the moment, we could only say, "Guess you like the booze more than scallops."

Mr. X taught us much as clinicians. Two years later, he began to hit bottom. We told him that outpatient treatment was out of the question and referred him to a 28-day, out-of-county rehabilitation center. Having brought his own portable TV, he left after 5 days because the clinical director refused to let him watch the football play-offs. We drove him back to the same program several months later in response to his desperate wife's pleadings. While we finalized arrangements for him with the clinical director, Mr. X called to notify us that he had returned via taxi to his home. Mr. X never did enter psychotherapy. Perhaps the interventions had some impact; AA clearly did. He has been sober now for over a year. With a sober cortex and the help of countless untrained clinicians, Mr. X's secondary narcissism has been transformed into a healthier self-esteem.

The scallop test has served us well in working with the substance abuser in denial. We modify it. We might blend it into the form of a simply hypothetical question: "Do you like scallops? Imagine that all the presenting problems that you've described involving your job, your marriage, could be resolved by giving up scallops...would you do it? Could you do without these scallops you love? Good. Now what about your poisonous scallops - your booze, your drugs?" Incredulous looks, laughs, and occasional anger are all patient reactions to our persistent, at times dramatic, attempts to strip-mine the denial.

We vary our strategies and interventions. Each clinician must make sure his or her interventions flow honestly and naturally from within. Substance abusers are most perceptive. They will respect, however, the clinician's courage to push on into the wastelands to which they have banished themselves and which have successfully warded off countless do-gooders. There are variations on the theme of insanity in this harsh land, where "fun ain't fun." Mr. X said it all with scallops!

VIGNETTE: "THE DRINKING RULES"

Clinician: "Tell me about your drinking."

Alcoholic: Well, I have it pretty much under control...occasionally, there are parties...sometimes the pressure builds up...you know how it is. I haven't had a drink now in almost 13-1/2 days...see, I rarely have more than two drinks at lunch; if I am playing racketball with the guys, I...."

Clinician: "Tell me about your pasta consumption."

Alcoholic: "I beg your pardon...."

Clinician to Nonalcoholic: "Tell me about your drinking."

Nonalcoholic: "I beg your pardon...could you clarify?"

Moral of the Story: Alcoholics have complicated response patterns that might be analogized to the complexity of chess rules. They have developed in the matrix of ongoing physiological need coupled with an equal rationalizing need to explain away that need. In accord with some of the obsessive-compulsive trends, the ingestion of the forbidden substance has to be counterbalanced very righteously with rules that place the alcoholic in compliance, while simultaneously striving to mesh with his or her ego ideals of what a good drinker should be. Much of this, at least for the defensive drinker or addict who has not yet hit bottom, will pour out at a rapid, almost unsolicited, verbal rate.

By contrast, when the denial has imploded, there is typically less verbal torrent and protection. Rather, hopelessness and *temporary* docility lead to "Doctor, what do I do now?" (Temporary is emphasized, for true surrender to the substance abuse process usually occurs most efficaciously in the confines of a rehabilitation center, something the outpatient clinician rarely witnesses.) Clinicians frequently misinterpret this phenomenon as representing progress out of a true desire to help, a lack of experience, and perhaps a tinge of grandiosity, only to be profoundly disappointed and disillusioned about working with substance abusers. Effective intervention requires honest understanding of what the clinician can influence, what he or she can't, and what the difference is. Elsewhere in this contribution, rehabilitation centers and self-help groups are discussed as important support systems to utilize on behalf of the patient. Remember, neither the clinician nor the patient has it "pretty much under control."

RARELY CITED QUICK SCREEN PATHOGNOMONIC INDICATORS

1. The Goodman Test (unpublished): Give patients any one of the substance abuse screening tests (e.g., MAST; Selzer, 1971). Add one final true-false item: "Did you cheat on this test?"
2. The Bryan Test (unpublished): Chronic substance abusers tend to position their feet wider apart when walking, for better balance.

3. Watch for convoluted logic: "Doc, if I stop using, people will think I had a problem."
4. "I have to do it myself, Doc" (inspired by underlying identification fantasies with *Bonanza's* Pa Cartright and John Wayne). This strategy provides both delay and disappointment.
5. "Once I get my marriage in shape, the drinking should fall in place." Strategy: Focus on any and all problems but the primary one!
6. "Doc, what do you think of vitamins?" Patients in denial seek wide ranges of diagnostic and treatment modalities: astrology, aerobics, and so on.
7. Clever patients sometimes even utilize spirituality: "Doc, it's a spiritual fellowship, AA is - right? I think I'll just pray instead."
8. "If I could just change: job, spouse, geography."
9. After spending thousands on a drug of preference: "I don't know if I can afford this (therapy)."
10. "I can't go to 'rehab' - the family (the boss) needs me" (to torture them more)!
11. "I went to that AA meeting, Doc; interesting, but (options):
    a. Have you seen the decor?"
    b. Not my kind of people (despite the probable mix from the professional to the unemployed)."
12. After spending at least 20 hours per week pursuing a drug of preference: "These meetings - 90 meetings in 90 days - hey, I have responsibilities."
13. Beware of the polyabuser (95% of substance abusers): "I only have a joint every now and then." Question. "Well, I have a little..." Question. "And a little..."
14. The "Megargee Substance Abuse Post-Dictive Predictor Test" (unpublished): When patients describe the first intoxicating, primary physiological reinforcement effect ecstatically: "I grew 2 inches, the world seemed rosy; it was a love affair."

EPILOGUE

Parenthetically, if the denial is massive and the rationalizations so entrenched, the clinician may have to tackle them directly. For example: "You have only one decision to make. Either you turn your marinated brain over to me or some other sober brain, or there will be one of three eventual outcomes: prison, a mental hospital, or the grave." Whatever the level of denial and resistance, the addiction process must be dealt with immediately. Whatever leverage is available to the clinician - family type, employer benefits, court order - should be constructively and tactfully used.

A CHINESE MENU TREATMENT PLAN

Effective help for the substance abuser requires a multifaceted approach which we have called a "Chinese Menu" treatment plan. The selection follows:

Column A:

Base line Assessment
Intervention

Column B:

4-6 Week Rehabilitation Center
Intensive Outpatient Program

Column C:

Individual Therapy
Family Therapy
Marital Therapy

Column D:

Chemotherapy

Column E:

Self-Help Groups

Column F:

Comprehensive Psychological Testing (3 months after being sober), preceding any intensive, insight therapy

At the Family Institute, after a period of 2 to 6 weeks, anyone who is still "using" is told they may be terminated lest they have the illusion of treatment. Prior to this, however, they would have gone through base line assessment consisting of clinical interviews, psychometric testing, and, if necessary, charting. Termination based on ongoing denial is very infrequent. First, great effort is spent building a rapport. The patient is encouraged to go to a self-help group to participate in his or her own diagnosis. He or she is told to identify rather than compare.

The intervention is usually routine insofar as clinical persistence can bypass the resistance. When this is not the case, the entire family set of influential friends, employers, and clergy, is invited to participate in an "intervention happening." Many of the staff at the Family Institute have a recovering background (though this is not essential), and self-disclosure may be blended with the intervention.

Typically, the active addict will be given two options: (a) preferably enroll in a 4-6 week inpatient rehabilitation program; (b) as a secondary and less preferred option, attend daily self-help group meetings in conjunction with individual therapy at least 3 to 5 times per week, depending upon needs and financial ability. Placement in conjunctive group therapy is also frequent. In response to protests about the strict regimen, it is clearly pointed out that the first option is clinically more efficacious as well as cost-effective. When a patient fails to take either option and, despite the constructive use of all leverage, continues to use a drug of preference, treatment is terminated. This is a rare event if confrontation and family involvement are vigorously pursued.

If treatment ends, it is important that the patient knows (a) exactly what his or her problem is upon termination, and (b) that he or she, rather than the treatment, failed. Usually the patient has failed to follow directions, for example, to go to AA meetings, or there have been major psychiatric problems interacting with the addiction process which can be very difficult to control on an outpatient basis. Such problems occur less frequently on an inpatient basis where there is greater opportunity for stabilization of both the client and the family, who must participate in treatment as co-alcoholics or addicts, or co-dependents.

The other components of the treatment plan involve individual and family therapy. At the Family Institute, we try to be flexible about treatment planning rather than forcing the alcoholic and co-dependents through a rigid outpatient program. Theoretically, we are eclectic, although by and large individual therapy is analytically oriented. Group therapy frequently takes on a Gestalt "hot-seat" format, and in family therapy much is borrowed from the structuralism of Minuchin (Minuchin & Fishman, 1981). Typically, the treatment of the family begins while the patient is in residence at a 28-day program. Depending upon the problems of family members, some individual therapy may be initiated, though it is often preferable to see the entire family together in order to break down the defensive structures which Kellerman (1980) describes so well in his pamphlet, *Alcoholism: Merry-Go-Round Named Denial.*

Upon the return of the alcoholic or addict from rehabilitation, for approximately the first 3 months the individual therapy is kept on a very directive and supportive, rather than uncovering, basis. It is most helpful to rely on self-help group members already in treatment to act as temporary sponsors to insure participation at fellowship meetings. It is very helpful for patients already in AA to facilitate the entrance of a newcomer, because this is an active expression of the spirit of the 12th step of AA and reinforces "getting out of oneself."

For approximately the first 3 months, therapy also focuses upon the individual's reaction to the self-help groups, and pockets of resistance are explored. This typically involves reservations about "spirituality" and "that God stuff," questions involving personal acceptance of alcoholism, frequency of AA meetings, and other matters. When resistance is particularly high, the individual is also placed in a group where the "older" members can serve as role models. The format of group therapy complements the AA discussion groups, where the rule is "Don't take the other person's inventory." Such a tradition makes sense (a) insofar as the sober neophyte begins to focus on himself or herself as "the problem" rather than on people, places, and things; and (b) in a situation where there is not necessarily a trained facilitator. However, feedback in group psychotherapy from others is also crucial to the neophytes who have been unknowingly trapped in the distorting sphere of their own self-centeredness. In short, one cannot emphasize enough the importance of reinforcing the ties to the self-help groups.

Depending upon the degree of ego strength and adaption to AA, the uncovering and more analytically oriented therapy can be undertaken anywhere from 3 to 12 months after the inception of sobriety. The same rule also applies to family members who have necessarily been the victims and have participated in a psychotic, chemically induced system of behavior. As alcoholics frequently say, referring to co-dependents, "I drank; what was your excuse for acting crazy?" Alanon and Naranon should be essential in the treatment programming.

All patients should be assessed as they would be for other disorders after there has been some period of sobriety in their lives. Not everyone needs therapy; the self-help groups represent a behavior modification program which alone is sufficient for many. As clinicians, we must remember that not all people, either because of motivation, finances, or the ability to introspect, are good therapy candidates. In turn, the effective clinician must be like a broken field runner, showing flexibility. Referring back to the combination Chinese Menu, our views are that Columns A and E are always essential. Column B (especially rehabilitation) is almost always necessary; Columns C, D, and F are less essential in that order.

SUMMARY

In summary, there are two basic points that we hope this contribution communicates to mental health practitioners. The first is that all clinicians need to be sensitive to the possibility that patients seen in the office may be suffering from the effects of alcohol, substance abuse, and addiction. The tendency to deny the presence of alcohol and substance abuse and its effects on peoples' lives is an ever present problem for patients and clinicians. It is imperative that clinicians have a mind set that helps them actively look for the presence of alcohol and substance abuse in their initial and ongoing sessions with patients, and not just passively wait for it to come up. Clinicians aware of the denial involved in addiction would not consider waiting for patients to tell them. The second point we hope this contribution communicates is that addiction is a disease, and that traditional forms of psychotherapy are at best ineffective and at worst facilitate the addiction process by creating an illusion that change is occurring. The treatment modalities advocated in this contribution are, when utilized, the most effective way to deal with addictions and ultimately to help these patients' lives change.

(Biographical material on the authors is included at the end of the next contribution, "Collaborating with Self-Help Groups for Substance Abusers.")

RESOURCES

Angyal, A. (1982). *Neurosis and Treatment: A Holistic Theory.* New York: Da Capo Press.

Big Book of Alcoholics Anonymous (3rd ed.). (1976). New York: Alcoholics Anonymous World Services.

Fenichel, O. (1945). *The Psychoanalytic Theory of Neurosis.* New York: W. W. Norton.

James, W. (1978). *The Varieties of Religious Experience.* Garden City, NY: Image Books.

Kellerman, J. (1980). *Alcoholism: A Merry-Go-Round Named Denial.* Center City, MN: Hazelden.

Kohut, H. (1982). *The Analysis of the Self.* New York: International Universities Press.

Milkman, H. (1979). Addictive processes, an introductory formulation. *Street Pharmacologist, 2*(4), 1-4.

Minuchin, S., & Fishman, H. C. (1981). *Family Therapy Techniques.* Cambridge, MA: Harvard University Press.

Ohlms, D. L. (1983). *The Disease Concept of Alcoholism.* Belleville, IL: Gary Whiteaker Co.

Pursch, J. (1978). *Alcohol, Pills, and Recovery.* Los Angeles, CA: FMA Film Production.

Rappaport, D. (1960). *The Structure of Psychoanalytic Theory, a Systematizing Attempt.* New York: International Universities Press.

Schuckit, M. (1972). A study of alcoholism in half siblings. *American Journal of Psychiatry, 18*, 1132-1136.

Selzer, M. L. (1971). Michigan Alcoholism Screening Test: The quest for a new diagnostic instrument. *American Journal of Psychiatry, 127*, 1653-1658.

Talbott, G. D. (1983, August). The disease of chemical dependence: From concept to precept. *The Counselor*, 18-19.

Talbott, G. D., & Cooney, M. (1982). *Today's Disease: Alcohol and Drug Dependence.* Springfield, IL: Charles C. Thomas.

Tiebout, H. M. (1954). The ego factors in surrender in alcoholism. *Quarterly Journal Studies on Alcohol, 15*, 610-621.

Valliant, G. E., & Milofsky, E. S. (1982). The etiology of alcoholism: A prospective viewpoint. *American Psychologist, 37*, 494-503.

COLLABORATING WITH SELF-HELP GROUPS FOR SUBSTANCE ABUSERS*

William Grady Ryan, Nancy J. Ryan,
Andrew Rosen, and Antonio R. Virsida

We believe that self-help groups can play a critical role in the recovery of substance abusers. In the preceding contribution, we have described key issues in professional intervention with substance abusers. Here we will address practical considerations in facilitating the effectiveness of self-help groups. If this contribution is to clarify the value of the self-help groups, it is first essential to review some of the historical and semantic issues that have formed the basis of a division between self-help groups and much of the professional mental health community.

DIVISIVE FACTORS

A superficial yet profoundly divisive issue between professionals and self-help groups is level of training. Frequently, we have encountered colleagues who regard Alcoholics Anonymous (AA) or Narcotics Anonymous (NA) people as well-intentioned fanatics who are equally misinformed about the miracles of modern chemistry and the breakthroughs of psychotherapy. It is inconceivable that anyone without the benefit of professional training should give advice - much less obtain results - often contradicting that of the professional. The AA or NA sponsors, however, can recount hundreds of examples of alcoholics and addicts who have inappropriately fallen prey to ECT, addicting drugs, and inhumane treatment such as aversive conditioning at the hands of such professionals. Without terming it as such, they have built up their own "internal predictive norms" about who will slip and who is responding well to treatment. Yet, all too frequently, as a result of remaining defiance and antiauthoritarian attitudes, addicts are blinded to the help that professionals can render.

We have found that an excellent way to draw upon the internal norms of all involved is to invite the AA or NA sponsor into the therapy situation with the patient, not only to bridge the above gap but to minimize destructive manipulation of communication channels by the newly sober person who has not yet made a full commitment to sobriety. A partial function of this contribution is to alert clinicians to advantages of coordinating their efforts with the self-help groups, thereby raising the base rates of recovery. For example, AA is a highly efficient, 24-hour-a-day, 7-day-a-week communication and support system that can buttress the 1 to 3 weekly outpatient hours spent with a patient. As clinicians, we sometimes cannot even get a message from our answering service, much less replicate the wide base of personal attention available in AA - a most important factor in early sobriety.

SPIRITUALITY AND RECOVERY

One controversial issue among professionals has been the role of spirituality in the recovery process. We prefer to view this issue in the context of values clarification. It is

---

important to minimize the injection of our own values, or when we do, to openly articulate that we are sharing our judgments, acting as philosophers rather than as psychologists applying science. However, many clinicians connotatively and subliminally inject their antispiritualism and induce in the patient a prejudice against anything philosophical or theological. Asking God for help has been considered an infantile projection of an ongoing wish for the perfect parent figure (Fromm, 1950). What many clinicians fail to see is the simple fact that whether there are levels of moral reasoning and whether humans do have projectional systems has nothing to do, per se, with the question of a separate ontological entity possessing creative intelligence. It merely demonstrates the philosophical axiom of St. Thomas Aquinas that "what is received is received according to the receiver." Accordingly, we believe that there is no correlation between the psychological issue of level of maturity and the philosophical issue of belief or disbelief in God.

As practical clinicians, however, we believe we should take into account the following realities: (a) Many of the people in AA do call their higher power "God," with some traditional trappings, and the self-help groups operate in a culture where the higher power or "God" is a central point of focus; and (b) at the onset of sobriety, the individual is riddled with self-hate and feelings of powerlessness and, of necessity, perceives the locus of change as external to himself or herself. It would seem absurd to the alcoholic who has tried every conceivable drinking schedule, from spritzers to martinis only on odd days and after 5:30 p.m., to initially conceive of any internal healthy resources. It is essential for the clinician to overcome any spiritual biases he or she may have and to avoid reinforcing the real problem - resistance to growth!

By working within the patient's framework, there can be a variety of conceptions of the "higher power." Phrases like "God works through people" are frequently found in AA groups. Accordingly, where appropriate we might state the relationship with God metaphorically as, "God is the solar source of power - you and your sponsor are like solar batteries." For the ambitious independent type, we might liken the relationship to that of a senior and junior partner in a firm; for the dependent type, communication with God could be compared to use of a hot line. For the affirmed agnostic, a humanistic equation of higher power and the Transactional Analysis (TA) "nurturing parent," the force of the group, or even "the Force" - á la Starwars - may fill the bill.

A final major issue dividing professionals and self-help members is one of semantics. Imagine the plight of the alcoholic who has decided to use all treatment resources. He or she goes to the psychologist who urges autonomy and self-actualization as the way to gain sobriety. The consulting psychiatrist talks about biochemical problems and notes that ultimately everything flows from a physiological substrate. The psychiatrist's solution is medication. Finally, the AA sponsor says the individual must surrender to a program of other people and turn his or her will and life over to some higher being. Even a nonmarinated cortex would have difficulty deciphering and sorting out these dysynchronous audio inputs. While each may agree on a final common goal, there is a clear problem in selecting pathways.

Many professionals have forgotten that systems can be translated, as Miller and Dollard (1941) illustrated some years ago. They have forgotten the basic reality that constructs are like conscious spider webs that do not capture the totality of the phenomena observed. The subjective reality of experience can only be approximated in the distorted mirrors of objectification that we call words. Yet clinicians naïvely take the words as reality and have fought over them with both their colleagues and patients.

Accordingly, in treatment, it is important to speak in terms consistent with what the patients will experience in self-help groups. Family Institute clinicians talk of acceptance and surrender rather than reality testing, the higher power rather than superego, interdependence rather than self-actualization, and inventory rather than analysis. This minimizes friction and enhances the probability of constructive self-help group participation.

THE ESSENCE OF SELF-HELP GROUPS

Having reviewed the previous mind sets, we shall briefly review the essence of the self-help groups (e.g., AA, NA, Alanon, Naranon, Alateen) which are included in the "steps." In doing so, it may be helpful to understand the psychological principles and sequencing of issues inherent in the "steps." Before doing so, the reader might first note the words of Herbert Spencer (cited in *Big Book of Alcoholics Anonymous*, 1976): "There is a principle which is a bar against all information, which is proof against all arguments and which cannot fail to keep a man in everlasting ignorance--that principle is contempt prior to investigation" (p. 570).

As a preface to the step analysis, it is important to point out that there is strong commitment by the individual and a quasi-religious aspect to AA, which itself becomes a possible substitute addiction according to Milkman (1979). The focus of our discussion, however, will be on what most AA and NA members believe to be the central mechanism in their behavior change (other than attending meetings and experiencing fellowship) - "working their program." These steps represent the abstracted experience of knowledgeable lay people who tried to specify what they had done to get and stay sober. This was the by-product of practical experience, influenced by the pragmatic spirit of William James (1978), whose *The Varieties of Religious Experience* and functional approach impressed early AA members, rather than the result of any theoretical-deductive model. A higher power, for example, was invoked simply because when it was, people got sober; it was not necessarily invoked out of any strong philosophical belief.

The AA step program is, of course, not the only possible approach to substance abuse. The movement appears to capture a relatively small percentage of substance abusers, but it has established a consistent and powerful tradition to which many will attest. Though not relevant to the steps per se, tradition with the AA program is that generally sponsors are of the same sex as the "pigeon." Frequently, closed groups are of the same sex. This may provide a role model that becomes internalized. Accordingly, self-help groups offer a nurturing environment that provides an opportunity for interdependence. They are not necessarily an addiction to "something to be gotten out of" once the patient gets "better."

The following is a section of Chapter V from *Big Book of Alcoholics Anonymous* (1976), which is read at all meetings and contains the steps after a motivational preamble:

Rarely have we seen a person fail who has thoroughly followed our path. Those who do not recover are people who cannot or will not completely give themselves to this simple program, usually men and women who are constitutionally incapable of being honest with themselves. There are such unfortunates. They are not at fault; they seem to have been born that way. They are naturally incapable of grasping and developing a manner of living which demands rigorous honesty. Their chances are less than average. There are those too who suffer from grave emotional and mental disorders, but many of them do recover if they have the capacity to be honest.

Our stories disclose in a general way what we used to be like, what happened, and what we are like now. If you have decided you want what we have and are willing to go to any length to get it--then you are ready to take certain steps.

Remember that we deal with alcohol--cunning, baffling, powerful: Without help it is too much for us. But there is One who has all power--that One is God. May you find him now!

Half measures availed us nothing. We stood at the turning point. We asked HIS protection and care with complete abandon.

Here are the steps we took, which are suggested as a program of recovery:

1) We admitted we were powerless over alcohol--that our lives had become unmanageable.
2) Came to believe that a Power greater than ourselves could restore us to sanity.
3) Made a decision to turn our will and our lives over to the care of God, as we understood Him.
4) Made a searching and fearless moral inventory of ourselves.
5) Admitted to God, to ourselves, and to another human being the exact nature of our wrongs.
6) Were entirely ready to have God remove all defects of character.
7) Humbly asked Him to remove our shortcomings.

8) Made a list of all persons we had harmed and became willing to make amends to them all.

9) Made direct amends to such people wherever possible, except when to do so would injure them or others.

10) Continued to take personal meditation to improve our conscious contact with God as we understood Him, praying only for knowledge of His will for us and the power to carry that out.

11) Sought through prayer and meditation to improve our conscious contact with God as we understood Him, praying only for knowledge of His will for us and the power to carry that out.

12) Having had a spiritual awakening as the result of these steps, we tried to carry this message to alcoholics, and to practice these principles in all our affairs.

Many of us exclaimed, "What an order! I can't go through with it." Do not be discouraged. No one among us has been able to maintain anything like perfect adherence to these principles. We are not saints. The point is, that we are willing to grow along spiritual lines. The principles we have set down are guides to progress. We claim spiritual progress rather than spiritual perfection. (p. 60)

It is important to note the mind sets that are encouraged in the first three steps prior to beginning the fourth step (usually after 6 months of sobriety). Psychotherapy is in some ways analogous to what is involved in steps four through seven, or at least four and five. To clarify and translate the issues, we draw loosely on a Transactional Analysis model where appropriate, because building new internal structures is essential for the substance abuser.

INCORPORATING THE AA MODEL IN TREATMENT

We tell patients that the "Twelve Steps" are a way to strengthen the TA Adult. In step one, stating that one is "powerless" over alcohol is merely a way of saying that when the critical parent and the crazy kid go 'round and 'round, the adult is nullified. This is inherent in the obsessive-compulsive trait. Reality testing demands a surrender and acceptance of the biochemical and psychological factors inherent in alcoholism. Sometimes the analogy of the medical-model reference to diabetes is helpful; for the sophisticated college student or professional, explanation of complicated habit hierarchies may suffice. Our clinical philosophy is to use whatever model we think will help the patient bypass the pseudo-moral dilemma of willpower in order to simply accept the reality that substance intake for him or her is like a tidal wave.

The first step is the only reference to alcohol, and the rest of the steps might be likened to a "Humans Anonymous Program." The second part of step one mentions unmanageability. The thrust is that it is important to recognize one's powerlessness over "people, places, and things," factors which may influence but never control the person. Time and time again members are urged to give up the illusion of control over these factors because it leads to unmanageability. Control means influence over 100% of the variance, while influence means less than 100% in any situation. The main emphasis on the control issue is made in step three, where the emphasis is on accepting personal responsibility for the way things are and avoiding denial. "I am the problem" is therefore emphasized from the beginning. We believe it is unfortunate when a therapist unintentionally colludes with the patient who looks at the spouse or job circumstances as the problem.

At this juncture in the therapy, we take the opportunity to do some root pruning and directly emphasize individuation. Active substance abusers have osmotic self-boundaries that we may diagram during treatment with a dotted line around "self," followed by a larger, solid circle encompassing "people, places, and things" outside the dotted line. The latter is psychologically incorporated only to produce the pains of unmanageability. Once detoxification and early sobriety have occurred, the issue of osmotic self-boundaries may well have to be dealt with - the extent depending upon the type of underlying character structure.

Steps two and three really involve the affirmation of access to healthy resources before any inner exploration is done. This is the affirmation of hope bolstered in the context of peer support. All too frequently therapists have the common experience that substance abusers seem to get worse rather than better in therapy. It is our contention that part of this, aside from the lack of training in the substance-abuse area, may be caused by the reinforcement of the unfulfilled secondary narcissism without the therapist providing the vision of healthy options.

The organismic personality theorist Andras Angyal (1982, p. 103) cleverly utilized the popular Gestalt visual illusion of the reversing figure-ground vase versus neurosis. Lines forming the sides of the vase or goblet were the same lines forming the outer profiles of the faces, on either side of the goblet, looking towards one another as the dark became the "figure" and as the white goblet receded into oblivion in the ground. Angyal's notion was that of antithetical healthy versus unhealthy strategies. Elaborating on this, we might symbolically view the addict as being trapped within the goblet of his or her own self-centeredness or secondary narcissism. The addict may have even described with mathematical accuracy to many therapists the precise dimensions of the goblet. By contrast, the healthy system needs to be activated by a perceptual shift of figure-ground, so the addict can envision attuning more interpersonally to the needs of others. With the help of treatment, and the AA steps, he or she needs to increase the frequency of "seeing the faces" throughout a day.

To use a more down-to-earth TA image, the patient has two systems much akin to a reverse-cycle air conditioner that is stuck on "heat" during a long, hot summer. The unhealthy resources of the critical parent and the crazy child, the neurotic core, predominate over an alternate system of the healthy resources of the nurturing parent (of which, depending on the patient's value system, there can be one or two: finite and infinite) and the healthy child orchestrated by the adult (who may be likened to Mickey Mouse/Stokowski orchestrating the waters in Fantasia - an image that seems to have appeal to substance abusers). We may suggest that the humanistically oriented patient paraphrase step two to read: "Came to believe that a power greater than my sick self could restore me to sanity." The issue here is that the alcoholic addict has locked him or herself in and repetitively searched the same room of self-hate without realizing that there indeed are other rooms within his or her own mansion. Without first knowing and affirming healthy options reflected in steps one through three, the psychotherapeutic task is merely an exercise in masochism based on an incomplete, one-sided understanding of human functioning.

Step two elaborates on control issues and offers in AA a description of self-centeredness. This is also discussed further in Tiebout's (1954) paper, "The Ego Factors in Surrender in Alcoholism," which could best be described as an experiential translation of Fenichel's (1945) handling of secondary narcissism. After first describing a controlling director, step two goes on to observe:

> Selfishness-self centeredness! That we think is the root of our troubles. Driven by a hundred forms of fear, self-delusion, self-seeking and self-pity, we step on the toes of our fellows and they retaliate. Sometimes they hurt us, seemingly without provocation but we invariably find that at some time in the past we have made decisions based on self which later placed us in a position to be hurt. (*Alcoholics Anonymous*, 1976, p. 62).

To the extent that other personality groupings may engage in the psychophysical illusion that much of life can be controlled rather than influenced, the frustration-aggression hypothesis becomes relevant. Garden-variety neurotics feel more guilt over their aggression; depressives may eat more cookies and watch more television; but the substance abuser runs the risk of becoming a tornado in his or her own life space. The equation becomes qualitatively different, however, when frustration leads to aggression which may be of an oral nature, and the factor of ingestion of mood- and mind-altering chemicals is added.

A key part of obsessive-compulsive problems is an inordinate need to control both internal and external environments in contrast to accepting or blending with them.

Angyal (1982) describes these as the two basic interactive and complementary personality forces, the strivings for autonomy versus homonomy. In the healthy person, there is a reciprocal and relatively even balance between the two. For the substance abuser, the obsessive-compulsive trait or patterns reflect a sterility and exclusion of intimate and warm feelings from both within and without. This actor or soloist patient typically tries to deny the very support of the stage upon which he or she stands.

The concept of the higher power is often a point of great resistance - sometimes more for the clinician than the patient. Yet, step two is an important one. The clinician must work flexibly here, remembering that cognitive assumptions, models, and beliefs are not chosen in a vacuum. They mesh with the years of feelings and emotions and provide a framework for change.

We frequently stress with patients the importance of the peace involved in the "God-experience" - the letting go of excessive control. Again, we care not what they label this power. From our perspective, the Moslem's experience of Allah, the born-again Christian's contentment in being saved, the humanist's experience of Thoreauian tranquility, and the AA member's experience of serenity with a higher power, are all probably overlapping psychological-physiological states which are interpreted and labeled differently by the subject.

Whether God exists or does not exist independently, clinicians need to understand the nature of linguistics and overcome their bias against referring their patients to a place where there is "God-talk" - but also a place where people get sober and straight! The AA program provides a cognitive behavioral prescription of what to do to get the "God-experience." It is contained in steps one and three which involve a sequence of first, acceptance, individuation, and detachment, and second, letting go of the excessive egoism, autonomy, or control. It is when this latter part occurs that there is a perceptual shift to that of harmony, followed by the consequent experience of serenity.

We remind patients of the usefulness of the popular serenity prayer - accepting the things you cannot change, having the courage to change the things you can, and finally the wisdom to know the difference. Patients, substance abusers or not, have found this to be a useful cognitive coping tool.

With the firm foundation of the first three steps, step four involves taking one's own inventory. For the new AA member, the practical question arises as to how psychotherapy differs from step four, and how the therapist is different from a sponsor. We typically respond to patients that they can only put in an inventory that of which they are consciously aware. The well-trained therapist should be able to identify those relevant unconscious factors that drive the patient's self-defeating behavior. By contrast, the AA sponsor may utilize practically developed internal norms to judge the patient's (or pigeon's) progress within the program.

A key element and focus of the fourth step is the identification of character defects - particularly resentment. AA (1976) notes ominously that "Resentment is the number one offender" (p. 64) when referring to relapses. Emphasis is placed on resentment toward loved ones, especially parents.

Alcoholics and addicts, perhaps due to past self-destructive behavior, talk more than other diagnostic groups of their lingering fears of success and assertiveness. It is only by coming to peace with the "parents in the back of our head" that the patient experiences serenity. In the fourth through seventh steps, one of the two forgotten needs of our modern era, "pulling your own strings," becomes critical - fulfilling the need to forgive. It is by the act of forgiving that we experience our own inner strength. Self-centered crazy kids do not have the capacity to forgive; nurturing parents orchestrated by the adult do. Forgiveness is a mechanism of health and strength that is too often forgotten in psychotherapy and certainly forgotten in almost all the self-help books that urge enlightened self-centeredness. Although the latter produces short-term benefits if one wants immediate gratification and justification of one's own viewpoint, the individual must also be ready to pay the price of long-term anxieties and fears that beset the oral character grasping at and incorporating all that appears pleasurable in the immediate environment. Aggression must be transformed into assertiveness; but the flip side of the coin of assertiveness must be the capacity to forgive, a trait valued in all religious systems - the original psychology. The tradition of forgiveness is nothing less than the distillation of the experience of the ages and should not be discarded lightly.

Step eight is an interpersonal extension of the intrapsychic or internal process occurring in steps four through seven. It involves the mental rehearsal of a shift from the crazy kid to the nurturing parent. Step nine represents an *in-vivo* behavioral form of implosion. Rather than just listening, imagining, and anticipating the response of the person hurt, and the possible retaliation from a real-life version of the critical parent, the AA member has the opportunity to extinguish the anxiety-producing cues. Behaviorally, the AA member, even in the face of rebuff, finds that the imagined retaliatory response probably was much worse than most victims' responses in real life; hence, the extinction effect and another context for the alcoholic or addict to work through these imagined lingering fears. The net result is that perfectionism and false pride can give way to reality-based humility. Step nine, if properly executed under a sponsor's or therapist's guidance, is an opportunity to reduce the effects of the introjections which have become more tyrannizing through the degrading, deteriorating process of substance abuse.

Step ten is a partial repetition of step four, and can provide immense relief to the perfectionist whose worst fear was the possibility of making a mistake. It further appropriately reinforces ongoing introspection and internal coordination geared for enhancing what the psychoanalyst might term the synthetic function of the ego. This might also be called the "working-through" step.

Step eleven includes the reinforcement and involvement of the nurturing parent or the positive reinforcement conferred by a now more flexible, loving superego. As with all learning, there is another element of repetition as the AA member learns to recue the "God-experience" within, developing more mastery over his or her internal maze.

Finally, step twelve brings the wheel full circle. What ends with getting out of oneself stands juxtaposed with the root pruning and individuation of step one. Step twelve focuses on the second of forgotten needs of forgiving and giving. Whether we refer to the "genital maturity" of Sigmund Freud, the brotherly love of Christ, or Fromm's (1956) *The Art of Loving*, a person's true fulfillment and potentialities are reflected in the capacity to give to others without strings attached.

SUMMARY

We believe that a beneficial cross-fertilization can take place between self-help groups and mental health professionals. Both have common goals: establishing and maintaining the alcoholics' or addicts' sobriety as well as enhancing their functioning in work, love, and play. The complementary aspects of self-help group step processes and the treatment process have been discussed.

Although it is helpful to think of the twelve steps of AA, NA, Alanon and Alateen, and the process psychotherapy as sequences, reality frequently interferes when we are planning treatment. The steps are viewed as reference points for both patient and therapist in a process of working through sobriety, interpersonal, and intrapsychic issues. Self-help groups offer an ever-present supportive and nurturing context that provides the alcoholic or addict an ongoing opportunity for interdependence and self-exploration, as well as inspiration. Finally, the interested professional could benefit from attending a self-help group meeting. The conceptual structure of a self-help approach can be more easily integrated through experience with self-help groups and their members. As one religiously oriented patient biblically described the experience, "You should know them by their deeds."

William Grady Ryan, PhD, is the Executive Director of the Family Institute of Broward and Palm Beach, Florida. He also serves on the Governor's Task Force for Substance Abuse - Project Freeway. He received his doctorate in 1969 from Adelphi University where he also taught on an undergraduate level; he has subsequently taught master's and doctoral students at Nova University in Florida. In addition to 14 years of private practice, he has consulted to the Olympic Training Center in Colorado Springs and has provided oversight to the South Florida Forensic Hospital and HRS alcohol and drug programs in Broward County. He co-authored a weekly column, "On Being Human," and has published and appeared in the media frequently. Dr. Ryan may be contacted c/o Family Institute, 1144 Southeast Third Avenue, Fort Lauderdale, FL 33316.

Nancy J. Ryan, MSW, JD, is currently the Forensic Director of the Family Institute of Broward and Palm Beach, Florida. In addition to her master's degree in social work, she holds a Juris Doctor in law. Dr. Ryan can be contacted c/o Family Institute, 1144 Southeast Third Avenue, Fort Lauderdale, FL 33316.

Andrew Rosen, PhD, is the Clinical Director of the Family Institute's Fort Lauderdale office. He received his doctorate from Hofstra University and his psychoanalytic training at Adelphi University's Post-Doctoral Program in Psychoanalysis and Psychotherapy. He has a Diplomate in Clinical Psychology, ABPP, and is Associate Professor at Nova University's Post-Doctoral Institute of Psychoanalysis and Psychotherapy. Dr. Rosen may be contacted c/o Family Institute, 1144 Southeast Third Avenue, Fort Lauderdale, FL 33316.

Antonio R. Virsida, PhD, is the Clinical Director of the Family Institute's Boca/Delray office. He is also Professor of Psychology and Supervisor at Nova University's Post-Doctoral Institute of Psychoanalysis and Psychotherapy. Following doctoral training at New York University, he completed psychoanalytic training at the Post Graduate Center for Mental Health. He is active in local and national professional organizations. Dr. Virsida may be contacted c/o Family Institute, One West Camino Real, Boca Raton, FL 33432

RESOURCES

Angyal, A. (1982). *Neurosis and Treatment: A Holistic Theory.* New York: Da Capo Press.
Big Book of Alcoholics Anonymous (3rd ed.). (1976). New York: Alcoholics Anonymous World Services.
Fenichel, O. (1945). *The Psychoanalytic Theory of Neurosis.* New York: W. W. Norton.
Fromm, E. (1950). *Psychoanalysis and Religion.* New Haven, CT: Yale University Press.
Fromm, E. (1956). *The Art of Loving.* New York: Bantam Books.
Gould, R. (1978). *Transformations.* New York: Simon & Schuster.
Hazelden Foundation: Box 176, Center City, MN 55012. Toll free telephone (800) 328-9000.
James, W. (1978). *The Varieties of Religious Experience.* Garden City, NY: Image Books.
Milkman, H. (1979). Addictive processes, an introductory formulation. *Street Pharmacologist, 2*(4), 1-4.
Miller, N. E., & Dollard, J. (1941). *Social Learning and Imitation.* New Haven, CT: Yale University Press.
Tiebout, H. M. (1954). The ego factors in surrender in alcoholism. *Quarterly Journal Studies on Alcohol, 15,* 610-621.

NEW DEVELOPMENTS IN PSYCHIATRIC DIAGNOSTIC TECHNOLOGY

Earl L. Loschen

Since the introduction of chlorpromazine in the early 1950s the practices of psychiatry, and secondarily those of the other mental health professions, have undergone dramatic change. Yet, we stand on the threshold of even greater change as a consequence of the advances of psychopharmacology and neurobiology. During the past 5 years we have seen the development of new investigative strategies that provide exciting insights into human brain functioning, and indirectly into human behavior.

This new technology is startling not only in terms of its results but also its complexity and cost. Many of the new techniques are possible only because of the ability of computers to analyze massive amounts of data and to construct a picture that we can understand and use. We must be concerned about the purposes of such technology given our restricted resources, so that we do not finally create technology only for technology's sake. On a practical level, the development of new technology in neurosciences can serve three important purposes in daily clinical practice. First, new techniques may be more powerful than available tests in uncovering organic lesions which either are causing the emotional and behavioral symptomatology or are complicating the treatment of the mental disturbance. Second, new strategies may allow us to develop practical biological measures of certain disorders which will allow us to be more accurate in our diagnoses and consequently more specific in our treatment. Finally, new measures may allow us to follow the progress of our treatment by measuring either the basic pathologic process or the treatment process itself. For clinical practice, if the new test or procedure does not assist us in one of these ways, then we cannot justify the cost of the procedure, no matter how minimal that cost may be.

In the following discussion, I will review several technological advances in psychiatry and neurosciences which have developed during the past decade or now are in evolution. First, I will discuss several physical disorders which may mimic mental illness and that new diagnostic techniques may assist in identifying. Then, I will outline new or recent laboratory and imaging techniques that may offer new diagnostic approaches to mental illnesses and to the evaluation and monitoring of treatment. Finally, I will briefly indicate some possible future directions in light of our present knowledge.

PHYSICAL ILLNESS AND EMOTIONAL SYMPTOMS

There are a variety of physical disorders which may provoke emotional or behavioral symptoms so similar to those of mental illnesses as to escape detection and lead to erroneous diagnosis and inappropriate treatment. Often the physical manifestations of these disorders are so subtle that they may be easily overlooked. Some of the recent developments in diagnostic medicine have allowed physicians to more adequately screen for many of these disorders and to start needed medical treatment earlier when expectation of success is greatest. Mental health professionals may actively assist in this process by assuring that all likely cases are thoroughly evaluated and by maintaining vigilance in their practices for possible undiscovered physical illness.

DEPRESSION

Depression is one of the most common complaints found in mental health practice. It also occurs frequently in association with a variety of physical disorders. Endocrine disorders involving the thyroid, parathyroid, and adrenal glands often cause treatment-resistant depressed mood. Other less common physical causes of depression may be metabolic or neurologic in origin, as well as certain tumors that are associated with such symptoms. A number of these causes are outlined in Tables 1 and 2.

TABLE 1: ENDOCRINE AND METABOLIC DISORDERS CAUSING EMOTIONAL SYMPTOMS

Disorder	Pathology	Common Emotional Symptoms
Endocrine		
hypothyroidism	inadequate thyroid hormone	depression
hyperthyroidism	excessive thyroid hormone	anxiety
parathyroid disorders	excessive or inadequate parathyroid hormone	anxiety and depression
Addison's disease	inadequate adrenocortical hormone	depression
Cushing's disease	excessive adrenocortical hormone	psychosis
hyperinsulinism	excessive insulin	anxiety
Metabolic		
pernicious anemia	vitamin B_{12} deficiency	depression
Wilson's disease	copper metabolism defect	depression, anxiety, or psychosis
acute porphyria	porphyrin metabolism defect	anxiety
chronic uremia	kidney disease	depression
Cardiopulmonary		
angina	ischemic heart pain	anxiety
cardiac arrhythmias	conduction deficits	anxiety
mitral valve prolapse	bulging of the mitral valve	anxiety
pulmonary emboli	blood clots or fat obstructing arteries	anxiety
emphysema	chronic damage to lungs	anxiety or depression

TABLE 2: OTHER DISORDERS CAUSING EMOTIONAL SYMPTOMS

Disorder	Pathology	Common Emotional Symptoms
Neurologic Disorders		
delirium	temporary loss of brain function	psychosis
dementia	loss of brain tissue	depression
myesthenia gravis	neuromuscular conduction disorder	depression
seizures	temporal lobe, or partial complex seizures	anxiety or mania
multiple sclerosis	scattered lesions in nervous system	hysteria
subdural hematoma	head trauma	depression
Neoplastic Disorders		
intracranial tumor	either primary or metastatic tumors	depression, psychosis
pancreatic carcinoma	especially of the tail of pancreas	depression
pheochromocytoma	tumor producing norepinephrine	anxiety
carcinoid tumor	tumor producing serotonin	anxiety
Miscellaneous Disorders		
infection	especially viral infections of the nervous system	depression, mania
lupus erythematosis	autoimmune disorder	psychosis

Drugs and drug therapy are commonly associated with emotional and depressive sequelae. This is a particularly troublesome problem since the cause of depression may go undiscovered, leading to addition of antidepressants to the treatment regimen. The resulting polypharmacy, in addition to being costly, also may result in dangerous drug interactions. Table 3 contains a list of commonly used drugs and prescribed medications and their likely emotional side effects. This particular cause of depression is important because no laboratory procedure now exists which can make the diagnosis; therefore, the cause must be discovered clinically.

TABLE 3:   DRUGS CAUSING EMOTIONAL SYMPTOMS

Drug	Examples of Uses or Drug Names	Usual Emotional Symptoms
alcohol	social drug	anxiety, depression
aminophylline	asthma	anxiety
anticonvulsants	epilepsy/phenobarbital	depression
antidiarrheal agents	Lomotil	depression
antihistamines	colds, allergies	anxiety, depression
antihypertensive agents	hydroDiuril, propranolol	depression
antiparkinsonian agents	Cogentin, Levodopa	depression, mania
caffeine	coffee, tea, soft drinks	anxiety
cocaine	drug of abuse	anxiety, psychosis
cytotoxic agents	treatment of cancer	depression
digitalis	heart disease	depression
disulfiram	Antabuse	depression
ephedrine and pseudoephedrine	cold preparations	anxiety
ginseng	ginseng tea, drug of abuse	anxiety
hormones	estrogens, steroids	depression, psychosis
insulin	diabetes mellitus	anxiety
nicotine	tobacco	anxiety
stimulants	amphetamines, methylphenidate	anxiety
thyroid preparations	hypothyroidism	anxiety
tranquilizers	neuroleptics, benzodiazepines	depression

ANXIETY

Anxiety symptoms are also commonly found in mental health clinical practice. Anxiety accompanies many medical illnesses, some of which may not be readily apparent to either the patient or the physician. Several of these disorders may now be diagnosed because of recent advances in technological aspects of medicine. For example, the recently well publicized association between anxiety and cardiac mitral valve prolapse can be investigated readily because of the development of echocardiography. In this technique, sound waves are analyzed by computer to create a moving picture of the heart and its valves. In mitral valve prolapse the valve may be clearly seen to bulge, thereby making the diagnosis.

Many other physical illnesses are associated with anxiety and several of these are summarized in Tables 1 and 2. Some of these disorders, like those which cause depression, may be hidden and not discovered unless an adequate physical and emotional evaluation is conducted.

As with depression, drugs and prescribed medications are commonly associated with anxiety. Several examples are shown in Table 3. Clinically, the most problematic of these are the over-the-counter medications which may not be discovered unless specific inquiry is made. Many people do not consider these to be medications and therefore will not reveal them unless specifically asked for the information.

HYSTERIA

Several physical disorders may produce such unusual and bizarre symptoms that physicians and mental health workers may suspect the person is being manipulative or at best is experiencing conversion symptoms. These disorders include hyperinsulinism, Wilson's disease, and acute porphyria, all of which may cause various vague somatic complaints, complaints of pain, and a labile mood. These disorders may be excluded rather easily by laboratory testing now available.

One disorder, multiple sclerosis, is not yet so easily excluded in all cases. Early in the disorder when permanent deficits are not pronounced, the shifting sensory and motor complaints combined with the typical labile and often euphoric mood may be indistinguishable from conversion symptoms. No definitive diagnostic technique is now readily available to help in the diagnosis but, as will be noted later, a new technique (magnetic resonance imaging) is about to offer us a major new diagnostic strategy.

PSYCHOSIS

Psychotic reactions may be the result of several different physical disorders and may occur rarely with the use of certain drugs. If the psychotic reaction occurs acutely, the differential diagnosis may be difficult to establish because of our inability often to get adequate history. In these instances the physician must often rely on the laboratory and other diagnostic techniques to establish the diagnosis. Several physical disorders which may present as psychotic reactions are listed in Tables 1 and 2. Table 3 lists some drugs which may also result in psychosis as a side effect. In many of these disorders, the advances in technology in the laboratory have allowed us to identify such individuals earlier, which often allows treatment to be more effective.

NEW DIAGNOSTIC TECHNOLOGIES

Many of the recent advances in medical technology have been helpful to psychiatry and other mental health professions because of the increased ability to rule out physical disorders as the cause for the presenting disturbed emotions and behavior. However, in several instances, new technological developments are offering us a possibility to explore and measure phenomena associated with mental illnesses. Consequently, we face a revolution both in our concepts of mental illness and in our approaches to the mentally ill. I will attempt to review several of these new biochemical and imaging techniques and to indicate some potential uses for them.

BIOCHEMICAL TESTS

Over the past two decades a multitude of new biochemical and laboratory techniques have been developed. In my discussion I will focus on five particularly relevant tests and techniques of interest in the care of the mentally ill.

Dexamethasone Suppression Test (DST). This is an example of a test procedure used widely in endocrinology which has been adapted for use in psychiatry. Certain persons with major depression have long been noted to also demonstrate abnormalities in the functioning of the pituitary gland - adrenal gland axis. Normally, steroid levels in the body as measured in blood vary during the day. In part, the adrenal gland secretion of steroids is under hormonal regulation of the pituitary gland by means of a negative feedback loop. As steroid levels rise in the body, the pituitary signals through hormone secretion that steroid secretion by the adrenal gland should slow or cease. Some depressed persons lose this negative feedback function. Consequently, more steroid does not decrease steroid output.

Dexamethasone is a powerful steroid which even in very small doses will precipitate a shutdown of adrenal production. To conduct the test, one milligram of dexamethasone is given by mouth at 11:00 p.m. Blood samples are taken at 4:00 p.m. and 11:00 p.m. the next day for measurement of circulating steroid levels. Normally, less than 4-5 micrograms per deciliter will be found at these times. In some depressed persons, however, much higher levels at one or both times will be found. This nonsuppression occurs in about 50% of major depressions.

The DST is positive not only in major depression but in a number of other circumstances. Carroll et al. (1981) outlined many of these confounding variables in their classic paper on the DST. These may include pregnancy, Cushing's disease, malnutrition, use of certain drugs such as Dilantin, major physical illness, and acute alcohol withdrawal. Certain persons with generalized anxiety disorder (Avery et al.,

1985) or with dementia may also demonstrate nonsuppression on the DST. Consequently, the DST is not specific to major depression and therefore has fallen into disuse in many clinical practices. Perhaps combining this test with other diagnostic strategies might improve its specificity and ultimately make it more clinically useful.

Thyrotropin Releasing Hormone Test (TRH Test). Some depressed persons demonstrate an abnormality in the regulation of the thyroid gland that does not create a state of hypothyroidism but nevertheless may be measured. This regulation is accomplished by the action of thyrotropin releasing hormone on the pituitary gland, thereby releasing thyrotropin or thyroid stimulating hormone (TSH). TSH then stimulates the thyroid gland to release thyroid hormone. The TRH test has been devised to measure this response. In certain conditions such as hypothyroidism, high levels of TSH are found in blood serum along with low levels of thyroid hormone. In pituitary disease, low levels of TSH and thyroid hormone are found. In the TRH test, a dose of TRH is given intravenously and measurements of TSH are taken serially over a 2-hour period. If TSH levels do not rise, the response is said to be blunted. This response is used along with thyroid hormone levels to make a diagnosis. Loosen and Prange (1982), in their excellent review, note that age, starvation, chronic renal failure, and certain drugs such as thyroid hormone actively interfere with the results of the test. In certain persons with major depression, the TRH test shows a blunted TSH response even though thyroid hormone levels will be within normal limits.

The TRH test has not achieved the same popularity as the DST in part, I think, because of the greater complexity of the test. The test requires that an open venous line be maintained for the duration of the test, a task in which many depressed patients are unable to adequately cooperate with the examiner. Still, further research is indicated to see if this test may be used alone or in combination with other strategies to assist in difficult differential diagnoses.

Serum Drug Levels. One of the problems in drug therapy for any disease is knowing what dosage of drug the physician must use to achieve the desired effects. In several instances in medicine, tests exist that measure the level of drug in blood or serum and the usual therapeutic range is known. Such tests are now available in psychiatry for two classes of drugs, lithium carbonate and tricyclic antidepressants.

Lithium, which is used for bipolar or manic-depressive disorder, has a very narrow therapeutic range before toxic reactions develop. The laboratory test for lithium level is straightforward, accurate, and readily reproducible. The test for tricyclic antidepressant level is somewhat more complex and not necessarily as clearly related to clinical outcome. Tests are commonly available for amitriptyline, nortriptyline, imipramine, desipramine, and doxepin. The tests for antidepressant levels are most useful when a patient remains depressed yet experiences no side effects. If the level is low, then the psychiatrist may decide to increase the daily dose of medication rather than change to another drug.

Chromatography. In both gas and high performance liquid chromatography, columns are used to separate out substances of differing sizes and weights. Although the technical aspects of the separation differ in the two methods, both allow the substances that are separated to be isolated and then identified and measured by means appropriate to each substance.

Chromatography has become critically important in neuroscience research because it allows various substances and neurotransmitters to be readily identified and measured. Much research has focused on measuring neurotransmitter metabolites in urine and cerebral spinal fluid, especially in depressed and manic patients. To date, consistent findings in any set or subset of depressed or manic persons have not been reported. However, if such a subset of persons with consistent abnormal findings could be identified, then this technique would be a valuable adjunct in diagnosis.

Radioimmunoassay. Radioimmunoassay is another technique that is highly useful in identifying substances and measuring levels of such substances in various fluids. It is useful, for example, in measuring drug serum levels. In this test, the substance to be measured is mixed with a known binding agent such as an immunoglobulin or a receptor. This mixture is next combined with a known amount of radioactive labeled substance.

The sample is then washed and the remaining radioactive substance measured. The amount of original substance can then be calculated from the known values.

This technique is widely used throughout medicine in a variety of tests including such routine measurements as thyroid hormone and drug levels. Besides measuring drug levels, the technique of radioreceptor assay is used in research to study the various aspects of drug activity in brain tissue. Many new applications in both research and clinical practice are likely to be developed in the future as we learn more about drugs and neuronal activity.

COMPUTERIZED AXIAL TOMOGRAPHY

Although x-ray examinations have been available for decades, the technique has been limited because the intensity of the x-rays obliterated the images of most tissue except for bone. Certain modifications were possible that allowed some better resolution. For example, pneumoencephalograms were such a modification. Air was introduced into the spinal cord canal and forced up over the brain. Because of the intense difference in density between air and brain tissue, resulting x-rays did show pictures of the conformation of the brain and the various sulci. However, this technique suffered from several substantial difficulties. First, the procedure often resulted in the patient experiencing severe and protracted headache. Second, by introducing a foreign substance (air) into the spinal and cranial cavities, a risk of infection was created. Finally, the older x-ray machines required a substantial exposure of radiation in order to do an adequate study.

With the advent of the microcomputer came the possibility of connecting microcomputers to various instruments and analyzing massive amounts of data almost instantaneously and on site. By coupling a computer to the process of tomography, a method of viewing internal soft tissues without invasion became possible. Tomography is a process of rotating a source of radiation and an opposing sensor around a point in such a manner as to give a clear picture of the tissue in the plane of the focus. Computerized axial tomography (CT scan) is simply this process carried out rapidly, recorded, and analyzed by the computer. The resulting image is then displayed on photographic film or on a monitor. This image not only displays various soft tissues but can do so at various levels in the body. The overall level of radiation used in CT scanning is no greater than in many other x-ray studies, and in some instances less.

The biggest impact of CT scans on mental health practice has been in the ease with which this technique can identify many disease processes in the cranium. Brain tumors larger than 1 centimeter are often clearly visible. Atrophy of the brain associated with Alzheimer's disease can be readily seen. Many other brain lesions which in the past were invisible to the available diagnostic techniques can now be visualized, making it possible to easily rule out many organic conditions in the differential diagnosis of disturbed emotion and behavior.

Brown and Kneeland (1985) provide an excellent review which outlines the different CT scan findings associated with various mental illnesses. All such studies have been carried out with carefully defined subsets of subjects and, therefore, the findings are not necessarily reproducible in clinical practice. In schizophrenia, cerebral ventricles have been found to be enlarged in certain chronic patients. Further, changes in density and distribution of brain tissue have been correlated with antipsychotic drug use and chronicity in schizophrenia. Unfortunately, these findings are often subtle and do not aid in diagnosis since enlarged ventricles do not mean that the person necessarily has schizophrenia. The findings are now best used in a research setting to identify certain subsets of schizophrenic subjects for studies that require uniform subject groups.

MAGNETIC RESONANCE IMAGING

When certain atoms are exposed to a strong magnetic force, parts of those atoms develop a net spin of very tiny magnitude. These tend to line up in parallel to the force field. If the magnetic force is then disrupted, for example by a radio frequency, certain events measured by changes in energy will occur. These can be measured, and from these measurements a computer can construct a picture of the different tissue densities because water (due to high hydrogen content) shows up well and is variably distributed throughout tissues. A more thorough but easily understood description of the process has been provided by DeMyer et al. (1985). In the resulting images, bone does not show up, but gray matter and white matter of the brain can be easily distinguished. Therefore, disease processes involving either gray or white matter can be distinguished.

Magnetic resonance imaging (MRI) has both advantages and disadvantages over other imaging processes. First, no external radiation source is used; therefore, the person is not exposed to radiation which may be harmful if large doses are accumulated. Although the question of the long-term safety of MRI has not been settled, there is little reason to suspect such ill effects. Second, when used to view the cranial cavity, the resulting images not only show soft tissues, but indeed may distinguish between different tissues, such as between gray matter and white matter. Several disease processes selectively attack one or the other of these tissues; therefore, MRI offers us a valuable new tool in diagnosis in these instances. Third, work is now underway to base the MRI process on elements other than hydrogen. The most exciting prospect lies in using phosphorus, which comprises a large part of the molecules in the energy cycle. In this instance, we could then observe and monitor metabolism in tissues such as brain. Deuel et al. (1985) have suggested that MRI may indeed serve the same role as positron emission tomography with much less difficulty and cost.

The disadvantages of MRI involve the equipment now in use. The magnets, because of the power needed, are large and bulky. This requires facilities that are specially built for the machine. Further, because of the tiny magnitude of the energies measured, a myriad of external events and machines can disrupt the test. Therefore, the room must be heavily shielded from such outside sources of energy as radios and other electronic equipment. Another disadvantage relates to the time required to initiate the process and to take readings. Because this is in the realm of minutes, the subject must lie quietly. However, motion is common in certain areas of the body such as the chest and abdomen where heart, lungs, and intestines are in constant motion. In these areas, MRI is significantly inferior to CT scans and other diagnostic techniques.

The MRI offers a major new technique to psychiatry and neurology. Because of the better resolution between white and gray matter, selective disease processes may be more easily visualized. For example, demyelinating diseases create lesions in white matter by destroying the myelin surrounding nerve cells in these areas. Multiple sclerosis is such a disease. Over years multiple small lesions are created in both brain and spinal cord white matter. These lesions show up distinctly in MRI, as opposed to CT scans where visualization of lesions is unusual. Since multiple sclerosis is a disease that early in its course is often misdiagnosed as hysteria or conversion reaction, MRI offers a major breakthrough in the differential diagnostic process in this area. MRI clearly visualizes the cortex of the brain; therefore, cortical atrophy as seen in Alzheimer's disease may be seen. The MRI may show not only the brain tumor itself, but also the surrounding mass effects, giving a clearer picture of the full extent of the neoplastic process.

Work on application of the MRI to functional mental illnesses in many instances is in preliminary stages, but early findings look promising. For example, DeMyer et al. (1985) have found that schizophrenic subjects may demonstrate a reversal of the brain's left hemisphere to right hemisphere ratio of tissue mass when compared to normals. They note similarities in these data to those provided by other techniques. Further, their results suggest a variation of frontal and parietal brain patterns in schizophrenic subjects. These results suggest that the MRI visualizes brain tissue in a way that allows for more subtle measurement and exploration of nervous system pathology, including that associated with the functional mental illnesses.

The potential development of phosphorus as a basis of MRI offers us an important new advance. Phosphorus is one of the prominent elements found in substances used by biological tissues in energy transfer and use. Consequently, an MRI based on phosphorus would visualize the metabolic rates of various tissues. Since neuron activity is seen as a fundamental aspect of many mental illnesses such as schizophrenia, depression, and mania, this technique could potentially offer dramatic new insights into these disorders.

Magnetic resonance imaging offers a valuable new tool even now useful in many neurological disorders. MRI units are now being installed in many areas of the United

States. However, its greatest promise may be in the yet largely uncharted areas of functional mental illness.

BRAIN ELECTRICAL ACTIVITY MAPPING

Just as the CT scan is an advance over x-ray made possible by the computer, brain electrical activity mapping (BEAM) utilizes aspects of the electroencephalogram (EEG) to collect data and then analyze and picture data using advanced computer programs. The EEG records electrical activity of the brain through electrodes placed on the scalp. Because these electrodes are relatively distant from neurons, the resulting EEG patterns show essentially random activity instead of specific neuronal activity. These patterns are highly useful diagnostically for such conditions as epilepsy, toxic states, and sometimes brain lesions. However, they tell us little about neuron functioning specifically, such as is seen in directed mental activity like seeing or hearing. A number of years ago, a technique called evoked potentials was developed. In this technique, a specific stimulus such as an auditory click is presented repeatedly to a subject who has an EEG attached and recording. By associating the repeated clicks with the EEG pattern, the investigator can progressively add the specific neuronal responses together until a new pattern called an evoked response emerges from the background activity. Aspects of this response have been investigated in a number of conditions such as schizophrenia. Certain distinctive patterns have been noted in schizophrenia. Evoked response testing is also valuable in evaluation of certain types of blindness, and recently in deafness in infants.

If aspects of the EEG and evoked response testing are combined and data entered into a microcomputer, patterns of specific neuronal activity (as opposed to random activity) can be derived. These patterns are known as brain electrical activity mapping. These patterns are developed by comparing responses between three points on the EEG serially and assigning values to each. Each value can then be assigned a color. These can then be displayed on a monitor as a picture of relative brain electrical activity.

The BEAM offers a bold new use of existing technology because of the ability of the computer to record and rapidly analyze massive amounts of data. The technique is noninvasive and uses no source of radiation or other external source of energy. It relies totally on recording natural biological phenomena, which means short- or long-term risk should be negligible. The procedure takes time and requires cooperation of the subject; consequently, it cannot easily be used in uncooperative or agitated persons. In marked contrast to other new techniques, BEAM is relatively inexpensive and easily set up.

BEAM measures electrical activity of brain tissue as opposed to looking at structure. Consequently, the images produced must be seem as maps of activity and not as evidence of structural change. This may be a disadvantage in that some lesions may have effects distant from the actual lesion site and other lesions may have little impact on electrical activity at all. This significantly detracts from BEAM as a neurological diagnostic instrument. However, because mental illnesses involve the functioning of neurons instead of gross structural change, BEAM offers an exciting new tool for psychiatry and neurosciences. Neuronal electrical activity is seen as a fundamental part of the functioning of the nervous system; this technique allows us to very directly observe this. This activity is not the same as that shown by positron emission tomography, which presumably measures metabolism. Metabolism and brain electrical activity are closely linked but are not synonymous. We may, therefore, view these two techniques as complementary views of brain activity.

Lesions of the brain that create mass effects either through stimulation of seizure-like activity or by displacement and slow wave activity may be pinpointed by BEAM. The resulting image will often demonstrate the area of involvement clearly as a focus of color not usually seen in such maps. In most instances, however, the CT scan and MRI can be expected to be of more assistance in diagnosis of brain lesions.

The great promise of BEAM lies in its applications in psychiatry. Many studies are now in progress investigating a variety of major disorders such as mania, depression, and schizophrenia. Morihisa (1985) has demonstrated increased delta activity in the frontal lobes of schizophrenic subjects in comparison to normals. Delta activity is slow activity and is generally interpreted as abnormal in waking states. Consequently, this finding would indicate abnormal functioning of the frontal lobes in schizophrenics. Morihisa notes that this finding has also been noted by investigators using positron emission tomography and cerebral blood flow studies.

Brain electrical activity mapping is a new technology that surely will provide many new insights into the mental illnesses. As more studies are done and compared to other techniques, patterns that may assist in diagnosis are likely to be identified, at least for some conditions such as schizophrenia. Since BEAM is relatively inexpensive, it may become an important part of the diagnostic process of the future.

REGIONAL CEREBRAL BLOOD FLOW

The measurement of regional cerebral blood flow was first accomplished in the 1940s by using inhaled nitrous oxide and analyzing blood samples from the internal jugular vein. Although some estimate of blood flow to various areas of the brain could be made in this way, the results were difficult to reproduce, and the technique was complicated by the invasive nature of the blood sampling. These problems have been overcome in part by the use of [133]Xenon instead of nitrous oxide.

The test using [133]Xenon, a radioactive substance, relies on three principles. First, [133]Xenon is an inert substance; therefore, it is not stored or metabolized by brain. Second, it is a gas which may be inhaled, and it is essentially cleared out of blood with one pass through the lungs. Last, regional cerebral blood flow is very closely related to the metabolic rate of the tissues in that region.

The testing equipment includes an inhalation apparatus and a scintillation counter which feeds data into a computer. The subject is fitted with a cap containing the counter terminals located over various areas of the head. The subject is asked to inhale [133]Xenon through the inhalation mask, and then counts of activity are made. These counts are analyzed by the computer, which creates a map of regional cerebral blood flow.

In his excellent review, Meyer (1978) outlined many of the factors that change regional cerebral blood flow patterns. Any activity arising out of neuronal activity in a specific region, speech for example, will cause an increase in cerebral blood flow to that region, presumably in response to increased metabolic demands there. Therefore, any type of arousal will affect the blood flow patterns. Other variables have been noted to include sex and handedness (R. C. Gur et al., 1982), and personality (Mathew, Weinman, & Barr, 1984). Consequently, regional cerebral blood flow studies must be carefully controlled so that valid comparisons between studies can be made.

Changes in regional cerebral blood flow have been extensively studied in a variety of organic conditions. Meyer (1978) reviewed the findings of a number of such studies. In stroke, flow is typically first dramatically reduced and then increased in areas subject to raised compensatory blood flow during recovery phases. Persons suffering from migraine headaches show, during the headache and some days afterward, increased flow in that segment of the test usually attributed to circulation flow to gray matter. This is in contrast to persons with muscle contraction or tension headaches, who show no changes in regional flow. Persons suffering from either Alzheimer's or multi-infarct dementia show reduced cerebral blood flow proportionate to the severity of the dementia. Increased regional flow has also been demonstrated in epileptics during seizure activity. The location of the activity has been correlated to the location of the epileptic focus.

Most of the psychiatric research utilizing regional cerebral blood flow has focused on findings in schizophrenic subjects. Unfortunately, the findings have been complex and sometimes contradictory. Ariel et al. (1983) found decreased cerebral blood flow in all regions of the brain in schizophrenic subjects. Further, they demonstrated a generalized decrease in anterior brain functioning which included a left-hemisphere frontal area loss. Their subjects were in a relaxed state. Mathew et al. (1981) demonstrated a similar finding for the right hemisphere only in one study. However, in a later study, Mathew et al. (1982) demonstrated reduced regional cerebral flow to both hemispheres in resting schizophrenic subjects. They found no differences between medicated or unmedicated subjects and different subtypes of schizophrenia. These results could not be confirmed by R. E. Gur et al. (1983). They found no differences between medicated schizophrenic and normal subjects in a resting state. However, upon activation as a consequence of task performance, the schizophrenic subjects showed patterns consistent with left-hemisphere overactivation. R. E. Gur et al. (1985) demonstrated that unmedicated schizophrenic subjects have patterns suggesting left-hemisphere overactivation in both resting and activated states. Consequently, no clearly verified pattern of change in schizophrenic subjects has yet been found.

Because the technique of regional cerebral blood flow is complex, slight variations in the test or even in subject selection can give quite varied results. Because the test is noninvasive and the cost is reasonable, further work and modifications seem to be appropriate. More work is indicated not only in schizophrenic subjects, but also in a variety of other conditions, before this test can be considered for any clinical applications.

POSITRON EMISSION TOMOGRAPHY

During the past 5 years, a new imaging technique has been popularized as an innovative approach to diagnosis in mental illness. This technique, called positron emission tomography, has been described as able to picture characteristic patterns for many illnesses. It is, however, still a research tool, and, because of many problems, not likely to assume clinical usefulness in the near future.

Positron emission tomography (PET) measures the utilization of glucose by means of a tracer. A molecule of glucose is labeled with an atom of radioactive fluorine. When tissue such as brain cells metabolizes the glucose, a reaction between a positron and an electron releases gamma rays which may then be detected by special detectors. This information is then analyzed by a computer which can construct a color map of the relative activities over the brain. At present, these activities are interpreted to indicate the rate of metabolism of the various regions of the brain. It is assumed that the metabolic rate of neurons is proportionate to overall neuronal activity.

Three major issues confront the further development of this technology. First, the safety of ingestion of the radioactive glucose has not been firmly established. The glucose utilized has a very short half-life and is, therefore, rapidly cleared from the body. One can assume that the short length of exposure will decrease long-term risk, yet this has not been demonstrated. The second major problem is directly related to the short half-life of the glucose. Because of this, the substance must be manufactured on site by use of a cyclotron, an exceedingly expensive and complicated piece of equipment. Thus the third problem relates to the great expense attached to purchase of equipment and construction of facilities which ultimately must be paid for by the users of this test.

Various findings in research populations have been outlined in a comprehensive review by Phelps and Mazziotta (1985). Two particularly interesting results for mental health professionals occur in affectively disturbed patients and in persons with Huntington's chorea. In depressed subjects a diffuse pattern of reduced glucose metabolism was noted over the brain. However, no changes when compared to normals were noted for hypomanic subjects. Baxter et al. (1985) confirmed these findings but also reportedly were able to differentiate between unipolar and bipolar depressed subjects. Kuhl et al. (cited in Phelps & Mazziotta, 1985) found a reduction in glucose metabolism in the striatum, that portion of the brain shown in autopsy to be severely affected by Huntington's disease. They further found that these PET findings were demonstrated much earlier than in CT scans. Consequently, in Huntington's chorea, PET may show some promise as a diagnostic instrument.

As in many other recent imaging techniques, much attention has been directed towards study of schizophrenic subjects. Buchsbaum et al. (1982) compared brain glucose metabolism of normal and schizophrenic subjects. In resting subjects, schizophrenic volunteers showed reduced levels of glucose metabolism in the frontal lobes when compared to normal subjects. They also found that the absolute metabolic rates over both frontal and temporal regions in untreated schizophrenic patients were lower than in normal volunteers. These results suggest that PET may offer some assistance in diagnosis of schizophrenia. However, one must be aware that these studies have been carried out using clearly diagnosed, chronically ill patients. We do not know if these findings occur in acutely ill persons experiencing their first episode of psychotic symptoms, where such information would be of greatest assistance.

Positron emission tomography is clearly an exciting new development in neuroscience research. Whether or not PET achieves some clinical utility remains to be seen.

THE FUTURE

It is a risky task to predict the future, especially in the biological sciences in light of the tremendous change we have seen even in the past 10 years. However, we can make some guesses that may guide our study and our attention.

In the immediate future I believe that we will see further development of several of the diagnostic techniques that have been discussed in this contribution. Those techniques that look at neuronal activity such as BEAM, MRI using ^{31}phosphorus, and PET seem to hold particular promise for psychiatry because our present view of mental illness points to aberrant neuronal activity as a mechanism in many illnesses. Clearly, much of our present research is focused on this area.

What else lies ahead? Although we may see other developments of yet unseen technology, the most probable advances will build on technology now in use. The most exciting possibility exists in recombinant DNA technology. In a recent paper Bird (1985) has outlined a possible new test using recombinant DNA technology in its development. This test would potentially identify persons who are destined to develop Huntington's chorea prior to the manifestation of symptoms. She highlights some of the procedural, ethical, and policy issues of such a test, yet concludes that such a test is possible and usable. If such technology can be used to develop specific tests for Huntington's chorea, it may likewise prove useful in the diagnosis of other illnesses thought to have genetic components. Such possibilities promise us an exciting future in mental health as new technology will provide us with innovative tools in our fight to conquer the major mental illnesses.

Earl L. Loschen, MD, is currently Assistant Chairman of the Department of Psychiatry, Director of Psychiatry Residency, and Associate Professor of Psychiatry at Southern Illinois University School of Medicine. He completed his training at the University of Nebraska College of Medicine. Along with clinical psychiatry, his interests are in medical education, community psychiatry, and rural mental health and he has published several articles on these subjects. Dr. Loschen may be contacted at SIU School of Medicine, P.O. Box 3926, Springfield, IL 62708.

RESOURCES

Ariel, R. N., Golden, C. J., Berg, R. A., Quaife, M. A., Dirksen, J. W., Forsell, T., Wilson, J., & Graber, B. (1983). Regional cerebral blood flow in schizophrenics. *Archives of General Psychiatry, 40,* 258-263.

Avery, D. H., Osgood, T. B., Ishiki, D. M., Wilson, L. G., Kenny, M., & Dunner, D. L. (1985). The DST in psychiatric outpatients with generalized anxiety disorder, panic disorder, or primary affective disorder. *Journal of Psychiatry, 142,* 844-848.

Baxter, L. R., Phelps, M. E., Mazziotta, J. C., Schwartz, J. M., Gerner, R. H., Selin, C. E., & Sumida, R. H. (1985). Cerebral metabolic rates for glucose in mood disorders. *Archives of General Psychiatry, 42,* 441-447.

Bird, S. J. (1985). Presymptomatic testing for Huntington's disease. *Journal of the American Medical Association, 253,* 3286-3291.

Brown, R. P., & Kneeland, B. (1985). Visual imaging in psychiatry. *Hospital and Community Psychiatry, 36,* 489-496.

Buchsbaum, M. S., Ingar, D. H., Kessler, R., Waters, R. N., Cappelletti, J., van Kammen, D. P., King, A. C., Johnson, J. L., Manning, R. G., Flynn, R. W., Mann, L. S., Bunney, W. E., & Sokoloff, L. (1982). Cerebral glucography with positron tomography. *Archives of General Psychiatry, 39,* 251-259.

Carroll, B. J., Feinberg, M., Greden, J. F., Tarika, J., Albala, A. A., Haskett, R. F., James, N. M., Kronfol, Z., Lohr, N., Steiner, M., deVigne, J. P., & Young, E. (1981). A specific laboratory test for the diagnosis of melancholia. *Archives of General Psychiatry, 38,* 15-22.

DeMyer, M. K., Hendrie, H. C., Gilmor, R. L., & DeMyer, W. E. (1985). Magnetic resonance imaging in psychiatry. *Psychiatric Annals, 15,* 262-267.

Deuel, R. K., Yue, G. M., Sherman, W. R., Schickner, D. J., & Ackerman, J. J. H. (1985). Monitoring the time course of cerebral deoxyglucose metabolism by 31p nuclear magnetic resonance spectroscopy. *Science, 228,* 1329-1331.

Gur, R. C., Gur, R. E., Obrist, W. D., Hungerbuhler, J. P., Younkin, D., Rosen, A. D., Skolnick, B. E., & Reivich, M. (1982). Sex and handedness differences in cerebral blood flow during rest and cognitive activity. *Science, 217,* 659-661.

Gur, R. E., Gur, R. C., Skolnick, B. E., Caroff, S., Obrist, W. D., Resnick, S., Reivich, M. (1985). Brain Function in Psychiatric Disorders. *Archives of General Psychiatry, 42,* 329-334.

Gur, R. E., Skolnick, B. E., Gur, R. C., Caroff, S., Rieger, W., Obrist, W. D., Younkin, D., & Reivich, M. (1983). Brain function in psychiatric disorders. *Archives of General Psychiatry, 40,* 1250-1254.

Harvey, A. M., Johns, R. J., McKusick, V. A., Owens, A. H., & Ross, R. S. (Eds.). (1980). *The Principles and Practice of Medicine.* New York: Appleton-Century-Crofts.

Jeresaty, R. M. (1985). Mitral valve prolapse: An update. *Journal of the American Medical Association, 254,* 793-795.

Loosen, P. T., & Prange, A. J. (1982). Serum thyrotropin response to thyrotropin-releasing hormone in psychiatric patients: A review. *American Journal of Psychiatry, 139,* 405-416.

Loschen, E. L. (1984). Psychiatric syndromes with physical causes. In P. A. Keller & L. G. Ritt (Eds.), *Innovations in Clinical Practice: A Source Book* (Vol. 3, pp. 41-54). Sarasota, FL: Professional Resource Exchange, Inc.

Mathew, R. J., Duncan, G. C., Weinman, M. L., & Barr, D. L. (1982). Regional cerebral blood flow in schizophrenia. *Archives of General Psychiatry, 39,* 1121-1124.

Mathew, R. J., Meyer, J. S., Francis, D. J., Schoolar, J. C., Weinman, M., & Mortel, K. F. (1981). Regional cerebral blood flow in schizophrenia: A preliminary report. *American Journal of Psychiatry, 138,* 112-113.

Mathew, R. J., Weinman, M. L., & Barr, D. L. (1984). Personality and regional cerebral blood flow. *British Journal of Psychiatry, 144,* 529-532.

Meyer, J. S. (1978). Improved method for noninvasive measurement of regional cerebral blood flow by [133]Xenon inhalation. *Stroke, 9,* 205-210.

Morihisa, J. M. (1985). Computerized topographical mapping of electrophysiologic data in psychiatry. *Psychiatric Annals, 15,* 250-253.

Phelps, M. E., & Mazziotta, J. C. (1985). Positron emission tomography: Human brain function and biochemistry. *Science, 228,* 799-809.

Wolkin, A., Jaeger, J., Brodie, J. D., Wolf, A. P., Fowler, J., Rotrosen, J., Gomez-Mont, F., & Cancro, R. (1985). Persistence of cerebral metabolic abnormalities in chronic schizophrenia as determined by positron emission tomography. *American Journal of Psychiatry, 142,* 564-571.

BORDERLINE PERSONALITY DISORDER: DEFINITION, DIAGNOSIS, AND ASSESSMENT*

William S. Pollack

THE "BORDERLINE" CONCEPT

For at least the past five decades, clinicians have been simultaneously fascinated and frustrated by a large, somewhat heterogeneous, and puzzling group of patients who did not fit neatly within traditional nosological categories of either the neuroses or psychoses. Nor did these patients' psychopathology respond well to classic psychoanalytic therapies or conventional treatment approaches. It is from within this baffling historical context that the clinical concept of Borderline Personality Disorder gradually emerged.

Early theorists drew attention to a group of patients who appeared diagnostically to belong on a *continuum* between the neuroses and psychoses (Glover, 1932; Oberndorf, 1930). Other clinicians were impressed by those patients who, when treated in more formal psychoanalytic therapies, manifested regressed transferences and primitive behavioral and emotional responses. Hoch and Polatin (1949) diagnosed such patients as suffering from "pseudoneurotic schizophrenia," while many of their contemporaries conceptualized this so-called "borderline" subcategory of patients as belonging to the schizophrenias, rather than placing them in the borderlands between the neuroses and psychoses. Stern (1938) was the first to use the term "borderline" as a distinct clinical phenomenon. He reported on a group of patients whose clinical presentation included disorders of narcissism, hypersensitivity to insult, a rigid personality, a sense of personal inferiority, and deeply rooted anxiety. Deutsch (1942) and Wolberg (1952) joined this argument, postulating that borderline patients were a distinguishable diagnostic entity with definitive, pathognomonic clinical symptoms.

Knight (1953) wrote a paper which came to represent a turning point in the conceptualization of this disorder. He postulated that the borderline patient suffered from severely weakened ego functions in the areas of secondary process thinking, realistic planning, adaptation to the environment, maintenance of object relations, and defending against primitive impulses. Knight suggested that among the etiological factors responsible for these impaired ego functions were constitutional development, disturbed early object relations, early traumatic events, and precipitating stress.

Knight proposed that the therapeutic goal in treatment with borderline patients was to strengthen the ego's control over the overwhelming impulses of the basic drives - aggression and sexuality. Like others, he suggested the need for special considerations within the psychotherapeutic transference due to borderline patients' vulnerability to severe psychological regression while in therapy (Knight, 1953). Indeed, regression in treatment manifested by the expression of overt dependency, angry (at times rageful) responses, and the expression of developmentally primitive needs in direct form had

*The author would like to acknowledge the help of the following colleagues in reviewing earlier preparations of this and the following contribution for publication: Arlene Frank, PhD; Marsha Padwa, PsyD; William Temby, MD, and Robert Waldinger, MD. Mrs. Fran MacNeil and Ms. Melinda Flood aided in the typing and editing of the work, and their support is gratefully acknowledged as well. The teaching and supervision of John Gunderson, MD, has been an invaluable resource in the author's understanding of BPD, and the author wishes to thank him for his ongoing support. The author gratefully acknowledges his colleagues for their ideas, suggestions, and support; the responsibility for the contribution, however, remains the author's alone.

already come to be seen as characteristic of such patients when they were engaged in treatment. The hospital treatment of borderline patients often led to a series of regressed and primitive behaviors, including highly self-destructive activity which left inpatient staffs feeling helpless and angry (Adler, 1985). The generation of countertransference experiences in both inpatient and outpatient settings became remarkable and definable characteristics of patients with borderline psychopathology.

Within the two decades following Knight's seminal paper, there was a proliferation of major research studies in the area of borderline psychopathology. Grinker, Werble, and Drye (1968) carried out a thorough and systematic collection of empirical data. Kernberg (1965, 1967) created a coherent and integrated theoretical and clinical perspective of *borderline personality organization*. Gunderson and Singer (1975) synthesized the descriptive and clinical lore as a first step in creating a bridge from borderline psychopathology as a syndrome (a heterogeneous group of symptoms and signs) to a definable and diagnosable clinical entity.

Grinker and his colleagues (1968) were the first to empirically investigate the clinical hypotheses generally attributed to the borderline patient. They postulated that what had previously been defined as the borderline syndrome was probably the consequence of a developmental arrest in childhood, resulting in adult deficits in ego functioning. Their controlled observations found that the borderline syndrome was definitely an enduring personality *trait* or disorder, rather than merely an affective *state* or mood. Statistical analysis revealed four subgroups within the borderline diagnosis: the psychotic character; the core borderline; the adaptive, affectless, compliant, "as if person"; and the "border with neurosis." Additional findings suggested four overall characteristics that were common to all groups: (a) anger as the main or only affect; (b) a defect in affectional relationships; (c) a deficient sense of self-identity; and (d) depressive loneliness (Grinker et al., 1968).

Kernberg (1967, 1975) conceptualized borderline illness from a psychoanalytic perspective as a pathology of internalized object relations; a disturbance of the intrapsychic ego structures of self and object representations (introjects). He delineated a group of patients with severe character pathology who were neither fully neurotic nor psychotic. He utilized the conceptual entity of *borderline personality organization* to differentiate these patients from those with other psychiatric disabilities. From his *structural* viewpoint there were three basic criteria for identifying borderline patients: (a) a diffuse and unstable sense of identity; (b) the use of more developmentally primitive defensive operations, particularly splitting and projective identification; and (c) generally intact reality testing with the capacity for transient regressions to primary process ideation under psychological pressure.

Gunderson's review of the literature and empirically derived diagnostic criteria have helped direct attention to the clinical treatment of the borderline patient, as well as to narrow the definition of borderline personality disorder (Gunderson & Kolb, 1978; Gunderson & Singer, 1975). Gunderson (1977, 1982, 1984) argues for a narrow, coherent, and delimited definition of borderline personality disorder.

The impact of these major studies, the growing clarity of both theoretical and empirical approaches, and the continued needs of borderline patients led to the development of a distinct diagnostic category in the most recent *Diagnostic and Statistical Manual of Mental Disorders (DSM-III): Borderline Personality Disorder* (APA, 1980; Spitzer, Williams, & Skodol, 1980).

DIAGNOSIS: PREVALENCE AND MORBIDITY

Although prevalence estimates are hard to achieve, it is clear that borderline personality disorder (BPD) may be the most frequent form of all the *DSM-III* personality disorders (Frances et al., 1984; Kass, Spitzer, & Williams, 1983; Koenigsberg et al., 1985, Koenigsberg, Kernberg, & Schomer, 1983). The best present estimate of the occurrence of BPD in the general population is 4% (report of the Institute of Medicine, 1985). When Kroll et al. (1982) utilized the Diagnostic Interview for Borderlines (DIB) to test consecutive inpatient admissions in both the United States and the United Kingdom, he found that between 15% and 20% of the inpatient population met the diagnosis for borderline personality disorder.

Of note is the degree to which the disorder appears to be more prevalent among women than men: the female to male ratio ranges from 2:1 to 4:1 depending upon samples (Gunderson, 1984). Kass and colleagues (1983) have discussed the possibility of sex bias in diagnostic criteria, but believe there are genuine differences between men and women. The findings of Pope et al. (1983), however, suggest the possibility that male patients with antisocial personality disorder may be reflecting similar developmental difficulties to female BPD patients. It has also been my clinical impression that male patients with moderate to severe personality disorders on the borderline - narcissistic axis tend to be diagnosed as having narcissistic personality disorder, while similarly disordered women are more often considered "borderline."

MORBIDITY

Although the major psychiatric illnesses diagnosed on Axis I, especially affective and schizophrenic psychoses, are usually seen as more serious than personality disorders, such an impression may be erroneous (Gunderson & Pollack, 1985). Many clinicians fail to recognize that personality disorders, especially BPD, may represent a serious risk of morbidity. There is evidence of a severe course of dysfunctional role performance, disabling anxiety and depression, and often suicide in those who go untreated or who are poorly treated. In a 3 to 5 year longitudinal study of matched samples of borderline and schizophrenic patients carried out under the auspices of the NIMH (Carpenter et al., 1977; Gunderson, Carpenter, & Strauss, 1975), there were surprising similarities in the course of borderline and schizophrenic patients in their unremitting symptomatology, evidence of sustained recidivism, poor employment functioning, and difficulty in social relations. Although it has been shown that the nature of these dysfunctions is different, the severity and toll upon the patient with BPD and upon the community cannot be underestimated. Pope et al. (1983) also provide evidence of the severely disabling aspects of BPD.

DIAGNOSTIC ISSUES: ASSESSMENT OF BORDERLINE PERSONALITY DISORDER

Controversies continue concerning the assessment and diagnosis of borderline personality disorder, most notably between descriptive clinical psychiatry (i.e., phenomenological symptom/syndrome approaches) and psychoanalytic psychology and psychiatry (emphasizing internalized dynamic structures and object relations). Nevertheless, reasonable clarity has been achieved concerning the diagnostic entity of borderline personality disorder in the *DSM-III* (APA, 1980). Although the diagnostic manual is in the process of ongoing revision (*DSM-III-R* and the proposed *DSM-IV*), and to some extent represents consensus and political negotiation as well as diagnostic research, it provides the most reasonable formulation for the diagnosis of borderline personality disorder.

In the *DSM-III* (APA, 1980) the "Borderline Personality Disorder" is diagnosed on Axis II (301.83) and characterized by a marked *instability* in the patient's functional, emotional, interpersonal, and intrapsychic capacities and activities. Consideration had been given to replacing the term "borderline" with "unstable personality disorder," but the original term was retained. However, one cannot overemphasize *instability* as a defining characteristic for patients with borderline psychopathology.

Patients with BPD are likely to have considerable interference with social and occupational functioning, may present complications of Axis I disorders (most notably, dysthymic disorder and major depression), and are more likely to be women than men. Where there is evidence of an "Identity Disorder" in a child or adolescent under the age of 18, that diagnosis would preempt the diagnosis of BPD.

For a patient to meet the diagnosis of BPD, at least *five* of the following eight problems must be present, be characterological in nature, and lead to functional impairment (vocational/social) and/or an ongoing sense of internal distress: (a) impulsivity or unpredictability in at least two areas that are potentially self-damaging; (b) a pattern of unstable and intense interpersonal relationships; (c) inappropriate, intense anger or lack of control over anger; (d) identity disturbance; (e) affective instability; (f) an intolerance of being alone; (g) suicidal enactment or physically self-damaging acts; and (h) a sense of chronic emptiness or boredom. For a full description of defining criteria, see the *DSM-III* (APA, 1980, pp. 321-323).

To give a more complete sense of how borderline patients may present themselves clinically, I have summarized some of the major dynamic aspects of BPD dichotomized along the axes of problems in and within the *Self*, and problems manifested along the lines of the *Self in Interaction with Others*.

THE SELF IN BPD

1. *Noncohesive sense of self, unstable identity.* One of the most striking characteristics of borderline patients is their developmental difficulty establishing a cohesive self (Kohut, 1971, 1977) and a stable sense of personal identity. Although such disturbances run deep and are central in the clinical case reports of patients with BPD, they remain difficult to objectively define. Also, one must be careful in using the criterion of an unstable or fragmented sense of self because patients with many other personality disorders (most notably narcissistic personality disorder), as well as younger patients in the midst of a normal developmental crisis, may manifest similar disturbances.

   Recently, theorists and clinicians have identified more specific disturbances within borderline patients that are related to a fear of *separation* from significant objects, probably resulting from faulty early parent-child interaction. The inability to tolerate feeling or being alone has been linked by Adler and Buie (1979) and Adler (1985) to the central core of borderline psychopathology. Consequently, such patients may be socially overactive or compulsively involved with others to avoid ever being without a primary object. Masterson (1971) noted a similar vulnerability of borderline patients to "abandonment depression," and Mahler (1971) related separation anxiety in adult borderlines to failures in the rapprochement subphase of separation-individuation in childhood.

2. *Transient psychotic experiences.* When under severe stress, borderline patients may experience episodes of severe dissociation, including derealization or depersonalization, thinking of a paranoid nature, or a host of primitive and regressive defenses. Such episodes of ego-dystonic psychosis are not necessarily pathognomonic for a BPD diagnosis, as many other patients, including neurotics, may have such experiences. In a borderline patient these experiences are almost always ego dystonic. They are *not* accepted by the patient as a consensual way of seeing the world, nor are they welcome. Often they are accompanied by massive anxiety and may be one of the reasons such patients seek treatment.

3. *Impulsive behaviors.* Linked with an unstable and noncohesive sense of the self is the equally striking impulsive behavior in borderline patients. Although impulsivity may manifest itself diversely as gambling, shoplifting, or massive changes in eating patterns, such specific behaviors must also be evaluated as possibly representing other discrete psychiatric disorders (e.g., eating disorder, bipolar affective illness, etc.). By far the most prevalent form of impulsive activity in borderline patients, especially in young adults, is the abuse of drugs or alcohol. Sexual promiscuity and deviance, utilized in an equally addictive manner, are also quite common in such patients. There is an ongoing debate over the etiology of such impulsive behaviors. Psychoanalytic clinicians tie them to the underlying sense of an unstable, noncohesive self and a need for self-soothing (Adler & Buie, 1979), but biologically oriented researchers use this same evidence to argue that borderline personality disorder may be part of an affective spectrum disease (Akiskal, 1981).

4. *Uncomfortable affect.* One of the most characteristic aspects of borderline patients (as well as one of the more problematic phenomena in the transference and countertransference experiences of clinicians treating them) is their expression of uncomfortable feelings such as anger and, at times, a painful emptiness. Patients

are likely to express their anger directly, sometimes in outbursts of rage, and at other times in ongoing bitterness or excessive demands on their primary objects. Virtually all empirical studies of borderline patients have identified negative or uncomfortable affect as a central component to the syndrome (Grinker et al., 1968; Gunderson & Kolb, 1978; Perry & Klerman, 1980; Spitzer, Endicott, & Gibbon, 1979). Often, the anger is a response to either past or present experiences of hurt and disappointment. Therapists are likely to discover a terrifying sense of depression, loneliness, and loss behind the rage.

Gunderson (1984) and Kernberg (1967, 1975, 1984) have stressed the sense of "badness" that patients may feel about themselves, which may get expressed as intense anger or severe, empty depression. The *DSM-III* diagnosis of BPD emphasizes this distressing affective state in such patients by noting "inappropriate, intense anger or lack of control over anger," as well as "chronic feelings of emptiness or boredom" and "affective instability" (APA, *DSM-III*, 1980, pp. 321-323).

THE SELF IN INTERACTION WITH OTHERS

1. *Unstable and intense interpersonal relationships.* No therapist who has worked with a borderline patient can mistake the characteristic pattern of unstable interpersonal connections in these patients' primary relationships. Authors have reported that such patients are likely to use *devaluation*, the discrediting and derogating of those upon whom they depend, and *manipulation*, subtle means of gaining support from significant others, usually through actions rather than words.

    Others (Stiver, 1985; Tolpin & Kohut, 1980), including this author, have questioned the language used to describe these relationships. Words such as "manipulative" often appear to be critical of the patients. Therapists should seek instead to understand how such patients' developmental difficulties and present anxieties cause them to crave and seek close, dependent relationships, while simultaneously defending against acknowledging any need for significant others by pushing them away. Such action may also be linked to past traumatic experiences, including abuse, incest, and other forms of exploitation.

2. *Self-destructive activity.* Borderline patients are likely to engage in a suicidal effort or gesture meant to cause significant others to intervene. Common manifestations of such interpersonally oriented suicide attempts are wrist slashing and overdosing. Grunebaum and Klerman (1967) have pointed out a group of patients who make repeated gestures, including acts of self-harm, as a dynamic expression of inner feelings. Some theorists have deemed such suicidal gestures "manipulative," a pejorative description of these patients' use of self-destruction in an attempt to engage those around them. However, there is also a serious risk of completed suicide; such activities represent one of the more dangerous actions of borderline patients. Suicide attempts are often the reason for therapeutic failure, therapist anxiety, and hospitalization of patients with BPD.

3. *Functional failures.* Although not directly described in the *DSM-III*, the inability of borderline patients to effectively apply their talents is an important consideration in the diagnosis of BPD. Such patients often show a significant potential for achievement which falls by the wayside, because of interferences in their functional capacity or the affective overloading of their cognitive skills.

    This important issue of *functional incapacity*, especially in vocational and occupational disabilities, helps in the differential diagnosis of BPD. BPD is not an appropriate diagnosis for those with problems related to cohesion of the self and affective stability, but who can function well with minimal support and intervention. Such patients are probably suffering from depressive disorders with characterological aspects, or less severe disorders such as a narcissistic personality disorder.

    One of the major motivations for treating borderline personality disorders is the tragic waste of these patients' talents and skills. Vocational rehabilitation is an important issue considered in more detail below.

ASSESSMENT: FURTHER CONSIDERATIONS

The descriptive characteristics of the *DSM-III* categories of borderline personality disorder and the dynamic constellations of *Self* and *Self in Interaction* should allow a trained clinician to make accurate diagnostic assessments. However, the overlap with other Axis I illnesses and the differential diagnoses of personality disorders require attention.

THE BORDERS OF BORDERLINE: SCHIZOPHRENIA AND AFFECTIVE ILLNESS

Although the term and category borderline were created originally to maintain a border between characterologically disturbed patients with severe dysfunction and psychotic patients with a schizophreniform disorder, evidence gathered over the years suggests no true connection between borderline personality disorder and schizophrenic illness. Borderline and schizophrenic patients differ from each other in significant ways. Borderline patients continue to have the potential for role performance, but their character impedes functioning; schizophrenic patients appear to experience a real diminution in role capacities. Also, the disruption of social connections and the inability to maintain close interpersonal relationships found in borderline patients results from their stormy affective situation and long history of difficulties connecting to others. By contrast, schizophrenic patients often present social isolation and a lifelong fear of any object connection. Family studies have also shown a lack of a familial genetic connection between borderline probands and any form of schizophrenic illness in their first degree relatives (Gunderson & Elliott, 1985).

On the border of *affective disorders*, there appears to be greater overlap between BPD and affective illness. For an excellent review of the relationship between BPD and affective illness, see Gunderson and Elliott (1985).

Briefly, a number of observers have discussed the possible relationship between BPD and affective disorders (Akiskal, 1981, 1983). Recently there has been note of unipolar depression as a form of affective disorder found in both borderline patients and their relatives. Although Pope et al. (1983) discovered that many bona fide BPD patients met concurrent criteria for a diagnosis of major affective disorder, the relationship between borderline disorders and affective disorders requires more examination by researchers.

It is important for clinicians to recognize that patients with BPD may also suffer from a major affective illness. The most likely forms are dysthymic disorder or a major depression without melancholia. One should, therefore, be aware of concurrent affective diagnoses and their need for treatment, but also careful not to abandon a diagnosis of BPD merely because the patient is also suffering from depression. When patients with an acute or episodic unipolar depression alone recover from a particular episode of the disorder, their functioning between phases of the illness will be quite different than depressed patients who continue to suffer from concurrent borderline personality disorder.

THE BORDERS: OTHER PERSONALITY DISORDERS

Differential diagnosis of BPD must also be made in relation to other *DSM-III* Axis II disorders. Pope et al. (1983) found that while BPD could be distinguished from affective illness and schizophrenia, it could not easily be distinguished from either histrionic or antisocial personality disorders. Pope and his colleagues have questioned whether these personality disorders are appropriately separate categories. Although research concerning the distinguishing personality characteristics goes on, the clinician can rest reasonably secure in making differential diagnoses of borderline personality disorder if the following clear distinctions in functioning are kept in mind.

1. *Schizotypal personality disorder*. The term "schizotypal personality disorder" was created to separate a small subgroup of patients within the larger group of borderline personality organization, and to distinguish them from those with borderline personality disorder, per se. Schizotypal patients are much more likely to have social isolation and emotional detachment, manifesting very suspicious

(almost paranoid) feelings about relationships. They are unlikely to use their affects to attempt to bring their primary objects closer, which is often characteristic of transference and countertransference experiences with borderline patients. If overlap does exist it is more likely among schizoid, schizotypal, and avoidant personality disorders, and with some of these disorders and certain types of psychosis.

2. *Antisocial personality disorder (ASPD).* Although ASPD patients may have a similar early background of parental failure in the holding environment, the clinical consequences can be quite different from those of borderline patients. The attempt to manipulate people into doing what one wants appears to be much more smooth, calculating, and successful in ASPD patients than in borderline patients. When borderline patients engage in acts that may be considered antisocial, they are likely to experience shame or remorse. Although they may need to justify such acts for the survival of the self, the behaviors are usually ego dystonic. Also, antisocial patients are likely to have much more of a sense of emotional aloofness and detachment from their objects, and fewer obvious dependent or demanding needs.

3. *Schizoid personality disorder.* Although there is clearly overlap between schizoid and schizotypal personalities, there should be no difficulty in the differentiation of BPD from a patient who is schizoid. Rather than engaging in intense, unstable relationships with uncomfortable affects, schizoid patients are usually quite socially isolated and unlikely to engage in an attempt to bring objects close to them. A major task in the therapeutic work with a schizoid patient is to help someone who has almost completely given up on object relations and feels hopeless. Borderline patients often are attempting to establish relationships, and continue to fantasize that relationships may be helpful to them.

4. *Histrionic personality disorder.* Pope et al. (1983) suggested that histrionic disorder is one of the most difficult personality disorders to differentiate from BPD. A good marker for such a distinction is functional disability. Patients with a histrionic personality disorder or the more classical hysterical neurosis are likely to perform at a much higher level than patients with at least moderate BPD. The histrionic patient also presents a more stable sense of self than the BPD. Also, sexuality appears to be a major modulator of self-esteem or success in histrionic patients, but it may play a less significant role in BPD. Specifically, where there is evidence of *repeated self-destructive activity* as a gesture for helping intervention, more serious *functional disability*, or ongoing dysphoric affect to the point of instability, one should suspect BPD rather than histrionic personality disorder.

5. *Narcissistic personality disorder.* Although both borderline and narcissistic patients require a primary object upon whom to depend, their expression of this need differs radically. Borderline patients are likely to be open in their needs for support; narcissistic patients tend to deny the nature of their dependency upon significant others. When in a supportive relationship, narcissistic patients may be able to perform effectively in their roles and maintain a stable sense of themselves in psychotherapy and social situations. Borderline patients, by contrast, are likely to have storms of affect that last much longer and are much more disorganizing; even in a supportive environment they continue to show major deficiencies in role performance and social relationships.

INTERNAL BORDERS: BORDERLINE PERSONALITY DISORDER VERSUS BORDERLINE PERSONALITY ORGANIZATION

Since Kernberg created a concept for the borderline syndrome separate from neurosis and psychosis, he has clung to the terminology of "borderline personality organization" (Kernberg, 1967, 1975, 1984). Kernberg believes that within the broad borderline concept one may fit a number of clearly linked but distinct subcategories. Although such a concept clearly has important developmental, psychoanalytic, and clinical meaning, it may blur distinctions between diagnostic groups. For example, Kernberg argues that the borderline personality diagnosis in *DSM-III* represents only one subsection of borderline personality organization (BPO) which he calls "infantile personality disorder." For

Kernberg, most patients with "as if" personality disorders, narcissistic, schizoid, cyclothalmic, impulse ridden, and antisocial personality disorders, as well as certain patients with histrionic, compulsive, or masochistic personalities, would all fit within the BPO category. Such an approach is designed to include almost all forms of severe character pathology and consequently may end up encompassing 25% to 30% of the general population or as much as 40% of the psychiatric population (Gunderson, 1984). Kernberg has suggested that the BPO category may include 15% of the general population (Kernberg, 1983)! Consequently, it seems more reasonable and clinically useful to make relatively clear distinctions among patients suffering from the diverse forms of severe character pathology.

ASSESSMENT: STRUCTURED INTERVIEWS

Although a full review of the empirical approaches for assessing BPD is outside the scope of this contribution, a brief description of some structured and semistructured interviews for diagnostic assessment of the borderline patient may be of use. For the beginning clinician or anyone reviewing borderline pathology within his or her practice, the use of such empirically based techniques may add a new perspective on the diagnostic and treatment issues with such patients. (For a full review of structured diagnostic and research instruments for BPD diagnosis, see Gunderson [1982, 1984] and Reich [1983]).

DIAGNOSTIC INTERVIEW FOR BORDERLINES (DIB)

The best known and probably most frequently used semistructured instrument for the diagnosis of BPD is the Diagnostic Interview for Borderlines (DIB) developed by Gunderson and his colleagues (Gunderson & Kolb, 1978; Gunderson, Kolb, & Austin, 1981; Kolb & Gunderson, 1980). Gunderson and his colleagues at McLean Hospital conducted a series of interviews with diagnosed BPD patients. Then they developed a 29-item semistructured interview for the identification of BPD. The original and most widely used format for the DIB included *five basic* sub-areas of functioning: social adaptation, impulse patterns, affects, psychotic symptomatology, and interpersonal relationships. Using the semistructured interview statements, the clinician makes inquiries into a number of specific and related areas and then generates subscores for the five hierarchical subsections and an overall DIB or diagnostic score. For patients with a total score of 7 points or above out of a possible 10, there is sufficient evidence to accept the diagnosis of borderline personality disorder.

The reliability of a diagnosis based on the total DIB score approaches .90 (Kolb & Gunderson, 1980; Kroll et al., 1981). Test-retest reliability has also been documented (Cornell et al., 1983), and the interview has been able to distinguish BPD from other Axis II personality disorders (Barrash et al., 1983).

I find that learning to do the interview helps to clarify one's diagnostic thinking and to refine one's clinical focus with all types of personality disorders. Gunderson has also devised a retrospective format of the DIB, called the DIB-R, which allows use of hospital chart material, one's own therapy notes, and so on, to make a retrospective diagnosis. A new edition of the DIB, which uses a more uniform and time-limited framework for the areas of psychopathology, is presently in preparation.

KERNBERG'S STRUCTURAL INTERVIEW

The Structural Interview is a clinical interview format designed by Otto Kernberg to delineate those aspects of borderline personality organization which he considers pathognomonic. As formulated by Kernberg and his colleagues (Kernberg, 1977, 1981, 1984), the structural interview measures how borderline patients respond to clarification, confrontation, or interpretation in ways which may allow discrimination from either psychotic or neurotic personality organization. Kernberg's interview focuses on here-and-now interactional features. It assumes that the interviewer's focus on the patient's main conflicts will induce a level of tension that reveals the patient's predominant ego defenses and internal "structural organization of mental functioning." The data obtained are organized into three categories of personality structure: (a) the degree of identity integration (or the integration of self and object representations in Kernberg's schema); (b) the type of defensive operations which predominate in the patient's personality (e.g., evidence of primitive defenses such as denial, splitting, and projective identification); and (c) the patient's capacity for reality testing.

Based on the results, the interviewer may classify the patient into one of three personality structures: borderline personality organization, neurotic, or psychotic organization. In the context of the interview, the clinician observes descriptive symptoms as "presumptive evidence of borderline personality organization." Evidence includes polysymptomatic neurosis, polymorphously perverse sexual trends, impulsive neurosis and addictions, the lack of an integrated identity, or the syndrome of identify diffusion. One particularly looks for the primitive defense mechanisms defined by Kernberg as denial, projection, projective identification, primitive idealization, and splitting. In addition, the interviewer looks for nonspecific manifestations of ego weakness such as the absence of anxiety tolerance, problems with sublimation or impulse control, a lack of superego integration, and the capacity for reality testing.

Some of the empirical results of structural interviewing have been reported by Kernberg (1981) and his colleagues (Bauer et al., 1980; Stone, 1980). However, given the range of interviewers and uncertainty in responses, reliability and validity will be harder to achieve than in more empirically oriented structured interviews. Nonetheless, this interview offers the clinician another opportunity to think cogently within a particular psychoanalytic object relations perspective, and to understand the patient in the interview context. A potentially more empirically valid self-report questionnaire version of Kernberg's BPD Interview is presently under development (Oldham et al., 1984).

OTHER MEASURES

Other measures for diagnosing borderline personality disorder or personality disorders in general include: the Schedule for Interviewing Borderlines (SIB) (Baron, Asnis, & Gruen, 1981); the Borderline Personality Disorder Scale (BPD Scale) developed by Perry (1984); the Structural Interview for the *DSM-III* Personality (SIDP) (Pfohl, Stangl, & Zimmerman, 1983); Spitzer's Item List (Spitzer & Endicott, 1979); and the Personality Disorder Examination (PDE) (Loranger et al., 1984).

Of recent interest has been an attempt to diagnose borderline personality disorder with self-report measures filled out by the patient alone. Most promising and interesting in this regard is Millon's Clinical Multiaxial Inventory (MCMI), a 175-item, forced choice, true/false self-report measure. The MCMI covers all 11 *DSM-III* Axis II personality disorders and is presently marketed as a computer scorable diagnostic test (Millon, 1981). The diagnostic categories in this measure, however, were developed prior to *DSM-III*, following a personality typology developed by Millon himself, and only later adapted to the *DSM-III* Axis II diagnostic categories.

There is also a Personality Diagnostic Questionnaire (PDQ) developed by Hyler et al. (1978). This 161-item questionnaire attempts to translate diagnostic criteria for 11 personality disorders on the *DSM-III* into true-false responses that can generate a personality disorder diagnosis. Recent research has shown that the specificity and sensitivity of the questionnaire for the diagnosis of BPD were higher than 60%, making it a potentially useful instrument for identifying borderline personality disorders (Hurt et al., 1984).

Recent research has suggested maintaining the *categorical* integrity of specific personality disorder diagnosis on the *DSM-III*, while utilizing a *dimensional* rating (or scoring) scale for identifying certain important personality traits within each patient. A 1- to 4-point scale is used for each personality disorder, with 1 being none or very few traits and 4 meeting the full *DSM-III* criteria. In this manner a clinician could identify a patient with several significant borderline traits requiring therapeutic intervention, but recognize that the patient did not meet full *DSM-III* criteria for BPD (Kass et al., 1985).

SUMMARY

The development of state-of-the-art clinical and empirical approaches to diagnosis have led us to discover within a reasonable degree of certainty who borderline patients are, what they are like, what they may be experiencing, and how we may be able to distinguish them from other patients. Now, the most important question for the clinician arises: How can we be of help? The next contribution, on the treatment of BPD, addresses that salient question in depth.

(Biographical material and resources for this contribution are included at the end of Dr. Pollack's other contribution, "Borderline Personality Disorder: Treatment Considerations," which follows.)

BORDERLINE PERSONALITY DISORDER: TREATMENT CONSIDERATIONS

William S. Pollack

GENERAL CONSIDERATIONS

Historically, the major modality for the treatment of Borderline Personality Disorder (BPD) has been a specialized or modified form of psychoanalytic psychotherapy. A variety of other treatment approaches have also been suggested, and a wide range of technical or structural considerations for treatment have been delineated (Adler & Buie, 1979; Frosch, 1983; Gunderson, 1984; Kernberg, 1967, 1975, 1984). There is a lack of agreement about a number of therapeutic issues. For example, how supportive, exploratory, or intensive should the process be; how empathic or confrontational should the therapist be; how often should therapy take place; how can medication be used effectively? This contribution cannot address all of these controversies in depth, and the reader interested in more detail should refer to Gunderson (1984), Adler (1985), and Kernberg (1984). My goal is to highlight several of the major psychodynamic therapeutic treatments for BPD. Also, I will briefly describe other pragmatic treatment approaches such as paradoxical interventions, family treatment, the therapeutic use of work, psychopharmacology, and cognitive-behavioral techniques.

Although a number of authors highlight prognostic indicators for the individual psychotherapy of borderline personality disorder (most notably Kernberg [1975, 1984]), the only clear and consistent *contraindication* for such treatment is an untrained or emotionally unavailable psychotherapist. I strongly agree with Gunderson's assertion (Gunderson, 1984) that a novice should not treat a BPD patient without intensive supervision. I also believe that psychotherapists who have not yet achieved substantial understanding of their own psychological functioning will not be therapeutically useful to such disturbed patients, and could well do extreme damage. The therapeutic work is difficult and frustrating, but can ultimately be quite rewarding for both patient and therapist if undertaken with an attitude of therapeutic flexibility and the realization that clinicians still have much to learn about BPD.

INTENSIVE EXPLORATORY VERSUS SUPPORTIVE PSYCHOTHERAPY

One of the greatest *nondebates* in the BPD treatment literature has been the development of the distinction between so-called intensive or exploratory (sometimes termed "insight-oriented") psychotherapy on the one hand, and supportive (nonintensive) psychotherapy on the other. Earlier researchers and clinicians, based upon their understanding of the fragile BPD ego structure, tended to suggest a more "supportive" approach. This involved less intensive and less frequent (usually once per week) meetings and a style of psychotherapy that tended *not* to uncover defenses, but to support them as coping styles (Friedman, 1975; Grinker, Werble, & Drye, 1968; Knight, 1953; Zetzel, 1971).

The "supportive" approach takes the stance that the creation of a sustaining and stabilizing therapeutic relationship will allow borderline patients to decrease their chaotic inner experiences and consequently gain greater stability in their daily life functioning. Given the possibility of regressive experiences in either a more intensive or less structured psychotherapy, such supportive treatment was believed to bolster the therapeutic alliance, decrease the possibility of unmanageable transference enactments, and minimize the possibility of self-destructive activity. Goals of such a treatment would be to decrease the possibility of suicide, lead to more functional work and social relationships, and allow for greater stability and emotional development in the patients' lives.

Kernberg, in contrast, has argued that such a "supportive" approach for borderline patients may lead to iatrogenic, toxic effects. His interpretation of data from the Menninger Psychotherapy Research Study suggested that even though patients with the weakest ego strength did poorly in *both* supportive and expressive treatments, borderline patients still required an *expressive* approach (Kernberg et al., 1972). This approach tended to focus more on clinical interpretation of the transference in psychotherapy, while utilizing hospital inpatient stays as adjunct to the psychotherapeutic treatment.

I have termed the distinction between "supportive" and "intensive" psychotherapy a nondebate for both clinical and empirical reasons. First, it is probably impossible to make any reasonable distinction between so-called supportive psychotherapies and intensive ones. Kernberg's argument itself is evidence of the fact that the intensity of the treatment may be a supportive adjunct for the patient. Wallerstein (1983), commenting on the same Menninger study, demonstrated that there was *not* a true differentiation between supportive and expressive therapy. Standard supportive techniques were found in the treatment interventions of insight-oriented or expressive psychotherapists. Wallerstein has also argued that the standard supportive treatments may have done more than merely bolster patients' defenses or decrease suicidal risk; they may have brought about internal structural changes that are usually ascribed only to intensive or expressive psychotherapy. Greenberg (1977), in a cogent clinical presentation on the supportive therapeutic approach for borderline patients, and Levine (1979), in a theoretical article on the "sustaining object relationship," have both argued for the importance of using therapeutic techniques which help borderline patients maintain their psychological equilibrium. Indeed, more recent approaches to intensive psychoanalytic psychotherapy for character neuroses have highlighted the importance of creating such a "holding environment" in both psychoanalysis and psychotherapy (Adler, 1985; Modell, 1976).

Clinical and common sense both indicate that an ongoing interpretive psychotherapy that does not help the patient stem the tide of chaotic, overwhelming feelings, or of suicidal enactment, will not be very therapeutic. Also, a sustaining supportive treatment which allows a patient to have more stable interpersonal relationships may eventually lead to some changes in internal psychological structure. Psychotherapists most likely blend supportive and interpretive techniques to react flexibly to the varying needs and levels of functioning of a particular borderline patient. Even Kernberg (1984) has recently changed his attitude toward supportive treatments, now seeing them as a useful intervention for many borderline patients, although his definition of "supportive" may be quite different from that of other authors. I believe it is better to conceptualize the nature of the psychotherapeutic intervention by the frequency of the sessions and the theoretical treatment approach, rather than by differentiation on a supportive-expressive axis which has little practical meaning.

PSYCHOTHERAPEUTIC TREATMENT
OF BPD: TWO PARADIGMS

Next, I will briefly describe two of the major treatment paradigms for borderline patients' individual psychotherapy: Kernberg's ego psychological and object relations approach, and Adler and Buie's developmental, therapeutic "holding environment" approach (based upon Winnicott and Kohut). I will then summarize some of the benefits and drawbacks of each of these paradigms and integrate the more eclectic approach of Gunderson, as well as the results of some recent research on normal development.

There are several other major approaches to the treatment of borderline personality disorder (BPD) which will not be discussed. For those who are interested in alternative psychodynamic formulations and approaches, it would be worthwhile to explore the work of Masterson (1976), Rinsley (1982), Frosch (1970), Stolorow and Lachman (1980), and Brandchaft and Stolorow (1984), among others (e.g., Giovacchini, Boyer, and Chessick).

KERNBERG'S EGO PSYCHOLOGICAL AND OBJECT RELATIONS APPROACH

Although Kernberg conceptualizes his theoretical outlook and clinical approach from the perspective of human object relations, his basic assumptions about BPD appear to be derived from more classic drive psychology, most notably the work of Melanie Klein. Kernberg (1967, 1975, 1984) conceptualizes BPD as a pathology of internalized object relations. He views it as a disturbance within the self, particularly in the intrapsychic ego structures of self and object representation (introjects). These inner mental representations are viewed as symbolic of the early mother-child relationship; with BPD, the pathology from this early relationship later generalizes to difficulties in adult relationships.

Kernberg has postulated that normal development of internalized object relations through mental representations (introjects) moves in the direction of the healthy cognitive development of the baby through increased *differentiation* and *integration*. The earliest memory representations are more undifferentiated and occur conglomerated in "self-object-affect units." If interaction with the caretaking environment goes well, then the baby and later the toddler will internalize a series of images which include the supportive human environment, especially the primary caretaker, the self in interaction with this primary person, and an affective coloring for both the object image and the self-image.

Central to Kernberg's theory is that the affective coloring of these memory images of the self and of the self in interaction with the early supportive other will come under the influence of "the drive representative present at the time of the interaction" (Kernberg, 1976, p. 29). The memories will be affectively colored either with libidinal energy, or with components of the aggressive drive. These "constellations of affectively integrated and cognitively stored perceptions" (Kernberg, 1967, p. 87) start to become structures in the young child's mind by being differentiated as those self-object units which are "good," meaning invested with libidinal or positive energy, and "bad," meaning connected with negative affects and strong aggressive content. Through the mastery of the separation-individuation phase of human development described by Mahler and colleagues (Mahler, 1971, 1972; Mahler & Kaplan, 1977), the child will eventually differentiate the images of self from the images of objects, and further subdivide mental contents into so-called good and bad *self* representations versus good and bad *object* representations. From Kernberg's perspective, this is the stage that is described as "part-object relations." The "part" refers to the fact that although self and other are somewhat differentiated, the good and bad aspects are kept apart. Finally, in Kernberg's schema of human psychological development, the integration and consolidation of the good and bad aspects will produce whole self-representations and whole object representations. In the healthy developing child and adult, the mixed affective colorings of both a positive and negative valence can become integrated into more complete and whole self and object representations.

In Kernberg's schema, borderline psychopathology occurs as a result of a developmental fixation or a regression to the stage of part-object relations. Most central for a clinical understanding of Kernberg's interventions is his argument that the primary etiology of this defect in the integrative aspect of the patient's ego is a predominance of *pathological aggression* and aggressive drive derivatives. Therefore, excessive rage, quite possibly congenital in its origin, is the basic cause implied by the distortions in ego functioning that lead to borderline psychopathology. For Kernberg, this overabundance of aggression results in a predominance of negative memory representations of both the self and other, so-called "bad" introjects.

Further, Kernberg argues that although this problem may begin as a deficiency in ego development, it is maintained defensively as a regression to an earlier level of functioning to avoid a certain type of pain. Consequently, Kernberg believes that these defective structures of all good or all bad senses of the self and others are ultimately maintained for defensive purposes. That is, what may once have been a *defect* in the functioning of the person's self eventually became a defense mechanism - *splitting*. The psychological process of splitting, according to Kernberg's formulation, is used to keep apart those introjects of opposite emotional valence (the good and the bad) so that the person can preserve the limited available good memories. To preserve all good memories, the BPD patient must split these off from any negative sense of the self or the other. In this sense, Kernberg feels that borderline patients are using a primitive defense to avoid noticing their own extremely angry feelings toward their primary objects.

The mechanism of splitting sets in motion other primitive defense mechanisms of the ego which, in turn, effect further nonintegration of the developmental emotional and cognitive processes (Kernberg, 1967, 1975). These other cognitive, emotional, and clinical dysfunctions are referred to by Kernberg as "nonspecific manifestations of ego weakness," and include primitive free-floating anxiety with concomitant lack of anxiety tolerance, lack of impulse control, lack of developed sublimatory channels, and weakness in cognitive functioning which may lead to occasional breakthroughs of primary process thinking.

In summary, then, Kernberg views borderline personality organization (BPO) as an object relations disorder, or a pathology of internalized object relations. This pathology is brought about primarily as a result of excessive aggressive drives. Although Kernberg notes the developmental concepts of Mahler and the separation-individuation phase of human development, he virtually ignores the environmental context in understanding the etiology of the patient's disorder. Thus, his model is primarily a classic conflict-drive theory in which borderline psychopathology is the consequence of intrapsychic conflict, usually over the binding of an excessive amount of aggression and rage, which is sometimes congenital in original.

Clinical Implications. Kernberg's theoretical perspective on borderline psychopathology has certain clinical implications. In addition to the so-called *nonspecific signs* of ego weakness and the major defense of *splitting* good and bad representations of the self and others, one expects to find other "lower level ego defenses" such as *denial*, *projection* (particularly Klein's formulation of *projective identification*), *idealization*, and *devaluation*. As a result, such patients are likely to experience contradictory part-identities, a form of *identity diffusion*, rather than a sense of a coherent self. A severe impairment of relationships is also likely because such patients will be unable to tolerate mixed feelings toward others and others' mixed feelings toward themselves.

Kernberg stresses that in the psychotherapeutic situation with borderline patients one is likely to experience a "premature activation in the transference of very early conflict-laden object relations" (Kernberg, 1982, p. 472). He sees the conflicts that get played out, especially in the early transference relationship, as a "pathological condensation of pregenital and genital aims *under the over-riding influence of pregenital aggression*" (Kernberg, 1982, p. 472, italics mine). *Projective identification* as described by M. Klein (1946) becomes a major defense in the treatment setting. Kernberg believes that patients try to defend against recognizing their own negative affect, especially their aggression within themselves, by psychologically projecting it onto the therapist. Then, patients may unconsciously identify with this partial representation of themselves - now seen as a quality of the therapist - through aggressive enactment. Consequently, Kernberg describes the transference as being manifest initially with intense distrust and fear of the therapist, who is often seen as a potent "attacker." Kernberg's approach emphasizes the need to *control* transference acting out. He recommends limiting the patient's enactment to protect the ongoing psychotherapy, while interpreting the need for such limits from the perspective of the transference relationship.

For BPD, Kernberg recommends an intensive psychoanalytic therapy paradigm with three to four weekly face-to-face sessions. The therapy is organized around three technical essentials: (a) interpretation, (b) the maintenance of technical neutrality, and (c) transference analysis.

Kernberg argues (1975, 1984) that *interpretation* must remain the central and fundamental technical tool in the psychoanalytic therapy of BPD. He feels that the therapist should not engage in any forms of suggestion or manipulation. The only exception to this should be the need for setting limits around acting out, which may require some additional external structuring of the patient's life. To accomplish this, the therapist may use a clinical team approach to intervene in the patient's social network. Even such interventions, Kernberg feels, should eventually be interpreted and wither away.

Although he stresses *technical neutrality*, Kernberg argues that the therapist still may be empathic. However, he does not see empathy as the central aspect of the therapist's function. Kernberg emphasizes that the therapist must not only empathize from within the patient's experience, but also bring to light those aspects of the patient's inner life which may be walled off or unbearable. The understanding and feeling of the dissociated, usually negative, experience of the borderline patient which is not being expressed, and the reflecting of these split-off parts of the self through interpretation, can only be achieved through technical neutrality in treatment.

An active but limited use of *transference interpretation* is the third functional aspect of Kernberg's approach. He emphasizes interpretation of the transference in a way that supports the immediate reality of the patient's life and the ultimate treatment goals. It is through transference interpretation, according to Kernberg, that primitive part-object projections and developmentally arrested object relations are finally integrated into a more complete sense of one's self and others. Ultimately, this allows the BPD patient to tolerate ambivalent feelings for both. With this aim in mind, he recommends the interpretation of defensive constellations in the transference as the locus of therapeutic change. To accomplish this, Kernberg suggests that: (a) the predominantly negative transference of borderline patients be systematically elaborated and interpreted, but only in its present manifestations; (b) typical defensive constellations need to be interpreted as soon as they enter the transference, particularly the use of splitting or projective identification; and (c) limits must be set to stop any acting out of the transference and to maintain the neutrality of the therapist (Kernberg, 1984). He even believes that the therapist might choose to hospitalize the BPD patient to maintain limits on acting out, rather than modify the transference interpretation or the technical neutrality; he feels that too much deviation from such an approach could lead to an inability to create structural change in the patient.

Kernberg suggests not interpreting relatively positive aspects of the transference, but allowing them to be the basis of the growing therapeutic alliance. Again the focus is on the so-called aggressive primitive transference:

> With borderline patients the focus on interpretation should be on the primitive, grossly exaggerated idealizations that reflect the splitting of "all good from all bad" object relations. These must be interpreted systematically as part of the effort to work through the primitive defenses. The negative transference should be interpreted as fully as possible. This is the major vehicle for indirectly strengthening the therapeutic alliance while dealing directly with the primitive conflicts around aggression and intolerance of ambivalence characteristic of borderline patients. (Kernberg, 1984, pp. 105-106)

Kernberg suggests that all interpretations be clarified systematically. He advocates interpreting any current patient defenses which distort reality to make it feel more comfortable or soothing. It is essential that both therapist and patient acknowledge such distortions. Kernberg suggests that the stepwise analysis of transference with interpretation should lead the patient toward a more integrated sense of self and internal images of primary objects. This should heal the splitting and decrease the need to protect against internal aggression or to act it out in suicidal gestures. If therapy is carried out properly, less primitive transferences with a more neurotic flavor should emerge, replete with whole object relations. This permits later interpretation of oedipal material.

Kernberg stresses that he is aware of the importance of the role of the therapist in "holding" or "containing" borderline patients (Bion, 1967; Winnicott, 1960). However, he makes it clear that the therapist who goes too far in providing such a context of support may lose technical neutrality and damage the treatment by "gratifying" rather than "interpreting" the patient's needs. The therapist can be most empathic and humane by helping patients understand the nature of their developmental difficulties through transference and conflict analysis. Consequently, Kernberg recommends a classical analytic attitude of "abstinence."

Advantages and Disadvantages to Kernberg's Approach. Clinicians will recognize in Kernberg's theory and technique his capacity to create an environment in which the therapist may face the patient's aggression and rage head-on without either giving way to an overtly critical response or avoiding strong feelings. In addition, Kernberg's stringent demands for maintaining a stance of "neutrality" allow the clinician the inner peace necessary to maintain a calming and supportive environment in the treatment of patients who are often experiencing intense chaotic feelings expressed through enactment. Also, the application and modification of psychoanalytic technique to more severely disturbed patients lends the intervention a sense of theoretical stability and cohesiveness. I believe that Kernberg's therapeutic optimism, which is embodied in this approach, is admirable.

There are, however, a number of criticisms of Kernberg's approach to treatment of BPD. Some clinicians have been concerned about the "Olympian" nature of Kernberg's treatment techniques (Searles, 1979b). The requirement of "abstinence" and technical neutrality may demand more than a psychotherapist can provide with such severely disturbed patients, or may leave patients feeling unsupported, criticized, or hurt (Tolpin & Kohut, 1980). Also, Kernberg's emphasis on patients' *aggression* and his understanding of the major defenses of BPD as motivated by congenital and negative drive energy may leave some patients with the sense that they truly are "bad," because they are always seen as so angry. Indeed, other clinicians have viewed their patients' aggression as a legitimate response to trauma or hurt from parents or a defense against a deeper and more genuine feeling of loneliness or abandonment. They criticize Kernberg's approach as colluding with the patients' harsh superego in believing that they are bad and aggressive, when they may really be sad and lonely.

Another criticism is that some of Kernberg's recommendations may be impractical. His earlier suggestions that few supportive techniques ever enter into the psychotherapy, but that the patient should experience external support through the creation of a treatment team network or inpatient hospitalization, are sometimes impossible to achieve. Often the borderline patient's psychotherapist must remain the central or only therapeutic figure. Although the recommendations against becoming too personally entangled in such a role are well taken, it may be impractical geographically, clinically, or economically, to add any other than flexible modifications in the therapy. This is not to diminish the importance of Kernberg's admonition about the dangerousness of becoming too involved and enacting transference fantasies. Rather, it highlights the fact that for various practical and clinical reasons, often one must do *more than interpret* to help BPD patients improve.

HOLDING AND SOOTHING THE SELF: FACING THE ISSUES OF ALONENESS (ADLER AND BUIE)

The creative theoretical contributions of Winnicott (1953, 1958, 1965) and their clinical application to modern American psychoanalysis by Modell (1963, 1976, 1984), as well as the recent reformulations of human development by the *self-psychology* of Kohut and his colleagues (Kohut, 1971, 1977; Kohut & Wolf, 1978; Tolpin, 1971), have created a rich new framework from which to view the developmental nature of borderline psychopathology. In the recent work of Adler and Buie (1979) and Adler (1985), these creative theoretical and clinical advances have been crystallized into an effective therapeutic treatment of BPD.

Winnicott and Modell. Winnicott, in delineating the pre-stages of an object relationship during infancy and childhood, defined an intermediate area of experience between the baby's self and the mother's function of titrating the demands of the external world. This is the developmental way station of the so-called "transitional object." This interpersonal space of healthy illusion, protection, and safety could only be provided by the "good-enough mother." Psychologically as well as biologically, such a primary caretaker would provide the facilitating environment in which maturational processes, ego growth, and development could occur. This is accomplished through the task of "holding" the infant or child emotionally through time. The "holding environment" depends upon the caretaker's empathic immersion, and upon the *active* creation of a "live adaptation" to the child's needs from his or her environment. When this is provided, according to Winnicott, a healthy, cohesive, and competent self will develop (Winnicott, 1953, 1960, 1965).

This process of good-enough holding requires an emphasis upon the flexible and growth-promoting aspect of the caretaker's or therapist's adaptation. Clinicians who follow such a developmental approach in their treatment of borderline patients argue that good-enough therapeutic and adaptive holding can occur for severely disturbed patients in intensive psychotherapy. With such treatment, patients with early environmental failure might begin anew to pursue the natural maturational course, which had once gone awry or been stunted in earlier years. Eventually in such a treatment, the internalization of a holding introject, a soothing memory of the understanding therapist, should occur. Therapy facilitates the arduous and slow task of taking into the self the skill of holding one's feelings, holding one's memories, and indeed *holding* one's *self* together safely through time.

Winnicott (1975) has argued that a central focus in the psychotherapeutic treatment must shift when one takes on such an object relations view of the disorder. As he stated: "In the work I am describing, the *setting* becomes more important than the interpretation. The emphasis is changed from one to the other" (Winnicott, 1975, p. 97). It is the environment of therapeutic holding, the active empathic, responsive, and understanding treatment environment, that the clinician creates and that begins to take on a curative focus.

Modell (1976, 1984) has explained that "object relations theory describes intrapsychic processes in the context of a human *environment*" (Modell, 1976, p. 289, italics mine). This is an environment or treatment setting where the interactions, the actual events, and especially the affects shared between the caretaker and child, or the treater and patient, must take on poignant significance. It may be conceived of as "an open system joined by means of a communication of affects" (Modell, 1976, p. 290). Such communication emerges in the psychotherapy of borderline patients as treaters learn to wait, not to interpret prematurely, and consequently to understand the patient's "deepest anxiety" (Modell, 1976; Winnicott, 1975). The focus, then, has shifted from a totally internalized experience to a theory which emphasizes the *interpersonal* nature of the psychotherapeutic setting. Indeed, in such a developmental context the caretaking adult will be expected to protect the child from the environment; and within psychotherapy, the patient may experience the illusion of the therapist providing the same protection from the potentially harmful vagaries of reality. Holding, then, for the borderline patient may become a form of protection provided in the appropriate psychotherapeutic setting, and may be experienced as protecting the patient's self from internal as well as external dangers.

When the treatment proceeds correctly, the psychotherapeutic cocoon may slowly wither away as the patient increasingly tolerates affective frustration: "the individual can build up memories of experiences felt to be good, so that the experience of...holding the situation...becomes assimilated into the ego...the individual acquires an internal environment" (Winnicott, 1975, p. 271). As the therapist "holds the situation in time," an experience of inner growth occurs. The sense of *time* is as important as the holding itself, for there is a re-experiencing, an over-and-over again sense of a developing experience of self-efficacy: "the...technique enables...coexisting love and hate to become sorted out and interrelated and gradually brought under control from within in a way that is healthy" (Winnicott, 1975, p. 263).

This last statement emphasizes how a holding environment takes into account the patient's aggressive energy, affective outbursts, and potentially destructive acting out, but approaches their interpretation and understanding from a different perspective than Kernberg. The psychotherapist may at times be the object of "assault during phases of instinctual tension" (Winnicott, 1975, p. 266), but these are times when holding and understanding must be continued in psychotherapy without interpretive retaliation. If done properly, such passive perseverance and active attempt at understanding will lead over time to a sense of "ambivalence" on the patient's part, to resolution or management, and eventually to the introjection of holding, itself (Winnicott, 1975, p. 266). Survival of the therapist as a useful object without the need to resentfully limit the patient's expression of aggression provides the ultimate usefulness of the psychotherapist in the ongoing treatment.

In addition, one may understand patients' *crises* of discontent as more than the expression of defective affective regulation or poor ego integration. From the object relations perspective, crises may be the active expression of an original hurt, combined with a creative wish for cure. Just as the neurotic may create symptoms in a structured, unifying crucible as a maladaptive attempt to resolve early conflicts, the borderline patient may demand in distorted ways that the environment undo earlier damage, impingement, or misunderstanding. Acting out, then, is not necessarily only negative and regressive, but may involve a kernel of hope that therapeutic change is possible. This is a hope which Winnicott (1965) describes as "never becomes quite extinguished, that the environment may acknowledge and make up for the specific failure that did the damage." Consequently, the patient is "all the time liable to moments of hope, moments when it would seem to be possible to force the environment to effect a cure" (Winnicott, 1965, p. 207). Thus, the empathic therapist may be able to creatively understand the patient's repetitive crises of so-called "acting out" - rather than necessarily interpreting them as forms of primitive aggression or prematurely setting therapeutic limits.

Kohut's Contributions. Kohut's theoretical concept of the *selfobject* may broaden and deepen our sense of the holding environment and its centrality in therapeutic treatment of borderline personality disorder (Kohut, 1971, 1977; Kohut & Wolf, 1978). Kohut describes selfobject as an object which we may experience as part of ourselves. Consequently, the expected control over it is closer to the sense of control which an adult usually expects to have over his or her own body and mind, than to the kind of control we usually expect to have over others.

Embedded in this seemingly simple definition is an empathic understanding of the borderline patient's endopsychic life. Kohut understands a self-selfobject relationship to be the expression of a phase appropriate, *legitimately* expressed need in patients for support from others, which a fragile or incomplete internal self-structure does not provide. As he has stated: "The essential psychopathology...(in these patients) is defined by the fact that the self has not been solidly established, that its cohesion and firmness depend upon the presence of a...self-object transference,..." and that such patients respond "to the loss of a selfobject with simple enfeeblement, various regressions, and fragmentation" (Kohut, 1977, p. 137). The selfobject and set of selfobject responses, then, may make up for and developmentally be "the precursors of [internalized] psychic structure" (Tolpin & Kohut, 1980, p. 442).

Such a shift in theory and treatment focus also suggests a different pathway to mental health. Kohut argues that it is more important to create a therapeutic environment in which supportive selfobjects help to maintain the cohesion of the self, than to exhort patients to become *independent*. Separation-individuation, then, becomes less salient than affective connection or the subsequent storing of such positive memories of holding. Kohut explains that most mature adults will seek "a selfobject environment that is in harmonious contact with them, until...[they can] obtain what they need" (Kohut, 1980, p. 453). Indeed, for BPD patients the empathic matrix of intensive individual psychotherapy with its holding environment becomes a psychological necessity to maintain emotional equilibrium, to forestall psychotic regression, and eventually to internalize a sense of holding.

Kohut (1977) explains that, in the course of normal human development, we all need the opportunity to merge with a calming, soothing, or idealized object as a precursor to creating self-capacities for affective regulation and psychological growth. When early parental environments fail, we see patients who have never achieved such a cohesive, internalized psychic structure. Their selves are, therefore, vulnerable to disintegration anxiety, fragmentation, or a sense of chronic depressive boredom, called enfeeblement. In turn, such patients require the provision of a flexible selfobject matrix or holding environment, first to maintain the homeostatic balance of healthy ego functioning, and later to allow for its internalization.

In Kohut's work there is a great sensitivity to the patient's inner experiences of the treatment environment, with its intermittent crises. He suggests that because BPD patients depend upon others to provide self-equilibrium, they are likely to demand perfect empathy. When, of course, these needs cannot be met, rage may ensue. Kohut explains, however, that this anger is not necessarily untamed primitivism or congenital aggression, but an expression of a lost connection - the pulling of a life sustaining plug for psychological equilibrium which leads to a crisis or regression as its signal of distress. Kohut is clear, however, that this does not mean psychotherapists must demand of themselves to "perform superhuman feats of never failing, perfect empathy" (Kohut, 1977). Failures or "therapeutic derailments" are unavoidable in treatment. Nonetheless, it is important for the therapist to persist with efforts to empathically provide, within the holding environment, the opportunity for patients to learn to soothe themselves through the crisis, without either having to attack and blame themselves or be attacked by others. This, of course, will eventually allow for the creation of internalized psychological structures for holding and self-soothing.

Adler and Buie. Adler and Buie have pinpointed a core existential state of frightening and painful *aloneness*, which they argue is characteristic of borderline psychopathology (Adler, 1985; Adler & Buie, 1979; Buie & Adler, 1982). Such aloneness, they propose, is the result of a developmental deficit of the capacity (in times of distress) to recall in fantasy as in memory a sustaining, holding, or soothing object - the so-called "holding introject" or "holding selfobject." As a result of this sense of painful aloneness that cannot be assuaged by the self, borderline patients engage in the intrapsychic defenses, interpersonal distancing operations, and self-destructive activities for which they are well known.

Borrowing from the work of developmental psychology (Bell), cognitive structuralism (Piaget), psychoanalytic developmental psychology (Fraiberg and Tolpin), object relations (Winnicott), and self-psychology (Kohut), Adler and Buie integrate these theories into an etiological understanding of borderline psychopathology which traces itself to approximately the second year of life. At this age, according to the authors, patients who are likely to suffer from BPD undergo difficulties in their early caretaking environment which impede their capacity to learn how to use a *transitional object* to soothe themselves at times of distress. This interferes with the development of a very important affective and cognitive process known as *evocative memory*, which should develop during the child's second year. Having acquired a form of object permanence, the child becomes able to re-evoke the image of a soothing, calming, or helping parental object at times when the actual parent is absent, but the child is in need of emotional relief. The inability to achieve a solid form of evocative memory, or the incapacity to utilize evocative memory at times of severe distress, leaves potential borderline patients at an immense disadvantage in soothing or calming themselves when they are upset as adults. In addition, Adler and Buie point out that the rage and hurt which accompanies the sense of separation in such patients further damages their already fragile capacity to evoke a positively tinged memory of a supporting object, and consequently leaves them even further bereft at times of separation. *As a result, separation from a supportive person leaves borderline patients with a sense of hurt and trauma reacted to with rage which, in turn, further hinders them from using any form of positively tinged evocative memory and creates an intolerable sense of panic and aloneness at times of distress.*

The therapeutic interventions advocated by Adler and Buie (1979) and Adler (1985), follow this theoretical underpinning. Adler (1985) suggests intensive individual psychotherapy two to five times a week. He advocates a basically psychoanalytic approach to psychotherapy utilizing: (a) the developmental interpretation of transference, (b) free association, leading to further clarification, (c) interpretation in order to reach unconscious content, and (d) a working-through period to consolidate internal structural gains. To cure what Adler and Buie consider the "primary" sector of borderline psychopathology - the inability to sustain a holding or soothing memory at times of separation, anger, or distress - requires the *therapist to provide actual active selfobject* functions to facilitate and resolve the transference.

Adler and Buie suggest that if one begins the treatment by *not* disturbing the development of the transference, and if the patient is not in a state of acute panic at the outset, then the issues of aloneness should more *gradually* emerge as the psychotherapist listens and understands empathically. Soon the patient will realize that the therapist has a reliable and sustaining capacity. As a consequence, the patient may spontaneously begin to shed some of the distancing techniques used to keep people from getting too close in the past. Then he or she will come to consciously experience, or re-experience, the vulnerable sense of dependence upon significant others for soothing, especially when the panic of separation becomes manifest. When there is an *interruption* in the therapy, for example a vacation or weekend, the early felt needs for selfobject support will emerge, sometimes forcefully.

Adler and Buie explain that the first stage of aloneness may appear as a sense of joylessness or lack of meaning in life. Eventually it may well into a deep sense of emptiness or loneliness, and a concomitant rage at the whole environment, but particularly at the therapist for not providing the desired amount of continuous soothing. During times of separation in the psychotherapy, the patient's rage may become so extreme that all evocative memory capacity is lost. Even the memory of the soothing therapist in previous sessions may be forgotten or replaced with a more negatively tinged sense of an uncaring person. Therefore, the central therapeutic task becomes the creation of an environment in which interactions between therapist and patient can eventually lead to taking in and holding onto real memories of sustaining and soothing at times of aloneness. This, in turn, should provide the internal structure for patients eventually to soothe themselves at times of distress.

Adler has described three phases in the treatment of borderline patients. In the first phase, there is initial regression with the full emergence of rage around abandonment and separation, fears of the loss of any positive sustaining holding memories, and worry about getting too close to or far from one's primary objects. During this phase, the psychotherapist must be able to use clarification, interpretation, psychological "holding," and limit setting to protect the patient from overt self-destruction or ruining the possibility for ongoing psychotherapy. Also, the therapist may have to extend him or herself directly to forestall more pathological regression. This may include offering intermittent telephone calls between sessions, negotiation of extra appointments, or when the going gets extremely rough, brief periods of hospitalization to continue intensive psychotherapy. The therapist must attempt to mitigate the level of rage and consequent loss of holding memories, so that they do not completely overwhelm the patient and can still be explored therapeutically. The therapist's actions, up to and including an allowance of several phone calls per day, sustains in the patient a sense of the therapist's "good-enough" provision of a new holding environment, and allows recognition that the therapist can tolerate the patient's rage, hurt, and loneliness and can continue to be helpful (Winnicott, 1965).

One specific way that a therapist may enhance the patient's capacity to provide soothing, in his or her absence, is through the use of Winnicott's *transitional object*. Adler and Buie suggest that it may, at times, be appropriate to use and share objects affectively connected with a therapist to help sustain patients during times of need. For example, something on the therapist's letterhead, in his or her own handwriting, or some piece of material mutually valued as a content of the specific therapeutic work, may be given to the patient during times of separation from the therapist. Many patients, as Buie and Adler note, use their own creative forms of transitional objects such as journal diaries, tape recordings of sessions, and so on. If things go well during this phase, the patient will begin to use holding, soothing memories of the therapist in a more positive manner and may begin to recall other such memories from the past. Such partial identifications, however, are likely to be highly idealized.

In the second phase of treatment, the issue of "optimal disillusionment" (see Kohut, 1977) becomes a central function. Patients are gradually able to notice the reality of the selfobject transference and their need to idealize the therapist as a calming, omnipotent object. Consequently, they gain the capacity to gradually relinquish their idealized view of the psychotherapist. Each moment of seeing the therapist as he or she really is may help the patient integrate the soothing, calming qualities once imagined to exist only in the idealized other. In the third phase of the treatment, the therapist performs the selfobject functions of admiring and supporting the growing autonomous capacities of the patient. The patient's own sense of personal competence, of caring about and for oneself, and of holding oneself through time is recognized, supported, and understood. The selfobject function of recognizing the capacity and wish for being *separate* from the other, as well as *attached*, becomes the central thrust of the therapist's work. If all goes well, the patient eventually becomes able to admire and treat himself or herself, as well as the significant others in his or her life, with the same respect, admiration, understanding, and feeling once expected from the psychotherapy.

Advantages and Disadvantages. Clearly, one of the central strengths of Adler and Buie's "holding environment" approach to treatment is the capacity to empathically understand the existential pain of aloneness, which many borderline patients bring to psychotherapy. Also, their flexible support for an active and creative interactional approach to treatment, and recognition of the *legitimacy of the need for depending upon others*, which is so central to borderline patients, makes such a treatment effective for the BPD patient. This approach may also help avoid struggles over limits by allowing a more mutual therapeutic process.

One criticism of this approach is that it may confuse the real needs for support with the gratification of more libidinally or aggressively derived demands. In this case, instead of providing necessary selfobject support, an inappropriate type of addictive and collusive enactment between therapist and patient may ensue. It is my experience, however, that when carried out from a psychoanalytically oriented perspective, such an approach is unlikely to lead to this end in the hands of a qualified psychotherapist who seeks appropriate supervision or consultation. Another criticism of this approach is the idea that it does not directly face the patient's aggression and rage. Adler and Buie, however, would argue that rage is a central aspect of the treatment, which can be understood empathically as a response to loss of the supportive object. Their goal is to help patients understand and sympathize with their own anger as part of an ongoing process of internalizing the soothing qualities of the psychotherapist.

NEWER CLINICAL APPROACHES TO BPD

Although it is beyond the scope of this contribution to describe all the alternative treatments for BPD, it is important to note some other significant contributions. The integrative clinical and theoretical work of Gunderson (1984) deserves special mention. Gunderson's (1984) most recent book synthesizes much of the available research on borderline personality disorder and describes effective clinical approaches to the treatment of borderline patients. Gunderson's delineation of the phases of treatment and levels of borderline functioning is likely to be of use to any clinician involved in the intensive treatment of BPD. His suggestions for treatment of such patients fall between the more confrontational, limit setting, and aggression-oriented approach of Kernberg, and the more holding environment, soothing-selfobject approach of Adler and Buie.

THE ROLE OF FAMILIES IN TREATMENT

Although research on the role of borderline patients' families in psychotherapeutic intervention comes from the inpatient treatment of such disorders, the inclusion of the patient's family members is worthy of consideration (E. Shapiro et al., 1975; E. Shapiro, R. Shapiro, & Zinner, 1977). Gunderson and his research team at McLean Hospital have delineated two distinct family patterns in borderline patients: those characterized by overinvolvement and those characterized by abandonment and neglect. Gunderson (1984) suggests that overinvolved families be contained within the therapeutic environment of family treatment, while neglectful families not be involved as they are unlikely to achieve any therapeutic gain, and may indeed enact their rage in a harmful way. In my experience with outpatient psychotherapy of BPD patients, the level of the patient's autonomous functioning, his or her age, and his or her actual economic or emotional dependence on the family should be taken into account in the decision to involve family members in treatment.

Psychotherapy of the borderline family is an exciting and potentially useful task if carried out by an appropriately trained clinician. E. Shapiro and his colleagues (1975, 1977) advocate a rational organization of such a therapeutic approach for adolescents or young adults. They use conjoint weekly family therapy in conjunction with individual psychodynamic psychotherapy for the identified patient and ongoing couples treatment for the parents. The conjoint family treatment would be carried out in tandem by the therapist for the individual psychotherapy and the couple's therapist. If the borderline patient is older and married, or engaged in a significant relationship, ongoing couples treatment may be appropriate as an adjunct to the individual psychotherapy.

IMPROVING WORK SKILLS

In my experience, rehabilitation aimed at work skills represents one of the greatest untapped resources in the treatment of BPD. Often these patients are severely deficient in vocational functioning (Gunderson, 1977). Anthony (1977) has outlined a psychological approach to vocational rehabilitation of mental health patients, and we have had good experiences combining individual treatment with clinical vocational interventions at McLean Hospital. Success in the work place often enhances self-esteem and progress in treatment. Nonetheless, analytically oriented clinicians have been reluctant to make full use of such approaches (Pollack & Dion, 1985).

COGNITIVE-BEHAVIORAL AND PARADOXICAL TECHNIQUES

Bond (in press) has suggested an innovative paradoxical technique for helping borderline patients to motivate their more autonomous capacities, especially at times when they may be involved in negativistic regressions. He cites examples of several patients who demonstrated their distress by avoiding any additional responsibilities in their lives. Rather than engaging in a senseless and negativistic struggle, he helped therapeutic staff to "join" the patients by accepting the severity of their problems and then overdramatizing just how incapable the patients were. As the therapist or staff overestimated patients' inabilities to function competently and began to suggest perhaps doing even less, patients would paradoxically begin to assume increased responsibility for their lives, and improve despite the staff's underestimation of them.

Levendusky (Berglas & Levendusky, 1985; Levendusky et al., 1983; Levendusky & Dooley, 1985) have structured an entire treatment regimen for severely disturbed character disordered patients which centers around a modification of cognitive behavioral techniques. A therapeutic contract, group feedback, and structured cognitive behavioral planning have helped borderline patients take increased responsibility for their lives and begin to cope with the anxiety which ensues when they attempt greater social interaction or higher levels of vocational functioning. Of particular interest is the use of (a) assertiveness training skills to help patients who feel downtrodden but become overly aggressive to meet their needs, (b) mood monitoring to help patients understand their affective lability while connecting it to external events, and (c) a basic form of group social skill training to support the acquisition of new behaviors through group cohesiveness and peer confrontation. To be effective, such a program must be planned by a skilled clinician who understands the realities of BPD.

GROUP PSYCHOTHERAPY

Horwitz (1977, 1980) has summarized many of the basic advantages of group psychotherapy with borderline patients. He suggests that (a) the intensity of transference and countertransference reactions can be positively diluted through use of multiple therapeutic objects in the group; (b) peer members in the group aid in the direction of reality testing and supporting appropriate social interaction; (c) the need for social and emotional distance may be titrated in a healthy manner by peers within the group; (d) peer pressure in the group may help patients who have difficulties with their anger to find more reasonable outlets than they might find in individual psychotherapy alone; (e) there are opportunities for multiple identifications if the patient has more than just the healthy capacities of one therapist to internalize or identify with; and (f) the group interaction must focus eventually on issues such as jealousy, competition, and narcissistic defenses in a way that can be quite powerful and therapeutic.

My own experience also indicates that patients are likely to accept confrontations and interpretations from other patients earlier in treatment than they would with individual psychotherapy. Consequently, issues of negativism toward authority or of a sense of being controlled are less likely to emerge among peers in the group.

Kibel (1980) as well as Roth (1980, 1982) suggest careful evaluation procedures before placing borderline patients in groups, including intensive pregroup screening and diagnostic evaluation. Wong (1980) feels strongly that groups should be heterogeneous in terms of diagnosis. Also, he advocates combining individual and group therapy conducted by the same therapist for patients with BPD. Stone and Weissman (1984) believe borderline patients do better when they are in groups that have other borderline members, to avoid risks of isolation and early termination. Macaskill (1982) notes the importance of the group therapist or group itself functioning along the lines of Winnicott's "holding environment" and being the "good-enough mother." Macaskill also stresses the capacity to provide soothing interpretations while instilling hope as important prognostic indicators for therapeutic efficacy in group psychotherapy for BPD.

PSYCHOPHARMACOLOGY

Some researchers and clinicians advocate various psychopharmacological interventions as a central or adjunctive treatment for BPD. Medications suggested include: (a) low dose antipsychotics (Brinkley, Beitman, & Friedel, 1979; Serban & Seigal, 1984), (b) heterocyclic antidepressants (Akiskal, 1981; Liebowitz, 1983), (c) MAO inhibitors (Klein, 1977), (d) lithium (Rifkin et al, 1972), and most recently, (e) Pemoline or Methylphenidate (Wood et al., 1976; Wender, Reimherr, & Wood, 1981), and (f) Carbamazepine (Tegretol) (Schatzberg, 1983). The choice of drug, of course, relates to the theoretical connection postulated between BPD and other more biologically linked illnesses. For example, one group of researchers connect aspects of borderline personality disorder with the affective disease spectrum and recommend a series of psychopharmacological treatments that have worked in unipolar and atypical depressions (see Gunderson & Elliott, 1984). Others see aspects of minimal brain dysfunction or a residual attention deficit disorder in some adults with BPD (Andrulonis et al., 1981). Still another group identifies some of the symptoms of BPD with syndromes commonly associated with limbic discharge disorders. Cole and Sunderland (1982), Liebowitz (1983), and Gunderson and Elliott (1984) have described the current psychopharmacological treatment regimens for borderline patients.

Although it is currently somewhat confusing to identify an appropriate pharmacological treatment for a borderline patient, there are several rules of thumb for the clinician. First, one should consider the possibility that patients with borderline personality disorder may also suffer from an affective illness - most likely unipolar depression (Gunderson & Elliott, 1984; Pope et al., 1983). These depressions may respond to psychotherapy alone, but they may also require medication. Clinicians who are used to treating depression psychopharmacologically may overlook an underlying personality disorder which will interfere with progress. However, therapists who tend to eschew medication may miss an opportunity to aid borderline patients by relieving biologically based depressive symptomatology.

Another aspect of psychopharmacology as an adjunct to the psychotherapy of BPD is the psychodynamics involved in prescribing "pills." The nature of the transitional object transference to both medication and to the prescribing treater (Adelman, 1985; Gunderson, 1984) must be understood and addressed. The use of medication in psychotherapy is bound to have its repercussions within the treatment environment and sometimes outside of it. Clinicians should consider the underlying meaning of giving pills to patients with a yearning for closeness and need for early parenting, and should proceed with caution and flexibility.

The need for a strong therapeutic alliance between patient and therapist or patient and prescribing physician is extremely important with BPD. In the absence of such an alliance, patients are likely either not to use the medication or to use it in a self-destructive manner. Part of such an alliance must be an open discussion of the meaning of the medication for the particular patient. If the prescribing physician and the psychotherapist are two different people, it is important to maintain frequent contact to avoid any "splitting" of these two helpers. Prescribing medication that is *least likely to be lethal*, and, at times, limiting the number of pills per prescription, may be necessary in the early psychopharmacological treatment of a borderline patient with suicidal impulses.

SPECIAL ISSUES IN TREATMENT

HANDLING AGGRESSION

A therapist's approach to aggression will no doubt be integrated into his or her theoretical and clinical approach to the overall psychotherapeutic treatment of the borderline patient. Kernberg's approach is to confront, limit, and interpret the patient's expression of aggression or rage from the beginning of treatment. As suggested above, this may be experienced by the patient as a sense of strength and capability on the therapist's part. At other times it may be experienced by patients as a form of invalidating the genuineness of their anger.

Adler and Buie view rage as a legitimate signal of a hurtful sense of disconnection or separation. Increasing rage may decrease the capacity for remembering the therapist as soothing or calming, leading the patient to feel even more distressed. Consequently, they advocate an empathic response and increased support during times of stress or separation from the therapist. Transitional objects are one mechanism they use to aid the process.

Gunderson (1984), in an attempt to find an intervention for borderline patients' aggression somewhere between the "confrontation" and "holding" camps, advocates an "ego psychological approach" to anger. He feels that one does an injustice to the borderline patient by either legitimizing the anger or by interpreting it quickly as a distorted, unrealistic response to the environment. His approach suggests joining with the patient to mutually explore the meaning of rageful experiences on a cognitive ego-psychological level. He also stresses discussion of the interpersonal meaning of the anger within psychotherapy. This should allow for enough ongoing expression to deepen the therapeutic transference, while limiting the severity when it threatens the therapy. In this way, Gunderson feels that one can recognize the patient's inner sense of "badness" and guilt, while continuing to help patients to "own up" or take responsibility for their rageful responses.

In my experience, BPD patients are almost always able to sense whether their therapist is comfortable with their aggression, can tolerate its affective expression, and is able to let them know when things are getting out of hand. In general, when one is able to achieve a balance of tolerating patients' genuine affect while setting limits on feelings that may lead to destructive actions, patients will feel increasingly secure to share a whole range of feelings, in addition to aggression. This should deepen the treatment and ultimately lead to patients' genuine tolerance for their own internal feeling states.

COUNTERTRANSFERENCE: THE THERAPIST'S OWN AGGRESSION

A major component of deep and intensive psychotherapy with BPD patients is the therapist's own hateful countertransference experiences which become mobilized in treatment. Whether one assumes this is an aspect of projective identification created by the patient's engendering of negative affects in the psychotherapist (see Kernberg, 1984) or believes the therapist is feeling hurt and angry because he or she is accused of being an inadequate selfobject or deficient holding environment, the therapist must remain aware of his or her own rage and hate which are likely to emerge in the treatment (Madow & Pollack, under review; Maltsberger & Buie, 1974). All countertransference experiences, especially those of being enraged at patients or wishing to hurt them, or feeling love for them and wishing to rescue them, should be monitored because either course may prove inappropriate.

Adler and Buie (1972) have pointed out the misuses of confrontation with borderline patients. Most often, these involve so-called clarifications or interpretations that are not really aimed at making psychological change but at appealing to a sense in patients that they have been "bad" and should desist. If therapists engage in such interpretations either by error or as a form of unconscious aggression, they may increase their patients' self-hate and engender self-destructive behavior. One cannot underestimate the borderline patient's capacity to unconsciously understand the therapist's anger and act out in a suicidal manner. To forestall such events, therapists should follow Winnicott's (1975) suggestion to accept and bear their own experiences of hate toward the patient (Winnicott, 1975) without enacting them. Therapists who are angry and unaware may confront a borderline patient at a time when he or she is *struggling to survive*, with disastrous results.

If one's own countertransference hate is either not conscious, or appears to be "leaking out" in the psychotherapy, consultation with a senior colleague is appropriate. Another technique I have used sparingly is to discuss with extremely angry patients who are engendering a great deal of hate the idea of one's own limits. I have found that under the right circumstances, with an already established alliance, sharing with the patient the fact that "if you continue to be as rageful and as negative as you have been, it may make me less able to be empathic," usually allows the patient to recognize the extremity of their position and to modify it to maintain the integrity of the therapist and the psychotherapy.

SELF-DESTRUCTIVE BEHAVIORS

Treatment of BPD requires the therapist's awareness of the possibility of suicide gestures. The difficult balance in treating the BPD patient requires the therapist to tolerate suicidal wishes and fantasies, while being active enough to intervene when actual suicide threatens. Although the two treatment paradigms we described above differ in their understanding of the patient's aggression and how it should be handled, there is a consensus that rage and hurt may reach a point where self-destruction appears to patients as their only way out. Also, patients with BPD may deal with the intolerance of their strong affect through minor forms of self-harm (cutting, minor accidents, hand banging, etc.), or they may have the need to "soothe themselves" for long periods of time with fantasies about death. One should not prematurely intervene in such activities if they are not seriously self-destructive and represent the patient's means of maintaining a psychological equilibrium.

What the therapist must always do in these circumstances is take the patient's feelings, thoughts, and plans *seriously.* Gunderson (1984) suggests that there are basically two classes of self-destructive activity in borderline patients. One occurs as a connection to a primary object and should be understood within the interpersonal milieu of therapist and patient. Here patients may be expressing their anger, hurt, or disappointment with the present therapeutic arrangement. They may be stating through their action, "Please change things for me, or help me differently." Such gestures can usually be understood within the context of psychotherapy, and clarified during the therapeutic hours. If crisis intervention is necessary, the therapist should be understanding and supportive until the issues can be discussed in a safe environment.

The other type of self-destructive activity, according to Gunderson, occurs following an experience of abandonment by a primary object or a severe derailment in psychotherapy. Here we see the aspects of the growing aloneness panic described by Adler and Buie. Patients may need to harm themselves in small ways to gain a sense of numbness or expel their bad feelings. Otherwise, this may escalate quickly into a guilty or empty sense which leads to self-destruction. The discussion of such feelings, the signals of their occurrence, or the description of clear plans to hurt oneself under these conditions should alert the therapist to a *serious suicide risk.* Sometimes psychotherapists mistake such desperate discussions as attempts to "manipulate" more time and effort. If such needs are not responded to quickly and directly, they well may lead to a *completed suicide.* Under these conditions the therapist should do everything in his or her power to provide the necessary additional organization and structure for the patient, including additional sessions, phone calls, or if necessary, acute hospitalization.

In general, therapists should be aware that with borderline patients suicide is always a possibility. In the early phases of treatment and before an alliance is established, one should be careful to inquire after missed appointments, perhaps telephoning the patient should there be any suspicion of concern. When patients discuss their suicidal wishes or plans, one should inquire actively about what they might mean, helping to differentiate a cry for help from a sense of despair that requires active intervention. However, both forms of experience need to be responded to appropriately.

If the patient appears to be floundering or unable to use additional therapeutic support (e.g., phone calls, additional sessions), hospitalization should be utilized. *Hospitalization does not necessarily mean a failure of psychotherapy.* The therapist's inner experience of anxiety may serve as a benchmark for the level of distress in his or her patient. Should a therapist's anxiety become so extreme that he or she is always worried about the patient's safety, therapy and patient are in jeopardy. This must be discussed with the patient and worked through with either additional structural supports (e.g., hospitalization) or a change in the structural arrangements of the psychotherapy. If one is seriously concerned about the patient's safety, it is better to act to create a secure environment first, and then to discuss what has occurred with the patient. There will be little use for limit setting or a therapeutically "neutral" approach if the patient is no longer alive!

WHEN ENOUGH IS ENOUGH: HOSPITALIZATION AND CONSULTATION

When intensive outpatient psychotherapy cannot stem the tide of the BPD patient's self-destructive acting out, inpatient hospitalization is indicated. The attempt to maintain outpatient psychotherapy at all costs is likely to cost too much. If patients are aware that their therapists do not believe in hospitalization or will not utilize it, they may have an unconscious need to push limits to the brink in a dangerous way. Short-term inpatient hospitalization is indicated when (a) active structural additions to outpatient psychotherapy do not stop the self-destructive enactment, (b) the therapist's level of anxiety about the patient's safety reaches a point where reasonable comfort in a psychotherapy is no longer possible, (c) the abuse of substances, eating difficulties, or other self-destructive personal activities require a structured environment for detoxification, or (d) countertransference experiences become so intense that patient and therapist need a breather in a setting where other skilled clinicians can help (see Gunderson, 1984; Madow & Pollack, under review).

A day treatment center or day hospital setting is an excellent alternative to inpatient hospitalization. Not only is such a therapeutic approach more cost-efficient and flexible, but it may provide the proper balance between a holding environment, and the capacity for separation and autonomy so necessary for borderline patients (Pollack, 1983a). In either active day treatment or short-term hospitalization, the psychotherapist should feel comfortable with the philosophy of the treating unit. If a sense of mutual trust between therapist and hospital setting does not exist, it is unlikely that a successful result will ensue. When outpatient psychotherapists feel that they have had enough, they should be candid about their wish to terminate with the patient while the patient is in the hospital. Under these conditions, the hospital staff may be helpful in finding an alternative psychotherapeutic arrangement.

Long-term, intensive inpatient hospitalization as the primary intervention for BPD has been reviewed elsewhere (Frosch, 1983; Gunderson, 1984). Generally, it seems advisable to reserve such intensive, long-term inpatient treatments of BPD for those patients who have shown an inability to sustain reasonable functioning in intensive outpatient psychotherapy. For patients who are hospitalized, it seems reasonable to consider their discharge when they appear able to sustain themselves in intensive outpatient psychotherapy without the need of the secure inpatient environment.

When less acute psychotherapeutic impasse occurs, *consultation* on an outpatient basis should be considered. Often psychotherapists feel wary of opening their treatments to colleagues, especially when this occurs under the somewhat angry or negative demands of dissatisfied patients. However, it is important to be flexible in seeking peer consultation when working with BPD patients. As long as the consultation is discussed openly with the patient, this process may model for them the possibility of problem solving with appropriate input from others. I recommend that both the therapist and patient talk to the consultant. Sometimes patients experience the use of a consultant as an important adjunct to the therapy and request that it be available on an ongoing basis. As long as such a process is not misused, it has many benefits for the therapist and patient alike.

BALANCING AUTONOMY AND AFFILIATION

Some psychotherapeutic paradigms for the treatment of BPD stress the importance of separation or individuation (Kernberg, 1984; Mahler, 1971); others highlight the importance of human interconnection (Adler, 1985; Adler & Buie, 1979; Kohut, 1977). Yet there is growing evidence to suggest that it is the *balance* of *autonomy* and *affiliation* - both within oneself and between oneself and one's social system - that supports normal, healthy human development. I have argued elsewhere (Pollack, 1982, 1983a, 1983b; Pollack & Grossman, 1985) that for healthy child development and normal parental response the capacities to experience and sustain an independent sense of oneself (*autonomy*) and an interconnected relation with others (*affiliation*) should be flexibly balanced. The Boston University Pregnancy and Parenthood Project (Grossman, 1985; Pollack & Grossman, 1985) has also supported the idea of an autonomy-affiliation balance as essential in normal individual and family development. The historical emphasis on autonomy as a measure of mental health may well reflect a masculine bias.

The integration of a better understanding of female development with object relations theory, normal childhood development, and parental functioning throughout the life cycle leads to important clinical implications. As Stiver (1985) has suggested elsewhere, we may be too preoccupied with the negative aspects of so-called "dependency" and not aware enough of normal, healthy needs to remain dependent on significant others or our social network. In the treatment of BPD, such dependency needs are paramount. Often, therapists stress the importance for individuation or autonomy building without maintaining an equal valuation of affiliative connection. In my own practice, it has become clear that severely disturbed or character disordered patients are not suffering from "overdependency" as much as from inability to recognize the legitimacy of their needs to depend on others and build an *interdependent* network of support.

The achievement of structural change in the psychotherapy of BPD is likely to require a capacity for interdependent mutual support as well as for enhanced autonomous functioning. The ability to tolerate aloneness must be balanced with the wish to tolerate togetherness. Psychotherapists must carefully consider this issue in their treatment of BPD patients.

SUMMARY

Treatment of BPD presents the clinician with stimulating but sometimes frightening dilemmas, as well as a myriad of potential satisfactions. The ability to accurately diagnose borderline personality disorder, and to utilize the knowledge gained for the in-depth therapeutic repair of long-standing emotional damage in such patients, provides the psychotherapist with the ultimate satisfaction of knowing that one has truly helped another human being. Knowing one's own limitations about such helping, and experiencing one's own feelings of hurt, disappointment, hate, and love, also are the invariable by-products of any such successful treatment.

In reviewing the current state of knowledge about the diagnosis and treatment of BPD, however, one becomes humbly aware of how much is yet to be learned. Consequently, the clinician should be able to tolerate a great deal of uncertainty, and to recognize the need for a great deal of creative flexibility in applying the principles outlined above. Work with the borderline patient takes us to the geographical and emotional *borders* of our own experience and, at times, to the limits of our emotions and strengths. Those of us willing to undertake the task must be equally willing to assume the attitude of explorers at the border or frontier: cautious optimism coupled with therapeutic flexibility.

William S. Pollack, PhD, is currently Psychologist-in-Charge of Codman House III, McLean Hospital; Director of Continuing Education in Psychology, McLean Hospital; and Instructor in Psychology, Department of Psychiatry, Harvard Medical School. His training is in clinical psychology. He has done research and published in the areas of personality disorders and treatment approaches to severe psychopathology, as well as in the fields of parent-child interaction; the interrelationships between object relations/self-object psychoanalytic theories; and group, organizational, and family processes. In addition to his clinical, research, and consultation duties at McLean, he teaches Harvard Medical School residents in psychiatry and interns in psychology. He also maintains a private practice in psychotherapy and organizational consultation. Dr. Pollack may be contacted through McLean Hospital, 115 Mill Street, Belmont, MA 02178.

RESOURCES

Adelman, S. (1985). Pills as transitional objects: A dynamic understanding of the use of medication in psychotherapy. *Psychiatry, 48,* 246-253.

Adler, G. (1985). *Borderline Psychopathology and Its Treatment.* New York: Jason Aronson.

Adler, G., & Buie, D. (1972). The misuses of confrontation with borderline patients. *International Journal of Psychoanalytic Psychotherapy, 1,* 109-120.

Adler, G., & Buie, D. (1979). Aloneness and borderline psychopathology: The possible relevance of child development issues. *International Journal of Psychoanalysis, 60,* 83-96.

Akiskal, H. (1981). Sub-affective disorders, dysthymic, cyclothymic and bipolar II disorders in the borderline realm. *Psychiatric Clinics of North America, 4,* 25-46.

Akiskal, H. (1983). The relationship of personality to affective disorders. *Archives of General Psychiatry, 40,* 801-810.

American Psychiatric Association. (1980). *Diagnostic and Statistical Manual of Mental Disorders: DSM-III* (3rd ed.). Washington, DC: Author.

Andrulonis, P., Glueck, B., Stroebel, C., Vogel, N., Shapiro, A., & Aldridge, D. (1981). Organic brain dysfunction and the borderline syndrome. *Psychiatric Clinics of North America, 4,* 47-66.

Anthony, W. A. (1977). Psychological rehabilitation: A concept in need of a method. *American Psychologist, 32,* 658-662.

Baron, M., Asnis, L., & Gruen, R. (1981). The schedule for interviewing borderlines (SIB): A diagnostic interview for schizotypal features. *Journal of Psychiatric Research, 4,* 213-228.

Barrash, I., Kroll, J., Carey, K., & Sines, L. (1983). Discriminating borderline disorder from other personality disorders: Cluster analysis of the diagnostic interview for borderlines. *Archives of General Psychiatry, 40,* 1297-1302.

Bauer, S., Hunt, H., Gould, M., & Goldstein, E. (1980). Personality organization, structural diagnosis and the structural interview. *Psychiatry, 43,* 224-233.

Berglas, S., & Levendusky, P. G. (1985). The therapeutic contract program: An individual oriented psychological treatment community. *Psychotherapy, 22,* 36-45.

Bion, W. R. (1967). *Second Thoughts: Selected Papers on Psychoanalysis.* New York: Basic Books.

Bond, T. (in press). Paradoxical intention in the treatment of borderline patients. *Psychiatry.*

Brandchaft, B., & Stolorow, R. (1984). The borderline concept: Pathological character or iatrogenic myth? In J. Lichtenberg, M. Bornstein, & D. Silver (Eds.), *Empathy, II* (pp. 333-357). Hillside, NJ: The Analytic Press.

Brinkley, J., Beitman, S., & Friedel, R. (1979). Low-dose neuroleptic regimens in the treatment of borderline patients. *Archives of General Psychiatry, 36,* 319-326.

Buie, D., & Adler, G. (1982). The definitive treatment of the borderline personality. *International Journal of Psychoanalytic Psychotherapy, 9,* 51-87.

Carpenter, W., Gunderson, J., & Strauss, J. (1977). Considerations of the borderline syndrome: A longitudinal comparative study of borderline and schizophrenic patients. In P. Hartocollis (Ed.), *Borderline Personality Disorders: The Concept, the Syndrome, the Patient* (pp. 231-253). New York: International Universities Press.

Cole, J., & Sunderland, P. (1982). The drug treatment of borderline patients. In L. Grinspoon (Ed.), *Psychiatry* (Vol. 1 of *Psychiatry* update, pp. 456-470). Washington, DC: American Psychiatric Press.

Cornell, D., Silk, K., Ludolph, P., & Lohr, N. (1983). Test - retest reliability of the diagnostic interview for borderlines. *Archives of General Psychiatry, 40,* 1307-1310.

Deutsch, H. (1942). Some forms of emotional disturbances and their relationship to schizophrenia. *Psychoanalytic Quarterly, 11,* 301-321.

Frances, A., Clarkin, J., Gilmore, M., Hurt, S. W., & Brown, R. (1984). Reliability of criteria for borderline personality disorder: A comparison of DSM-III and DIB. *American Journal of Psychiatry, 141,* 1080-1083.

Friedman, H. (1969). Some problems of inpatient management with borderline patients. *American Journal of Psychiatry, 126,* 299-304.

Friedman, H. (1975). Psychotherapy of borderline patients: The influence of theory on technique. *American Journal of Psychiatry, 132,* 1048-1052.

Frosch, J. (1970). Psychoanalytic considerations of the psychotic character. *Journal of the American Psychoanalytic Association, 18,* 24-50.

Frosch, J. P. (1983). *Current Perspectives in Personality Disorders.* Washington, DC: American Psychiatric Press.

Gilligan, C. (1982). *In a Different Voice.* Cambridge, MA: Harvard University Press.

Giovacchini, P. (1979). *Treatment of Primitive Mental States.* New York: Jason Aronson.

Glover, E. (1932). A psycho-analytic approach to classification of mental disorders. *Journal of Mental Science, 78,* 819-842.

Greenberg, S. (1977). *The Supportive Approach to Therapy.* Unpublished manuscript, McLean Hospital, Belmont, MA.

Grinker, R., Werble, B., & Drye, R. (1968). *The Borderline Syndrome: A Behavioral Study of Ego Functions.* New York: Basic Books.

Grossman, F. K. (1985). Autonomy and affiliation: Parents and children. *Conference Paper Series.* Washington, DC: NICHD.

Grunebaum, H., & Klerman, G. (1967). Wrist slashing. *American Journal of Psychiatry, 124,* 524-534.

Gunderson, J. (1977). Characteristics of borderlines. In P. Hartocollis (Ed.), *Borderline Personality Disorders: The Concept, the Syndrome, the Patient* (pp. 173-192). New York: International Universities Press.

Gunderson, J. (1982). Empirical studies of the borderline diagnosis. In L. Grinspoon (Ed.), *Psychiatry* (Vol. 1 of *Psychiatry* update, pp. 414-437). Washington, DC: American Psychiatric Press.

Gunderson, J. (1983). Discussion of Chessick, R.: Problems in the intensive psychotherapy of the borderline patient. *Dynamic Psychotherapy, 1,* 33-34. (a)

Gunderson, J. (1983, December). *Interfaces Between Psychoanalytic and Empirical Studies of Borderline Personality Disorder.* Unpublished paper presented at the annual meeting of the American Psychoanalytic Association, New York. (b)

Gunderson, J. (1984). *Borderline Personality Disorder.* Washington, DC: American Psychiatric Press.

Gunderson, J., Carpenter, W., & Strauss, J. (1975). Borderline and schizophrenic patients: A comparative study. *American Journal of Psychiatry, 132,* 1257-1264.

Gunderson, J., & Elliott, G. (1985). The interface between borderline personality disorder and affective disorder. *American Journal of Psychiatry, 142,* 277-288.

Gunderson, J., & Englund, D. (1981). Characterizing the families of borderlines. *Psychiatric Clinics of North America, 4,* 159-168.

Gunderson, J., & Kolb, J. (1978). Discriminating features of borderline patients. *American Journal of Psychiatry, 135,* 792-796.

Gunderson, J., Kolb, J., & Austin, V. (1981). The diagnostic interview for borderline patients. *American Journal of Psychiatry, 138,* 896-903.

Gunderson, J., & Pollack, W. (1985). Conceptual risks of the axis I-II division. In H. Klar & L. J. Siever (Eds.), *Biological Response Styles: Clinical Implications.* Washington, DC: American Psychiatric Press.

Gunderson, J., & Singer, M. (1975). Defining borderline patients: An overview. *American Journal of Psychiatry, 132,* 1-10.

Horwitz, L. (1977). Group psychotherapy of the borderline patient. In P. Hartocollis (Ed.), *Borderline Personality Disorders: The Concept, the Syndrome, the Patient* (pp. 399-422). New York: International Universities Press.

Horwitz, L. (1980). Group psychotherapy for borderline and narcissistic patients. *Bulletin of the Menninger Clinic, 44,* 181-200.

Hoch, P., & Polatin, P. (1949). Pseudoneurotic forms of schizophrenia. *Psychiatric Quarterly, 23,* 248-276.

Hurt, S. W., Hyler, S. E., Frances, A., Clarkin, J. F., & Brent, R. (1984). Assessing borderline personality disorder with self-report, clinical interview, or semistructured interview. *American Journal of Psychiatry, 141,* 1228-1231.

Hyler, S. E., Rieder, R., Spitzer, R. L., & Williams, J. B. W. (1978). *Personality Diagnostic Questionnaire (PDQ).* New York: New York State Psychiatric Institute.

Institute of Medicine. (1985). A report of the board on mental health and behavioral medicine: Research on mental illness and addictive disorders: Progress and prospects. Supplement to the *American Journal of Psychiatry, 142,* (July, 1985).

Kass, F., Skodol, A. E., Charles, E., Spitzer, R. L., & Williams, J. B. W. (1985). Scaled ratings of DSM III personality disorders. *American Journal of Psychiatry, 142,* 627-630.

Kass, F., Spitzer, R. L., & Williams, J. B. W. (1983). An empirical study of the issue of sex bias in the diagnostic criteria of DSM III Axis II personality disorder. *American Psychologist, 38,* 799-801.

Kernberg, O. (1965). Countertransference. *Journal of the American Psychoanalytic Association, 13,* 38-56.

Kernberg, O. (1967). Borderline personality organization. *Journal of the American Psychoanalytic Association, 15,* 641-685.

Kernberg, O. (1971). Prognostic considerations regarding borderline personality organization. *Journal of the American Psychoanalytic Association, 19,* 595-615.

Kernberg, O. (1975). *Borderline Conditions and Pathological Narcissism.* New York: Jason Aronson.

Kernberg, O. (1976). *Object-Relations Theory and Clinical Psychoanalysis.* New York: Jason Aronson.

Kernberg, O. (1977). The structural diagnosis of borderline personality organization. In P. Hartocollis (Ed.), *Borderline Personality Disorders: The Concept, the Syndrome, the Patient* (pp. 87-121). New York: International Universities Press.

Kernberg, O. (1981). Structural interviewing. *Psychiatric Clinics of North America, 4,* 169-195.

Kernberg, O. (1982). Supportive psychotherapy with borderline conditions. In J. Cavenar & H. Brodie (Eds.), *Critical Problems in Psychiatry* (pp. 180-202). Philadelphia, PA: Lippincott.

Kernberg, O. (1983, February). Cited in *Medical World News.*

Kernberg, O. (1984). *Severe Personality Disorders: Psychotherapeutic Strategies.* New Haven: Yale University Press.

Kernberg, O., Burstein, E., Coyne, L., Appelbaum, A., Horwitz, L., & Voth, H. (1972). Final report of the Menninger Foundation's psychotherapy research project: Psychotherapy and psychoanalysis. *Bulletin of the Menninger Clinic, 34,* 1-2.

Kibel, H. (1980). The importance of a comprehensive clinical diagnosis for group psychotherapy of borderline and narcissistic patients. *International Journal of Group Psychotherapy, 30,* 427-440.

Klein, D. (1977). Psychopharmacological treatment and delineation of borderline disorders. In P. Hartocollis (Ed.), *Borderline Personality Disorders: The Concept, the Syndrome, the Patient* (pp. 365-384). New York: International Universities Press.

Klein, M. (1946). Notes on some schizoid mechanisms. *International Journal of Psychoanalysis, 27,* 99-110.

Knight, R. (1953). Borderline states. *Bulletin of the Menninger Clinic, 17,* 1-12.

Koenigsberg, H., Kaplan, R. D., Gilmore, M. M., & Cooper, A. M. (1985). The relationship between syndrome and personality disorder in DSM III: Experience with 2,462 patients. *American Journal of Psychiatry, 142,* 207-212.

Koenigsberg, H., Kernberg, O., & Schomer, J. (1983). Diagnosing borderline conditions in an outpatient setting. *Archives of General Psychiatry, 40,* 49-53.

Kohut, H. (1971). *The Analysis of the Self.* New York: International Universities Press.

Kohut, H. (1977). *The Restoration of the Self.* New York: International Universities Press.

Kohut, H. (1980). From a letter. In A. Goldberg (Ed.), *Advances in Self-Psychology.* New York: International Universities Press.

Kohut, H., & Wolf, E. (1978). The disorders of the self and their treatment: An outline. *International Journal of Psychoanalysis, 59,* 413-425.

Kolb, J., & Gunderson, J. (1980). Diagnosing borderline patients within semi-structured interviews. *Archives of General Psychiatry, 37,* 37-41.

Kroll, J., Carey, K., Sines, L., & Roth, M. (1982). Are there borderlines in Britain? A cross-validation of U.S. findings. *Archives of General Psychiatry, 39,* 60-63.

Kroll, J., Sines, L., Martin, K., Lari, S., Pyle, R., & Zander, J. (1981). Borderline personality disorder: Construct validity of the concept. *Archives of General Psychiatry, 38,* 1021-1026.

Levendusky, P. G., Berglas, S., Dooley, C. P., & Landau, R. J. (1983). Therapeutic contract program: A preliminary report on a behavioral alternative to the token economy. *Behavior Research and Therapy, 21*, 137-142.

Levendusky, P. G., & Dooley, C. P. (1985). An inpatient model for the treatment of anorexia nervosa. In S. Emmett (Ed.), *Theory and Treatment of Anorexia Nervosa and Bulimia -- Biomedical, Sociocultural and Psychological Perspectives* (pp. 211-233). New York: Brunner/Mazel.

Levine, H. B. (1979). The sustaining object relationship. *The Annual of Psychoanalysis, 7*, 203-232.

Liebowitz, M. (1983). Psychopharmacological intervention in personality disorders. In J. Frosch (Ed.), *Current Perspectives on Personality Disorders* (pp. 68-93). Washington, DC: American Psychiatric Press.

Loranger, A. W., Oldham, J. M., Russakoff, L. M., & Susman, V. L. (1984). *Personality Disorder Examination: A Structured Interview for Making DSM-III Axis II Diagnoses (PDE)*. White Plains, NY: The New York Hospital - Cornell Medical Center, Westchester Division.

Madow, M., & Pollack, W. S. (under review). *Countertransference and Inpatient Psychiatry*.

Macaskill, N. (1982). Therapeutic factors in group therapy with borderline patients. *International Journal of Group Psychotherapy, 32*, 61-74.

Mahler, M. (1971). A study of the separation-individuation process and its possible application to borderline phenomena in the psychoanalytic situation. *Psychoanalytic Study of the Child, 26*, 403-424.

Mahler, M. (1972). Rapprochement subphase of the separation-individuation process. *Psychoanalytic Quarterly, 41*, 487-506.

Mahler, M., & Kaplan, L. (1977). Developmental aspects in the assessment of narcissistic and so-called borderline personalities. In P. Hartocollis (Ed.), *Borderline Personality Disorders: The Concept, the Syndrome, the Patient* (pp. 71-86). New York: International Universities Press.

Mahler, M., Pine, F., & Bergman, A. (1975). *The Psychological Birth of the Human Infant*. New York: Basic Books.

Maltsberger, J. T., & Buie, D. H. (1974). Countertransference hate in the treatment of suicidal patients. *Archives of General Psychiatry, 30*, 625-633.

Masterson, J. (1971). Treatment of the adolescent with borderline syndrome (a problem in separation-individuation). *Bulletin of the Menninger Clinic, 35*, 5-18.

Masterson, J. (1976). *Psychotherapy of the Borderline Adult*. New York: Brunner/Mazel.

McGlashan, T. (1983). The borderline syndrome, II: Is borderline a variant of schizophrenia or affective disorder? *Archives of General Psychiatry, 40*, 1319-1323.

McGlashan, T. (1984). The Chestnut Lodge follow-up study, II: Long-term outcome of borderline personalities. *Archives of General Psychiatry, 41*, 586-601.

Meissner, W. (1978). Theoretical assumptions of concepts of the borderline personality. *Journal of American Psychoanalytic Association, 26*, 559-578.

Millon, T. (1981). *Disorders of Personality, DSM III*. New York: John Wiley & Sons.

Modell, A. (1963). Primitive object relationships and the predisposition to schizophrenia. *International Journal of Psychoanalysis, 44*, 282-291.

Modell, A. (1976). The holding environment and the therapeutic action of psychoanalysis. *Journal of the American Psychoanalytic Association, 24*, 285-308.

Modell, A. (1984). *Psychoanalysis in a New Context*. New York: International Universities Press.

Oberndorf, C. (1930). The psycho-analysis of borderline cases. *New York State Journal of Medicine, 30*, 648-651.

Oldham, J., Clarkin, J. F., Appelbaum, A., Carr, A., Kernberg, O., Lotterman, A., & Haas, G. (1984). *A Self-Report Instrument for Borderline Personality Organization*. White Plains, NY: The New York Hospital - Cornell Medical Center, Westchester Division.

Perry, J. (under review). The borderline personality disorder scale: Reliability and validity. *Archives of General Psychiatry*.

Perry, J., & Klerman, G. (1980). Clinical features of the borderline personality disorder. *American Journal of Psychiatry, 137*, 165-173.

Pfohl, B., Stangl, D., & Zimmerman, M. (1983). *Structured Interview for DSM-III Personality Disorder (SIDP)*. Iowa City, IA: University of Iowa Medical School, Department of Psychiatry.

Pollack, W. S. (1982). *"I"-ness and "We"-ness: Parallel Lines of Development.* Unpublished monograph, Boston University, Boston, MA.

Pollack, W. S. (1983). *The Day Hospital as a Therapeutic Holding Environment.* 1982 Proceedings of the annual conference on Partial Hospitalization, Boston, MA. (a)

Pollack, W. S. (1983). Object-relations and self psychology: Researching children and their family systems. *The Psychologist-Psychoanalyst, 4,* 14. (b)

Pollack, W. S., & Dion, G. (1985). *Functional Disability, Severity of Illness and DSM III Diagnosis: The Creation of a Scale.* Unpublished manuscript, Harvard Medical School, Belmont, MA.

Pollack, W. S., & Grossman, F. K. (1985). Parent-child interaction. In L. L'Abate (Ed.), *The Handbook of Family Psychology and Therapy* (pp. 586-622). Homewood, IL: Dorsey Press.

Pope, H., Jonas, J., Hudson, J., Cohen, B. M., & Gunderson, J. G. (1983). The validity of DSM-III borderline personality disorder. *Archives of General Psychiatry, 40,* 23-30.

Reich, J. (1983). *Instruments Measuring DSM-III Axis II Personality Disorders.* Unpublished manuscript, Yale University Medical School, New Haven, CT.

Rifkin, A., Quitkin, F., Carrillo, C., Blumberg, A., & Klein, D. (1972). Lithium carbonate in emotionally unstable character disorder. *Archives of General Psychiatry, 27,* 519-523.

Rinsley, D. (1982). *Borderline and Other Self Disorders.* New York: Jason Aronson.

Roth, B. (1980). Understanding the development of a homeogeneous identity-impaired group through countertransference phenomena. *International Journal of Group Psychotherapy, 30,* 405-426.

Roth, B. (1982). Six types of borderline and narcissistic patients: An initial typology. *International Journal of Group Psychotherapy, 32,* 9-27.

Schatzberg, A. (1983). *Brain Imaging in Atypical Depressions.* Unpublished paper presented at the McLean Hospital Symposium on Atypical Depressions, held in New York City, NY.

Searles, H. (1979). *Countertransference and Related Subjects: Selected Papers.* New York: International Universities Press. (a)

Searles, H. (1979). The countertransference with the borderline patient. In J. Leboit & A. Capponi (Eds.), *Advances in Psychotherapy of the Borderline Patient* (pp. 347-403). New York: Jason Aronson. (b)

Serban, G., & Seigal, S. (1984). Response of borderline and schizotypal patients to small doses of thiothixene and haloperidol. *American Journal of Psychiatry, 141,* 1455-1458.

Shapiro, E., Shapiro, R., & Zinner, J. (1977). The borderline ego and the working alliance: Indications for family and individual treatment in adolescence. *International Journal of Psychoanalysis, 58,* 77-87.

Shapiro, E., Zinner, J., Shapiro, R., & Berkowitz, D. (1975). The influence of family experience on borderline personality development. *International Review of Psychoanalysis, 2,* 399-411.

Siever, L., & Gunderson, J. (1983). The search for a schizotypal personality: A review. *Comprehensive Psychiatry, 24,* 199-212.

Spitzer, R., & Endicott, J. (1979). Justification for separating schizotypal and borderline personality disorders. *Schizophrenia Bulletin, 5,* 95-104.

Spitzer, R., Endicott, J., & Gibbon, M. (1979). Crossing the border into borderline personality and borderline schizophrenia: The development of criteria. *Archives of General Psychiatry, 36,* 17-24.

Spitzer, R., Williams, J., & Skodol, A. (1980). DSM-III: The major achievements and an overview. *American Journal of Psychiatry, 137,* 151-164.

Stangl, D., Pfohl, B., Zimmerman, M., Bowers, W., & Corenthal, C. (1985). A structured interview for the *DSM-III* personality disorder. *Archives of General Psychiatry, 42,* 591-596.

Stern, A. (1938). Psychoanalytic investigation of and therapy in the borderline group of neuroses. *Psychoanalytic Quarterly, 7,* 467-489.

Stiver, I. (1985). The meanings of "dependency" in female male relationships. *Work in Progress Series, Stone Center.* Wellesley, MA: The Stone Center for Developmental Services and Studies at Wellesley College.

Stolorow, R. D., & Lachman, F. M. (1980). *Psychoanalysis of Developmental Arrests: Theory and Treatment.* New York: International Universities Press.

Stone, M. (1980). *Borderline Syndromes.* New York: McGraw-Hill.

Stone, M., & Weissman, R. (1984). Group therapy with borderline patients. In N. Slavinka-Holy (Ed.), *Contemporary Perspectives in Group Psychotherapy.* London: Routledge & Kegan Paul.

Tolpin, M. (1971). On the beginnings of a cohesive self: An application of the concept of transmuting internalization to the study of the transitional object and signal anxiety. *The Psychoanalytic Study of the Child, 26,* 316-354.

Tolpin, M., & Kohut, H. (1980). The disorders of the self: The psychopathology of the first years of life. In S. I. Greenspan & G. Pollack (Eds.), *The Course of Life* (Vol. 1, pp. 425-442). Adelphi, MD: NIMH.

Wallerstein, R. (1983, October 29). *Psychoanalysis and Psychotherapy: Relative Roles Reconsidered.* Unpublished paper presented at the Boston Psychoanalytic Society and Institute Symposium, held in Boston, MA.

Wender, P., Reimherr, F., & Wood, D. (1981). Attention deficit disorder (minimal brain dysfunction) in adults - Replication study of diagnosis and drug treatment. *Archives of General Psychiatry, 38,* 449-456.

Winnicott, D. (1953). Transitional objects and transitional phenomena. *International Journal of Psychoanalysis, 34,* 89-97.

Winnicott, D. (1960). The theory of the parent-infant relationships. *International Journal of Psychoanalysis, 41,* 585-595.

Winnicott, D. (1965). *The Maturational Process and the Facilitating Environment.* New York: International Universities Press.

Winnicott, D. (1975). Hate in the countertransference (1947, ch. XV, pp. 194-203) and The depressive position in normal emotional development (1954, ch. XXI, pp. 262-277). In *Through Paediatrics to Psychoanalysis.* New York: Basic Books.

Wolberg, A. R. (1952). The "borderline" patient. *American Journal of Psychotherapy, 6,* 694-710.

Wong, J. (1980). Combined group and individual treatment of borderline and narcissistic patients: Heterogeneous vs. homogeneous groups. *International Journal of Group Psychotherapy, 30,* 389-404.

Wood, D., Reimherr, F., Wender, P., & Johnson, G. (1976). Diagnosis and treatment of minimal brain dysfunction in adults. *Archives of General Psychiatry, 33,* 1453-1460.

Zetzel, E. (1971). A developmental approach to the borderline patient. *American Journal of Psychiatry, 128,* 867-871.

COGNITIVE-BEHAVIORAL TECHNIQUES IN MARITAL THERAPY*

Stephen E. Schlesinger and Norman B. Epstein

In this contribution, we focus on recently developed marital treatments based on cognitive-behavioral principles. These approaches embody the principles of the cognitive mediation and social learning models of individual treatment, and integrate them with systems theory concepts for application to the interactions of couples.

Cognitive-behavioral approaches to individual treatment have sprung from a number of sources, particularly the works of cognitive theorists such as Aaron Beck (see, e.g., Beck, 1976 and Beck et al., 1979), Albert Ellis (see, e.g., Ellis, 1962), Michael Mahoney (see Mahoney, 1974) and Donald Meichenbaum (see Meichenbaum, 1977), and social learning theorists such as Bandura (see Bandura, 1969, 1977).

More recently, these techniques have been adapted to marital and family treatment (see, e.g., Epstein, 1982; Jacobson, 1981; and Jacobson & Margolin, 1979). These efforts have produced a new, multidimensional approach to the conceptualization and treatment of marital dysfunction.

THEORY AND MODEL OF MARITAL DYSFUNCTION

Some marital theories emphasize intrapsychic processes, others, an individual's environment as the pre-eminent influence on the marital relationship. While each plays a role from the cognitive-behavioral perspective, neither is sufficient to account for marital dysfunction or its remediation. The cognitive-behavioral approach bridges the two quite nicely. It posits that marital dysfunction is due to the interaction of two individuals' behavioral and cognitive responses; consequently, treatment involves an integration of behavioral and cognitive techniques. A clear implication of this integration is that a cognitive-behavioral perspective of marital functioning differs both from a pure behavioral view that focuses on environmental determinants of an individual's responses and from psychodynamic views that emphasize internal personality factors.

A behavioral model of marital interaction (e.g., Stuart, 1980) posits that marital satisfaction is a function of ratios of positive to negative behaviors exchanged between spouses. Although behaviorists traditionally have focused on overt behaviors exchanged by spouses, in recent years they have moved toward a cognitive-behavioral model which takes into account the idiosyncratic cognitive appraisals spouses make of each other's behaviors. Whether a person experiences his or her partner's behavior as positive or negative depends on the particular meaning that he or she attaches to that behavior. Spouses attach meaning to each other's behavior through an active process of cognitive appraisal. That appraisal, in turn, influences both the behavioral and emotional responses of the person to the partner.

Cognitive-behavioral approaches also differ from psychodynamic approaches. Psychodynamic views of marital interactions stress two complementary and dysfunctional intrapsychic processes which, when combined, lead to dysfunction in the relationship. According to this model, individuals form marriages that recreate unresolved conflicts

---

*The authors contributed equally to this article.

from earlier (i.e., family of origin) relationships. In this sense, each partner's historical material, rather than current interactions, is the primary focus of treatment. In contrast, several foci are important for the cognitive-behaviorist. Historical (i.e., family of origin) material, experiences in past intimate relationships (friendships and romances), general thinking styles, beliefs about relationships engendered by the culture as a whole, and the nature of the current interactions between the partners are all important targets of assessment and treatment.

Cognitive-behavioral approaches to marital dysfunction use both behavioral interventions and cognitive restructuring techniques to change behaviors and cognitions. Changes in behavior are used to facilitate cognitive changes and vice versa. To the behavior exchange paradigm are added the intervening cognitive processes. Figure 1 illustrates such an interactive model in which two sets of processes are important. The first, depicted by the solid arrows, concerns interactions between the two partners. The second, depicted by the broken arrows, focuses on internal feedback loops within each partner. Interpersonally, each spouse's emotional and behavioral responses simultaneously *result from* his or her own cognitive appraisals of the partner's responses and, in turn, *serve as stimuli* that will be appraised by the partner. Intrapersonally, each partner's emotions, behaviors, and cognitions interact. A person appraises his or her own emotions and behaviors as well as those of a partner; in this process cognitions, emotions, and behaviors can be altered independently of any interaction with the partner. These intrapersonal feedback loops have an important impact on marital interactions.

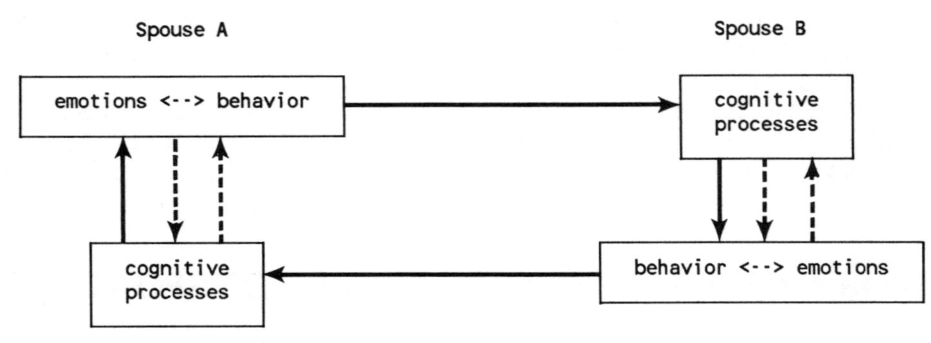

Figure 1

The cognitive-behavioral model described above identifies two categories of factors which influence marital interactions and therefore can be targets for treatment: internal cognitive and overt behavioral responses. In the following sections we shall describe each of the categories of factors, discuss ways of assessing them, and present strategies for modifying them.

COGNITIVE FACTORS

As described in the model of marital dysfunction we presented above, the cognitions of interest to the marital therapist are those that contribute to each spouse's subjective dissatisfaction with the marriage. Although marital partners' appraisals of their relationships can reflect unpleasant realities, there are a number of cognitive factors that can distort perceptions of interactions in a negative manner, thereby exacerbating conflict.

Beliefs about Relationships. Cognitive theorists such as Beck (1976) and Ellis (1962) have emphasized how an individual's dysfunctional emotional and behavioral responses to life events commonly are tied to basic underlying beliefs and assumptions that the person holds about the world and his or her place in it. These beliefs, generally in the form of "should" statements (e.g., "In order to be a worthwhile person, I should achieve great things"), are usually learned early in life, particularly in one's family of origin, but they may also come from other sources such as the mass media. They become standards by which a person judges many aspects of life (e.g., own and others' work performance, quality of friendships and marital relationships, success in roles such as parenthood). Concerning marital relationships, people's basic beliefs generally include ideas about role performance ("A good husband should..."), qualities of love ("Being in love feels like..."), and qualities of good marital interaction ("The way to communicate is...").

When a person's basic beliefs about an aspect of life are extreme or unrealistic, they can be sources of considerable distress. For example, Epstein and Eidelson (1981) found that the degree to which spouses held beliefs such as "disagreement between spouses is destructive," "partners should be able to mind read each other's needs and desires," and "partners cannot change their relationship" was positively correlated with their level of marital distress and desire to end their marriage.

Although some relationship beliefs are learned directly from sources such as parents, others can be developed as reactions to perceptions of faults in others' unhappy relationships. For example, a person who grows up in a family marked by tension and minimal communication may develop a belief that a good marriage is characterized by uncensored sharing of all of one's thoughts and feelings. When this extreme standard is applied later to the person's own marriage, it can lead to hurt and disappointment if the partner does not self-disclose fully or when the person who holds the belief fails to use tact when criticizing the other.

Expectancies. In contrast to the global beliefs that often pre-date marriage, partners develop specific expectancies about the nature of interactions with their mates. Based on past experiences with the person, the individual develops estimates of the probabilities that the partner will respond in particular ways in specific situations (e.g., "If I suggest a new activity in love-making, he will most likely become anxious and defensive"). Expectancies can be either positive or negative, and they can vary in their accuracy. Those that are based on accurate observation of past marital interaction patterns can help partners anticipate consequences of their behaviors toward one another and thereby enhance cooperation and conflict resolution. On the other hand, distorted expectancies that a partner will react negatively can inhibit a person from taking constructive action or can lead to defensiveness or aggression in anticipation of a negative response.

Thus, based on a combination of general beliefs about relationships and a set of specific expectancies developed within the current relationship, marital partners approach their interactions with pre-conceived notions about what "should" occur and what "will" occur. This cognitive template is likely to serve as a set of standards for evaluating marital interaction, a "filter" that produces selective attention to behaviors that are relevant to the individual's beliefs and expectancies (and inattention to other behaviors), and a guide for the individual's responses toward his or her spouse. For example, assume Mr. Jones holds a belief that a good relationship is characterized by uncensored expression of needs and feelings but has an expectancy that Mrs. Jones will not communicate all her feelings to him. When he greets her at the end of a work day, he may try to coerce her to share all the experiences of her day. Unfortunately, his coercive style may lead her to be defensive and to withhold information, creating a self-fulfilling prophecy consistent with Mr. Jones's initial cognitive set.

Causal Attributions. People tend to make inferences about the possible causes of pleasant and unpleasant events that occur in their interpersonal relationships. The tendency to make causal attributions has been theorized to result from a desire for predictability in one's life (Berley & Jacobson, 1984). Recent research studies (e.g., Baucom, Bell, & Duhe, 1982; Fincham & O'Leary, 1983; Holtzworth-Munroe & Jacobson, 1985) have indicated that members of distressed couples are more likely than nondistressed spouses to attribute negative actions of their partners to global, stable characteristics such as negative personality traits (e.g., "She is selfish"), as well as to negative intent (e.g., "He was trying to hurt me"). In contrast, when spouses make causal attributions for pleasant events that occur between them, the opposite of the above pattern holds. Distressed individuals are more likely than nondistressed individuals to discount their partners' positive acts by attributing them to specific, unstable characteristics that are not predictive of future pleasant marital interactions (e.g., "She was nice to me because she was glad to be on vacation"). Nondistressed individuals are more likely to attribute such behaviors to stable, global characteristics and positive intent.

Although most of the studies conducted to date have used structured questionnaires to elicit spouses' attributions, our clinical experience suggests that the attributional patterns found in those studies are representative of at least some of the inferences people make naturally about their marital interactions. Also, Holtzworth-Munroe and Jacobson (1985) found similar attributional patterns when they gave spouses the opportunity to generate their own causal attributions with open-ended questions.

Even when a person's inference that his or her partner's negative acts reflect a pattern that has been fairly consistent over a period of years, such global, stable attributions do not take into account any variation in the other's behavior that might be a basis for constructive change in the relationship. This style of "all-or-nothing" thinking has been described by Beck (1976) as characteristic of depressed individuals, but it can also be quite problematic for distressed spouses (Epstein, 1985). Just as such dichotomous thinking exacerbates depression by restricting an individual's perceived options (e.g., "Either I am a success or a failure"), it impedes change in marital problems when spouses perceive each other in all-or-nothing terms (e.g., "He is *always* stubborn, so there is no use in trying to negotiate with him"). These negative cognitive sets based on biased attributions are countertherapeutic. They often pose a problem for the marital therapist early in treatment when they decrease spouses' motivation for treatment ("Why try?"), and later in therapy when one partner's constructive behavior change is discounted by the other as fleeting or illusory ("He'll go back to his old ways").

Fincham (1985) has noted that the attributions most strongly related to marital satisfaction include those in which a person draws inferences both about who is responsible for marital problems and about the significance of the problematic behaviors for the overall status of the relationship. The first type of attribution is reflected in the common tendency for people to blame their spouses rather than themselves for relationship problems. In the second attributional process, people infer from specific behaviors the degree to which the marriage provides for their very basic needs such as love, affection, security, and respect. The significance that spouses attach to even small daily actions through this attributional process can account for many of the fights over "trivia" that couples present to the marital therapist.

The strong tendency for distressed spouses to assess blame for problems means that couples are unlikely to conceptualize mutual causality in their interactions. Consequently, one of the early therapeutic tasks is to broaden the clients' attributional models to include circular causality. Strategies for achieving this goal are described in the section on intervention below.

In summary, cognitive factors such as beliefs, expectancies, and attributions not only influence a couple's current level of distress, but also can exacerbate problems and impede therapeutic efforts to improve an unsatisfactory relationship. Consequently, these constitute important variables for assessment and treatment in marital therapy.

BEHAVIORAL FACTORS

Based on social learning and behavior exchange principles, behaviorally oriented marital therapists (e.g., Epstein & Williams, 1981; Jacobson & Margolin, 1979; O'Leary & Turkewitz, 1978; Weiss, Hops, & Patterson, 1973) have identified both behavioral deficits and behavioral excesses that influence marital adjustment. On the one hand, deficits in basic skills such as communication, problem solving, assertiveness, and negotiation limit the extent to which members of a couple can make their needs known to one another and resolve any conflicts that may develop between them. On the other hand, there is substantial research evidence to support clinical observations that distressed couples use an inordinate amount of aversive stimulation (e.g., criticism, threats) in their attempts to influence each other, and such excesses are common targets for modification in therapy. Behavioral marital therapy consists of a variety of learning-based procedures for building relationship skills and decreasing the rate of aversive exchanges between spouses. The following is a description of the major behavioral factors that have been implicated in marital distress and that have become the foci of treatment.

Communication Skill Deficits. Some couples lack basic skills for communicating their thoughts and feelings to each other, and as a result they experience misunderstandings or a lack of information necessary if they are to provide for each other's needs. Therapists who work with marital communication problems focus on the skills of both parties to a communicative act: the sender of a message and the receiver. Marital therapists commonly use Guerney's (1977) Relationship Enhancement program to teach spouses expressive skills and empathic listening skills, and a program developed by Gottman et al. (1976) to teach skills designed to maximize the degree to which a person's intended message has the desired impact. Both programs identify spouses' deficits in the ability to be clear, specific, and brief, and the ability to phrase messages in a manner that will minimize defensiveness (e.g., by prefacing a request with a statement demonstrating empathy for the other person's position). The therapist looks for communication patterns that interfere with the clear transmission of information (e.g., general deficits in the amount of self-disclosure, lack of skills for initiating and maintaining conversations, use of vague terms, failure to use words describing feelings, frequent shifts in topics) and targets these for skill training.

Guerney (1977) provides specific guidelines for empathic listening skills. These involve paying close attention to the subjective experience the other person is attempting to describe and restricting one's feedback to an accurate reflection of the expresser's message, in a manner similar to a Rogerian therapist. The empathic listener's feedback must be clear, specific, and free of evaluative statements. When the therapist identifies deficits in these skills, he or she must determine whether the individual has difficulty paying attention to the partner, difficulty understanding the partner's messages, or difficulty expressing an understanding of those messages. The intervention will vary, depending on the particular type of deficit.

It is important to note at this point that a person's failure to exhibit particular skills in conversations with a partner may not indicate a general skill deficit, but rather a deficit in performance of skills with the partner that he or she may use with others. Failure to use a skill in one's marital relationship may stem from cognitive factors described earlier (e.g., a belief that a loving partner should be able to mind read one's needs) or from a strong emotional response to the partner (e.g., anxiety, anger) that interferes with normal skill development.

Assertiveness Skill Deficits. Some spouses have deficits in their ability to influence their marital interactions by assertively expressing their preferences (either making a request of their partner or refusing to comply with the partner's request). Similarly, deficits sometimes exist in the assertive giving or receiving of compliments (a common unassertive response to a compliment is "Don't be silly!"). Some assertive skill deficits are based on cognitive factors, including concerns about the potential negative consequences of acting assertively (e.g., "She won't love me any longer") and misunderstanding of the difference between appropriate assertion and socially disapproved (coercive and aversive) aggression (Epstein, 1981). Other assertiveness deficits may be based on unfamiliarity with effective phrasing of requests and refusals (e.g., use of "I" statements).

Problem-Solving Skill Deficits. A number of writers (e.g., Jacobson & Margolin, 1979; Stuart, 1980) have identified specific steps that facilitate dyadic problem solving. These include operational definition of the problem (and breaking a larger problem into manageable components when necessary), generation of a list of potential concrete solutions, evaluation of the costs and benefits of each possible solution, selection of a mutually acceptable solution, and monitoring of each spouse's performance of his or her role in the solution. Because many couples fail to take a systematic approach to solving their problems, identification of such deficits and training in problem-solving skills often reduce conflict and increase marital satisfaction.

Negotiation Skill Deficits. For some couples, problem solving breaks down when it reaches the stage where the spouses have to negotiate a solution, either by means of compromise or an agreement to adopt one person's plan for the present topic. Negotiation involves bargaining skills and the ability to generate creative compromise solutions, without being distracted by tangential discussions of other relationship issues. Deficits in these areas may be the result of inadequate prior learning, but in some cases an individual may have failed to generalize skills to marriage that he or she knows and uses effectively in other settings, such as work.

Excesses of Aversive Behavior Exchange. As noted earlier, marital interactions can suffer not only from deficits in skills but also from excesses in certain behaviors exchanged by spouses. Treatment often involves increasing use of a constructive skill while decreasing frequencies of behaviors that impede conflict resolution and elicit marital distress. For example, a deficit in assertiveness skills often is combined with excessive use of aggressive behaviors that alienate the partner and further decrease the person's fulfillment of his or her needs in the relationship. Similarly, deficits in problem-solving skills often exist in combination with excesses of criticism and descriptions of long lists of past and present relationship problems ("kitchen sinking"). This not only decreases spouses' cooperativeness but also makes it quite difficult for them to focus their attention on any one problem.

E. J. Thomas (1977) has provided a detailed description of how a variety of excesses and deficits in verbal communication can be problematic. Examples of behavioral excesses that are either distracting or distressing include providing too much or redundant information, excessive agreement or disagreement, excessive questioning, negative talk surfeit (such as frequent negative evaluations of others, the world, and events), topic content persistence, and quibbling over details. Clearly, it would be difficult to apply a fixed standard of normality in judging how much of any behavior constitutes an excess for a particular couple; such a conclusion must be based on an assessment of the consequences that certain rates of behaviors have for that pair.

ASSESSMENT

Development of procedures for the assessment of cognitive and behavioral factors in marital distress still is in its early stages, but there are a number of instruments that have proved to be reliable, valid, and useful in clinical practice. The following is a survey of these measures, with references for the reader who wishes to obtain more information.

The major methods for assessing the variables of interest are self-report questionnaires, clinical interviews, and systematic observation and coding of behavioral samples. In general, self-report questionnaires are the simplest to administer. Although many of them are valid measures of the constructs they were designed to assess, they can be subject to response biases and should be interpreted with caution. Interviews permit more flexibility in data gathering, because the clinician can inquire about a wide range of topics, tailor the inquiry to the particular characteristics and presenting problems of the individual couple, and follow up on "leads," such as a spouse's parenthetical remarks that point to additional relevant information. The interview shares with the questionnaire the potential for bias in the respondent's reports.

In contrast to questionnaires and interviews, behavioral observation procedures potentially provide an objective view of marital interaction through the use of trained coders. This reduces the difficulty that spouses face when asked to be participant-observers of their own relationships. On the other hand, behavioral observations necessarily are restricted to small samples of a couple's interactions, collected in the office, laboratory, or home. Such a sample may not be representative of the range of interactions the couple has at other times, and the process of being observed may influence the spouses' behaviors. Nevertheless, research studies have demonstrated that behavioral observation systems reliably discriminate distressed from nondistressed couples and are sensitive to changes in their behavior due to therapy. Although the coding systems used by researchers often will be too time-consuming and expensive for clinicians, much can be gained from careful observation of behavioral interactions recorded on videotape. Not only can the clinician identify specific behaviors that impede communication and conflict resolution, but he or she also can use videotape or audiotape feedback to illustrate to a couple what behaviors should be targeted for change. Tapes of marital interaction also are useful for demonstrating circular causality to spouses who tend to attribute responsibility for problems in terms of unidirectional causality.

ASSESSMENT OF COGNITIVE FACTORS IN MARITAL DISTRESS

Until recently, available cognitive measures focused on a person's beliefs and attributions about his or her individual functioning in the world. For example, Jones's (1968) Irrational Beliefs Test (IBT) assesses 10 basic beliefs that Ellis (1962) identified as central in a wide range of dysfunctional emotional and behavioral responses to life events (e.g., the belief that one must have the approval of others in order to be worthwhile and the belief that one must strive for and achieve perfection in one's life). Although Ellis and Harper (1975) described how these beliefs can interfere with marital adjustment, Epstein and Eidelson (1981) argued that the focus on individual functioning limits their relevance for assessing potentially dysfunctional beliefs that people hold about the nature of intimate relationships. Consequently, the Relationship Belief Inventory (RBI; Eidelson & Epstein, 1982) was devised to assess five beliefs theoretically related to relationship problems: disagreement between spouses is destructive; loving partners should be able to mind read each other's thoughts, feelings, and needs; partners cannot change; one should be a perfect sexual partner; and systematic differences between the sexes account for communication problems and conflict. Research results have indicated that relationship-oriented beliefs assessed by the RBI are more strongly associated with marital dysfunction than are the individually oriented beliefs measured by the IBT, although IBT scores also are related to marital distress. Administration of both scales can aid in the identification of extreme beliefs that may pose problems for spouses by setting unrealistic standards and reducing hope for change.

Recently, a number of self-report scales have been developed to assess spouses' causal attributions about positive and negative events in their marriages. Baucom, Bell, and Duhe (1982) constructed the Dyadic Attributional Style Inventory (DASI) to assess the extent to which an individual attributes hypothetical positive and negative relationship events to internal versus external, global versus specific, and stable versus unstable causes. For each hypothetical event, the individual is asked to imagine that the event actually has taken place with his or her partner and then rates its perceived causes on a scale for each attributional dimension. A similar instrument was constructed by Fincham and O'Leary (1983).

A somewhat different approach was used by Pretzer, Fleming, and Epstein (1983), whose Marital Attitude Survey (MAS) focuses more on the content of marital attributions than on dimensions such as global-specific, assessed by other scales described above. A goal of the MAS is to give respondents an opportunity to describe attributions about their relationship in more familiar terms. Consequently, items on the questionnaire ask the individual to report the causes of actual problems in his or her own marriage in terms of six subscales: attribution to one's own personality; partner's personality; own behavior; partner's behavior; partner's malicious intent; and partner's lack of love. Two additional scales measure expectancies regarding change in the relationship: the degree to which partners have the ability to change and the degree to which they *will* change.

All of the above attribution scales are easy to administer and score, and they have been demonstrated consistently to measure cognitions associated with marital distress. When used in clinical practice, they can stimulate productive discussion with spouses on an item-by-item basis, in addition to providing scores that can be compared to norms.

Clinical interviews are another rich source of information about spouses' beliefs, expectations, and attributions. Basic cognitive therapy interview procedures (Beck et al., 1979) can be used to probe for the "automatic thoughts," or stream-of-consciousness thinking, that occur when a spouse becomes upset with his or her partner. The idiosyncratic meanings that the partner's behavior (e.g., arriving home late, with no warning) have for the person often involve attributions about the causes of that behavior (e.g., "She doesn't love me"), expectancies (e.g., "She is going to ignore me and may leave me"), and hints of basic underlying beliefs (e.g., "A loving partner is always there when you need him or her"). The task of the clinician is to observe changes in the spouses' emotions and behaviors and then inquire about thoughts that were occurring when those shifts took place. Some clients initially will not be skilled at monitoring their cognitions, but with practice most can report relevant thoughts linked to dysfunctional marital interactions.

Because the initial cognition that a client reports may not be the most relevant one, the interviewer can search for other meanings the person attaches to the partner's actions by asking a series of questions in the form of, "Then if that were so, what would that mean?" Following the person's line of reasoning from implication to implication, one can often discover a "bottom line" cognition that is the most upsetting. This is a useful way of uncovering basic beliefs that a person may otherwise have difficulty identifying or articulating. Another strategy for determining dysfunctional beliefs is to look for common themes in the range of situations and associated cognitions that upset the individual.

The covert nature of cognitions necessitates that assessment rely heavily on self-report methods, but a potentially less reactive way of eliciting spouses' cognitions about one another is to have them interact in an open-ended way with or without the clinician present. When the couple is taped while discussing their relationship, they often forget that they are being observed and become quite involved in their interaction. The content of their communication in such a situation can reveal a great deal about their attributions and beliefs.

ASSESSMENT OF BEHAVIORAL FACTORS IN MARITAL DISTRESS

Both self-report and behavioral observation methods have been used widely in the assessment of couples' behavioral interactions. The following are some of the more commonly used measures, with comments regarding their advantages and limitations.

Self-Report Measures. Questionnaires with which spouses report the quality and quantity of behaviors exchanged between them vary in their specificity. At the more general end of the continuum, the Primary Communication Inventory (PCI; Locke, Sabagh, & M. Thomas, 1956) asks the respondent to make fairly broad observations, such as, "Do you and your spouse talk over things disagree about or have difficulties over?" Scores on this scale tend to correlate significantly with marital satisfaction, but the imprecise nature of the item content limits the information one gains about the specific behaviors that occur. Concerning the sample item noted above, for example, it is not clear *how* the spouses "talk over" things.

Somewhat greater specificity is obtained with the Verbal Problems Checklist (VPC) developed by Chavez, Samuel, and Haynes (1981). This is a self-report version of the checklist that E. J. Thomas and his associates (E. J. Thomas, 1977) developed to code instances of dysfunctional marital communication. The respondent rates the frequency with which his or her partner exhibits each of 27 problematic behaviors, such as "talks too much, tends to dominate the conversation," "criticizes you in an unhelpful manner", and "refuses to discuss a topic." Total scores on the VPC correlate highly with level of marital distress, but the strength of this association may be due at least in part to the subjectivity of the items and the degree to which they may tap a global evaluation of one's marriage. For example, all of the sample items listed above involve subjective judgments about the partner's behavior, and high ratings of one's partner may reflect a negative "halo effect." Thus, both the PCI and the VPC provide useful information about a couple's communication but should not be interpreted as totally objective measures.

A daily log of the pleasing and displeasing behaviors emitted by a person's partner can be obtained with the Spouse Observation Checklist (SOC; Weiss, Hops, & Patterson, 1973; Weiss, 1978). This inventory consists of a list of 400 spouse behaviors that the developers categorized as pleasing or displeasing. Each spouse rates his or her partner on the SOC each day, indicating which of the behaviors occurred, as well as how beneficial the person finds these acts to be. The partner also rates how costly it would be to perform each behavior the spouse finds pleasing. Research studies (e.g., Birchler, Weiss, & Vincent, 1975) have indicated that ratios of pleasing to displeasing behaviors reliably differentiate nondistressed and distressed couples. The clinician must weigh the advantages of obtaining the detailed behavioral information that the SOC provides against the time and effort (and potential associated client noncompliance) involved with this procedure.

Clinical Interviews. Clinical interviews also can be used to collect detailed reports about marital interactions. The goal is to conduct a "functional analysis" in which both the antecedent stimuli and consequences of any problematic behavior are identified. For example, once a couple has noted that spouse A criticized B, the interviewer inquires about the events immediately preceding the critical remark and the events that followed it. The result is a sequential analysis that reveals how each person's behaviors stimulate and reinforce or punish the other's behaviors, and how this pattern involves circular causality. It is crucial that this analysis be restricted to concrete observable behaviors.

Behavioral Observation. A number of reliable coding systems have been devised by which trained observers record the occurrence of specific categories of positive and negative spouse behaviors. As noted earlier, these systems lend a factor of objectivity that self-reports lack, but they also are time-consuming for clinical practice. Among the major systems are the Marital Interaction Coding System (MICS; Weiss, Hops, & Patterson, 1973), the Couples Interaction Scoring System (CISS; Gottman et al., 1976), and the communication coding scheme devised by Raush et al. (1974). Systems such as the MICS tend to be more reliable when the categories are lumped into broader classifications of positive and negative behaviors.

TREATMENT

In this section, we cover four techniques of treatment: discrimination training, communication training, problem-solving training, and cognitive restructuring techniques with couples. These are not mutually exclusive techniques; marital treatment usually combines these into a treatment regimen. Generally, we present concepts and techniques to couples much as we describe them here.

DISCRIMINATION TRAINING

Discrimination training refers to a technique of helping couples monitor their behavior, both positive and negative, and their observations of each other, both objective and subjective, as a way of evaluating the accuracy of appraisals and attributions they make regarding each other's behavior. Typically, distressed partners particularly monitor, or track, their spouses' negative behaviors and formulate global, negative impressions and attributions of each other based on untested assumptions. These negative impressions and attributions lead to a further narrowing of the person's focus to the partner's negative behaviors exclusively. Initial observations sometimes are influenced by partners' emotional states and usually are generalized beyond their applicability. Overgeneralization obscures the couple's ability to see appropriately the links between behaviors and their consequences and to highlight the cause-effect relationships between behaviors each spouse exhibits. Monitoring frequently helps couples counteract distorted observations by bringing to bear collected and balanced data.

Monitoring frequently takes the form of homework assignments after a model of a couple's attributions is constructed in a treatment session. Homework typically consists of maintenance of a journal in which are entered observations each member makes of the other's behavior and attributions about the other's intent. Journal instructions provide for the recording of both positive and negative events and for an assessment of how each journal entry improves or detracts from the spouse's marital satisfaction. Spouses then can ask each other to increase the number of specific satisfying behaviors which, in turn, begin to increase the amount of global satisfaction in the relationship in fairly short order (Liberman, Wheeler, & Sanders, 1976).

For example, the wife in one couple came to treatment reluctantly after her husband cajoled her participation. Dysfunctional as the couple was, she made one thing quite clear practically from the outset: She did not trust his intentions either in the relationship or in coming for treatment. "He won't change. He's been horrible to me. Well, I guess he didn't beat me, so it could be worse. But it's been bad enough. I never see him. He likes his buddies better than me. He doesn't understand me, and I don't think he wants to change or can."

The husband's first reaction was to her final two statements. He took issue with her conclusions that he did not understand her, and that he neither cared to change nor could. Though the homework after this session involved monitoring for both partners, for illustrative purposes let us examine the portion concerned with these attributions.

The wife was asked to maintain a journal in which her daily entries would concern her observations of her husband's behavior, both positive and negative, as it related to her perception of his understanding of her. Confusing as it first seemed, she was able to produce 26 journal entries before the next weekly session. At that time, the journal (along with other facets of the homework assignments we have not discussed) was analyzed for data she found compelling that either supported the negative attribution or refuted its basis in fact.

The difficulty which such negative attributions and beliefs cause throughout treatment is that they interfere with a couple's rational ability to evaluate their observations of each other. They frequently constitute shorthand descriptions of untested - and faulty - conclusions about each other. Even when they reflect some degree of reality, they often are so extreme as to preclude any perceived potential for change.

COMMUNICATION AND ASSERTIVENESS TRAINING TECHNIQUES

In the earlier section on behavioral factors in marital distress, we distinguished between communication problems that focus on difficulties in transmission of messages and assertiveness problems that involve faulty methods of making and refusing requests. In this section, we shall consider the treatment of these difficulties together because they share common premises and procedures.

We usually begin working on couples' communication problems by focusing on expressive and listening skills. Guerney's (1977, 1983) relationship enhancement techniques provide spouses with a highly structured framework of education and experiences designed to help them learn to listen accurately, to communicate their accurate comprehension of their partner's messages, and to reinforce their respect for their partner's integrity. Because they are so structured, Guerney's techniques are adapted nicely to groups of couples. Therapists are very active in guiding couples through communication exercises, providing feedback to them on their performances, and modeling effective communication strategies. Homework is frequently assigned in the belief that frequent practice of new communication skills strengthens not only partners' mutual respect but also the couple's ability to meet and resolve future difficulties.

The techniques described by Gottman et al. (1976) focus on reducing misunderstanding in a couple's communication and on increasing the sense each partner has of the other's good will. The sense of good will is related in part to the willingness each partner exhibits to persist in treatment beyond an initial period of discomfort. Attentive listening and feedback by partners on the accuracy of the listener's understanding are keys to reducing misunderstanding and increasing each partner's sense that his or her thoughts and feelings are valued by the spouse, quite apart from the question of whether spouses agree on matters between them. The book that describes the ingredients of this approach (Gottman et al., 1976) is both an excellent source for therapists and a valuable resource for couples.

Having taught couples these expressive and listening skills, we typically move next to assertiveness skills. Assertiveness training techniques teach couples to speak directly to each other in a manner which is brief and to the point. It follows from the assumption that complicated communication which either misses the point or buries it in a confusing array of conversation is ineffective and unproductive. Such communication not only hinders identification and resolution of marital problems but likely perpetuates them. Assertiveness offers many couples another communication option.

The assertiveness training techniques we describe here are designed to help couples simplify their communication and avoid some of the pitfalls we describe later. The process begins with the acknowledgment that, when we speak to each other, we do so automatically on two levels. The *verbal* level refers to what we say with the words we choose. The *nonverbal* level refers to what we say with our bodies. The latter is variously referred to as the paralinguistic or body language factor in communication.

Effective communication, one goal of treatment, is accomplished when we give another person the same message nonverbally as we do verbally. When we give mixed messages, we give the other person a choice about which message we intend. Given such a choice, our listener will most often choose the nonverbal message. Typically, it is this level of communication about which partners are least aware, so we tend to model examples of consistencies and inconsistencies between verbal and nonverbal communication channels.

Next comes the task of building a model of the components of assertive communication. It begins with a discussion of nonverbal components. Although spouses initially may not be able to identify these components consciously, they are indeed sensitive to them in their partners' communication. We encourage couples to start listing components, and we offer help if they run out of items. Typically, six nonverbal components emerge. They are eye contact (we explain that it is important to have someone's eye contact if we are to have their attention; we assume that others are not interested in what we say when they look away, and they assume the same when we are talking), facial expressions, body posture (in which are included posture, grooming, dress, distance, and general appearance), gestures (of the extremities, head, and neck), tone of voice, and timing. Timing refers to the idea that, because it is difficult for each of us to entertain more than one thought in our mind at a time, we maximize the chance that our message will be heard when we time our communication to correspond to a moment when the other person's mind is as clear as possible of his or her own thoughts. This involves some thought and observation, and it precludes interrupting the other person.

The verbal portion of the assertiveness model has three components. Each represents an important part of communication, and we encourage partners to use this model to organize their thoughts before they talk. Because an important goal of assertive communication is to be brief and to the point, we encourage partners to allocate one sentence to each component. Early use of this model frequently generates a series of three-sentence messages:

1. Step one of the three-step verbal model is to tell the other person the issue, topic, or situation on which you want him or her to focus. We explain that just because we might have been thinking about a particular matter for some time and it may be very important for us, we cannot assume either that another person is thinking about the same issue or that he or she knows its importance for us. For that reason, we have to tell that person what the issue or topic is.
2. Step two is to tell the other person about one's emotional reaction to the topic, issue, or situation. A problem sometimes presents itself at this stage. There is a linguistic anomaly in the American dialect of the English language. People often use the word "feel" when they mean "think." For the cognitive-behaviorist, this is no small distinction. We suggest a helpful rule of thumb for couples to test whether that which they plan to say at this stage is truly a feeling, or a thought in emotional disguise. Take a sentence with "I feel" in it and substitute the words "I think" or "I believe." If the sentence still makes sense grammatically, then the notion is a thought, not a feeling. If it does not, then the person likely has described a feeling. The following are two examples. Applying the above rule to the sentence "I feel it's time to stop this," we make the substitution and get "I think it's time to stop this." That sentence makes sense grammatically, and it is a statement of a thought or opinion. In contrast, "I feel angry" becomes "I think angry," which does not make sense. It, therefore, is a feeling, and it is appropriate to include it in step two.

    The rule of thumb is not infallible, however. It is important to help couples distinguish between feelings, and cognitions which might pass the test as feelings. For example, consider the phrase "I feel hopeless." Applying the rule of thumb suggests that this phrase expresses a feeling. More accurately, however, this phrase is the result of an appraisal and is a cognition, not an emotion. As an adjunct to the rule of thumb, we help couples test whether such phrases are emotions or cognitions by helping them explore whether they are accompanied by gut level feelings with physical sensations. If not, we suggest couples consider whether they are appraisals of their current situations.
3. Step three is the point at which people ask for what they want. By this time, they have brought their partner's attention to some matter and told the partner about an emotional reaction to it. It is now time to tell the partner what one wants.

The three-step model can reduce hostile verbal interchanges by requiring each spouse to state explicitly what his or her reactions are to specific situations, and allowing a mechanism for specific communication of partners' respect for each other's positions, as Gottman et al. (1976) describe.

For example, in one couple the husband discussed a particular annoyance related to their social life. He was a salesman for a large supply house and had agreed previously to discuss his weekly sales report with his wife. They agreed to this arrangement in order to settle his wife's previous concern that she did not know enough about family finances and felt vulnerable to the ups and downs of his income.

The couple had attended two parties during which she had made his sales record part of the social discourse. He was annoyed, but, for a number of reasons, unsure how to bring it up with her. Using the verbal model, he worked out this approach: "You discussed my sales figures at Helen and Bill's party last week. I felt embarrassed. Please don't discuss them in public in the future." His response was brief, to the point - and perhaps somewhat awkward initially. More important than feeling awkward at first, we stress to our clients, is the value of hearing themselves speak succinctly and directly to others. That is the substance; the form can be adjusted later for personal comfort.

When asked for sample situations with which to rehearse assertiveness skills, couples frequently offer the negative. That is, they suggest a matter in which one partner has reacted negatively and wants the other to *stop* something. This is an appropriate application of assertiveness training, but another point is sometimes overlooked. Improving marital communication involves both asking others to do *less* of what we do not like and giving them positive feedback by asking them to do *more* of what we *do* like. A partner's expectations of what can reasonably be expected from his or her spouse are related in part to what he or she asks for directly.

Part of assertiveness training is an introduction to several ancillary techniques. Three are described briefly below. The first two concern ways to deal with responses to assertive messages. We stress that changing communication styles provides no guarantee of success. Just because one formulates and delivers a well-crafted, assertive message, we caution, does not guarantee that others will appreciate and respond to these efforts in the manner one desires. Sometimes people - including, perhaps, one's spouse - will ignore the assertive efforts.

For this eventuality, we offer the first ancillary technique, the "broken record" technique (Smith, 1975). This technique gets its name from a phonograph record which has a nick or scratch on it. When the phonograph needle hits the scratch, it jumps back a groove, and we end up hearing the same thing over and over again. The broken record technique is applied analogously. When one partner's assertive message is met by a change of topics by the other, the sender is encouraged to use the concept of timing, to wait until the other completes the response (the spouse can entertain only one thought at a time) and to acknowledge the other's thought. The sender is taught then to provide a summary of his or her understanding of the partner's reply using the techniques of Relationship Enhancement described by Guerney (1977, 1983). At the point at which the partner acknowledges that the sender has understood his or her reply accurately, the sender is encouraged to restate the original three-step message ("I understand that; however..."). This brings the focus back to the original topic and allows both partners to feel satisfied that they have not been misunderstood.

Sometimes in dysfunctional couples, however, responses to assertive messages may be tangential but a good deal more hostile, perhaps in the form of personal insults or verbal attacks. In this case, the insult frequently is offered as bait to derail communication on a particular issue and deflect it to a nonproductive direction. The response to this is the second ancillary technique, and it involves a modification of the broken record. Senders are encouraged to acknowledge such insults or replies (a difference is stressed between acknowledging and accepting them) as the receiver's opinion, then to return to the original message. A typical response might start with: "It may seem that I'm inept, but...(original message)."

After reviewing the assertiveness model with couples, we engage the couple in a number of exercises to illustrate its application. These exercises seem to be most fruitful when they focus on incidents which have occurred recently and which have been stressful for the couple. They provide an opportunity to apply - and, through homework assignments, to rehearse further - new ways of talking to one another, with feedback from the therapist(s). Role-play re-enactments of prior incidents in which communication resulted in strife allow the couple to hear themselves speaking directly and differently to one another in a manner which allows each to be heard accurately.

Epstein (1981) and Epstein and Eidelson (1981) suggested that beliefs about possible negative consequences of assertive expression of thoughts and feelings may reinforce a partner's reluctance to talk openly with his or her spouse. Attributions concerning the spouse's capacity to accept the open communication ("He's insensitive"; "He doesn't care") may inhibit the partner's attempts as well. As communication becomes more direct and productive, however, it affects each partner's cognitive construal of his or her spouse's attitudes and capacity for change. For example, the spouse who considers his or her partner to be "insensitive" and who therefore has restrained attempts to be heard may change that view in the context of a new-found technique which allows the partner to be understood.

The third ancillary technique is applied to step three of the verbal model. It is called the "workable compromise" (Smith, 1975). This helps couples view step three as an opportunity to open negotiations with each other by offering (or responding with) suggestions of compromise in an effort to resolve what might otherwise develop into an impasse. An important application of the workable compromise technique is to help couples develop flexibility in their communication and avoid becoming rigid in an assertive manner. Negotiation is the goal, and compromise is its key.

Part of communication training involves identifying several problems for couples. These include interrupting each other, diverting conversations in unproductive directions, mind reading, and predicting that communication efforts will be fruitless, each of which was mentioned earlier. At this stage we help couples practice avoiding these communication pitfalls by modeling effective communication alternatives, coaching couples in their use, and providing feedback about their trials.

Problem-Solving Training. Distressed couples often suffer from an inability to make sense of their problems in an organized manner. As components of their difficulty contaminate one another, partners are left with an impression that the problematic façade of their relationship is impregnable, and with feelings of helplessness and hopelessness. Problem-solving training addresses itself to these feelings and their sequelae.

We apply problem-solving training to the treatment of marital dysfunction within a general three-step model. Step one helps partners operationalize - or define clearly - their problems. Step two helps them learn to brainstorm for possible solutions. Step three concerns the choice of an agreed-upon solution. The material we cover along the way is consistent with the work of Platt and Spivack (1975), among others.

Step 1 - Operationalizing Problems. Problem solving begins with adequate problem definition. For many couples, however, this is an elusive goal. We stress several tasks in this step. First, we encourage partners to identify and tell each other about feelings associated with the problem as they are aware of it. In some couples, partners' feelings guide their reactions but infrequently are identified concretely. Sometimes feelings can become too intense, however, and themselves become the focus of the couple's interactions. Consequently, we work to compartmentalize the feelings and stress the need to approach problem solving as a cognitive task.

Second is the task of helping couples distinguish between facts - those things they know about through one of their five senses - and opinions - second-order conclusions reached, sometimes irrationally, after assembling (sometimes unidentified) facts. Successful problem solving relies on accurate perception of *facts*. Dysfunctional couples, however, frequently lead with their *opinions*.

The third task in learning to define problems is to develop adequate observational skills. This includes both practice in asking questions directly to get information from one's spouse and the explicit recognition that people have different likes and dislikes and respond differently in the same situation. The belief that differences of opinion are destructive itself can impede effective cooperation between spouses to solve their mutual problems. Divergence is encouraged because it is helpful later, as couples brainstorm to generate possible solutions to their problems. Emphasizing convergence of thought at this point may destructively limit a couple's options.

The fourth component of step one emphasizes communication styles. For those couples who need them, exercises for practicing nonverbal communication are appropriate. These might include role-plays by each spouse in which a particular emotion is communicated nonverbally, with specific feedback from the partner and from the therapist concerning the concrete variables which led the other to "read" a particular emotion. These exercises are important because *mis*reading each other's emotions may channel an attempt to solve a problem in a direction not intended by the other partner.

Step 2 - Generating Possible Solutions. Problem solving rarely yields a perfect outcome. Couples who do not solve problems well frequently are tempted to settle for the first - and often inadequate - solution. Several tasks are important to circumvent this tendency and its opposite - inaction. First is the need to teach couples to stop and give themselves time to think before making a decision. Each spouse is coached to use internal dialogue about the decision-making process itself ("We don't have to jump to conclusions. We can take time to make a good decision."), and then to share their internal dialogues with each other. Second, in order to encourage couples to view problem solving not as the search for *the* solution but as a choice among several possible solutions, couples are urged to think out loud with each other. Private decision making - that is, partners thinking through mutual problems independently - hobbles the process and robs it of the richness of ideas so crucial to adequate problem solving.

Third, as they think out loud, couples are encouraged to generate and write down alternative solutions that occur to them. We stress in this initial step that couples ought not to censor their thoughts as they generate alternatives. ("Mention them, write them down, but do not judge them at this stage. Make the list of alternatives as exhaustive as you can.")

Because there are not perfect decisions (only relatively better or worse ones), couples need some framework within which to evaluate the potential solutions they generate and, ultimately, to choose and implement the (relatively) best one among them. A couple's *goal* is the cornerstone of that framework, and it is the goal which helps the partners evaluate alternatives for the instant circumstance and for their relationship. One couple with severe problems informed their therapist at this stage that their goal was to make the best of their relationship. Divorce was out of the question and was quickly stricken from their list of alternatives as they began to evaluate it in light of this goal. Another couple eschewed a "tough love" response to their errant teenage son after they defined a central goal as: "The family must end up living together, come what may."

Once the goal is established, the list of alternatives can be culled and entries eliminated which either seem ridiculous on their own merit or which are inconsistent with the defined goal. The next step is to define the consequences (good and bad) for the remaining entries.

Step 3 - Choosing a Solution. Choosing a solution is the next step. No choice is perfect, and none need necessarily be cast in stone. A choice must be rational and reached by consensus of both partners. Rational refers to its having been developed with other alternatives, evaluated against the couple's goals, and paired with its good and bad anticipated consequences. Consensus refers to its acceptance by the couple as the best solution among available options.

We encourage couples to choose solutions which make sense at the time, but to remain observant and flexible enough to change them or try new ones if they do not work. *Adaptation* through problem solving, rather than repair of static traits of relationships, is the most desired outcome.

COGNITIVE RESTRUCTURING TECHNIQUES

Techniques of cognitive restructuring apply to marital treatment in ways analogous to their applications in individual treatment. To some degree, they may be identical, in that it may be necessary sometimes for spouses to define individual cognitive processes as they may bear on relationships. For example, one couple's path was blocked by the husband's fear of change which, on closer examination, was rooted in a set of beliefs about himself concerning failure and incompetence. However, with couples, cognitions that concern relationships themselves are of prime importance.

Restructuring techniques emphasize cognitive rather than behavioral interventions. They focus on two general areas: beliefs each partner has about the relationship with his partner and beliefs each has about the nature of relationships generally.

Beliefs are important in relationships because they define a set of criteria against which partners evaluate the state of their marriage. Beliefs are often a set of lessons or conclusions drawn implicitly from a number of experiences or influential persons in partners' lives. Dysfunctional couples frequently have generated erroneous or extreme beliefs.

This is not to suggest that we have a set of standard, healthy beliefs to which we steer couples. Quite the contrary. We encourage each couple to evaluate each partner's beliefs idiosyncratically. We do, however, press for a logical analysis of beliefs.

Logical analysis begins with an elicitation of the system of beliefs which sustains the relationship and characterizes the dysfunction. To evaluate a system of beliefs is first to evaluate the evidence - pro and con - which pertains to the beliefs. Evidence consists of facts, or observations of specific behavior. ("He ignores me" is not sufficient; "When I came home last Thursday, he had already eaten" is better.) When they must test them concretely, the couple then can evaluate their beliefs by looking at concrete evidence.

In addition, as beliefs are made specific, the advantages and disadvantages of holding each can be illuminated. We evaluate these next. The husband who believed his wife was insensitive, and responded by withdrawing, conveniently avoided a degree of intimacy with her which, on reflection, had been difficult for him since his teens. His withdrawal from intimacy both encouraged her (erroneous) belief that he was insensitive and provided a haven for her against a fantasized re-enactment of an earlier exploitive relationship. While both saw the effect of their beliefs as disadvantageous (isolation), the belief each had was maintained in part by its advantage (protection from feared intimacy).

Each partner is unlikely to be motivated to change a basic belief unless its disadvantages clearly outweigh its advantages. When an existing belief has distinct disadvantages, the therapist can help its owner construct a modified (usually softened) belief that is palatable and involves fewer disadvantages than his or her original extreme standard or assumption.

Tied to this system of beliefs about a particular relationship are the beliefs each partner has about relationships in general. Frequently, partners' beliefs about the characteristics of well-functioning marriages are vague and poorly formulated (O'Leary & Turkewitz, 1978). Similarly, predictions of poor functioning often tend to be global and ill-defined. One husband's belief that "relationships are doomed if one person shows some insensitivity" had a major impact on the problems experienced by the couple, whose system of beliefs involved *mutual* assessments of the other's insensitivity. We help partners recognize the role played in their relationship by these more generic beliefs and help each test the current applicability of them for their present lives. For some couples, it is helpful to encourage partners to trace the origins of these generic beliefs so that they can see how such views may even have been realistic in a past situation (e.g., as a child) but are no longer valid.

More important than illuminating beliefs is facilitating the spouses' acknowledging them as a set of persuasive expectations in their relationship, and evaluating them in the context of the marriage. Of prime concern in this regard is the implicit nature of these expectations. Sager (1976) suggested that marital dysfunction arises in part when a partner's implicit set of expectations is violated by his or her spouse. The partner's reaction to this violation may be incomprehensible because of the implicit nature of the expectations. It is important, therefore, for the therapist to help the couple make explicit and concrete the implicit expectations and contracts they have with each other ("I'll do A in this relationship and get B in return"). Once the gap between spouses' implicit expectations and the nature of their actual marital interactions has been made explicit, the therapist can facilitate modification of either the expectations or the behavioral patterns.

OBSTACLES TO GETTING STARTED

Our discussion so far in this contribution has rested on the assumption that both partners have come to treatment ready to understand and resolve their problems, whatever the outcome for their relationship. Couples must be engaged in treatment - often by helping them reduce quickly some of the hopelessness and frustration they feel - and although this typically takes some time, the techniques we have described are successful only to the degree that partners agree to engage themselves in treatment.

In some cases, engagement in treatment is blocked by the residuals of prior trauma experienced by one partner, who attributes the suffering to actions by (and possible bad faith of) his or her spouse. In such cases, participation in treatment may be pre-empted by the effects of the trauma. We will review now a model suggested by Schlesinger (1984) for helping the victimized spouse come to terms with the obstacles to his or her engagement in treatment using cognitive principles. We have chosen to focus on one type of trauma - an extended drinking career of one spouse - as a case in point.

3 Rs in the Marital Treatment of Alcohol Abuse. Few people challenge the view that drinking imposes tremendous financial, social, and emotional burdens on drinkers' families. For spouses, as for drinkers, the trauma caused by the abusive behavior frequently lingers when the drinking stops. It may accompany the couple to treatment and impede the progress of therapy.

In their excesses, drinkers often engender in their spouses a set of "prior issues" to treatment, a number of specific expectations which clamor for attention. These expectations seem to resolve themselves into three basic components. The first is a fantasy of *retribution* harbored by nondrinkers for past sufferings inflicted by their spouses. The second is an expectation of *restitution* for their pains. The third is a quest for *refuge* from future disruptions, some insurance against a possible return to abusive drinking. We would like to consider each of the 3 Rs briefly in turn.

Retribution. Nondrinking spouses often come to treatment nurturing the fantasy of inflicting pain on their spouses commensurate with their own suffering during the period of heavy drinking. For two reasons, this fantasy is often elusive and difficult to elicit in treatment. First, people are loath to come to terms openly with their vengefulness. Many people see vengeance as "not nice," and they shun the hint of it in themselves. Second, when recognized, such inclinations are hard to fulfill. The feeling of retribution is often expressed in vague terms which do not translate easily to appropriate means of execution. In some cases, however, the fantasy may play itself out in rather demonstrative fashion.

Consider this case as a rather dramatic example. When he and his wife were referred for marital treatment, Mr. G had been increasing his drinking steadily for 11 years. Three months before referral, he had been treated in an alcoholism treatment program, and he was attending Alcoholics Anonymous (AA) meetings regularly. Mrs. G had been attending Alanon meetings since her husband's enrollment in alcoholism treatment. They had asked for marital treatment because they were interested in resolving some chronic marital difficulties which were independent of, though exacerbated by, Mr. G's drinking.

Cognitively oriented treatment commenced after three evaluation sessions, but progress was very arduous. Mrs. G directed most of the attention of the early therapy sessions to her husband's past drinking escapades and particularly to their effects on her and their two adolescent children. Soon, Mr. G complained that she "always harp(ed) on things which I can't change now and I told you I was sorry for." He was frustrated that his replies did not mollify his wife. Her husband's apologies merely seemed to incite Mrs. G, who repeated that it was "easy for you to say that now. You didn't go through what we went through." Mr. G opened the eighth session with a challenge to his wife to explain incontrovertible "evidence I have that you're having an affair" with a man she had met at work some years before. Mrs. G conceded that, indeed, she had been quite indiscreet in their meetings over the previous 3 weeks.

By the end of the session, both were very angry, and Mr. G made an elaborate point of telling his wife "how hurt I am that you would do this to me." In the following session, they talked about the genesis of Mrs. G's affair in her overwhelming "need to get back at you. You hurt us so much I couldn't bear it." The need was satisfied, she said, when she was sure he had found out about the brief affair.

In general, efforts to resolve retribution fantasies usually are most productive when they focus on reducing the issue to its concrete implications. This usually is a two-step process. Initially, spouses evaluate whether retribution is possible, first by considering what form it would have to take to be satisfying and then by contemplating how it could be accomplished. This examination usually leads to the conclusion that retribution is not possible as fantasized, however compelling the fantasy may be. Later, aggrieved spouses consider whether retribution is *desirable*, especially in light of the chance that it could have a further destructive impact on the marital relationship. Often the conclusion is that retribution is undesirable (and/or impossible to obtain), and it is resolved by "writing off the pain," perhaps in return for acknowledgment of its legitimacy and some protection against its recurrence. In couples in which the feelings of vengeance could not be resolved effectively, the stability of the marriage immediately has come to the fore as the primary focus of treatment. When such feelings *have* been resolved, they are usually succeeded by the second of the triad of expectations.

Restitution. Nondrinking spouses often present an expectation of repayment for their sufferings. Unlike the issue of retribution, this expectation is usually fairly easily elicited in treatment. While the wish for repayment may be clear, however, it is usually expressed in vague emotional terms which cannot be reduced to a specific currency. As a result, ex-drinkers often express frustration that the ill-defined expectation cannot be met. One woman described her husband's expectation as "demands I can't meet. How can I pay you for what you went through? What's the price? It's like blackmail, emotional blackmail," for which a ransom cannot be defined concretely. Ultimately, this couple resolved the issue by working out a set of agreements about their mutual contributions to each other's future needs. That process, the husband later said, helped him in two ways. On the one hand, he could "expect things to improve emotionally in the future." On the other, he was able to "end my futile search" with the conclusion that ultimately he could not be repaid for his past sufferings; the emotional means for meeting his expectation simply did not exist.

Refuge. The desire for refuge against future disruptions occasioned by a spouse's return to drinking comes to the fore when spouses move past the frustration of the two previous fantasies. Following resolution of those fantasies, nondrinking spouses then usually insist upon some assurance that their immediate future be fairly secure from major disruption before they will commit themselves to treatment. Especially in cases in which the ex-drinker has suffered lapses in the past, protection may be a primary concern to the nondrinking spouse. Indeed, for some, it is the initial *sine qua non* of treatment.

Protection is elusive though. The ex-drinker cannot offer much more than a promise that (s)he will not start drinking again. For many couples, promises are not impressive commodities. The A's, however, took such a promise a step further.

Mr. A had been drinking for 17 years when he entered a detoxification and rehabilitation program. He did so after promising his wife, in front of the judge officiating at the divorce hearing she had initiated, that he would seek treatment for his drinking problem. His wife agreed to postpone that proceeding if he met one condition: In her words, "I need some protection." He assented, and the following week they signed an agreement, prepared by her attorney, which provided that he would automatically forfeit claims to the house and family car and to custody of the children, and that the divorce proceedings would be reinstated automatically, if he took even one drink after he entered treatment. Though this agreement is among the more extreme we have seen, it allowed Mrs. A some comfort in the knowledge, expressed to her husband, that "at least I know you have something riding on it if you decide to go back to the booze. You know, your word hasn't been worth much in the past. I can't really trust you about your drinking. Maybe this will make you think." The agreement allowed Mrs. A to proceed with treatment with at least a modicum of confidence that she was "protected" from a repeat of her sufferings.

In the main, the issue of refuge usually does not present itself in such stark proportions as it did with the A's. The "Catch-22" quality, however, usually does - "I require a guarantee from you, but I can't trust any guarantee you give me." The resolution for most couples is to reach a willingness to live with some uncertainty, both in their relationship and, initially, in the treatment.

We do not mean to imply that this triad of expectations is to be found exclusively in couples in which drinking has been problematic. Certainly they may be brought to treatment by couples in which other traumas have affected the marital relationship. While in one respect trauma is trauma when it comes to its impact on the couple, perhaps these three issues are more readily articulated when drinking has been a problem, because the trauma in these instances can be identified so clearly. These traumas seem more accessible to treatment because they are so clear and specific. It seems that marital treatment proceeds apace only after the issues presented by the 3 Rs have been resolved.

The techniques we have discussed represent relatively recent developments in the field of marital treatment. Current research and advances in theory suggest that the coming years will see further developments in the area of cognitive-behavioral marital treatment. The future of these approaches seems very promising indeed.

Stephen E. Schlesinger, PhD, is currently a staff psychologist at the Edward Hines, Jr. VA Hospital, Assistant Professor in the Department of Psychiatry at Loyola University School of Medicine, and a private practitioner in Oak Park, Illinois. His training is in clinical psychology with areas of specialization in marital treatment and treatment of addictions. He has published numerous articles in clinical psychology, and his latest book is entitled *Stop Drinking and Start Living*. Dr. Schlesinger may be contacted at 1010 Lake Street, Suite 107, Oak Park, IL 60301.

Norman B. Epstein, PhD, is currently an Assistant Professor in the Department of Family and Community Development at the University of Maryland, College Park. Prior to this position he was Director of Research at the University of Pennsylvania School of Medicine's Center for Cognitive Therapy. His doctoral degree is in clinical psychology. He has published extensively concerning marital assessment and therapy, with a focus on the integration of cognitive and behavioral approaches. His interests also include family therapy, as well as the etiology and treatment of depression. Dr. Epstein can be contacted at the Department of Family and Community Development, University of Maryland, College Park, MD 20742.

RESOURCES

Bandura, A. (1969). *Principles of Behavior Modification*. New York: Holt, Rinehart and Winston.

Bandura, A. (1977). *Social Learning Theory*. Englewood Cliffs, NJ: Prentice-Hall.

Baucom, D. H., Bell, W. G., & Duhe, A. D. (1982). *The Measurement of Couples' Attributions for Positive and Negative Dyadic Interactions*. Paper presented at the annual meeting of the Association for the Advancement of Behavior Therapy, Los Angeles.

Beck, A. T. (1976). *Cognitive Therapy and the Emotional Disorders*. New York: International Universities Press.

Beck, A. T., Rush, A. J., Shaw, B. F., & Emery, G. (1979). *Cognitive Therapy of Depression*. New York: Guilford Press.

Berley, R. A., & Jacobson, N. S. (1984). Causal attributions in intimate relationships: Toward a model of cognitive behavioral marital therapy. In P. Kendall (Ed.), *Advances in Cognitive-Behavioral Research and Therapy* (Vol. 3, pp. 1-60). New York: Academic Press.

Birchler, G. R., Weiss, R. L., & Vincent, J. P. (1975). A multi-method analysis of social reinforcement exchange between maritally distressed and nondistressed spouse and stranger dyads. *Journal of Personality and Social Psychology, 31*, 349-360.

Chavez, R. E., Samuel, V., & Haynes, S. N. (1981). *Validity of the Verbal Problems Checklist*. Paper presented at the annual meeting of the Association for the Advancement of Behavior Therapy, Toronto, Ontario, Canada.

Eidelson, R. J., & Epstein, N. (1982). Cognitions and relationship maladjustment: Development of a measure of dysfunctional relationship beliefs. *Journal of Consulting and Clinical Psychology, 50*, 715-720.

Ellis, A. (1962). *Reason and Emotion in Psychotherapy*. New York: Lyle Stuart.

Ellis, A., & Harper, R. A. (1975). *A New Guide to Rational Living.* Englewood Cliffs, NJ: Prentice-Hall.

Epstein, N. (1981). Assertiveness training in marital treatment. In G. P. Sholevar (Ed.), *The Handbook of Marriage and Marital Therapy* (pp. 287-302). New York: Spectrum.

Epstein, N. (1982). Cognitive therapy with couples. *American Journal of Family Therapy, 10,* 5-16.

Epstein, N. (1985). Depression and marital dysfunction: Cognitive and behavioral linkages. *International Journal of Mental Health, 13,* 86-104.

Epstein, N., & Eidelson, R. J. (1981). Unrealistic beliefs of clinical couples: Their relationship to expectations, goals and satisfaction. *American Journal of Family Therapy, 9,* 13-22.

Epstein, N., & Williams, A. M. (1981). Behavioral approaches to the treatment of marital discord. In G. P. Sholevar (Ed.), *The Handbook of Marriage and Marital Therapy* (pp. 219-286). New York: Spectrum.

Fincham, F. (1985). Attribution processes in distressed and nondistressed couples: II. Responsibility for marital problems. *Journal of Abnormal Psychology, 94,* 183-190.

Fincham, F., & O'Leary, K. D. (1983). Causal inferences for spouse behavior in maritally distressed and nondistressed couples. *Journal of Social and Clinical Psychology, 1,* 42-57.

Gottman, J., Notarius, C., Gonso, J., & Markman, H. (1976). *A Couple's Guide to Communication.* Champaign, IL: Research Press.

Guerney, B. G., Jr. (1977). *Relationship Enhancement.* San Francisco: Jossey-Bass.

Guerney, B. G., Jr. (1983). Marital and family relationship enhancement therapy. In P. A. Keller & L. G. Ritt (Eds.), *Innovations in Clinical Practice: A Source Book* (Vol. 2, pp. 40-53). Sarasota, FL: Professional Resource Exchange, Inc.

Holtzworth-Munroe, A., & Jacobson, N. S. (1985). Causal attributions of married couples: When do they search for causes? What do they conclude when they do? *Journal of Personality and Social Psychology, 48,* 1398-1412.

Jacobson, N. S. (1981). Behavioral marital therapy. In A. S. Gurman & D. P. Kniskern (Eds.), *Handbook of Family Therapy* (pp. 556-591). New York: Brunner/Mazel.

Jacobson, N. S., & Margolin, G. (1979). *Marital Therapy: Strategies Based on Social Learning and Behavior Exchange Principles.* New York: Brunner/Mazel.

Jones, R. G. (1968). *A Factored Measure of Ellis' Irrational Beliefs System with Personality and Maladjustment Correlates.* Unpublished doctoral dissertation, Texas Technical College, Lubbock, TX.

Liberman, R. P., Wheeler, E. G., & Sanders, N. (1976). Behavioral therapy for marital disharmony: An educational approach. *Journal of Marriage and Family Counseling, 2,* 383-395.

Locke, H. J., Sabagh, G., & Thomas, M. (1956). Correlates of primary communication and empathy. *Research Studies of the State College of Washington, 24,* 116-124.

Mahoney, M. (1974). *Cognition and Behavior Modification.* Cambridge, MA: Ballinger Publishing Co.

Meichenbaum, D. (1977). *Cognitive-Behavioral Modification: An Integrative Approach.* New York: Plenum Press.

O'Leary, K. D., & Turkewitz, H. (1978). Marital therapy from a behavioral perspective. In T. J. Paolino & B. S. McCrady (Eds.), *Marriage and Marital Therapy: Psychoanalytic, Behavioral and Systems Theory Perspectives* (pp. 240-297). New York: Brunner/Mazel.

Platt, J. J., & Spivack, G. (1975). *Manual for the Means-End Problem-Solving Procedure (MEPS): A Measure of Interpersonal Cognitive Problem-Solving Skill.* Philadelphia: Hahnemann Community Mental Health/Mental Retardation Center.

Pretzer, J. L., Fleming, B., & Epstein, N. (1983). *Cognitive Factors in Marital Interaction: The Role of Specific Attributions.* Paper presented at the World Congress on Behavior Therapy, Washington, DC.

Raush, H. L., Barry, W. A., Hertel, R. K., & Swain, M. A. (1974). *Communication, Conflict and Marriage.* San Francisco: Jossey-Bass.

Sager, C. J. (1976). *Marriage Contracts and Couple Therapy.* New York: Brunner/Mazel.

Schlesinger, S. E. (1984, August). *3 R's in the Marital Treatment of Alcohol Abuse.* Paper presented at the 92nd annual convention of the American Psychological Association, Toronto, Ontario, Canada.

Smith, M. (1975). *When I Say No, I Feel Guilty.* New York: Bantam.

Stuart, R. B. (1980). *Helping Couples Change: A Social Learning Approach to Marital Therapy.* New York: Guilford Press.

Thomas, E. J. (1977). *Marital Communication and Decision Making: Analysis, Assessment and Change.* New York: The Free Press.

Weiss, R. L. (1978). The conceptualization of marriage from a behavioral perspective. In T. J. Paolino & B. S. McCrady (Eds.), *Marriage and Marital Therapy: Psychoanalytic, Behavioral and Systems Theory Perspectives* (pp. 165-239). New York: Brunner/Mazel.

Weiss, R. L., Hops, H., & Patterson, G. R. (1973). A framework for conceptualizing marital conflict, a technology for altering it, some data for evaluating it. In L. A. Hammerlynck, L. C. Handy, & E. J. Mash (Eds), *Behavior Change: Methodology, Concepts and Practice* (pp. 309-342). Champaign, IL: Research Press.

THE EFFECTIVE USE OF HUMOR IN PSYCHOTHERAPY

Waleed A. Salameh

As we travel through life with all its tribulations, the experience of humor comes to replenish and heal us. We enjoy the innocent laughter of children, the zestful effervescence of youth, and the wise smile of maturity. We value the company of those friends who seem to possess an invigorating sense of humor that can brighten our day. And we may have wondered about how the refreshing potency of humor can be channeled into our everyday psychotherapeutic work. While some clinicians have commented upon the positive value of humor as a therapeutic tool, a review of the existing literature (Salameh, 1983) offers little direction on how humor can be used in psychotherapy apart from general remarks and interesting clinical vignettes.

This contribution presents a systematic, five-phase training approach used in workshops conducted by the author to help train therapists in the psychotherapeutic application of humor. The training focuses on expanding the clinician's skills in using humor effectively in psychotherapy, and includes the following five facets: (a) a rationale for using humor, (b) therapist traits that help optimize the effective use of humor, (c) creative uses of absurdity, (d) Humor Immersion Training, and (e) ethical considerations.

A RATIONALE FOR USING HUMOR

> "If you're not allowed to laugh in heaven,
> I don't want to go there." - Martin Luther

The first issue to be addressed is, why is humor of therapeutic import? In my view, five attributes of the humor experience can be therapeutic:

1. *Humor Is Emotionally Therapeutic Because It Is an Invitation to Emotional Freedom Coming from the Therapist to the Patient.* It can change a patient's constricted emotional perspective by helping him or her to be open to feelings, humorous and otherwise. Since a major goal of psychotherapy is to help decongest patients emotionally, humor can serve as the junction leading to the freeway of emotional unblocking. If therapist and patient can laugh together, then they can share other intimate feelings as well. Humor may also bring balance and a sense of proportion to those instances in which the emotional world is chaotic, warped, or unduly stunted.

2. *Humor Is Cognitively Therapeutic Because It Activates a Patient's Creative and Problem-Solving Abilities and Helps the Patient Reframe Problems So That New Solutions Can Emerge.* In this sense, humor invites a more exploratory attitude in dealing with seemingly stalemated issues. It unstructures or deconstitutes rigid defensive postures, while facilitating their replacement by more adjustive ones. Moreover, the matching of humor with insight around particular issues establishes a positive preventive link in the mind, so that humor enters at critical moments to remind the person that "Here I go back to...," when old patterns strike again. The resulting detachment can help patients devitalize dysfunctional patterns and attain a wider, more adaptive life perspective.

3. *Physiologically, the Humor Reaction May Be Described As a Mini-Workout Akin to "Stationary Jogging."* As reviewed by Fry (1986), the beneficial physiological effects of humor that have been established thus far include activation and stimulation for those muscles involved in the humor-mirth-laughter response spectrum coupled with relaxation for other body muscles that do not partake in the humor response (this initial response pattern is then followed by relaxation of tension in all body muscles); increased heart rate with stimulation of both arterial and venous blood circulation; amplified respiration with enhancement of oxygen intake and increase in carbon dioxide discharge; and enhancement of catecholamine production leading to a heightening of alertness for both therapist and patient. In summary, the physiological findings clearly indicate that humor is an invigorating form of exercise which involves significant muscular, circulatory, respiratory, and hormonal participation. Furthermore, in comparison to other sports, humor exercise has the added advantages of accessibility and higher frequency potential: One can engage in humor exercise at any time throughout the day and with greater frequency than more strenuous forms of exercise.

4. *Humor Is an Economical Mode of Interaction, Allowing the Therapist to Crystallize Interpretive Feedback in Lieu of a Rambling Interpretation That Might Be Too Difficult or Threatening for Patients to Digest.* A good instance of the economical properties of humor occurred when I was working with a young married couple. The husband reported in a marital therapy session that his wife had recently complained about him ignoring their relationship due to his unending pre-occupation with money and business trips, which resulted in a marked qualitative and quantitative deterioration of the couple's sexual life. After listening for some time to the wife's justified concerns and the husband's half-defensive replies, I turned to the man and said, "Well, it sounds like the best way for you to get more invested in your sex life is to make it *tax deductible!*" My comment triggered much laughter, yet also registered with the husband as a simple and tangible description of his skewed motivational investments. The subsequent changes in his behavior patterns and in the couple's relationship started, I believe, at the very moment he responded with laughing acknowledgment to my humorous interpretation. In addition, the "tax deduction" theme was used as a stem to create other therapeutic jokes in working with this couple.

5. *As a Form of Human Communication, Humor Can Be a Refreshing, Relaxing, Attention-Getting, and Motivation-Boosting Contact Medium.* The therapist's appropriate use of humor promotes a constructive tone of interaction, fostering a positive working alliance and helping to avert a solemn mode of approaching oneself or one's problems. Moreover, humor can further a climate of openness wherein new options may be explored without provoking undue patient resistance. Like guided daydreams, psychodrama, or role-playing, humor can sometimes be an indirect form of communication that disarms patients' resistances and encourages them to make cognitive and emotional sense of what is being communicated. By tailoring an answer for themselves out of the communication, patients come to feel that they *own* the alternative suggested by the therapist's humorous interpretation. The feeling of self-approbation for having decoded the humorous message on one's own, combined with the "Aha!" reaction following the uncovering of a new alternative to an old problem, can often lead to a shift in perspective and behavior.

THERAPIST TRAITS THAT HELP OPTIMIZE
THE EFFECTIVE USE OF HUMOR

"The biggest problem with self-analysis
is the countertransference." - Anonymous

The personal characteristics that therapists bring into the consulting room can exert an important influence on the course and nature of psychotherapy. The research conducted by Carkhuff and his associates (e.g., Carkhuff, 1969; Carkhuff & Berenson,

1967) has identified the following important core facilitative traits of the effective therapist: empathy, respect, genuineness, concreteness, self-disclosure, immediacy, and confrontation. Both the existing evidence regarding the therapeutic uses of humor (Chapman & Foot, 1976, 1977; Goldstein & McGhee, 1972; McGhee & Goldstein, 1983; Salameh, 1983, in press-a, in press-b; Fry & Salameh, in press) and clinical experience allow us to postulate that humor is another facilitative trait of effective therapists that is most constructive when used in conjunction with the traits specified by Carkhuff.

An important part of training therapists to use humor consists of presenting and defining the above traits, and discussing (with role-play illustrations) how humor can be facilitative as well as empathic, respectful, genuine, concrete, and so on. I have constructed a five-point Humor Rating Scale (Salameh, 1983, pp. 72-74) to rate the facilitative level of therapist humor. The scale ranges from Level 1 which refers to destructive humor to Level 5 which describes outstandingly helpful humor responses. Each higher level is assumed to add to and surpass the preceding level on the therapeutic humor dimension.

In addition to its research applications, the Humor Rating Scale is used as an operational tool in training therapists to rate recorded segments of humorous interventions. This process allows therapists to gain a greater awareness of the level of humor they are using and to assess the degree of improvement in their use of humor subsequent to Humor Immersion Training. In my experience, most individuals can be trained to use humor at least up to Level 3 (Minimally helpful humor response) of the Humor Rating Scale. The scale also makes clear that humor, like any other powerful communication tool, can be abused to convey nontherapeutic or vindictive messages at Levels 1 and 2. The Humor Rating Scale is presented in Table 1 below. An illustrative clinical vignette is included for each of the five levels of therapist humor. The written version of these vignettes may not completely reflect their full "live" impact as they occurred during psychotherapeutic work and within the context of patient statements, but I hope the essential flavor of the intervention will still be conveyed.

TABLE 1: HUMOR RATING SCALE*

Level of Therapist Humor	Clinical Vignette
Level 1 - Destructive Humor Therapist humor is sarcastic and vindictive, eliciting patient feelings of hurt and distrust. Therapist abuses humor to callously vent his or her own anger toward patients or the world and is consequently insensitive to and unconcerned with the impact of his or her humor on patients. Therapist humor may judge or stereotype patients; its caustic quality denigrates patients' sense of personal worth, leaving them with a typical "bitter aftertaste" reaction. Since the therapist's use of humor is destructive and retalia- tory in nature, it tends to significantly impede patient self-exploration and divert the therapeutic process.	Therapist to patient who reports feelings of inadequacy related to negative self-image: "Well, you obviously have much to be modest about; your face could sink a fleet, and on top of it you have the IQ of a tree. On the other hand, being stupid could help you qualify for disability payments."
Level 2 - Harmful Humor Therapist humor does not manifest the blatant patient disrespect found at Level 1, but is still not attuned to patients' needs. Therapist mixes the irrelevant use of humor with its abuse, at times introducing humor when it is not applicable to the issues at hand. The therapist may follow-up his or her abuse of humor with a "redemptive communication" that essentially acknowledges the inappropriateness of the previous abusive comment and attempts to make verbal or nonverbal amends for it. Over all, therapist humor is harmful and incapable of facil- itating therapeutic process since it is indiscrimi- nate and invalidated by either missed timing or the attempt to redeem derisive comments.	Patient states that he is confused about his goals in life and unable to understand him- self. Therapist replies, "Here you go off on a fishing pole again! It's almost like your mind is full of wallpaper." Patient, with a nervous titter: "So I guess I should be per- fect! Asking confusing questions can lead me astray, right!" Therapist, now self-conscious: "Well, uh, I'm like that too sometimes. Some- times I can't think straight." Therapist goes on to explain about his own periods of con- fusion, indirectly apologizing. Attention is gradually shifted away from the patient's experiencing.

Level of Therapist Humor	Clinical Vignette

Level 3 - Minimally Helpful Humor Response
Therapist humor <u>does not</u> question the essential worth of individuals and is adequately attuned to patients' needs. Therapist uses humor for and not against patients as a means of reflecting their dilemmas in a concerned yet humorous manner. Therapist humor promotes a positive therapist-patient interaction, yet remains mostly a reaction to the patients' communication rather than an active or preferred therapist-initiated mode of communication.

A married couple is reporting to the therapist that their sexual contacts have gradually decreased in frequency and are presently relegated to rare "special occasions" instead of being a continuous element of the relationship. Therapist: "So I guess it's (sexuality) now like the good old Christmas tree. It's a hassle to get it from the attic and set it up. It's nice while it lasts, but it only gets turned on once a year!"

Level 4 - Very Helpful Humor Response
Therapist humor is substantially attuned to patients' needs and to helping them identify new options. Therapist humor may expose or amplify specific maladaptive behaviors yet simultaneously conveys a respect for patients' personhood. It facilitates patients' self-exploration while inciting them to recognize and alter dysfunctional patterns. The educational, comfortable, and enjoyable nature of therapist humor stimulates a positive and candid patient-therapist relationship. Nevertheless, therapist humor still lacks some of the intensity, timing, and graphic language characteristic of Level 5 humor responses.

Obsessive patient constantly rejects interpretations with the statement, "No, that's not my bag." Therapist: "So what is your bag, or rather, what's your briefcase?"

Level 5 - Outstandingly Helpful Humor Response
Therapist humor conveys a profound understanding of patients, is characterized by spontaneity and excellent timing, and challenges patients to live to their fullest potential. Therapist humor reflects his or her emotional and cognitive freedom used to facilitate patients' emotional arousal and cognitive restructuring. It generates significant self-exploration and accelerates the process of patient change by defining problems, condensing and symbolizing therapeutic process material, identifying new goals, and promoting constructive alternatives. The creative nature of therapist humor can elicit decisive existential insights and encourages patients to develop their own humor along with other attitudinal changes.

During a group therapy session, a manipulative patient is recounting to the group his repeated failings at achieving honest nonmanipulative communication with others. Although he tries, others don't seem to believe or respond to his "authentic" self-revelations. Therapist: "You know your situation reminds me of a corrida scene with the bull and toreador. We don't know whether you're the bull for whose slaughter we should feel sorry or the toreador whose courage we ought to admire." Another group member: "But he's really not the bull; he sets other people up as being bulls." Patient, laughing: "So I end up being the toreador. I give my coup de grace and demand my Olé!" Group members, in unison: "Olé!"

<u>Note</u>: This author's observational data indicate that physical responses to Levels 1 and 2 humor are usually characterized by a preponderance of giggling, tittering, forced laughter, or short anxious laughs. Level 3, 4, and 5 humor usually elicits predominantly diaphragmatic or abdominal gut level laughter.

*From "Humor in Psychotherapy: Past Outlooks, Present Status, and Future Frontiers" by W. A. Salameh in <u>Handbook of Humor Research: Applied Studies</u> (Vol. 2, pp. 72-74) by P. E. McGhee & J. H. Goldstein (Eds.), 1983, New York: Springer-Verlag. Reprinted by permission of Springer-Verlag.

CREATIVE USES OF ABSURDITY: PARADOXICAL HUMOROUS PRESCRIPTIONS AS INDIRECT SUGGESTIONS

"After all, what was Medea? Just another
child custody case." - Frank Pierson

In Albert Camus' (1959) movie *Black Orpheus*, an intriguing scene presents a maintenance worker in a huge, record-keeping office building who decides to give up on sweeping papers off the floor: No matter how much he sweeps there are always more meaningless papers falling from the inundated files and cluttering up the office floors. A highly anxious patient made the startling announcement during a therapy session that he had decided to stop worrying and start taking things one day at a time because, "Behind every worry there's a worry, and behind that worry is another worry." These two experiences illustrate significant understandings which can result from a person's coming to grips with the ubiquitous absurdity of existence - the absurdity of things that do not have to be but are, of events that escape the human capacity for logical comprehension, of unexpected discoveries and chance happenings. Absurdity provides fertile soil for humor because humor builds on parasitical realities to drive home important messages.

In psychotherapy, the patient's zealousness for repeatedly applying maladjustive solutions to everyday problems may, at times, constitute an absurdly humorous scenario. Accordingly, the judicious therapist can make creative use of the absurdity theme to design indirect suggestions that address specific therapeutic issues with which the client is grappling. As Watzlawick (1978) has observed, indirect suggestions derive their potency from the paradoxical inference that they hide what they reveal: "There seems to be a tacit rule of communication that what is said without being said is 'not really' said, but somehow is communicated with particular power" (p. 86). Some strategic therapists are adept at constructing indirect paradoxical suggestions based on absurdity. For example, Erickson (cited in Watzlawick, 1978, p. 75) treated a sexually unresponsive woman by instructing her to imagine how she would go about defrosting her refrigerator: how she would deal with this situation, which shelf (top, middle, or bottom) to begin with, what to take out first, how she would tackle the thawing, what unexpected thoughts or memories might come up as she proceeded, in what order she would put things back, and so on. Throughout the interaction, myriad minute details of the defrosting chore where elicited.

In a parallel example, Madanes (in press) reported how Haley instructed a student intern who was overly worried about making mistakes under supervision to deliberately make three mistakes during a supervised psychotherapy session - two that Haley would be able to detect and one that he would not be able to discern. A second case reported by Madanes (in press) refers to a male patient who was concerned about being rejected by women. The patient's therapist gave him the assignment of "practicing rejection" by standing at a certain corner in front of a boutique and spending several hours during two weekends inviting young women to have a cup of coffee with him. It was explained to the patient that the women would refuse, and that he would, therefore, have the experience of being rejected and tolerating it. Unfortunately, so many women accepted the invitation that the patient did not really have the chance to experience rejection! Frankl (1963) used his technique of "paradoxical intention" to similar ends by asking a young physician who had a fear of perspiring to decide to deliberately show people how much he could sweat whenever his sweating reappeared. Frankl reported that the patient was able to extinguish the excessive sweating by telling himself whenever he met anyone who triggered his anticipatory anxiety, "I only sweated out a quart before, but now I'm going to pour at least 10 quarts!"

A common element in the interventions described above is the use of absurdly humorous prescriptions to redefine phenomenological reality. By redirecting the attentional flow regarding a given situation (through the use of confusion, distortion, deletion, and generalization devices), the normal boundaries of one's conceptualizations can be altered so that the core dilemma may be seen in a different light. Another example occurred during the treatment of a ruminating, obsessive man whom I asked to plan his worrying. The patient was instructed that since he was *very organized*, he could devote a specific time to his worrying. He was instructed to set a specific time to worry on Tuesday and Thursday evenings between 7 p.m. and 9 p.m. In this way, the rest of his time would be efficiently spent on other *secondary* pursuits. He was to mark in advance on his *organized* calendar the exact times and items he intended to worry about for a given week so that he would not forget to worry about important things: "Remember to save all your worries for this time and this time only, and forget about it for the rest of the week. Otherwise, you would be cheating on your program." The patient took the assignment to heart and started to worry at the specified times, but only at these times. This gave him ample time to engage in more productive or enjoyable activities for the rest of the week. Three weeks later, the patient requested that his "worry time" be reduced to one night per week because he was busy with other things. Four weeks later, the patient requested a further reduction of his worry time to 1 hour on Tuesday evenings. In pure paradoxical logic, he needed to be given permission to worry deliberately at specified times in order for him to stop worrying! Subsequently, the alleviation of tensions related to the patient's ruminations allowed for more interpretive work focusing on the origins and development of such ruminations in the patient's history.

In yet another case, a severely disturbed, antisocial patient with poor impulse control was constantly leaving group psychotherapy before the group's termination. Typically, he would come to the weekly group sessions, attend for about 10 minutes, then mutter some angry comment and storm out of the room. One day at the beginning of group, I stated to the patient in a serious tone, "I think you would probably want to sit pretty close to the door because you usually leave after a few minutes. That way it will be easier to leave when your time is up." I pointed to a chair for the patient to sit in that was actually the closest chair to the door but was also the closest to my own chair. The patient laughed and said, "Well, now if I leave it'll all be your fault!" However, he stayed in the group for a half-hour that day which was a record for him. Before leaving, he excused himself with the comment, "I'm leaving now, but it's not because of you. I just can't stay in one place for too long." During the next group session, he came on time and stayed for the duration of the session, adequately contributing to group process and sharing his favorite joke with group members. Over time, this patient became more friendly with others. Whenever the group met, he always chose to sit in the chair that I had originally assigned to him, closest to the door but also closest to my chair. His impulsivity decreased and his humor became less sarcastic. For instance, he once stated at the end of the Thursday group session, "I'll see you on the second Thursday of next week!" Other problems related to inadequacies in social functioning remained, requiring longer treatment, yet some emotional connection was made with the patient through the use of humor and paradoxical directives.

I will now describe the use of goal-directed humorous suggestions in psychotherapy. The term "suggestion" is used here in the general sense proposed by Kroger (1977), namely, the utilization of the patient's ability to respond experientially to the therapist. (For a fuller discussion regarding the use of humor as a form of indirect hypnotic communication see Salameh, in press-a). The suggestions discussed here have a humorous quality, a specific target, are indirect in nature, and are used to convey therapeutic messages. Since these suggestions are indirect by definition and may be subject to misinterpretation, I usually preface the use of any form of humorous intervention by relating the following to the patient during the first therapy session:

> It is important for you to know that I am your ally, totally on your side, and that we're cooperating, working together to tackle your problems. My orientation is not to judge you or tell you what to do but to help you clarify your available choices, where you are now and where you can go from here if you so decide. I respect the courage you have shown today by seeking treatment for intimate issues that are usually hard to talk about. I will do my best to support you and help you feel comfortable throughout our working together. I may sometimes use humor in working with you, not to make light of your problems but to point out patterns or help identify new options. I also encourage you to use humor because positive forms of humor can help us see things in new, refreshing ways. When I use humor at a certain point, I may ask you what I meant by using a joke or a story, and you might want to ask me what I meant as well so that things can make sense as we go along.

Statements similar to those mentioned above can prevent many misunderstandings and create a cognitive framework within which humorous interventions will not only be welcomed but will also receive favorable consideration. In this context, it is important that patients feel that humor is not at their expense and they can make sense of the message embedded in the humorous metaphor. Accordingly, I sometimes encourage patients' anchoring of solutions by asking, "Why are you laughing?" upon seeing the smile of recognition in response to a humorous intervention that I might have made: A patient's explanation of why he or she found what I said to be funny can help "lock in" an interpretive cycle which has been fermenting throughout the therapeutic work.

Given the aforementioned structure for using therapeutic humorous suggestions, therapists can practice developing paradoxical humorous prescriptions for patients by making creative use of the "absurd material" that inevitably emerges in psychotherapy. Table 2 offers some target-specific humorous suggestions and illustrates each with a pertinent clinical vignette.

TABLE 2: INDIRECT HUMOROUS SUGGESTIONS

Indirect Humorous Suggestion	Definition	Clinical Issue	Therapist Intervention
Restorative Suggestions	Replacing patient's negative sense of uniqueness by a positive sense of uniqueness with the overall goal of building self-esteem.	Patient reports that she was able to overcome her negative self-ruminations and ask for a well-deserved promotion, which was actually granted by her employer.	"So good to be driving up that freeway at sunrise, bright-eyed and bushy-tailed, your favorite song on the radio, taking in the sweet smell of early morning, happy as a lark, knowing that the best is yet to come, not a care in the world."
Self-Permission Suggestions	Encouraging patients to take reasonable (and sometimes unreasonable) risks in order to explore new ways of being that can be therapeutic for them.	Rigid patient prides himself on his maturity and "not engaging in childish acts," thus missing much of the excitement and happiness available to him.	"I know I can say this in strict confidence to a mature person like yourself: I believe that maturity has been overrated."
Hibernating Suggestions	Detecting a major recurring maladaptive pattern, describing it humorously, letting it hibernate, then going back to the same theme later on in therapy to verify that the issue is being dealt with appropriately.	Patient denies feelings (especially his own) about various situations by keeping himself busy with work. Following a long, drawn out divorce, he claims that he is "too busy to think about meaningless things like my divorce."	"Sounds like you just have not had time to enjoy your misery!" Patient picks up on this theme to describe his alienation from his feelings, and uses above statement in later sessions, "Well, again, I haven't had time to enjoy my misery this past week."
Ratification Suggestions	Expressing encouragement for new patient behaviors reflecting autonomy and healthy change.	Dependent patient reports, "Feeling a little better" by doing things that make her happy instead of her usual pattern of adopting only those behaviors that others usually condone.	"Feel better, feel better, that's all you think about! Some people have so much to be responsible for in this world, and all you're concerned about is feeling better."
Discarding Suggestions	Helping patients get rid of old carcasses by creating a humorous image representing the maladaptive pattern.	Patient imprisons himself within his own constrictions, then complains bitterly about his self-creating imbroglios.	"By the way, did I warn you about not swimming in wet cement pools anymore? To start with, it's bad for your skin. On top of that, it's not the kind of exercise activity that allows you free-flowing movement."

Indirect Humorous Suggestion	Definition	Clinical Issue	Therapist Intervention
Win/Win or Positive Double Bind Suggestions	Framing seemingly insolvable issues in such a way that no matter which part of the frame patients choose to focus on, they can still end up with a viable alternative that is preferable to their present stuckness.	Middle-aged patient reports that she has not been dating recently: "I have a UFO (ugly, fat, and old) syndrome. I feel like men don't find me attractive anymore."	"There are normally two answers to a scientific question of this kind: a blue answer and a green answer. The blue answer is that there are plenty of UFO men out there who come from that very same planet, and it's usually rather easy to recognize them. The green answer is just to leave your UFO behind, divorce ET, and find out why it is that you are afraid of getting close to <u>ordinary</u> men. I mean, just because you don't speak the dialect...."
Uncontested Contest Suggestions	Highlighting the untenableness of dysfunctional patterns by explaining them "from within" in paralogical ways.	Patient chooses to punish himself for "crimes" he did not commit, ends up "inexplicably dissatisfied" while ignoring simple solutions to his problems.	"You know, a masochist is a person who likes a cold shower in the morning, so he takes a hot one."
Sealing Suggestions	Locking in specific patient insights at the conclusion of a given interpretative cycle in therapy by providing a positive ambient environment within which the insight can be retained.	Patient comments that she is beginning to realize that it is acceptable for her not to be "perfect" because being perfect means there is nothing left for a person to learn in life.	"And <u>they</u> keep throwing monkey wrenches at you! Just when you're ready to graduate from the school of life, someone thinks up a new course."

HUMOR IMMERSION TRAINING*

"Even if you're on the right
track, you'll get run over if you
just sit there." - Will Rogers

We cannot prescribe humor for our patients unless we can accept humor in our own lives. It sometimes seems difficult for us as therapists to enter into the world of humor. Some therapists may feel that using humor discredits patients or may even discredit our own "professional" stance. Moreover, conventional training does not usually encourage a humorous perspective as we must often work against a background of the pessimistic outlook on life presented to us by many of our patients. While it is understandable why our patients are pessimistic (think of all the things *they* have had to worry about since learning that California is due for a major earthquake), it is not understandable why *we* cannot raise our humor quotient as we struggle with the stress of working with distressed individuals.

In this sense, humor is sometimes the best gift we can offer both our clients and ourselves in order to move from a negative view to a constructive one where problems are solvable. Consequently, I have developed Humor Immersion Training (HIT) and

---

*Humor Immersion Training is trade marked by the author.

currently offer it in a workshop format of one to several days for therapists and other individuals interested in raising their humor quotients. In HIT, workshop participants can boost their humorous abilities through exposure to mini-lectures on various psychological aspects of humor and through the active practice of specific humor generation techniques. Below are three important components of the HIT technology: Attitudinal Blocks, Prime Time, and Humor Creation Techniques.

ATTITUDINAL BLOCKS

Before looking at how one can be humorous, it is important to examine some of the attitudinal blocks to our sense of humor. For example, consider carrying out an experiment. First, go to the children's section in any department store and buy some *Fun Button Stickaroos*. Choose any number of stickaroos you like and stick them anywhere on your face as you wish. There is no need to feel bashful about this foolish and inappropriate behavior: You can always explain that you did it out of scientific curiosity after reading this contribution. Now find a mirror, look at your face for 5 minutes, and repeat, "Gooli-Googoo." If you were able to complete this experiment, you accomplished a very important undertaking. You crossed the barrier of what I call "Fear of the Non-Linear." Such fear is a major attitudinal block which frequently prevents us from being humorous. Other blocks include:

1. *Looking for One Big, Right Answer.* Gertrude Stein said, "There ain't any answer. There ain't going to be any answer. There never has been an answer. That's the answer."
2. *Playing a Judgmental or Status Assigner Role.* Oscar Wilde once commented that "Morality is simply the attitude we adopt towards people whom we personally dislike." Being judgmental ossifies us because it engenders an evaluative stance towards life. On the other hand, humor emanates from an appreciation and acceptance of the dilemmas inherent to the human paradox.
3. *Expecting to Be Liked By Everyone.* It is somewhat difficult to be humorous if we feel we must have total and unconditional acceptance from everyone we meet. In most democracies, it is possible to become president with less than 60% of the popular vote.
4. *Adopting the Attitude That Humor Is Frivolous or Childish and That It Discredits Our Professional Standing.* Part of this attitudinal formation is the mistaken belief that we must be solemn to be effective. Being humorous does not denote a lack of seriousness but rather a willingness to unburden ourselves of unnecessary solemnity. Giving up solemnity allows us to be more flexible, more responsive, less stifled, and generally more effective in our work. Moreover, it is not difficult to observe that individuals often joke about what is most serious to them: death, sex, anxiety, relationships, or other important topics.
5. *Confusing Humor with Sarcasm.* Healthy humor is not to be confused with sarcasm. As children or even as adults, we may have had negative experiences as victims of ridicule. The anxiety and bitterness resulting from these unfortunate experiences may still be prejudicing us against humor.
6. *Mutilating Humor.* We mutilate humor when we use it as a dumping ground for expressing anger or as a way of exhibiting racist or sexist tendencies.
7. *I'm Not Humorous.* This refers to an attitude toward oneself that blocks talent, experimentation, and the potential for new learning. As an exercise in self-discovery, take some time after reading this contribution and list on a piece of paper which of the above blocks, fears, or objections you have to being humorous. Read them again and see if they are really valid. Share them with your friends and ask for their feedback. Remember that undue fears sometimes cripple creativity.

PRIME TIME

In HIT, prime time refers to the skill of discerning when humor is welcome and when it would fall flat, depending on the sensitivities and emotional tone associated with any given situation. It is at times preferable to introduce humor into an interaction by using situationally related or self-directed humor (e.g., humor about the weather or about current events; humorous experiences in the therapist's own life that may be of relevance to the patient's issues), then proceeding to unobtrusive other-directed humor (humor related to the patient's own paradoxes, dilemmas, absurd patterns, maladaptive behaviors, etc.) as trust develops and the ambience becomes more relaxed. Timing is crucial in humor and takes time to cultivate.

HUMOR CREATION TECHNIQUES

If we can surpass the attitudinal hurdles delineated above, then we may access a state of *humorous readiness* which would in turn facilitate learning new humorous techniques. These techniques are not an end in themselves, but they serve as a key for gaining a humorous perspective. The following are some of the training methods used to help individuals open up to humor:

Overstatement, Incongruity, Understatement, and Reversal. Most humorous material can be subsumed under four general categories of humor creation.

1. Overstatement - making mountains out of molehills, taking an accurate fact and exaggerating it to absurdity. For example: (a) To a family in a psychotherapy session, "I don't mean to exaggerate the degree of discipline in your family. There are more disciplined contexts - Devil's Island, for example. The Wax Museum, the changing of the guards at Buckingham Palace, an interview with the Queen Mother." (b) To an unduly self-repressive patient, "Are you aware that having lunch with men friends when you are a married woman can constitute grounds for excommunication?" You can practice overstatement (as well as the other humorous techniques presented herein) by deleting the punchline in the above examples (Devil's Island, the Wax Museum..., excommunication) and filling in your own or adding new punchlines.
2. Incongruity - putting together two *non sequiturs*, as in connecting two events or experiences that are apparently unrelated but for which you can find an unexpected underlying humorous "fit." The ensuing joke was developed by using this system. The two *non sequiturs* are (a) the recent debate over capital punishment in our legal system, and (b) the religious belief in reincarnation in India. The joke (a + b): "A lawyer is trying to defend a capital punishment case in India. He appeals to the judge, 'Your Honor, I believe that my client deserves another chance. I submit that his sentence be reduced from death without reincarnation to death *with* reincarnation!'"
3. Understatement - the opposite of overstatement, consists in shrinking giants down to pygmies, and sizing down important happenings to benign proportions. Some examples are (a) "Depression is a low tolerance for euphoria," (b) "Death is nature's way of telling you to slow down," and (c) "Getting a divorce could ruin your whole day."
4. Reversal (or Paradox) - based on deviation from expectation; beginning with a concept, condition, or act in a straight line, then taking it out of its constitutional meaning to place it in a new "meaning loop." This new meaning loop is so atypical that it is experienced as humorous, yet it can still be *admissible* because it retains the ring of familiarity that feeds back to the concept's usual meaning. The pivotal element in creating reversals is knowing when to throw in a new meaning loop within a particular linguistic or interactive context in order to generate humor. One-liners provide an immediate natural channel for reversals, as in (a) "If you want to be a hypocrite, you might as well be honest about it"; (b) "It sounds like you just have not had time to enjoy your misery."

Beyond the above techniques, Table 3 (Salameh, 1983, pp. 76-78) defines and illustrates 12 therapeutic humor techniques practiced in HIT.

TABLE 3: THERAPEUTIC HUMOR TECHNIQUES*

Therapeutic Humor Technique	Definition	Clinical Vignette
Surprise	Using unexpected occurrences to transmit therapeutic messages.	Drilling noise outside office. Patient is talking about his domineering wife. Therapist: "Your wife is talking to you <u>now</u>!"
Exaggeration	Obvious overstatement or under-statements regarding size, proportions, numbers, feelings, actions.	To patient who romanticizes his depression while refusing to consider alternatives: "I could help you, but I guess that wouldn't do any good anyway. You know we all die eventually."
Absurdity	That which is foolish, non-sensical, insane, irrationally disordered. That which <u>is</u> without having any logical reason to be.	A young businessman is spending inordinately long hours at the office and on business trips. He reports that his wife has complained about his increasing lack of interest in their sexual relationship. Therapist responds: "It sounds like the best way for you to get more invested in your sex life is to make it tax deductible!"
The Human Condition	Refers to problems of living that most human beings encounter, viewed from a humorous perspective to stress their commonality.	Therapist to a perfectionist patient who worries that she is not being "totally honest" in communicating <u>all</u> her feelings to others: "As the holy books have indicated, it is difficult for mankind to be honest at all times. But if you want to be a phony, you should be honest about it."
Incongruity	Linking two or more usually incompatible ideas, feelings, situations, objects, and so on.	Oppositional male patient reacts to therapist interpretation by stating that he "has already entertained that possibility." Therapist responds: "You've entertained it, but you didn't go to bed with it."
Confrontation/ Affirmation Humor	Confronts patients' maladaptive and self-defeating behaviors while simultaneously affirming their personal worth as individuals. Assumes that patient confrontation is best digested by patients when coupled with affirmation.	A patient in group therapy is confronted by other group members regarding his compulsive nose-blowing behavior. He passionately defends his need to "breathe clearly." Therapist responds: "You know, we can all see that you've got a lot of intensity, but you don't have to blow it out your nose!"
Word Play	Using puns, double entendres, bons mots, song lines, and well-known quotes or sayings from popular culture to convey therapeutic messages.	Therapist to patient who keeps depriving herself of what she really wants: "You know what Oscar (Wilde) said, 'I can resist anything but temptation.'" To another woman who prevents herself from enjoying life or other people because she refuses to take small acceptable risks: "Mae West did say, 'When I choose between two evils, I always like to take the one I've never tried before."
Metaphorical Mirth	The use of metaphorical constructions, analogies, fairy tales, and allegories for therapeutic story telling to help patients assimilate new insights or understand old patterns.	Patient is talking about how her interpersonal communication is becoming less confused as she really listens to others and gives relevant feedback. Therapist: "It's like that lion you see at the zoo who always growls at you but you don't know what it means. And one day you go to the zoo and the lion smiles and says, 'Hi, there, I've been fixin' to talk to you.' And you talk to each other and become pen pals."

Therapeutic Humor Technique	Definition	Clinical Vignette
Impersonation	Humorously imitating the typical verbal response or maladaptive style of patients and of significant others they may bring up in therapy.	Patient repeats a characteristic "Fssss" sound with his tongue whenever he experiences sadness or other "vulnerable" emotions, so as to block the expression of such feelings. Therapist imitates this "Fssss" sound when patient displays it. Patient gradually shifts from suppression to acknowledgment of his feelings.
Relativizing	Contextualizing events within a larger perspective such that they lose their halo of absoluteness. Relativizing gives the message that: "Nothing is as serious as we fear it to be, nor as futile as we hope it to be" (Jankelevitch, 1964).	Patient recounts his painful struggle with his "weight problem," even though his physician informed him that he is only 3-5 pounds overweight. Therapist: "Well, I notice you've lost some weight behind the ears since last week."
The Tragi-Comic Twist	A delicate humor technique requiring almost surgical precision that consists of a transformation of patients' detrimental tragic energies into constructive comical energies. It begins with a well-timed implicit or explicit juxtaposition of the tragic and comic poles of a given phenomenon followed by a reconciliation of the two poles in a humoristic synthesis that triggers laughter.	Patient who has chosen depression and crying as a behavioral mode of response to any environmental stressor is crying during session about feeling rejected and tense. Therapist responds: "I guess you're trying to relax now." Patient's crying turns into frantic laughter as she replies: "That's one thing I do really well, I know how to cry." Therapist: "Maybe you can relax about crying." More laughter. Therapist asks patient why she is laughing. Patient: "I suppose there are other ways of releasing tension besides crying." The entire session then focuses on the above issue.
Bodily Humor	Using the entire body or specific muscle groups in physical activity aimed at imitating or creating nonverbal reflections of typical maladaptive mannerisms in order to encourage their extinction.	Patient exhibits a typical rotational hand movement to express disillusionment with others' behavior when it does not meet his "requirements." Therapist uses this same hand movement in therapy whenever patient is expressing disillusionment with therapist's behavior not meeting his expectations.

*From "Humor in Psychotherapy: Past Outlooks, Present Status, and Future Frontiers" by W. A. Salameh in Handbook of Humor Research: Applied Studies (Vol. 2, pp. 76-78) by P. E. McGhee & J. H. Goldstein (Eds.), 1983, New York: Springer-Verlag. Reprinted by permission of Springer-Verlag.

Resources for Facilitating Humor. A sense of humor can be facilitated by exposing yourself to humorous experiences from a number of sources. One source is *humorous books*. Examples of books that I find particularly humorous are *The Groucho Marx Letters* (Marx, 1975), *Titters: The First Collection of Humor by Women* (Stillman & Beatts, 1976), *How to Make Yourself Miserable* (Greenberg & Jacobs, 1966), and *Side Effects* (Allen, 1975). *Humorous records* by comics such as George Carlin, Lily Tomlin, Bill Cosby, and Bob Hope can also be a good source.

There are also many *humorous magazines and publications*. Examples include the *Journal of Polymorphous Perversity*, the *Journal of Irreproducible Results*, the *New Yorker* magazine, *Punch* magazine, *Laughing Matters*, and *Laughers Anonymous Newsletter* (published semi-annually by the author).

Comic performers can be seen in action at stand-up comedy clubs. Examples include "The Comedy Store" and "The Improvisation" clubs in Southern California, "The Holy City Zoo" in San Francisco, "Catch a Rising Star" and "Caroline's" in New York City, and others. Such performances can literally be a moving experience. A concerted effort can also be undertaken to locate quality comic movies, plays, and television shows.

Other Strategies for Adding Humor to Your Life. *Draw cartoons* (without worrying about their artistic value) about situations, persons, or events which you find to be particularly humorous. Create humorous collages. Take an art or photography catalog (or even your own family photo album) and *make up humorous captions* for each picture. When you come home every evening, try to *remember at least one funny event* that happened during the day. Write it down and share it with friends and family. Practice "International Dyslexia" by *creating new words or onomatopoeias* that cannot be found in dictionaries. Ask your friends to tell you their *favorite jokes* and tell them yours.

Find some time to be alone, sitting in your most comfortable position, relaxed, and breathing soundly. Close your eyes and bring up a humorous experience. Visualize the event as concretely as possible, and allow yourself to fully relive and enjoy it in all its details and with all the feelings you experienced at that moment. Make a date with yourself to repeat this experience on a regular basis by bringing up the same event, constructing a cassette tape of the experience, or picturing other humorous events you have been involved in. Keep in mind that all of us have had happy, humorous experiences, even if we are sometimes more prone to remember negative happenings.

List five facts or life situations you frequently experience and which you find to be absurdly humorous. For example, why can't public telephones return change, or why do some envelopes have a caption on the top right corner saying, "Place stamp here"?

Make written notes of *humorous car stickers* you notice as you drive. Some examples are "Plumbers do it with a flush," "Teachers do it with class," "Fishermen have all the angles," "Quilters do it warmly," "Chemists get better reactions," "Chess players are better at mating." Start your own "...do it with..." sequence.

Think of a problem that has been bothering you. Think of one sentence which you could use to define your problem in a humorous vein and write it down.

Don't be afraid to *share with others the spontaneous humorous associations or scenarios* that cross the freeways of your mind. Of course, some of what you find humorous may not be humorous to others because different individuals have predilections for different humorous genres. It is okay for some people to feel that some other people's humor is not okay.

With your co-workers, friends, or colleagues, *start a humor support group.* Your group can share jokes and success stories on the constructive applications of nondestructive humor used with oneself or others. Each group member can also share with the group an embarrassing episode that he or she has lived, simply relating what happened without censuring the event in any way. The sharing of embarrassing episodes promotes group cohesiveness, encourages members to be less self-conscious, and brings home the message that we are all imperfect human beings living in an imperfect world. Additionally, the group may enjoy experimenting with improvisational comedy sketches, miming, or other humorous performances.

Start the day with a zing. As soon as you get up in the morning, make a habit of calling up a good friend and exchanging humorous repartee with him or her. This will get you perked up and humorously ready for the day. You can also call any of your friends during the day (especially those who are unhappy and need to laugh) and leave humorous messages on their answering machines. Examples include imitating various dialects or funny advertisements, remembering private jokes, sharing new jokes, and so on.

Make funny lists to exaggerate, stretch, and spoof some of your own problems, fears, and behaviors. You may find that writing such comical lists is not only a lot of fun but can also help you deflate and gain perspective on hitherto insurmountable or disquieting concerns. And, who knows, you may find out about things you always wanted to know but were afraid to ask. Examples include "ten things I must remember to do to fail my exams," "twelve recommendations that would virtually squelch my chances of ever getting a promotion," "five things I must remember to do to spoil my relationships with others," "ten favorite anxieties I can't live without," "twelve worries I want to indulge in from now until death do us part," "five myths I want to keep believing about myself so I can enjoy depression," "seven myths and seven realities about my fear of success," and "three reasons why undue guilt is good for me."

You can also *take the Humorous Sentence Completion Blank test* which I have included on the next two pages.

TABLE 4: HUMOROUS SENTENCE COMPLETION BLANK

NAME____ SEX_____________ AGE______________ MARITAL STATUS _______________

PLACE____ DATE____

INSTRUCTIONS: Please complete the sentences below with the first spontaneous response that occurs to you. Since this is <u>not</u> a scholastic performance test, there are no right or wrong responses. The only requirement is that you make complete sentences and that your responses reflect your spontaneous reaction to each item below. Please wait for the signal to begin.

1. Although I realize roosters cannot lay eggs, I ____

____

2. While I know I cannot count all the raindrops, I ____

____

3. Although it is vain to build castles in Spain, I ____

____

4. Given that winter follows fall and summer follows spring, I still _______________________

____

5. Squirrels store their nuts, and I ____

6. When the lights are on but nobody is home, I ____

____

7. While it is apparent that chickens do not have lips, I ___________________________________

____

8. It is widely known that tickling provokes pleasant vibrations, yet I _____________________

____

9. Bankers do it with interest, and I do it ____

10. Martial artists do it for kicks, and I ____

11. Although others make hay while the sun shines, I still ___________________________________

____

12. Every dog has his or her day, and every frog ____

____

13. When I am as happy as a lark, I ____

____

14. While research has proven that real men or women don't eat quiche, I _____________________

____

15. Athletes go for the gold, and I ____

16. Due to the fact that I remember some people's names, I _________________________________

____

17. The early bird gets the worm, and I ____

____

18. When I wake up in the morning, I insist ____

____

19. Although I acknowledge that a stitch in time saves nine, I _________________________________

____

20. Some dress for success, yet I ____

21. When all else fails, my saving grace ____

____

22. If misery is optional, then joy ____

23. Since I stopped going to the circus as often as I used to, I _________________________________

____

24. If Virginia is for lovers, New York for muggers, and Los Angeles for uncertains, then _________________

____

25. If I could be either John Wayne, Mae West, Elvis Presley, Tarzan, or Lily Tomlin, I _________________

____

26. When I'm singing in the rain, I ____

____

27. The most important difference between pirates and buccaneers is _________________________________

____

28. When my mother calls to inquire about my last visit to the zoo, I _________________________________

____

29. When I think about counting all the hairs in some people's beards, I _________________________________

____

30. Although I abhor swimming in wet cement, I ____

____

31. All good things must come to an end, yet at this moment my heart _________________________________

____

LIMITATIONS AND ETHICAL
CONSIDERATIONS IN USING HUMOROUS APPROACHES

"Humor distorts nothing, and only false gods are laughed
off their earthly pedestals." - Agnes Repplier

The purpose of this section is to examine some of the limitations and ethical dimensions related to the therapeutic uses of humor. First, it is important to clearly differentiate between therapeutic and destructive humor. What has been discussed throughout the various sections of this contribution is a wholesome, therapeutic form of humor which covers a wide range of positive experiences and affect. Such forms of humor would exclude sarcasm, scorn, mockery, and other abuses of humor commonly known as "putdowns" which can usually be detected by the "bitter aftertaste" they trigger. Table 5 (Salameh, 1983, p. 84) summarizes some of the differences between therapeutic and harmful humor.

TABLE 5: THERAPEUTIC VERSUS HARMFUL HUMOR*

Therapeutic Humor	Harmful Humor
Concerned with impact of humorous feedback on others.	Unconcerned with impact of comments on others.
Has an educational, corrective message.	May exacerbate existing problems.
Promotes the onset of a cognitive-emotional equilibrium.	Prevents the onset of a cognitive-emotional equilibrium.
May question or amplify specific maladaptive <u>behaviors</u> but does not question the essential worth of all human beings.	Questions sense of personal worth, such as in racist jokes.
Implies self- and other awareness.	Implies self- and other blindness.
Has a gentle, healing, constructive quality.	Has a callous, "bitter aftertaste," detrimental quality.
Acts as an interpersonal lubricant; constitutes an interpersonal asset.	Tends to retard and confound interpersonal communication; constitutes an interpersonal liability.
Based on acceptance.	Based on rejection.
Centered around clients' needs and their welfare.	Reflects the perpetuation of personal dysfunctional patterns.
Strengthens, brightens, and alleviates.	Restricts, stigmatizes, and retaliates.
Aims to reveal and unblock alternatives.	Aims to obscure and block alternatives.

*From "Humor in Psychotherapy: Past Outlooks, Present Status, and Future Frontiers" by W. A. Salameh in <u>Handbook of Humor Research: Applied Studies</u> (Vol. 2, p. 84) by P. E. McGhee & J. H. Goldstein (Eds.), 1983, New York: Springer-Verlag. Reprinted by permission of Springer-Verlag.

Subsequently, an important component of HIT consists of training participants (through various role-play situations depicting nontherapeutic versus therapeutic humorous interventions) to clearly differentiate between the therapeutic use of humor and its harmful abuse. The Humor Rating Scale (see Table 1) can also provide a useful reference point to help discriminate between destructive and helpful forms of therapist humor.

In this respect, it is important to indicate that therapeutic humor is gentle and respectful, even when it confronts clients' defenses. It is not fueled by anger but rather by joy and by an authentic commitment to help clients change in healthy ways. Therapeutic humor is also well-timed, taking into account the patient's specific needs at the moment when a humorous intervention is considered. Moreover, the judicious therapist is aware of when *not* to use humor, depending on the therapeutic material and the patient's level of absorption.

Furthermore, it is evident that the use of humorous approaches is not sufficient for achieving constructive therapeutic results, because humor is only one element in the successful synthesis of factors which make a therapeutic experience effective. What the therapist seems to need in conjunction with humor is a sound theoretical frame of reference, a clear process model coupled with an intervention strategy to implement a specific method of treatment, a certain emotional maturity, and a cluster of therapist characteristics similar to those specified previously. It is under such conditions that the therapist's humor can have an optimally therapeutic effect. Fry and Salameh (in press) introduce current perspectives on the productive uses of humor in psychotherapy with different patient populations using several theoretical orientations.

CONCLUSION – THE COURAGE TO BE HUMOROUS

"He who has the courage to laugh is almost
as much master of the world as he who
is ready to die." - Italian Proverb

In a world threatened by violence, fraught with distrust and alienation, and full of events we find hard to accept, humor becomes a courageous affirmation of the continuity and resiliency of human life. In effect, both courageous and humorous acts generally represent adaptive responses reflecting the human quest for meaning in the face of what may be called the swarming absurdity of existence. Accordingly, humor symbolizes the courage to persevere, to strive for something better or, barring that possibility, to accept the unpleasant with a smile and continue the human struggle.

The purpose of psychotherapy is not to change life and its inevitable cycles but rather to provide a more resourceful vision, a fresh perspective regarding swarming absurdities. Such a perspective assumes that individuals can experience less distress and more joy, can value caring relationships, and can learn to distinguish between what is really important for them and what constitutes an unnecessary burden to be unloaded at the nearest Burden Recycling Center. Therapeutic humor helps us accomplish these goals in two ways: First, humor emphasizes relationship in that it constitutes a nonthreatening bonding experience between therapist and patient. In this regard, humor makes caring visible, taking both helper and helpee beyond the realm of the superficial, into the realm of the significant. Second, humor can be seen as a radiant meditation, a higher form of seriousness which goes to the headwaters of the human condition and makes them potable.

The ultimate aim in developing the technology of therapeutic humor presented in this contribution and elsewhere is to contribute to the unfolding of a new understanding of psychotherapeutic work whereby clinicians can transcend the wall of unresponsiveness in order to move toward a more responsive and more humorous therapeutic stance. Humor is a legitimate therapeutic tool that models flexibility for the patient while infusing psychotherapeutic interactions with energy and hopefulness. The humorous self awaits within, ready to be catalyzed in the services of change. It all begins with a simple smile.

Waleed A. Salameh, PhD, is a licensed clinical and consulting psychologist in private practice in San Diego, California. He obtained his BA degree from the University of Michigan, his MA from Duquesne University in Pittsburgh, and his PhD in clinical psychology from the University of Montreal in 1981. He is the author of numerous professional articles and presentations and three book chapters in the area of psychotherapy. He is co-editor (with W. F. Fry, Jr.) of the forthcoming book *Handbook of Humor and Psychotherapy: Advances in the Clinical Use of Humor.* Dr. Salameh's clinical practice focuses on using the psychotherapeutic approach he has developed, Integractive Short Term Psychotherapy (or ISTP) in working with individuals, couples, families, and groups. Dr. Salameh may be contacted at 1335 Hotel Circle South, Suite 316-17, San Diego, CA 92108-3487.

RESOURCES

CITED REFERENCES

Carkhuff, R. R. (1969). *Helping and Human Relations: A Primer for Lay and Professional Helpers* (Vols. 1 & 2). New York: Holt, Rinehart, & Winston.

Carkhuff, R. R., & Berenson, B. G. (1967). *Beyond Counseling and Psychotherapy.* New York: Holt, Rinehart & Winston.

Chapman, A. J., & Foot, H. C. (Eds.). (1976). *Humor and Laughter: Theory, Research, and Applications.* London: Wiley.

Chapman, A. J., & Foot, H. C. (Eds.). (1977). *It's a Funny Thing, Humour.* Oxford: Pergamon Press.

Frankl, V. (1963). *Man's Search for Meaning.* New York: Pocket Books.

Fry, W. F., Jr. (1986). Humor, physiology, and the aging process. In L. Nahemow, K. McLuskey-Fawcett, & P. E. McGhee (Eds.), *Humor and Aging* (pp. 81-98). New York: Academic Press.

Fry, W. F., Jr., & Salameh, W. A. (Eds.). (in press). *Handbook of Humor and Psychotherapy: Advances in the Clinical Use of Humor.* Sarasota, FL: Professional Resource Exchange, Inc.

Goldstein, J. H., & McGhee, P. E. (Eds.). (1972). *The Psychology of Humor.* New York: Academic Press.

Jankelevitch, V. (1964). *L'ironie.* Paris: Flammarion.

Kroger, W. S. (1977). *Clinical and Experimental Hypnosis in Medicine, Dentistry, and Psychology* (2nd ed.). Philadelphia: J. B. Lippincott.

Madanes, C. (in press). Humor in strategic family therapy. In W. F. Fry, Jr. & W. A. Salameh (Eds.), *Handbook of Humor and Psychotherapy: Advances in the Clinical Use of Humor.* Sarasota, FL: Professional Resource Exchange, Inc.

McGhee, P. E., & Goldstein, J. H. (Eds.). (1983). *Handbook of Humor Research* (Vols. 1 & 2). New York: Springer-Verlag.

Salameh, W. A. (1983). Humor in psychotherapy: Past outlooks, present status, and future frontiers. In P. E. McGhee & J. H. Goldstein (Eds.), *Handbook of Humor Research: Applied Studies* (Vol. 2, pp. 61-88). New York: Springer-Verlag.

Salameh, W. A. (in press). Humor as a form of indirect hypnotic communication. In M. Yapko (Ed.), *Hypnotic and Strategic Interventions: Principles and Practice .* New York: Irvington Publishers. (a)

Salameh, W. A. (in press). Humor in integractive short-term psychotherapy (ISTP). In W. F. Fry, Jr. & W. A. Salameh (Eds.), *Handbook of Humor and Psychotherapy: Advances in the Clinical Use of Humor.* Sarasota, FL: Professional Resource Exchange, Inc. (b)

Watzlawick, P. (1978). *The Language of Change.* New York: Basic Books.

HUMOROUS RESOURCES

Allen, W. (1975). *Side Effects.* New York: Random House.

Bentley, N. (Ed.). (1958). *The Pick of Punch.* New York: E. P. Dutton & Company.

Copans, S., & Singer, T. (1978). *Who's the Patient Here? Portraits of the Young Psychotherapist*. New York: Oxford University Press.

Ewers, M., Jacobson, S., Powers, V., & McConney, P. (Eds.). (1983). *Humor: The Tonic You Can Afford*. Los Angeles: Andrus Volunteers, Ethel Percy Andrus Gerontology Center, University of South California.

Franklin, J. (1979). *Joe Franklin's Encyclopedia of Comedians*. New York: Citadel Press.

Greenberg, D., & Jacobs, M. (1966). *How to Make Yourself Miserable*. New York: Random House.

Journal of Polymorphous Perversity, G. C. Ellenbogen, Editor, Wry Bred Press, Inc., 20 Waterside Plaza, Suite 24-H, New York, NY 10010.

Laughing Matters, J. Goodman, Editor, Sagamore Institute, Saratoga Springs, NY 12866.

Laughers Anonymous Newsletter, published semi-annually by W. A. Salameh, San Diego, CA.

Marx, G. (1975). *The Groucho Marx Letters*. New York: Manor Books.

Stillman, D., & Beatts, A. (1976). *Titters: The First Collection of Humor By Women*. New York: Collier Books.

Witty, S. (1983, August). The laugh-makers. *Psychology Today*, pp. 22-29.

HUMOR IMMERSION TRAINING (HIT)

Humor Immersion Training (HIT) Workshops are conducted by the author on a regular basis in San Diego, CA, and nationally. For more information on registering for an HIT Workshop or arranging for a workshop to address specific organizational needs, please contact the author or call (619) 260-1014. The following materials are used in the HIT training workshops:

Salameh, W. A. (1984). *Humor and Your Mental Health*. Cassette tape #HAO1 ordered at above address.

Salameh, W. A. (1985). *Relaxation Through Humorous Suggestions*. Cassette tape #HAO2 ordered at above address.

Salameh, W. A. (in press). *Humor Immersion Training (HIT) Manual*.

THE THERAPLAY TECHNIQUE FOR CHILDREN

Ann M. Jernberg

Theraplay is a restitutive method of child therapy. It is based on the knowledge gleaned from the practice of adult psychotherapy that individuals must have had certain experiences as infants and small children if they are to grow into confident adults capable of engendering confidence in others. This theory, in line with that of Kohut (1971, 1977), Miller (1981), Robertiello (1975) and others, takes account of the impact of life experiences, particularly interactions with parents, upon the self-esteem of the small child. Whether parents proudly place on the kitchen wall the drawings brought home by their kindergarten artist or whether they crumple them into a ball and drop them in the wastebasket, for one example, and whether they make a big deal of birthdays or ignore them, for another, will influence how those children come to value themselves. Self-esteem rises and falls over a lifetime of being the object of others' valuing or discounting behaviors. The object of Theraplay is to provide the individual such a high level of self-esteem that, to the greatest extent possible, he or she will be rendered immune to most of life's confidence-lowering experiences.

In the best of all possible worlds, it is by means of the natural, day-to-day interactions between a wholesome mother and her infant that the child comes to be convinced of his value, his uniqueness, his specialness, not for what he can do for her, but in his own right. (At this point in time, it is still the mother not the father, who usually does the early primary, though increasingly less exclusive, infant caretaking in the majority of households.) For purposes of clarity, the parent will from here on be referred to as "she" and the child, to differentiate between parent and child, as "he." Her squeals of delight as she "discovers" him in his crib each morning; her joy as she counts his toes or finds his freckles; her empathic affirmation of his enjoyment in mastery; her investment of emotion and energy as she engages with him in the little things that make his life worthwhile; these all attest to how extraordinary and splendid a child he is. The reader need only picture a scene devoid of these marvelous reactions, then ask the question, "If I were that child, growing up in a family where, rather than using every activity as an opportunity for playful, personal, empathic interchange, activities like diapering, feeding, and bathing, for example, were carried out with utilitarian efficiency in an atmosphere more like a railway station than a lover's tryst, how would I come to feel about myself and, for that matter, how would I come to feel about the world?"

ESSENTIAL PARENT-CHILD ACTIVITIES

The playfulness, the vigorous engagement and empathy, in the best of all possible nurseries, provide the context within which four different kinds of parent-child activity typically take place at one time or another. These are: Structuring, Challenging, Intruding, and Nurturing (SCIN).

The parent *structures* when she communicates to the child clear boundaries between real and unreal, acceptable and unacceptable, here and there, early and late, mine and yours, and so on. She also structures when she delineates his body parts and differentiates for him where he leaves off and the rest of the world begins. She structures not so much through pedantic teaching as through play, casual chatter, and physical experience.

The parent *challenges* when she encourages the child to stretch, to exert himself, to strive, not with driven ambition, but to move himself just a little beyond the point at which he is at this particular moment. Again, she does not do this as though she were a high school teacher, but rather through spontaneous play and games such as "peek-a-boo," and "how big is the baby?" and by placing his rattle just slightly out of his reach in his play pen. Later she challenges by allowing him to search for just a moment for the word he is seeking rather than jumping in to provide it for him. It goes without saying that the sensitive mother will do all of this challenging within the limits of what it is feasible for her particular child to accomplish at each stage of his individual development. She will never do it according to standards set by her neighbor's children or by the books of child norms on her bookshelf. Nor will she do it for purposes of having an accomplished child whom she can show off in order to raise her own self-esteem.

The parent *intrudes* when she impinges on the child's space, his rituals, his body, and so on. Mothers in the nursery intrude on their children all the time, and it is the intrusions which offer the opportunity for some of the most pleasurably exhilarating moments between them. When the adult, standing at the foot of the changing table, conceals her face between the supine baby's tightly closed, vertically held legs and then suddenly separates his legs to reveal her face, that is intrusion. When she runs her fingers up his tummy saying, "I'm coming to get you," one of Daniel Stern's International Baby Games (Jernberg & Stern, 1984), that is intrusion. When she puts her nose to the baby's nose and he hears a loud "beep," that is intrusion, as it is also intrusion when she blows on his belly button. More than any other of the four SCIN dimensions, intrusion is full of delightful surprises and fun. Given that it is appropriate in timing, intensity, frequency, and to her infant's temperament, intrusion, more than any other dimension, is what makes the baby giggle and indicate he is asking for more.

The parent *nurtures* not only when she feeds and cuddles or strokes, powders and lotions, but also when she empathically listens. Listening to the pre-verbal child sometimes requires more skill and patience than does listening to a verbal child. Yet the good mother will know how to tune in to what the child is trying to say and respond in such a way as to be in sync with his message.

Again, in families where interpersonal activities include all four SCIN dimensions and where these take place in a context which is playful, personal, empathic, and appropriate, children will more likely grow up feeling confident about themselves and eager to explore their world. Children whose lives have been devoid of these experiences will more likely grow up doubting both themselves and others. The Theraplay method, as I have described elsewhere (Jernberg, 1976, 1979, 1982a, 1982b, 1982c), is designed to fill this void. "We learn how to treat patients," writes Winnicott (1965), "from watching mothers of very young children." Depending on where the deficit occurred, Theraplay seeks to provide the missed experience at the appropriate developmental level. If his mother had been in perfect sync, playful, empathic, and providing all SCIN experiences to the child when he was a newborn, but was incapable, for whatever reason, of sustaining these interactions into his infancy or toddlerhood, then Theraplay will gear its activities beginning with the infant or toddler level of development.

A child's psyche cannot be expected to endure without a solid foundation any more than a house can. For a child the necessary foundation is attachment. Without the kind of relationship described above, attachments tend to be shaky and impermanent. And without firm attachment the child grows into an adult who lacks a necessary core of certainty of himself as a person (cf. Winnicott's, 1965, description of the "false self," pp. 140-152), a necessary direction to his life, and the capacity for an enjoyable and reciprocal relationship with another human being.

These are the individuals who appear as adults in the therapeutic consulting room. Often they are highly successful in their professions but report feelings of emptiness and fraud. Often they have been programmed to achieve but never to feel valuable in their own right. Only insofar as they were effective in making *their* parents feel good about *themselves* did they appear to be valued by others. Thus it will evolve in the course of adult therapy that as children these successful individuals achieved not in their own self-interest, but because becoming superb violinists, or swimmers, or journalists offered the hope of enhancing the self-esteem of their parents. Adult psychotherapists themselves, in fact, often began life as little therapists to their parents, again with the unstated intention of making the parents, not the children, feel good about themselves. It should be noted that the child is more likely to be exploited in this latter way when the exploiting parent has no other source of supplies, as when his or her adult partner is unempathic or absent or when his or her own parent was emotionally unavailable in childhood. Thus it is developmental, psychodynamic, and family systems theories, more than any others, which underlie Theraplay.

THE THERAPLAY METHOD

The Theraplay method consists of a two-part sequence: diagnosis followed by intervention.

DIAGNOSIS

Diagnosis consists of (a) the intake interview and (b) the Marschak Interaction Method (Marschak, 1960, 1969, 1973a, 1973b, 1973c, 1979; Jernberg et al., 1982, 1983). In general, the initial Theraplay interview follows the format of the traditional intake interview. As the parents (or parent in the case of single parent families) discuss their child, the therapist listens, formulates hypotheses, and asks questions. The questions cover the full range of the child's development beginning with the years prior to his conception (i.e., the parents' own childhoods, their courtship, their marriage) and ending with parental future expectations for him. The hypotheses the therapist formulates as the interview progresses determine further questions (e.g., "Father seems so hostile toward his son," the therapist might think, "and so intolerant of his physical frailty and emotional sensitivity. I wonder if his own father had ambitions for him which *he* failed to fulfill?"). These internal dialogues are all just hunches. They are to be confirmed or refuted by a series of further questionings. These questionings, in turn, lead to the formulation of further hypotheses. Slowly a clear picture emerges. Gradually it becomes apparent what it must have been like to be this particular child entering into and then growing up in this particular family. Thus it becomes apparent how this child has come to view himself and what he says to himself about the world around him. It has probably also become apparent what resolves he has had to make to himself from early on (in terms of behaviors and attitudes) in order to best insure his survival.

Having completed the intake interview, appointments are arranged for the next step in the diagnostic process: the Marschak Interaction Method (MIM). One focus of the MIM is to round out the information gathered in the intake interview and to affirm or refute the hypotheses generated on that occasion. Another is to provide feedback to parents regarding their relationship with their child. A third purpose is to use the conclusions drawn from the MIM observations in planning the upcoming Theraplay sessions.

The MIM permits the therapist to observe firsthand what happens when parent and child are engaged in short-term interaction with one another. The interaction is structured (a) to encompass the usual facets of the typical parent-child interaction and (b) to allow the therapist to focus on particular aspects of the relationship about which he or she has specific questions. It is assumed that, even though the MIM situation is a contrived one, the interactions evoked between parent and child are more likely to be representative than otherwise. MIM tasks, like Theraplay activities, generally fall into discrete dimensions. MIM tasks elicit degrees of one or another (although on occasion there may be some overlap) of the following kinds of behavior: Adult alerts child to the environment and child alerts to the environment. Adult guides purposive behavior and child shows purposive behavior. Adult reduces stress and child shows reduced stress. Adult enhances attachment and child shows attachment.

The MIM administration requires the adult and child to sit side by side at a table (or, for infants, the adult sits leaning against a backrest; the child lies alongside on a mat). A stack of seven or eight index cards is placed in front of the adult. These cards contain the selected tasks the adult and child are to perform. Each task provides information being sought by the therapist. The adult reads each card aloud and then proceeds to engage the child in carrying out the directions. Thus an "alerting" card may ask the adult to "show dolly's eyes, ears, nose, and hands." The observer takes notes of both the adult's style of alerting and the child's response. Is the adult clear or confusing, dull or enticing; is the child engaged or uninterested? A "purposive behavior" card may instruct the parent to "build a tower with blocks. When you are finished say to the child, 'Now *you* build one just like mine.'" Some adults are supportive, free-wheeling, and encouraging of their child's creative independence. Some children conform timidly; others may sabotage. A stress-reducing task may consist of the adult handing a sealed bottle containing candies to the child, saying, "If you can open it, you may have them." The therapist observes whether the adult (a) sits by impassively, (b) rushes to try to open the bottle, (c) places an arm on the child's shoulder while the child attempts the task; reassures, comforts, and perhaps offers a substitute from his or her pocket, or (d) finds some other way to help the child cope with the inevitable frustration. Attachment-enhancing cards may ask the adult to "tell child about when he or she was brand new." Examples of adult behaviors run the gamut from child-focused ("You were adorable. You had a dimple on each cheek. Let me see. Yep. You still have them. And sparkling eyes. And a funny little way of chuckling to yourself when you were alone in your crib or splashing in your bathtub") to self-focused ("I'll try to remember. Oh yes. I wore my green dress. I had just ironed it and it looked real pretty. And my hair was brushed long." This latter commentary was given by a mother who was only recently reunited with her 8-year-old son, having abandoned him shortly after giving birth.) The task, "Adult leaves the room for 1 minute" (Marschak, 1960), can vary in its execution from abandonment to symbiosis. Depending upon the hypotheses to be tested, card selections will place a heavier emphasis on one or another facet of adult-child interaction.

The therapist observes and records both verbal and nonverbal interactions between each of the two participants. If available, a videotape recorder is of immeasurable value. In two-parent families a subsequent session is scheduled for the other parent, again in interaction with the same child. Following both sessions, the protocol is analyzed, conclusions are drawn, and, where appropriate, a report is written. Then the parents are called back in for a feedback session. This session often serves as the introductory intervention session, for it is here that the therapist first confronts the parents with the overt behaviors and covert implications of what goes on when they and their child find themselves in direct interaction with one another. "Did you notice," the therapist might ask a parent, "that sometimes he moves toward you and you move away? I wonder what makes you two behave like that?" Or, "I notice that you do those lovely things for her. You smile at her and do just what a child her age should love to have done to her. In fact, you really knock yourself out to engage her. Yet she keeps turning her head away, avoiding eye contact, and so on. That must feel devastating sometimes. Does it?" This latter observation is not an uncommon one, incidentally, in the MIMs of older adopted children and other children who suffer from "failure to attach." Thus it can be seen from the two examples that the feedback session will (a) offer the opportunity for self-observation and (b) offer support. For the next 8 weeks, both experiences will become two of the hallmarks of the parental side of the family Theraplay equation.

INTERVENTION TECHNIQUES

In the four weekly half-hour sessions that follow the feedback session, an interpreting therapist sits with the parents in the viewing room as they watch the child's therapist play with the child in the Theraplay room. The interpreting therapist will (a) explain the reasons for what is happening right now (e.g., "He is cradling Johnny in his arms like that to make good eye contact"); (b) support the parents of the difficult or unattached child ("It often makes parents, especially the mother, feel so discounted when unattached children treat them that way. Often other people like friends and family, or even their husbands, don't have that same view of the child and can't understand the mother's pain [Koller, 1981]. Is it like that for you sometimes?"); (c) ask for descriptions of recent difficult interactions and for triumphs of the week preceding; and (d) make specific Theraplay recommendations for the week to come (e.g., "Right now he needs an inordinate amount of nurturing. Let's see if we can think of ways you might provide it for him when you're at home this week"). Between-session phone calls for emergencies are always invited, but very seldom are they made.

The four sessions subsequent to these initial four will follow the same format for the first 15 minutes. For the last 15 minutes, however, the parents will enter the Theraplay room and join in with whatever the child and the therapist are doing. During these periods the parents will be helped to focus on the child's positive (but not achievement-oriented) attributes, to engage in eye contact and other appropriate intimacies, to listen to and be empathic with the child's overt and covert communications, to set appropriate limits, and so on. Often it is in these sessions that parents learn to discover and to care for the little scrapes and bruises so common to the bodies of children who have been encouraged to become prematurely independent.

The Theraplay session itself uses activities and interactions reminiscent of the nursery - interactions which are structuring, challenging, intruding, and nurturing, always in a context which is self-esteem enhancing, playful, and highly personal. The proportion of SCIN dimensions used for each particular child is initially determined by the MIM profile and intake information (e.g., Has he had too little structure? Has she been kept at too early a level [usually to meet somebody else's needs]? Has he managed to tune out all but the most intrusive of stimuli? Is nurturing difficult for her to accept?). Later it is the evolution of the child's development from one session to the next which determines the planning for each subsequent session. Examples for activities in each of the SCIN dimensions include the following:

Structuring: Simon Says, Mother May I, drawing full body or head or foot outline.

Challenging: Thumb or leg wrestling, pillow pushing, pillow balancing, bean blowing, hide and seek, singing "rounds."

Intruding: "Where are you? I can't find you" (as child is carried upside down over therapist's back). "Look! You've got 11 toes...1, 2, 3, 4, 5 on your right foot and, let's see, 10, 9, 8, 7, 6 on your left foot. Five plus six makes 11. You've got 11 toes! Did you know that?" Activities which interrupt a ritual, momentarily disrupt body part expectations, or playfully interfere with the child's space in one way or another are intrusive. Even peek-a-boo can be an intrusive activity.

Nurturing: Feeding yogurt, baby bottle, and so on; cuddling, applying lotion, stroking, rocking, singing to, and similar activities.

It is important to note that each of these activities is conducted in such a way that a therapist is always able to feel that a normal child would enjoy these activities. Even so, therapists must be extremely sensitive to the child's reaction; they must be able to determine whether the child's rejection of an activity is born of genuine discomfort or whether, and this is most often the case, it is one more tyrannical effort to "call the shots." Above all else, therapists must be ever-vigilant as to whose need is being met by instituting and persevering at a particular activity. Is it the child's need? For the child's ultimate optimum development, is this particular activity going to prove helpful? Or is it the therapist's need to serve some conscious or unconscious purpose of his or her own? If it is the latter, the activity must be terminated instantly.

PHASES OF THERAPY

Children tend to approach the sessions in a predictable sequence. It helps if the therapist is prepared for each phase:

1. The introduction phase spells out, albeit quite informally, what the sessions will be like (e.g., directed by the therapist, action oriented, and clearly delineated as to time and space, etc.).
2. The exploration phase allows the therapist and child to get to know the salient features of one another (e.g., size of feet, curliness of hair, giggliness, etc.).
3. The tentative acceptance phase is the step at which the child appears cooperative and seems to be "going along with the gag." Yet this is a pretense only. It would be premature for him at this point to feel engaged, relaxed, and trusting.

4. The negative phase may produce accompanying negativistic behavior at home or at school. It is important that parents and teachers be prepared. In children referred because of their withdrawn behavior, this negative phase may take the form of open defiance and teachers may rue the day they ever made the referral. In children who are aggressive and overactive, the negative phase may take the form of depression. After a few more Theraplay sessions the behavior of both kinds of children will indicate a growing trust and joy in the relationship, as well as interpersonal engagement that is more typically normal. Figure 1 depicts the sequence:

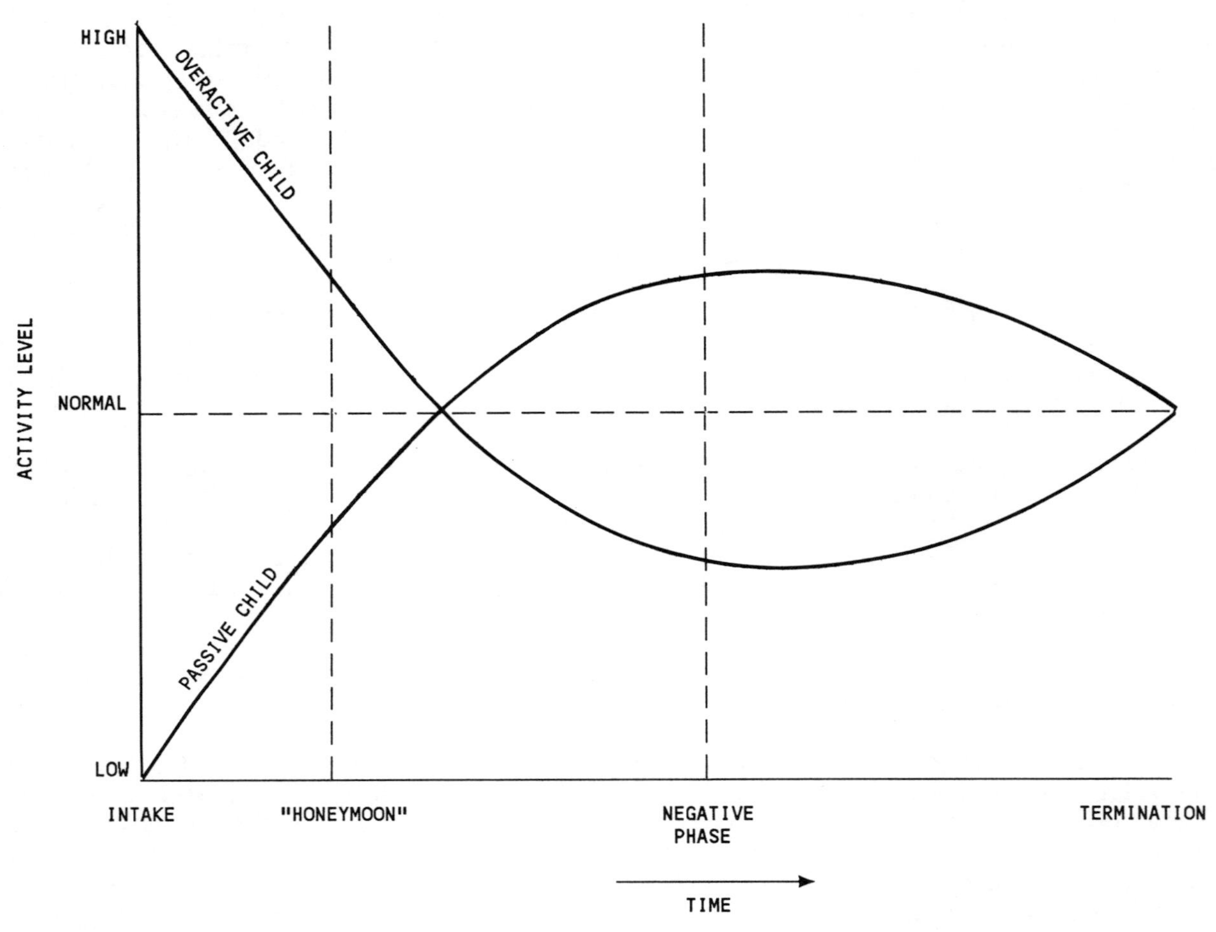

Figure 1. The effect of Theraplay on overactive and passive children.

Of course, not all children in Theraplay consistently follow this pattern. Yet it happens often enough that a word of caution to parents and teachers is generally appropriate.

5. The beginning of the growing and trusting phase marks the onset of that period in which the child has the kind of experiences which redress the issues that brought him into treatment in the first place. It is now that he first genuinely feels pleasure in the sessions and joy in the relationship with his therapist.

Termination in Theraplay begins at about the next-to-last session. In this session the child and his therapist plan the "goodbye party" which is to take place at their next and final meeting. In this session the child and therapist take stock of the child's growing beauty, strength, skill, height and weight, and so on. The child's wall chart showing his height at the outset is taken off the wall, and new measurements are added to it, as well as to his "freckle chart," for example. Child and therapist usually have a rollicking good time together during this last session and also find time to talk softly together about what lies in store for the child's immediate future.

Parents enter the Theraplay room and join in for the last 15 minutes. The therapist may share with them his or her observations as to how the child has grown. It is important to note that this should never be in performance terms (e.g., "He's learned his ABCs"), only in qualities intrinsic to the child himself or herself ("You know, Dad, she giggles so musically now when she's happy; have you noticed?" or "Mom, I bet he never showed you these new muscles he's grown. Look at these. Go on, feel them."). Quarterly "checkup visits" are scheduled for the next year, and annual ones are planned thereafter. Phone calls, as before, are invited, as are interim visits if indicated.

CASE ILLUSTRATION

Jeremy, a little boy of 4, was referred by a nursery school teacher for help with his withdrawn behavior. He was described as not initiating, not participating, not speaking, and not interacting with other children. Jeremy attended two nursery schools: a Montessori school in the mornings and another school in the afternoons.

In the intake interview his parents echoed his teacher's concern but said they themselves noticed nothing about Jeremy which was out of the ordinary. His mother did say that, growing up as an only child, she herself had always had a fantasy companion. When Jeremy was born he became her companion. His father reported that since he and his son had constructive talks and "intelligent" times together, he saw no cause for alarm.

Jeremy's parents were loving, well-meaning individuals, yet both appeared lacking in spontaneity and optimism themselves, and neither seemed to consider that there might be genuine unhappiness in their son. The MIM was geared to assess each parent's capacity for attachment-promoting. Since infantile attention would seem to have been lacking in these parents' repertoire, attachment-promoting appeared to be what a child like Jeremy would need. Thus MIM situations were selected to include tasks like feeding, powdering, applying lotion, and telling Jeremy about when he was a baby. In addition, we wanted to see how these parents would handle tasks (e.g., build a tower, draw a picture, teach the child something) which tap the ways in which they probably too often guide purposive behavior in their child. One task will be chosen to illustrate the behavior most typical for each parent.

FATHER-SON MIM

Task: Teach Child Something He Doesn't Know

<u>FATHER</u>	<u>CHILD</u>
I'm going to teach you about weight.	(nods)
Shall I teach you about weight?	(nods)
Well, some things are heavy and some things are light,	(nods)
but all things have *some* weight.	(nods)
Take my shoes and put them on that scale.	(silently does so)
How much do they weigh?	Three pounds (haltingly).
No. They weighed 2-1/2 pounds.	
All things have weight, see?	(nods)
Now bring me that garbage over there.	(does so in silence)
No. Bring me the whole thing, not just the bag.	(does so)

This one task, excerpted here out of consideration for the reader, took a good 10 minutes. Only toward the end did Jeremy express his impatience by placing his arms behind his back and turning his body slightly away from his father's.

Interpretation: This father engages with his son in the only way he knows. Very likely his interactions with his wife and with his legal colleagues are not too different. Yet his particular style allows Jeremy no leeway, provides him no opportunity for experimentation with the out of the ordinary, leaves him no room for 4-year-old spontaneity. Nothing is done to fit the boy's own interests. Nothing about it conveys that life (or learning) can be fun. Whereas some fathers have chosen to teach their sons to tap dance, or how to fly paper airplanes or write their names in sand, this father has chosen to teach his son the universality of gravity.

If Jeremy were asked, "As a result of your interaction with your father on this task, how have you come to view yourself?" he might answer, "A disappointment to him; I never do seem to get things just right enough to please him; a poor substitute for the intellectual partner he needs." In other words, the interaction has done little to raise Jeremy's self-esteem.

Keeping in mind that an interaction is a two-way street and that a similar question could therefore be asked of his father he, in turn, might answer, "Jeremy makes me feel bad. He never acts as though I matter to him. In spite of the inordinate amount of effort I put forth to try to engage him, he seldom responds. He makes me feel like a dud, not a Dad."

MOTHER-SON MIM

Task: Feed Each Other M & Ms

<u>MOTHER</u>	<u>CHILD</u>
Here. Jeremy. Let's construct a scene with these (emptying candies from envelope).	(nods)
Shall we make a picture that tells a story (lays out elaborate pattern of "trees" and "paths" and "animals")?	(nods)
Well, here is the little girl (taking one M & M) leaving her house after breakfast. OK?	(nods)
She walks out into the fields and she hums. She's so happy. She's thinking about the deer she's going to meet in her favorite field. And the bird in her favorite tree. And so she walks and she walks. And she gets a little thirsty so she stops at the brook here and she has a drink of water. Then she walks some	(watches table top)
more. And now she's tired so she lies down in the soft grass..........................	(looks on, by now barely interested)

This feeding task is designed to encourage just that: feeding. Yet at no point is Jeremy invited to eat even *one* M & M. The drama about the little girl continues for so long that the observer has to enter the testing room to interrupt the task, which is not typical observer behavior.

Interpretation: His mother, like his father, fails to read Jeremy's signals, subtle as these are. She too has her own agenda. Nor does she do anything at all, in this task, to make Jeremy feel good about himself. She never tells him how special he is or how much she enjoys nurturing him. Except for her occasional perfunctory "OK?" she makes no effort to engage him.

If he were asked, "As a result of your interaction with your mother on this task, how have you come to view yourself?" Jeremy might well answer, "As a presence, not much more. An accommodating presence." Again, there is no evidence of enhancement of self-esteem.

If she were asked for a description of how this interaction has contributed to her view of herself, she might answer, "I had such good ideas, ideas that I truly thought would entice him to engage with me. But what did I get from him? Nothing. He made me feel like a person from Mars, talking a foreign language, playing a foreign game. He made me feel unfamiliar and alienated."

In the feedback sessions, sample tasks were reviewed in depth. Parental reactions to, and feelings about, their child were given as serious attention as their behavior toward him. Tentative direction was also given; for example, "What do you think might have happened if you'd just held him in your arms and gently popped the M & Ms into his mouth?" The feedback session avoided criticism, using praise and understanding as a backdrop to the specific suggestions.

With no formal introduction, the first Theraplay session began with his therapist, Charles West, greeting Jeremy in the reception room by swooping him off the hassock. Grabbing one of his hands and breaking into a run with Jeremy in tow, he announced, "I'll race you." Once down the corridor and into the Theraplay room, Mr. West seated Jeremy on the gym mat and said, "WOW! You *are* a good runner. I kind of figured you would be. A boy with a good, strong name like Jeremy. I knew you'd be a good runner. And now that I look at you and I see those nice white teeth and those great sparking eyes, I just know you must be some real neat kid to play with. Let's go look in the mirror so you can see your teeth and your eyes too."

Behind the observation mirror both parents sat with an interpreting therapist who pointed out, for example, "Notice how the therapist is so delighting and what he has to offer is so delight*ful* that Jeremy can't help but peek at him and even shyly smile at him, in spite of himself. Notice too, though, the lengths to which Jeremy will go to try to avoid engaging with him. When you two notice that happening with you at home, what could *you* do to try to help him come out of it?"

After the fourth session his parents were prepared to wear comfortable clothing because they would be joining Jeremy in the Theraplay room, for the latter part of his next session. As they approached the halfway mark of their fifth visit, the interpreting therapist advised them, "Now when you go into the room, Jeremy's going to be hiding - see, you can see his therapist hiding him now - don't take *too* long at it because he's little and he can't wait, but *do* let him know how really eager you are to hunt and find him. Then go about 'discovering' different parts of him: an ear maybe, or a toe, or a giggle you hear. OK. Go." From then on the session was exuberantly focused on Jeremy exclusively. Everybody admired him, physically engaged him, delighted and surprised him and, toward the end of the session, gently cuddled and tenderly sang to him, "Twinkle twinkle little star, what a handsome boy you are." (In his final session he joined them in singing this song about himself.)

Each successive session was an expansion and a variation of the previous session. Increasingly Jeremy shared more openly, and did less concealing of the joy he was experiencing. His parents were good students and eager to keep the momentum going, so they learned readily to show their appreciation of him at home, not for what he could do for them, but for the wonderful person he was.

The sixth and seventh sessions repeated the format of the fifth.

At the termination (eighth) session, all four participants - Jeremy, his mother, his father, and his therapist - had a party. It was here that he showed off his muscles, and how his nose could go "beep" whenever he wanted it to, and how far he had grown on the chart labeled "Jeremy" hanging on the cork board. He put party hats on everyone and streamers around their necks, and everyone had a turn to feed him his yogurt sundae.

Feedback from his teachers was enthusiastic: "He plays with others and speaks spontaneously," they reported.

Jeremy returned for quarterly checkup visits and for annual visits thereafter. Seven years later, in an unexpected telephone call, his father provided further follow-up. "I heard The Theraplay Institute is going to be on television. Jeremy's in sixth grade now. He has friends and is doing really well in school. I know he'd love to be on TV with you and tell the audience all about his experience with Theraplay."

CLIENT CONSIDERATIONS

Theraplay is a useful method of therapy for many different kinds of children, yet Theraplay therapy is not for everyone. There are children for whom it would be inappropriate, some who will not benefit, and some, although not as many as we are inclined to believe, for whom it could be potentially harmful.

Theraplay can be most beneficial for children who are "tyrants" of one kind or another. Children who need to call the shots are adamant about maintaining this position and fearful, to varying degrees, of abdicating their despotic roles. Among the most rigidly tyrannical are autistic children, and perhaps next-most tenacious are obsessive-compulsives. Children who have vowed never to attach will go to unbelievable lengths to deny Theraplay's pleasures and to turn a deaf ear to the offers of intimacy. The extent of resistance to Theraplay seems often to be a measure of the extent of the underlying need for it (as seen by the degree of change made in the process).

Children who should not as a rule be seen in Theraplay include those who have been recently traumatized and those who are sociopathic. A handful of children, but only a handful, whether because of temperament or early life experience, are truly fragile and frightened. Recently traumatized children need the opportunity to relive the experience in a trustworthy atmosphere. They need a compassionate ear, and the chance to re-enact over and over again, if necessary, the dreadful experience with dolls or clay or crayons. They need the reassurance that they did not make it happen, even though they might have wished it would (e.g., in anger), and the knowledge that, from now on, they themselves will be safe and cared for. They may be helped by the nurturing of Theraplay (e.g., a cup of hot chocolate, a lap to sit on while talking, or an arm around the shoulder), but any other of the SCIN dimensions, such as intrusion, challenging, or structuring, would be inappropriate.

Sociopathic children enjoy Theraplay. They appear eagerly for each successive session, yet nothing ever changes. The interpreting therapist, sitting with the parents in the viewing room, may soon come to understand why. As the parents describe the child's antisocial antics of the prior week, their facial expression, tone of voice, choice of words, or sentence construction may belie any genuine concern or worry about the child's future or even about the self-destructive nature of his or her actions. Careful exploration from the outset may reveal that the problem is a concealed marital one, the child conveniently serving as scapegoat. Theraplay with the child in this case, of course, will not heal the damaged marriage. A referral for marital therapy is the appropriate course of action.

Ann M. Jernberg, PhD, is currently Clinical Director of The Theraplay Institute. She was on staff at Billings Hospital (University of Chicago) and Michael Reese Hospital, Chief Psychologist at the LaPorte County Comprehensive Mental Health Center in Indiana, and Director of Psychological Services for the Chicago Head Start program. She is the author of the book *Theraplay* and has published numerous articles and chapters in others' books. Other interests include treatment of the "fraudulant" achiever, couples therapy, adoption, parents-to-be and their attitudes and behaviors toward the fetus, and parent-infant relationships. Dr. Jernberg may be contacted at The Theraplay Institute, 333 North Michigan Avenue, Chicago, IL 60601.

RESOURCES

Jernberg, A. (1976). Theraplay technique. In C. Schaefer (Ed.), *The Therapeutic Use of Child Play* (pp. 345-349). New York: Jason Aronson.

Jernberg, A. (1979). *Theraplay: A New Treatment Using Structured Play for Problem Children and Their Children and Their Families.* San Francisco: Jossey-Bass.

Jernberg, A. (1982). Therapeutic use of sensory motor play. In C. Schaefer & K. O'Connor (Eds.), *Handbook of Play Therapy* (pp. 128-147). New York: John Wiley. (a)

Jernberg, A. (1982). Theraplay: History and method. In E. Nickerson & K. O'Laughlin (Eds.), *Helping Through Action: Action-Oriented Therapies* (pp. 150-162). Amherst: Human Research Development Press. (b)

Jernberg, A. (1982). Theraplay: The nursery revisited. In L. Abt & I. Stuart (Eds.), *The Newer Therapies* (pp. 171-180). New York: Van Nostrand Reinhold. (c)

Jernberg, A., Albert, A., Koller, T., & Booth, P. (1982). *MIM Manual: Adult-Preschooler.* Chicago: The Theraplay Institute.

Jernberg, A., Albert, A., Koller, T., & Booth, P. (1983). *MIM Manual: Adult-Infant.* Chicago: The Theraplay Institute.

Jernberg, A., & Stern, D. (1984). *Start with a Hug...and a Huggies.* Neenah, WI: Kimberly-Clark. (Parent-infant interaction chart developed for Huggies Diapers.)

Kohut, H. (1971). *The Analysis of Self.* New York: International Universities Press.

Kohut, H. (1977). *The Restoration of the Self.* New York: International Universities Press.

Koller, H. (1981). *Older Child Adoptions: A New Developmental Intervention Program.* Paper presented at the annual meeting of the American Psychological Association, Los Angeles, CA.

Marschak, M. (1960). A method for evaluating child-parent interaction under controlled conditions. *Journal of Genetic Psychology, 97,* 3-22.

Marschak, M. (Producer). (1969). *Nursery School Child-Mother Interaction* [Film]. Chicago: The Theraplay Institute.

Marschak, M. (Producer). (1973). *Patterns of Parenting in Israel* [Film]. Chicago: The Theraplay Institute. (a)

Marschak, M. (Producer). (1973). *Two Climates of Childhood in Israel* [Film]. Chicago: The Theraplay Institute. (b)

Marschak, M. (Producer). (1973) *Selma Fraiberg: Epilogue to Two Climates of Childhood in Israel* [Film]. Chicago: The Theraplay Institute. (c)

Marschak, M. (1979). *Parent-Child Interaction and Youth Rebellion.* New York: Gardner Press.

Miller, A. (1981). *Prisoners of Childhood.* New York: Basic Books, Inc.

Robertiello, R. (1975). *Hold Them Very Close, Then Let Them Go.* New York: Dial Press.

Winnicott, D. (1965). *The Maturational Processes and the Facilitating Environment.* New York: International Universities Press.

BEHAVIORAL ASSESSMENT AND TREATMENT OF FACIAL PAIN*

Robert M. Malow and Ronald E. Olson

Health practitioners are becoming increasingly aware of temporomandibular joint (TMJ) pain and dysfunction as a health problem affecting an estimated 24% of the population. The disorder was originally conceptualized as a structural problem associated with malocclusion of the teeth, malformation or degeneration of the condyle, fossa, or meniscus of the temporomandibular joint. This led dentists to treat the problem with mechanical means which were reversible (e.g., biteplates to adjust the occlusion) or irreversible (e.g., equilibration of the occlusion by removing tooth enamel, or surgery to correct the suspected defect in the temporomandibular joint or meniscus).

Recent evidence, however, has strongly suggested that the majority of patients complaining of TMJ pain and dysfunction do not have a structural problem but rather are experiencing stress which leads to tension which leads to muscle hyperactivity, pain, and dysfunction. Laskin (1969) has termed this disorder Myofascial Pain Dysfunction Syndrome (MPDS) which is characterized by pain in and around the temporomandibular joint, tenderness to palpation of the muscles of mastication, joint clicking or popping sounds when opening the mouth, and limitation of movements of the mouth. In addition, the diagnosis is based on a lack of any clinical, radiographic, or biochemical evidence of organic pathology.

MPDS has been conceptualized as a psychophysiological disorder that is promoted by psychological factors such as anxiety, depression, and fatigue or interpersonal conflicts within the family, circle of friends, or work environment. It is also promoted by oral habits such as clenching or grinding the teeth; cheek, lip, or nail biting; excessive gum chewing; or biting on the stem of a pipe; and so on. Several lines of research generally support this conceptualization (see Malow, Olson, & Greene [1981] for a comprehensive review).

First, personality tests, tests of family dynamics, evidence of illness behavior, and secondary gain all indicate that MPDS patients differ both from other dental patients and from normal individuals, but are similar to patients with tension-related psychophysiological disorders. Many of these differences are associated with difficulties in coping with stressful life situations and with an individual's perception of and reaction to pain.

Second, compared to a normal population, MPDS patients are more likely to have other psychophysiological disorders. These include low back pain, neck and shoulder pain, ulcers, migraine or tension headaches, dermatitis, and asthma.

Third, MPDS patients are under more psychological stress and are more anxious than normal individuals. MPDS patients have higher than normal urinary concentrations of catecholamines and 17-hydroxysteroids, two substances associated with emotional stress. They also show significantly greater masticatory muscle activity than normal individuals when subjected to experimentally induced stress. It has been shown that chronically heightened muscle activity can lead to masticatory pain and dysfunction.

Fourth, MPDS patients are highly responsive to a variety of physical (e.g., drugs, occlusal adjustment, biteplates) and psychological (e.g., biofeedback, relaxation training,

---

*Supported in part by grant DE 06946 from USPHS awarded to Daniel M. Laskin, DDS, MS.

individual and group psychotherapy) treatments. What may be common to all effective therapies is simply the reduction of muscle tension.

TYPICAL CASE HISTORY

Janice Smith (a fictitious name) is a 38-year-old housewife and mother of two. For the last 4 years she has had episodes of jaw pain. She describes this pain as a dull, persistent ache in the cheek area in front of her right ear, which she notices upon rising in the morning and which continues for the whole day. In the late evening, it usually subsides and she is able to sleep at night. She reports that the pain is worse if she eats any chewy foods like steak, hard rolls, carrots, apples, and so on. Sometimes the pain is so bad that it hurts to talk. She states that she has this pain once or twice a week. She currently is concerned and seeking treatment because she has noticed that she is not able to open her mouth very wide and fears that the disorder is becoming progressively worse. When asked how she has coped with the problem for 4 years, she states that when in pain she either does not eat or eats very soft foods. She also has found that a hot, wet face cloth applied to the painful area in combination with two aspirins sometimes helps. She reports under questioning that she has been experiencing more life stress in the past several years since her husband got a new job and they moved to a larger home. Her children are getting older and also require a lot of her time ferrying them around and participating in a number of school-related activities.

Janice's case is similar to that of 12 million Americans, about 80% women, who have MPDS. The chief complaint is pain, usually on one side of the face. The pain is most often described as a dull ache but sometimes as sharp or shooting. Generally, the pain occurs in the cheek area just in front of the ear, but occasionally extends to other areas of the head, neck, and shoulders. In addition, some patients complain of general headaches, dizziness, sinusitis, and ringing in the ears. The multiplicity of symptoms often makes the diagnosis difficult, leading some practitioners to label MPDS the "Great Impostor."

THERAPEUTIC MANAGEMENT

MPDS has been treated in the past by many radical, costly, and irreversible procedures, including temporomandibular joint surgery, injection of sclerosing agents into the joint, extracting all the teeth and making dentures, capping all the teeth, and equilibrating the bite. However, recent research has led to a new treatment philosophy. MPDS is viewed increasingly as a stress-related, functional disorder rather than a morphologically caused problem. This reconception leads to a redefinition of the goals of treatment. Instead of seeking underlying morphological aberrations and correcting them, it has become important to understand and manipulate the complexities of stress, neuromuscular dysfunction, pain cycles, illness behavior, and the psychological aspects of the treatment situation. As a result, the pendulum of treatment philosophy has swung from irreversible to reversible treatment; hence, the goals of clinical treatment involve pain control and restructuring environmental systems and habits to alleviate stress.

ASSESSMENT

Excluding Possible Organic Dysfunction. Initially, an individual must be evaluated for organic causes of pain and dysfunction. Systemic disorders such as rheumatoid arthritis may affect the temporomandibular joint, and some cases of MPDS may be caused or influenced by local irritating factors. Assessment of several of these factors is discussed by Malow et al. (1981).

While most patients with MPDS do not have significant co-existing occlusal problems, the possibility exists that such correlations can occur. Any history of recent bridgework, partial dentures, or other major dental work that coincides with the onset of MPDS symptoms should lead the clinician to suspect an iatrogenic occlusal problem. Treatment of the MPDS problem in such patients should include the management of these occlusal problems by the simplest means possible. Extensive dental procedures should be avoided until pain symptoms are under control.

Questionnaire. To rule out the possibility of other disorders, to establish a diagnosis of MPDS, and to determine the functional relationship of various parameters to MPDS requires a comprehensive history and complete oral exam. In obtaining a history, we have found it helpful to employ two questionnaires which the patients are sent upon requesting an appointment and which they complete at home before being seen (Malow et al., 1981).

The first questionnaire deals with prior care. It is not uncommon to find that patients with MPDS have had numerous consultations with health professionals such as dentists, neurologists, psychologists, psychiatrists, chiropractors, and ear-nose-throat specialists. It is important for the practitioner to be aware of these previous contacts to avoid repeating extensive diagnostic evaluations or unsuccessful therapy, to help rule out the possibilities of other disorders, and to clarify the patient's expectations of how the present treatment will differ from previous treatments. Medication use also is explored in order to avoid previous unsuccessful treatment and to avoid dangerous drug interactions.

A number of questions in the second questionnaire (see Patient's Health Questionnaire on pages 198-199) concern other psychophysiologic disorders which may relate to MPDS, such as headaches, ear pain, stomach troubles, ulcer, lower back aches, joint swelling, and so forth. This information aids in arriving at a final diagnosis. For example, the existence of tension headaches would make a diagnosis of MPDS more likely because muscle tension is common to both disorders. Other questions assess psychological aspects of patient functioning related to emotional stress. These factors are important in that they often lead to dysfunctional oral habits such as bruxism, excessive gum chewing, or biting of the nails, tongue, cheeks, or lips, all of which can lead to muscle fatigue and spasm. From items on the questionnaire, it is also determined whether the patient is suffering from the cardinal symptoms of MPDS - pain in or around the TMJ, tenderness to palpation of the muscles of mastication, limitation of jaw movement, and clicking or popping sounds in the TMJ.

Interview. While a questionnaire may be economical in reducing patient contact hours by providing information about possible etiological and concurrent factors, it cannot completely substitute for an interview. This can involve a brief history of pain onset, duration of pain, and time of occurrence. What was going on in the patient's life when the pain began? Was there a loss or death? Was there a change in employment, lifestyle, environment, or marital status? As the interview proceeds along these lines, stress areas are usually identified and elaborated. Basically, the interviewer is interested in the patient's manner of coping with stress. Does the patient become tense or clench his or her teeth, and if so, how quickly? Are teeth clenching and self-destructive oral habits related to any specific stress activity, for example, freeway driving? Does the patient awaken with facial pain? An affirmative response to this question may suggest nocturnal bruxism. The interview often can reveal stresses in the environment that may have led to the symptoms of MPDS. Next, the present pain is discussed with attention to oral habits that are elicited by stress, the nature of these stressors, and the relationship between stress and pain. If the patient has difficulty recalling what was happening when the pain occurred, it is often useful to obtain hourly, daily, or weekly records of pain, along with significant accompanying events. Such records should include who was with the patient, what was said before and during the pain episode, how long the pain lasted, what seemed to relieve the pain, and so forth.

Often patients are unaware of what situations produce muscle tension. Such information may be obtained by observing the patient during the interview. Does the patient clench his or her teeth? Does the patient bite his or her lip, tongue, or cheek? If so, simple habit retraining through positive practice or biofeedback may be sufficient to eliminate the problem. Often, however, the activities related to stress-induced muscle tension cannot be readily detected in the clinic, either because they occur only in specific outside situations, or because they are not visually observable in the clinic. For clinical assessment, Rugh (1977) has suggested the use of an electromyographic (EMG) diagnostic procedure outside of the lab.

In this procedure a small, portable, inexpensive EMG unit, which can be worn inconspicuously by the patient during normal daily activities and during sleep, is used. When the patient's muscle tension exceeds a pre-set threshold, a tone will go off in an earphone. Thus, the patient can monitor the stress-induced activity that produces an increase in muscle tension and keep a record of such activities.

Research has indicated that patients with MPDS fit a broad spectrum of personality types. Accordingly, Olson (1983) has stated that personality assessment does not appear to aid in the diagnosis or treatment of a particular individual. Hence, while there are indications that MPDS patients as a group are more tense and anxious than normal individuals, sophisticated tests do not appear to contribute information beyond that which can be obtained from a thorough assessment such as that described above.

TREATMENT

Education and Self-Management. There is a continuing need throughout the diagnostic assessment and at the beginning of the therapeutic intervention to explain the role and requirements of being a patient, the sequence of treatment, and the rationale for the suggested procedures. Even before the first clinic contact, it is recommended that patients receive a written description of the clinic, its procedures, and costs.

Once a diagnosis has been established, a comprehensive explanation of the philosophy of treatment is given to the patient during the first treatment session. It is explained that MPDS is not a problem of the joint, the nerves, or the blood vessels, but rather of excessive muscle tension related to stress in the patient's life. Patients must understand the importance of taking responsibility for treatment success by working hard to follow the suggested treatment regimen. If the patient has trouble accepting this, treatment is likely to be difficult. Some patients want the doctor to do something to them or give them a pill that eliminates the pain, rather than relaxing and actively attempting to reduce life stress. If this is the case, considerable effort ought to be directed at reshaping these patients' expectations. The relationship of stress and anxiety to the development of muscle tension and pain must be discussed in a clear and detailed manner. Analogies and comparisons to other psychophysiological disorders, such as lower back pain and tension headaches, are helpful in aiding patients' appreciation of this idea. Along these lines, it can be explained that treatment will focus upon stopping the pain, relaxing the muscles, and restoring normal mandibular functioning. A final point to be made is that treatment is usually successful, and if one treatment is not completely successful, there are several others available.

As in all treatment endeavors, it is important to establish a therapeutic context in which fear and anxiety relating to the pain is reduced, hope is aroused, an expectation of improvement is developed, and a motivation for the client to get well is cultivated. This is especially important when the disorder is related to muscular tension accompanying emotional reactions. These characteristics of the therapeutic climate are often collectively referred to as manifestations of the placebo effect, and they can be enhanced when the practitioner shows both confidence in treating the disorder and an understanding of the disorder. Facial pain can be a particularly anxiety-producing experience, and adopting a caring and concerned attitude will do much to reduce the patient's anxiety. Rugh and Solberg (1976) have pointed out that a staggering variety of treatments have been successfully employed in treating MPDS (i.e., hypnosis, TMJ surgery, muscle exercise, counseling, electrical stimulation, biofeedback, tranquilizing drugs, corticosteroids, muscle relaxants, placebo drugs, psychoanalysis, group psychotherapy, occlusal adjustment, and a variety of occlusal splints). Regardless of the treatment, however, "clinicians who are successful demonstrate a 'psychologic awareness' and accept the necessity of listening to the patient's problems" (p. 24).

After being given an explanation of their disorder, many patients may be able to effectively treat themselves. Patients often are able to re-examine their life patterns, to become increasingly aware of those emotional reactions leading to muscle tension, and to make appropriate therapeutic changes in their habits. Cobin (1969) has suggested that patients with MPDS should think about whether they frequently keep their teeth clenched together. Many will find that their upper and lower teeth are clenched most of the time. If this is happening, a conscious effort should be made to control the habit. The patients also should try to find out from their spouses or roommates if audible grinding or clenching of the teeth occurs at night. Such unconscious nocturnal habits may be difficult for patients to eliminate entirely. Sometimes the awareness of these habits, in addition to some form of relaxation training, enables them to control excessive parafunctional activity. The voluntary muscle relaxation techniques described by Jacobson (1970) as well as modern biofeedback techniques Dohrmann and Laskin (1978) are examples of how active patient cooperation can aid in controlling bruxism and muscle tension.

In addition to changing habits and life patterns associated with stress, patients can treat themselves by the application of moist compresses, altering oral and sleep habits, adopting a diet of soft food, and restricting jaw function. Such measures may interrupt the pain cycle long enough to allow the sensitized muscle tissue time to return to normal. After the painful symptoms have been alleviated, the patient can be treated by prescribing specific jaw exercises to help in regaining the full range of normal jaw functioning.

Secondary Treatment. The majority of MPDS patients will show significant improvement after 2 to 3 weeks of educational and self-management therapy. For those individuals who are nonresponsive, a second level of treatment should be initiated either alone or in combination: exercise, drugs, relaxation training, stress management, biteplates, and so on. Because all of these forms of therapy are highly successful and none of them have been shown conclusively to be more effective than any other, the treatment chosen is somewhat arbitrary. The choice probably will depend upon the practitioner's specialty (psychology, dentistry, pharmacology, physical therapy, etc.). Because certain procedures may turn out to be more effective for specific patients, treatment optimally should take place in a multidisciplinary clinic employing dentists, pharmacologists, psychologists, physical therapists, psychiatrists, neurologists, surgeons, and others. Treatment should be escalated to more intense, less cooperative measures only when simpler procedures are unsuccessful.

Psychopharmacology. Many different drugs have been used in the treatment of MPDS. In addition to the nearly universal use of analgesics for control of pain, clinicians have prescribed anti-inflammatory agents, sedatives, muscle relaxants, tranquilizers, vitamins, and antidepressants. Other medications have been administered by injection either into the joint (e.g., steroids, hyaluronidase, anesthetic agents, and normal saline) or into the masticatory muscles (anesthetic agents, steroids, and hyaluronidase).

Within the psychophysiological framework, the goals of chemotherapy are threefold. First, stop the pain. Because muscular pain has the distinction of being self-perpetuating or cyclic, the pain cycle needs to be interrupted long enough to permit recovery of muscle tissue to normal. Second, decrease muscle tension that leads to spasm, masticatory hyperactivity, and pain. Third, reduce the psychophysiological factors that may be operating to produce muscle tension. We believe that these goals are best accomplished using a combination of an analgesic and minor tranquilizer. The minor tranquilizer is superior to a pure muscle relaxant because it both reduces muscle tension and reduces psychophysiological response to stress. However, the minor tranquilizer should not be used alone because it does not directly reduce pain. For this purpose an analgesic is best.

Following several years of clinical experimentation and use, the TMJ center at the University of Illinois has found a combination of diazepam (5 mg three or four times a day) plus enteric coated sodium salicylate (600 mg three or four times a day) to be most effective for the treatment of pain associated with MPDS (Greene & Laskin, 1973). The sodium salicylate is used rather than conventional aspirin to further the placebo effect and also to lessen gastric irritation. This regimen of medications should be taken regularly for 2 to 6 weeks, depending on the response obtained, after which the medication should be withdrawn gradually (decreasing doses for 2 weeks). These drugs should not be taken randomly or only when the pain occurs, because this does not eliminate the pain cycle. For many patients, this combination of medications, taken properly, will provide adequate or total relief from painful MPDS symptoms and permit the return of normal function. Much of the success of these medications, however, depends on proper communication and patient cooperation. Because of the addictive quality of diazepam, caution must be exercised in prescribing it so that it is not abused.

Reduction of Muscular Hyperactivity with Biteplates. The most widely used method for reducing muscle activity has been, and still is, some type of intraoral appliance or biteplate. Despite the many variations of concept, material, design, and use, there are four tangible features that nearly all such appliances have in common. They are devices of acrylic and wire, can be inserted and removed by the patient, alter the proprioceptive input from the mouth to the muscles, and passively stretch the elevator muscles of the mandible. In effect, the biteplate alters the load on the TMJ by elevating the plane of occlusion, thereby allowing the masticatory muscles to work smoothly and without resistance, reducing joint trauma.

Transcutaneous Stimulation. Transcutaneous electrical nerve stimulation (TENS), which refers to electrical stimulation of the skin over major sensory nerves, has been widely used and has received much publicity as an effective treatment for clinical pain. According to the gate control theory of pain, which has had enormous influence on the conceptualization and treatment of pain, TENS is presumed to activate a spinal "gating" mechanism that blocks or attenuates painful sensation produced by peripheral stimulation. A recent study by Malow and Dougher (1979), using signal detection measurement procedures, confirmed the assumption that TENS does reduce sensation. A number of clinical reports and experimental investigations also indicate that it reduces verbal reports and physiological indices of pain. It has been used and found effective in treating MPDS patients.

Physical Therapy. Nearly all of the physical therapy techniques commonly used for muscle and joint problems have been applied to the treatment of MPDS problems. Included among these are dry and wet heat applications, ultrasound, diathermy, refrigerants, and several different types of exercise. The latter is by far the most commonly employed physical therapy procedure. Exercise serves both the function of relaxing tense muscles and of restoring the full range of normal function. By stretching the muscles through exercise, they become more flexible and clicking noises may be minimized.

Complete instructions for performing jaw exercises have been provided by Kraus (1963). These exercises must be done regularly over a period of several weeks, and it is wisest to begin them only after the pain has subsided. Immediately prior to performing the exercises, it is helpful to apply moist heat to the affected areas to warm them up and improve circulation. The exercise routine includes actively moving the jaw through a prescribed regimen, passively moving the jaw with the hands, and trying to open the jaw against pressure from the hands.

Psychological Approaches

Psychotherapy. For patients to relax muscles, they often must learn how to deal with emotions that can contribute to muscle tension. Suppressed anger, agitation, and feelings of depression are examples of such emotions, and they can be addressed with conventional psychotherapy or by using various behavior therapy techniques. Nevertheless, psychotherapy is not the first treatment of choice for MPDS patients because it is more time consuming and expensive than other procedures. Moreover, MPDS patients usually are coming to a dentist or physician with what they consider a physical rather than a psychological problem, and they may resent a suggestion to seek psychotherapy. For those patients who are nonresponsive to usual treatment approaches, however, short-term individual psychotherapy may be indicated, and it frequently can be helpful. The therapist can focus on those situations that precipitate or co-exist with the symptoms of MPDS and help the patient explore new ways of dealing with these situations to reduce tension.

Time-Limited Group Psychotherapy. Group psychotherapy has also been used to treat those patients who are nonresponsive to more conventional treatment approaches. Patients in groups typically deny psychological aspects of their problems in initial group meetings, but they can benefit from sharing the descriptions of their symptoms with others similarly affected and becoming aware that they are not unique. As patients share this material, the therapist can provide information, support, and reassurance. As group cohesiveness emerges and allows patients to begin exploring emotional concerns, the therapist can become more probing and challenging. Marbach and Dworkin (1975) found social isolation and withdrawal associated with chronic depression to be the issues most often revealed in the later sessions of group therapy. They also found dependency on the group to be an issue at termination. Nonetheless, 60% of their patients showed symptom improvement.

Family Therapy. Minuchin and others (Liebman, Minuchin, & Baker, 1970; Minuchin, 1974) have found that many individuals suffering from a variety of psychophysiological disorders come from dysfunctional families. Such "psychosomatogenic" families usually demonstrate the characteristics of enmeshment, overprotectiveness, rigidity, and lack of conflict resolution. Recent research by the authors (1984) indicates that MPDS patients come from similar dysfunctional families.

In such cases, structural family therapy methods, such as those reported by Minuchin, have been found useful. These methods emphasize changing a family's interactional patterns. Recent research suggests that family dynamics play an important role in the patient's illness behavior, overuse of medication and the health care system, and the expression of pain. Failure to consider family dynamics has been shown to significantly reduce the effectiveness of treatment programs.

Relaxation Therapy. Jacobson (1970) developed a method of progressive muscle relaxation to provide tension control for use in the treatment of anxiety neurosis and phobias. His method can be adapted for use with patients with MPDS. They can be trained to become increasingly aware of their muscle sensations, especially in the head and neck region. They learn to counteract habitual muscular contraction patterns that cause their pain. Patients learn to tense and relax muscle groups, and to pay close attention to the sensations that are generated. Clenching the teeth and opening the jaws with control are practiced. This technique has proved successful as a treatment approach, especially in conjunction with electromyographic biofeedback. Patients have also learned tension control by listening to cassette tapes designed to teach progressive relaxation or by participating in group tension control training sessions (Olson & Malow, in press).

Electromyographic Biofeedback. As in relaxation therapy, investigators who use muscle biofeedback believe that patients who are made aware of the tension level in their jaw muscles and trained to relax these muscles will get relief from pain. Indeed, improvement has been reported in the majority of patients in from 3 to 28 sessions. Patients sit in a comfortable, semireclining position, and surface electrodes usually are attached to the masseter muscle on the side of the face where the patient experiences discomfort. Electromyographic information is transduced into a sound or light which the patient can hear or see. When a sound is used, the patient learns to slow the frequency of the beeps and lower the pitch as much as possible. Instruments are equipped with gain control settings with increased sensitivity that require the patient to relax more deeply to keep the tone low and slow. Therapy may be facilitated by having the patient rent or buy biofeedback equipment to practice at home. In addition, the therapeutic effect may be further enhanced by training the patient to induce relaxation without the machine. Finally, the effectiveness of biofeedback may be enhanced by providing concurrent short-term psychotherapy with the goal of identifying stressors for the individual and exploring alternative means of handling this stress. This involves helping the patients understand how stress reactions develop and how they are maintained. Furthermore, patients can use both cognitive and behavioral coping skills to deal with the stress, and they can learn to restructure belief systems that may contribute to maintaining stress (Olson, 1977).

Assertiveness Training. Several reviewers have indicated that MPDS patients have difficulty expressing frustration and aggression. Such unassertive behavior is likely to result in poor psychosocial adjustment in family and employment situations. This is likely to lead to a greater willingness to remain in the role of a patient and a less favorable prognosis and response to treatment. Where patients lack assertiveness skills, it may be helpful to provide them with an assertiveness training program.

Hypnotherapy. The standard relaxation training tapes use a form of hypnotic induction to produce deep levels of relaxation. If the practitioner is comfortable using hypnosis, it can prove quite effective in treating MPDS patients.

Treatment Failures. There are certain patients with MPDS who do not respond to any type of conservative treatment within a reasonable time. Although some of these nonresponsive patients may have been diagnosed incorrectly, the reason for most treatment failures relates to the personality and behavioral characteristics of the patient. A significant number of these patients are depressed. Rugh and Solberg (1976) have observed that nonresponsive patients are ones who report the most emotional reactions from their symptoms and who have stress-related disorders occurring at several body sites. Schwartz, Greene, and Laskin (1979) found that nonresponders have less healthy MMPI personality profiles than responders. Using measurement procedures that yield scores for sensitivity and response bias, Malow and colleagues (Malow, Grimm, & Olson, 1980; Malow & Olson, 1981) investigated differences in pain perception between normal subjects, patients who responded to treatment, and patients who did not respond to treatment. They found that, after treatment, nonresponsive MPDS patients had lower pain thresholds, showed less sensitivity to different levels of painful stimulation, and had a greater tendency to report pain. By comparison, responsive patients were more like normal subjects in their reactions to painful stimulation.

In the past, it was common for dentists and physicians to escalate the intensity of therapy for nonresponders. Recent research has shown, however, that nonresponders to conventional therapy show no greater improvement from subsequent aggressive physical treatment than similar patients who discontinue all treatment. There are various alternatives for nonresponders. The most promising results have been obtained with time-limited individual psychotherapy. One study showed that nearly two-thirds of such nonresponders displayed considerable improvement following psychotherapy. Other investigations reported similar results with group psychotherapy as well as with antidepressant medication. Good results have also been reported with various relaxation training methods such as biofeedback, guided imagery, and progressive relaxation.

Another reason for treatment failure relates to the environmental contingencies that patients face. For example, if the patient is in therapy to please someone else, then he or she is unlikely to improve and may resist therapy. Resistance to therapy is often seen when there are secondary gains for the patient to remain ill. Secondary gains are rewards a patient may obtain for being in pain (e.g., excuses from responsibility, unemployment insurance, sympathy from others, or added attention from spouse or doctors). The contribution of secondary gain to treatment failure may be particularly potent when the patient is receiving some form of monetary compensation that will be terminated upon improvement.

A final form of resistance to treatment can be seen in patients whose disorder is one part of their overall adjustment to life stress. In a very real sense their symptoms have come to serve a function in their life situation and mental economy, even though they would function better without these symptoms. Sternbach (1978) has described this type of "loser" pattern in patients with chronic lower back pain. By far, the most successful approach for dealing with such resistant patients is the operant conditioning approach proposed by Fordyce (1976). His framework for analyzing chronic pain patients is derived from Skinner's work on conditioned responses and learning theory. Fordyce regards chronic pain behavior as a series of operants, or actions, which elicit a response from other people in the patient's environment. Many of these responses may serve to reinforce the particular operant (e.g., a grimace of pain on walking brings sympathy), and thus the behavior has more and more to do with learning, and less and less to do with the original pathologic stimulus.

The concept of operant pain behavior has led to an operant conditioning approach to treatment in which patients receive feedback from trained personnel while hospitalized for chronic pain therapy. The behavioral objectives of chronic pain management programs include (a) learning and accepting the concept of a useful and satisfying existence in spite of pain; (b) increasing programmed activity and efficient self-care; (c) gradually reducing the pain medication; and (d) improving family relationships.

Although the use of the inpatient, behavior modification program described by Fordyce has not been reported for MPDS patients, its success in treating similar patient populations warrants its use in treating nonresponding MPDS patients.

CONCLUSIONS

MPDS is currently considered to be a psychophysiologic disorder because of its mixture of physical symptoms and psychological factors. While the condition is located primarily in the muscles of mastication, it is clearly influenced by stress, emotional states, and personality traits, and its treatment is affected by many psychological aspects of the doctor-patient relationship.

There is no single personality style that typifies the patient with MPDS. A number of different methods of coping with life can result in this condition. In general, most of these patients would not be classified as pathologic or exhibiting serious emotional illness. Nevertheless, an individual's difficulties in resolving stress can produce tension, promote chronic hyperactivity in the masticatory muscles, and lead to a predisposition to develop the symptoms of MPDS. Furthermore, these patients are similar to other patients with chronic pain; they suffer similar emotional reactions, such as depression, anxiety, and anger. Because MPDS is a psychophysiological disorder, both the psychological and physical components of this problem must be treated. Pain and dysfunction are alleviated with any treatment that relaxes the masticatory muscles. If the dentist or physician is warm, empathic, and reassuring, patients gradually understand and accept the psychological component of their disorder. A healthier psychological state results from knowledge about the relationship between emotional stress and physical tension. Pain can be reduced when the knowledge and relevant skills are integrated into the treatment.

PATIENT'S HEALTH QUESTIONNAIRE[*]

Name____Age____________Sex__________Date________________________

    If you can answer YES to the question asked, put a circle around YES. If the answer is NO to the question asked, put a circle around NO. Answer all questions and fill in blank spaces when indicated. If you are not sure, guess.

1. Are you being treated by a medical doctor at present?   YES   NO

    If yes, for what? ____

2. Do you suffer from any chronic (long-standing) diseases?   YES   NO

    If yes, list them. ____

3. Do you regularly take any medication or pills? If yes,   YES   NO

    what are they? ____

4. Do you suffer from headaches?   YES   NO

5. Do you have any allergies?   YES   NO

6. Do you have chronic ear pain or infection?   YES   NO

7. Do you suffer from stomach troubles or ulcers?   YES   NO

8. Are you suffering from rheumatism or arthritis?   YES   NO
    If yes, circle what kind: rheumatoid   degenerative   traumatic   gout

9. Do your muscles and joints ever feel stiff or swollen?   YES   NO

10. Do you ever experience muscle aches or spasms?   YES   NO

    If so, where? ____   YES   NO

11. Do you have frequent diarrhea?   YES   NO

12. Have you ever had any serious accidents or injuries?   YES   NO

13. Have you ever been hospitalized for any serious illness or operation?   YES   NO

    If so, what was the problem?____

14. Do you have any oral habits such as grinding or clenching your teeth,   YES   NO
    cheek- or lip-biting, or biting on hard objects?

15. Have you ever had a nervous breakdown, counseling, psychotherapy,   YES   NO
    or psychoanalysis?

16. Do you take sedatives, tranquilizers, nerve medicine, sleeping pills,   YES   NO
    or medicine to relax?

17. Do you have trouble sleeping?   YES   NO

18. Do you ever have dizzy spells?   YES   NO

19. Do you suffer from low back pain?   YES   NO

20. Do you have, or have you ever had, ileitis or colitis?   YES   NO

21. Do you have any eye problems?   YES   NO

22. Do you have any sinus problems?   YES   NO

23. Do your saliva glands ever hurt or swell?   YES   NO

24. Do you ever have dental pain or infection?   YES   NO

25. Have you ever had your wisdom teeth removed?   YES   NO

26.   Do your teeth feel loose?   YES   NO

27.   Does your bite feel comfortable?   YES   NO

28.   Does your jaw ever snap or lock?   YES   NO

29.   Does your jaw crack or pop?   YES   NO

30.   Does your jaw ever feel stiff?   YES   NO

31.   Does eating make your jaw hurt?   YES   NO

32.   Do you get swellings or sores in your mouth?   YES   NO

33.   Do you ever get swollen glands?   YES   NO

34.   Are you frequently confined to bed by illness?   YES   NO

35.   Are you always in poor health?   YES   NO

36.   Do you come from a sickly family?   YES   NO

37.   Has pain made work impossible for you?   YES   NO

38.   Are you constantly made miserable by poor health?   YES   NO

39.   Do you have to lie down and rest often because of pain?   YES   NO

40.   Does pain bother you so much you have to keep moving?   YES   NO

41.   Has pain interfered with your sex life?   YES   NO

42.   Are you unable to do the things you want because of pain?   YES   NO

43.   Do you find that all you can think about is your pain?   YES   NO

44.   Do doctors seem to have failed you?   YES   NO

45.   Do you keep looking for a specialist to solve your case?   YES   NO

46.   Do you have trouble getting doctors to take you seriously?   YES   NO

47.   Have some doctors said your pain is imaginary?   YES   NO

48.   Do you secretly think your case may be hopeless?   YES   NO

49.   Do you have, or have you ever had, any other significant medical   YES   NO
      problems that were not mentioned above?

      If yes, what are they? ____

      ____

50.   My last medical examination was on ____________________________________

      My last dental examination was on ______________________________________

      The name, address, and telephone number of my physician are:

      ____

      The name, address, and telephone number of my dentist are:

      ____

Robert M. Malow, PhD, is currently staff psychologist at the Veteran's Administration Medical Center, New Orleans and Assistant Professor in the Department of Psychiatry and Neurology at Tulane Medical School. Prior to his present position he was a psychologist in the Temporomandibular Joint and Facial Pain Research Center in the College of Dentistry at the University of Illinois at Chicago. His training is in clinical psychology and he has published numerous articles on the subject of facial pain. Other interests include chemical dependency and psychopathology. Dr. Malow may be contacted at 1601 Perdido Street, New Orleans, LA 70146.

Ronald E. Olson, PhD, is currently Professor of Psychology in Occupational Therapy and the Assistant Dean for Research in the College of Associated Health Professions at the University of Illinois at Chicago. Prior to his present position he was the chief psychologist in the Temporomandibular Joint and Facial Pain Research Center in the College of Dentistry at the University. His training is in clinical psychology and he has published numerous articles on the subject of facial pain. Other interests include disordered thinking in schizophrenia. Dr. Olson can be contacted at 1919 W. Taylor, Room 325, Chicago, IL 60612.

RESOURCES

Cobin, H. P. (1969). Treatment of the temporomandibular pain-dysfunction syndrome. *New York State Dental Journal, 35,* 552-554.

Dohrmann, R. J., & Laskin, D. M. (1978). An evaluation of electromyographic biofeedback in the treatment of myofascial pain-dysfunction syndrome. *Journal of the American Dental Association, 96,* 656-662.

Fordyce, W. F. (1976). *Behavioral Methods for Chronic Pain and Illness.* St. Louis, MO: C. V. Mosby.

Greene, C. S., & Laskin, D. M. (1973). Therapeutic effects of diazepam (Valium) and sodium salicylate in myofascial pain-dysfunction (MPD) patients. *IADR Program and Abstracts, 50,* Abstract 193.

Jacobson, E. (1970). *Modern Treatment of Tense Patients.* Springfield, IL: Charles Thomas.

Kraus, H. T. (1963). Muscle tension and the temporomandibular joint. *Journal of Prosthetic Dentistry, 13,* 950-955.

Laskin, D. M. (1969). Etiology of the pain-dysfunction syndrome. *Journal of the American Dental Association, 79,* 147-153.

Liebman, R., Minuchin, S., & Baker, L. (1970). The use of structural family therapy in the treatment of intractable asthma. *American Journal of Psychiatry, 131,* 535-540.

Malow, R. M., & Dougher, M. (1979). A signal detection analysis of the effects of transcutaneous stimulation on pain. *Psychosomatic Medicine, 41,* 101-108.

Malow, R. M., Grimm, L., & Olson, R. E. (1980). Differences in pain perception between myofascial pain dysfunction patients and normal subjects: A signal detection analysis. *Journal of Psychosomatic Research, 24,* 303-309.

Malow, R. M., & Olson, R. E. (1981). Changes in pain perception after treatment for chronic pain. *Pain, 11,* 65-72.

Malow, R., & Olson, R. E. (1984). Family characteristics of myofascial pain dysfunction syndrome patients. *Family Systems Medicine, 2,* 428-431.

Malow, R., Olson, R., & Greene, C. (1981). Myofascial pain dysfunction syndrome: A psychophysiological disorder. In C. Golden, S. Alcaparras, F. Strider, & B. Graber (Eds.), *Applied Techniques in Behavioral Medicine and Medical Psychology* (pp. 101-133). New York: Grune and Stratton.

Marbach, J. J., & Dworkin, S. F. (1975). Chronic MPD, group therapy and psychodynamics. *Journal of the American Dental Association, 90,* 827-833.

Minuchin, S. (1974). *Families and Family Therapy: A Structural Approach.* Boston: Harvard University Press.

Olson, R. E. (1977). Biofeedback for MPD patients nonresponsive to drug and biteplate therapy. *Journal of Dental Research, 56,* B61. (From *Special Issue B,* Abstract No. 40)

Olson, R. E. (1983). Behavioral examinations in MPD. In D. Laskin, W. Greenfield, E. Gale, J. Rugh, P. Neff, C. Alling, & W. A. Ayer (Eds.), *President's Conference on the Examination, Diagnosis and Management of Temporomandibular Disorders* (pp. 104-105). Chicago, IL: American Dental Association.

Olson, R., & Malow, R. (in press). The effects of relaxation training on myofascial pain dysfunction syndrome patients. *Clinical Journal of Pain.*

Rugh, J. (1977). A behavioral approach to diagnosis and treatment of functional disorders: Biofeedback and self control techniques. In J. D. Rugh, D. B. Perlis, & R. I. Disraeli (Eds.), *Biofeedback in Dentistry: Research and Clinical Applications* (pp. 95-112). Phoenix, AZ: Semantodontics.

Rugh, J. D., & Solberg, W. K. (1976). Psychological implications in temporomandibular pain and dysfunction. *Oral Sciences Review, 7,* 3-30.

Schwartz, R. A., Greene, C. S., & Laskin, D. M. (1979). Personality characteristics of patients with myofascial pain-dysfunction (MPD) syndrome unresponsive to conventional therapy. *Journal of Dental Research, 58,* 1435-1439.

Sternbach, R. A. (1978). *The Psychology of Pain.* New York: Raven Press.

CONSTRUCTING AND INTERPRETING GENOGRAMS: THE EXAMPLE OF SIGMUND FREUD'S FAMILY

Randy Gerson and Monica McGoldrick

Genograms are diagrams of family trees used by many clinicians as a core component of family assessment. Usually, the initial interview is organized around making sense of a client or family's presenting problem in relation to the three-generational patterns that are depicted on genograms. The genogram has been developed primarily in the fields of family therapy (Bowen, 1978; Bradt, 1980; Carter & McGoldrick, 1976; Guerin & Pendagast, 1976, Hartman, 1978; McGoldrick, 1980; N. Paul & B. Paul, 1974; Wachtel, 1982) and family medicine (Jolly, Froom, & Rosen, 1980; Medalie, 1978; Mullins & Christie-Seely, 1984; Rakel, 1977). In this contribution we have summarized our basic approach to genogram construction and interpretation, using the family of Sigmund Freud as an illustrative example. For a more complete explanation of the use of the genogram, the reader is referred to *Genograms in Family Assessment* (McGoldrick & Gerson, 1985).

Genograms are appealing to clinicians because they are tangible and graphic representations of a family. They allow the clinician to map the family structure clearly and to note and update the family "picture" as it emerges. The genogram provides an efficient clinical summary, allowing a therapist unfamiliar with a case to grasp quickly a large amount of information about a family and to have a view of potential problems. While questionnaire answers or notes written in a chart may become lost in a clinical record, genogram information is immediately recognizable and can be added to and corrected at each clinical visit as more is learned about the family.

Genograms make it easier for a clinician to keep in mind family members, patterns, and events that may have recurring significance in a family's ongoing care. Just as language potentiates linear thinking and thus organizes our thought processes, family diagrams may potentiate circular thinking by mapping interconnected relationships and patterns of functioning, and thus may help clinicians think systemically about how events and relationships in their clients' lives are related to patterns of health and illness.

The information on a genogram is best understood from a systemic perspective. The genogram interview should be seen as one part of a comprehensive, systemic, clinical assessment. There is no measurement scale by which the clinician can use the genogram in cookbook fashion to make clinical predictions. Rather, the genogram is an interpretive tool with which the clinician can generate tentative hypotheses for further systemic evaluation.

We will use the family of Sigmund Freud as an illustrative example of the genogram construction process. This historical family was chosen because of (a) available biographical and genealogical information on the family, and (b) a general interest in Freud as an historical personality who greatly influenced the mental health field. Neither Freud nor his biographers ever did extensive research into his family, and the details of his family life are sketchy. This is interesting considering the huge amount of literature on Freud's life. Systemic history is hampered by nonsystemic biographers. Freud himself destroyed much information; as his biographer, Ernest Jones, has pointed out, "Freud took elaborate measures to secure his privacy, especially concerning his early life. On two occasions he completely destroyed all his correspondence, notes, diaries and manuscripts" (1953, 1, p. xii). This lack of information is common in constructing genograms. When little is known about early life and previous generations, much can often be made of the bare facts.

CONSTRUCTING THE GENOGRAM

The genogram is usually constructed as part of a general clinical interview. This is typically done in the first interview as an initial assessment and revised as new information becomes available. We will discuss the genogram interview and the actual drawing of the genogram separately.

THE GENOGRAM INTERVIEW

The process of gathering family information is similar to casting out a metaphorical information net in larger and larger circles to capture relevant information about the family and its broader context. The net spreads out in a number of different directions: (a) from the presenting problem to the larger context of the problem; (b) from the immediate household to the extended family and broader social systems; (c) from the present situation to an historical chronology of family events; (d) from easy, nonthreatening queries to difficult, anxiety-provoking questions; and (e) from obvious facts to judgments about functioning and relationships to hypothesized family patterns.

The Presenting Problem and the Immediate Household. The family usually comes in with specific problems, which is where we begin. From there, it usually makes sense to ask about the immediate household, that is, the immediate context in which the problem occurs.

A fictional interview with the Freud family might go something like the following (the date is 1896; in the room are Sigmund and his wife, Martha):

Clinician:	How can I be helpful?
Sigmund:	I am the problem. I am quite depressed. I feel self-absorbed, trying to analyze things all the time.
Clinician:	Who else has noticed this?
Martha:	I have. He seems to have no time for his children or even me.

The clinician gathers information about the presenting problem and how the problem is affecting each member of the household. From this comes information about the different members of the household. The name, age, and sex of each person in the household is asked in order to sketch the immediate family structure. The immediate Freud household consists of Sigmund, Martha, their six children, and Minna, Martha's sister.

The Family Situation. Next, the clinician asks about the current family situation:

Clinician:	How long has this been going on?
Sigmund:	It's been particularly bad over the last year.
Clinician:	What's been happening to you and your family over the last year?
Sigmund:	Nothing very much, but my work has been very interesting.
Martha:	Well, Anna, our youngest, was born and my sister moved in. Other than that, I can't think of anything.

It is important to ask about recent transitions as well as anticipated changes in the family situation, especially exits and entrances: births, marriages, divorces, deaths, and so on.

The Wider Family Context. At some point, the clinician looks for the opportunity to widen the scope of family information gathered.

Clinician: I would like to ask you something about your background to help make sense of your present problem.

Sigmund: That makes sense. What would you like to know?

Clinician: Let's start off with your own family. You are which one of how many sisters and brothers?

The clinician goes on to get the names, sex, and ages of Sigmund's siblings and parents. Then the previous generation is explored: Sigmund's aunts, uncles, and grandparents. The goal is to get information on at least three generations. Sigmund had even done a genealogy as a child, but is reluctant to give any but the most minimal information about his parents' families. Interestingly, we find out that Sigmund's father died in the last year, a fact that was not mentioned when the current situation was discussed, suggesting that it was an emotionally loaded issue for him. Then, information on Martha's family is explored, though here the information is more scanty.

The information gathered should extend beyond the biological and legal structure of the family to encompass common-law and cohabiting relationships, miscarriages, abortions, stillbirths, foster and adopted children. Sometimes, when the family reacts negatively to questions about extended family or complains that the questions are irrelevant, the clinician returns to the present problem until the connections between the present situation and other family relationships or experiences can be made.

The Social Context. Inquiries should be made regarding friends, clergy, caretakers, teachers, doctors, and so on, who are important to the functioning of the family. We find that Sigmund has a very important colleague and friend named Fleiss with whom he corresponds regularly and who is his most important confidante. It appears that he is rather isolated within his own medical community.

The Historical Perspective. As the clinician gathers more and more "facts" about family events, certain gaps will appear in the history, which can have great significance in understanding the family. For example, in our fictional interview, Sigmund mentions that his father, Jakob, had a previous wife and two sons from that marriage. However, the fact that Jakob had a third wife, sometime between his first wife and Sigmund's mother, is never mentioned by any family member. This should clue the clinician to explore Jakob's early marriages and the events leading up to Sigmund's birth. The time around Sigmund's birth seems to be particularly critical: the beginning of a new family, the death of an infant son, the emigration of two sons from an earlier marriage, the death of Jakob's father, and the moving of the whole family to Vienna.

The aim is not only to track important family events, but also to locate the family's development in historical time. The migrations of the Freud family make more sense when seen as part of the migratory patterns of the Jews of that time, just as Sigmund's anxiety about recognition and advancement must be seen in the context of the anti-Semitism in Viennese society as well as the academia of the period.

Tracking Family Relationships and Roles. More difficult, but equally important, are inquiries and judgments about the different types of relationships among family members and the functioning and roles of each person in the family. Inquiries about family relationships, functioning, and roles can touch sensitive nerves in the family and should be made with care.

Clinician: When you were courting, how did you get along with each other's family?

Martha: Sigmund didn't want me to listen to my family at all. He told me that I had to choose between them or him. He still doesn't want to have much to do with my brother, Eli, or his sister, Anna, ever since they got married.

Sigmund: It was your family that made you move even after we were engaged and kept you away from me for years.

The clinician should get as many perspectives on family relationships as possible. In addition, from such responses, information on family roles starts to emerge:

Clinician:	So how did you work out the question of the in-laws?
Martha:	I chose Sigmund.
Sigmund:	I think a wife should side with her husband and take care of things at home first. She has a family to bring up.

Difficult Questions about Family Functioning. Finally, there are questions about issues such as alcohol abuse, chronic unemployment, and severe symptomatology. It often takes careful questioning to clarify the true level of functioning, because family members often cover up their difficulties. Questions about individual functioning must be approached with sensitivity and tact. The clinician needs to judge the degree of pressure to apply if the family resists discussing such problems. Four areas should be covered: (a) serious problems, (b) education and work history, (c) drugs and alcohol, and (d) trouble with the law.

In the Freud family, serious problems might include a discussion of Sigmund's migraines and neurotic fears, his mother's tuberculosis, and his suggestion that his father may have been incestuously involved with one of his sisters. A thorough education and work history would uncover the long period it took Sigmund to get his medical degree, his career uncertainties, and his current isolation within the Viennese medical community. Exploring drug and alcohol use would reveal Sigmund's previous use and sometimes dependence on cocaine. The only known legal problems were during Sigmund's mandatory service in the military, when he tended to leave duty without permission.

Setting Priorities. One of the most difficult aspects of genogram assessment is the problem of setting priorities for inclusion of family information on a genogram. The clinician cannot explore every area that comes up in a family assessment interview. In a later section, we will discuss some basic interpretive categories for analyzing family patterns on the genograms. We have found that an understanding of these patterns helps the clinician set priorities in gathering and organizing family information.

DRAWING THE GENOGRAM

As information is gathered on a family, it is mapped on a sheet of paper. First the family structure is drawn. The backbone of a genogram is this graphic depiction of how different family members are biologically and legally related to one another from one generation to the next. The genogram is a construction of figures representing people and lines delineating their relationships. Figure 1 on the next page depicts a standardization of the symbols used to draw genograms.

Figure 2 on page 208 is an illustrative genogram of Sigmund Freud and his family. Sigmund is the Index Person, whose figure is doubled and lowered out of his sibling line. The spouses of the siblings are drawn slightly smaller and placed a bit lower than the siblings, to keep sibling patterns clear. The family is shown as of 1896, the date of our fictional interview, as is indicated at the lower right. The current members of the Freud household are encircled by a dotted line. At times it may be useful to construct a genogram for a different moment in the past, such as the point of symptom onset or a critical life change for a family, to better understand the way changes have occurred in a family.

Demographics, Functioning, and Critical Events. Beyond mapping the basic family structure, three other types of information are included on the genogram: demographics, functional information, and critical life events. Demographic information includes age, dates of birth, marriage, divorce, and death, location, occupation, and educational level. Functional information includes more or less objective data on the medical, emotional, and behavioral functioning of different family members. Indications of high or low functioning should be included where possible or relevant. Critical family events include important transitions, relationship shifts, migrations, losses, and successes. These give a sense of the historical continuity of the family and of the effect of the family history on each individual. Critical events not listed as part of the demographic information are recorded either in the margin of the genogram, or, if necessary, on a separate attached page.

(If Index Person is child place in G3, if couple, do separate genogram for each spouse with note to other genogram and place each spouse in G3)

A. Symbols to Describe Basic Family Membership and Structure. (Include on genogram significant others who lived with or cared for family members - place them on the right side of the genogram with a notation about who they are.)

Male: □   Female: ○   Birth Date ⟶ 43-75 ⟵ Death Date

Index Person (IP): □ ○   Death = ⊠
or Identified Patient

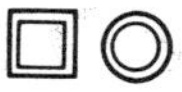

Marriage (give date)
(husband on left, wife on right): 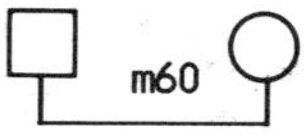 □ m60 ○   Living Together Relationship or Liaison: □ L 72 ○

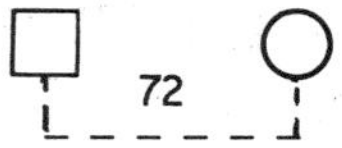

Marital Separation (give date): □ s70 ○   Divorce (give date): □ d72 ○

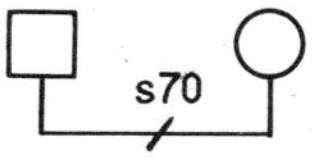

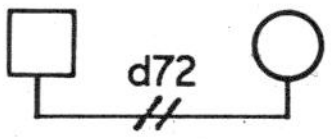

Children: List in birth order, beginning with oldest on left: 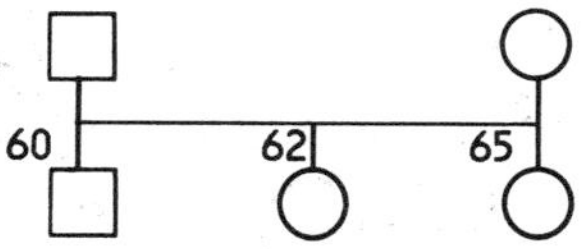 60 62 65   Adopted or Foster Children:

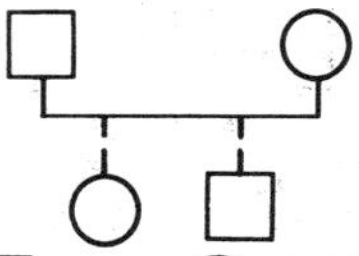

Fraternal Twins: 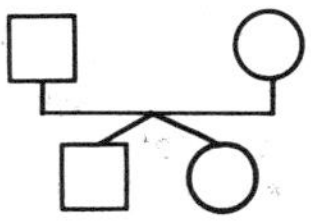   Identical Twins: 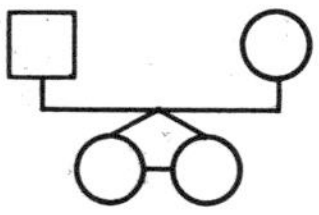   Pregnancy: △ 3mos.

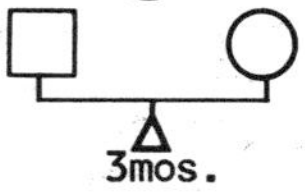

Spontaneous Abortion: 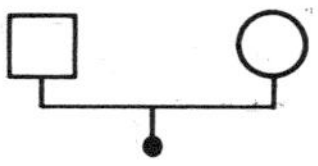   Induced Abortion: 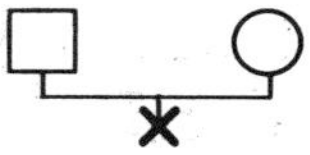 ✗   Stillbirth:

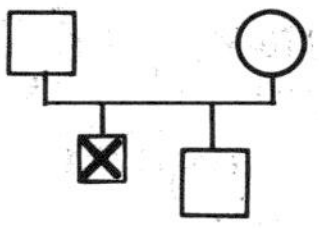

Members of Current IP Household (circle them):

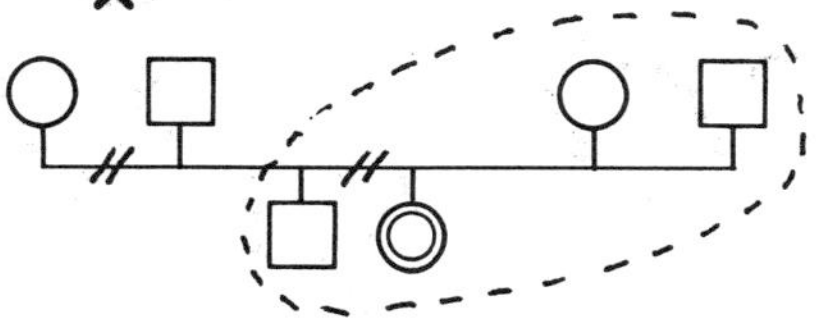

Where changes in a child's living arrangements have occurred, please note:

B. Family Interaction Patterns. The following symbols are among the least precise information on the genogram, but can be key indicators of relationship patterns the clinician wants to remember:

Very Close Relationship: 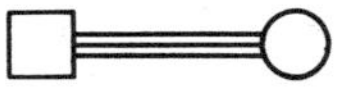   Conflictual Relationship:

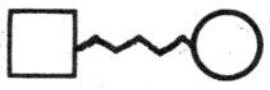

Emotionally Distant Relationship: 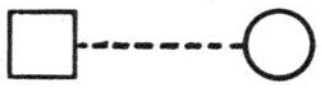   Estrangement or Cut-Off (give dates if possible): Cut-off 62-78

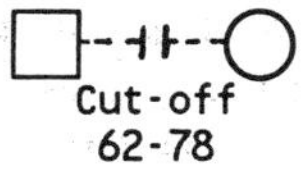

C. Medical History. Since the genogram is meant to be an orienting map of the family, there is room to indicate only the most important factors. Thus, list only major illnesses or chronic medical problems. Include dates in parentheses where feasible or applicable. Use <u>DSM-III</u> categories or recognized abbreviations where available (e.g., Cancer: CA - Stroke: CVA).

D. Other Family Information should, when appropriate, be noted on the genogram with dates, if possible.

1. Ethnic Background
2. Religion or Religious Change
3. Education
4. Occupation or Unemployment
5. Trouble with Law
6. Physical Abuse or Incest
7. Obesity or Anorexia
8. Dates When Family Members Left Home: LH '74
9. Current Location of Family Members

E. Alcohol or Drug Abuse. Please darken top half of square or circle and give dates. ◧ ◓

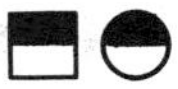

F. Other Key Information. This would include anniversary dates, concurrent events, nodal events, changes in the family constellation since the genogram was made, hypotheses and other notations of major family issues or changes. These notations should always be dated, and should be kept to a minimum, since every extra piece of information on a genogram complicates it and therefore diminishes its readability.

Figure 1. Genogram format

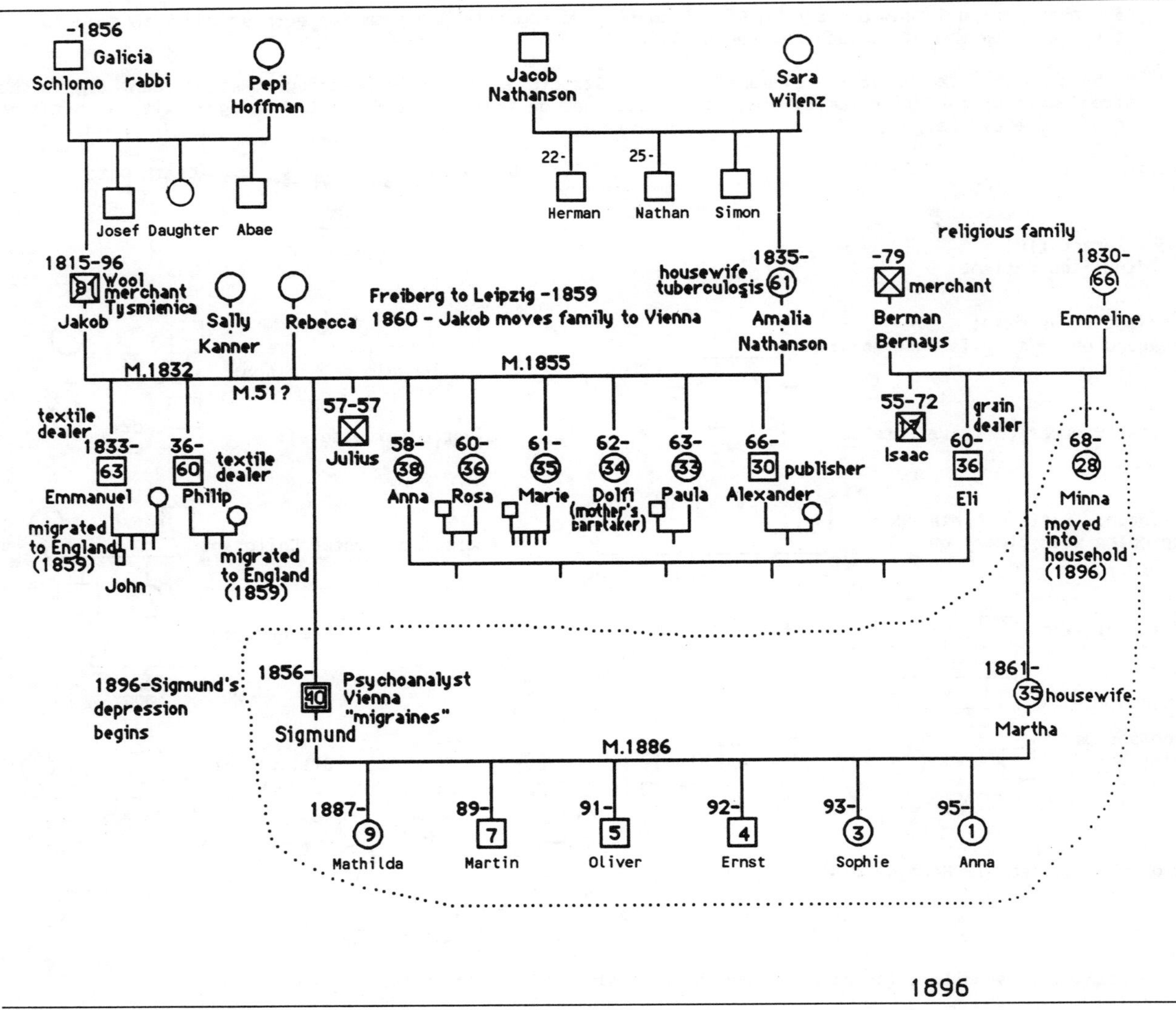

Figure 2. Sigmund Freud's family.

We have included on the Figure 2 Freud genogram the three types of information. As is evident, only the most important data can be included. There is always more information available than can be included on a single page; extra information will make the genogram cluttered and unreadable. When only partial, but critical, information is unearthed, it should be included, as with the marriages of Sigmund's father. We know that he was married three times and that he had two sons with his first wife, Sally Kanner, but little is known about her, and less about his second wife, Rebecca (Clark, 1980; Glicklhorn, 1969). We do not even know what happened to her, whether they divorced or she died. The third wife, of course, was Sigmund's mother, Amalia Nathanson.

The Family Chronology. We generally keep a family chronology with the genogram. This is a listing in order of occurrence of important events in the family, as can be seen in part on Figure 3 (p. 209) for the Freud family. An individual chronology may also be useful for tracking a particular family member's life course (symptoms, functioning) within the context of the family. Figure 4 (p. 209) shows Sigmund's illnesses in relation to other life events.

Showing Family Relationships. Finally, we show on the genogram important family relationships. This level of genogram construction is the most inferential. It involves delineating the relationships between family members. Such characterizations are based

```
1854       Sigmund's nephew, John, born
1855       Niece, Pauline, born
07/29/55   Jakob and Amalia are married
02/21/56   Schlomo Freud, Jakob's father, dies (Jakob is 40)

05/06/56   Sigmund born in Freiberg, Moravia (now Pribor, Czechoslovakia)
04/57      Julius Freud, Sigmund's brother, born
12/57      Julius dies
12/58      Anna Freud, Sigmund's sister, born
1859?      Sigmund's nursemaid leaves - arrested for theft, reported by Sigmund's half brother, Philip
1859       Emmanuel  and Philip emigrate with their families,  including Sigmund's nephew,  to whom he  is
           very attached
1859       Freud family moves from Freiberg to Leipzig (?) because of economic reversals for Jakob
1860       Family settles in Vienna
03/60      Rosa, Sigmund's sister, born
03/61      Marie (Mitzi), Sigmund's sister, born
07/62      Dolfi, Sigmund's sister, born
05/63      Paula, Sigmund's sister, born
04/66      Alexander, Sigmund's brother, named by Sigmund, born
06/17/82   Sigmund and Martha engaged
1883?      Minna engaged to Ignaz Schonberg, friend of Sigmund
06/14/83   Martha's mother moves with her daughters to Wandsbek
10/83      Eli Bernays and Sigmund's sister Anna are married.   Sigmund does not attend,  nor even mention
           the  wedding in letter to Martha (at least not in published correspondence.   Apparently only a
           small part of this correspondence has been published).
1884       Jakob Freud having business problems
04/85      Sigmund destroys all his papers
06/85      Schonberg breaks engagement to Minna
02/86      Schonberg dies of TB, diagnosed in 1883
09/14/86   Sigmund and Martha are married, as a result of a gift from Martha's aunts
10/87      Mathilda, Sigmund and Martha's first child, born (named for friend Breuer's wife)
12/89      Martin, the second child, born (named for teacher, Charcot)
02/91      Oliver, the third child, born (named for Sigmund's hero, Oliver Cromwell)
04/92      Ernst, the fourth child, born (named for teacher Ernst Brucke)
11/92      Eli to America
1893       Eli returned and took family to US with him (? 2 daughters Lucy and Hella stayed with  Freud's
           family for 1 year).  Sigmund gave Eli some money for the trip.
04/93      Sophie, the fifth child, born (named for teacher Hammerschlag's niece)
1894       Sigmund writes of having heart problems; trying to give up smoking; depression, and fatigue
01/95      Fleiss  operates on Sigmund's nose.   (Fleiss is apparently treating Freud for a  pseudocardiac
           condition - Mannoni, 1968, 1971.)
11/95      Minna comes to stay with Freud family
12/95      Anna, the sixth and last child, born (named for Hammerschlag's daughter)
04/96      Sigmund writes of migraines, nasal secretions, fears of dying
05/96      Sigmund writes of the medical community isolating him
10/23/96   Jakob Freud dies (Sigmund is 40)
```

Figure 3. Freud family chronology.


```
1919       Martha has bad case of pneumonia
1919       Sigmund and Minna go together to a spa for a "cure."  Martha does not come along because she is
           already at another sanitorium.
1920       Daughter Sophie catches pneumonia and dies
05/23      Sigmund goes to friend Felix Deutsch for diagnosis and his first cancer operation
06/19/23   Favorite  grandson  dies of TB.   Sigmund weeps for first time.   He is never to get over  this
           loss, which follows so shortly his own illness
10/04/23   Second operation
10/11/23?  Third operation (over next 16 years Sigmund has 30 more operations)
1923       Eli dies in New York.   Sigmund writes bitterly about his money and suggests that maybe now his
           sister, Anna, will do something for her four indigent sisters
```

Figure 4. Chonology of Freud family illnesses.

on the report of family members and direct observations. Different lines are used to symbolize various types of relationships between family members. Although such commonly used relationship descriptors as "fused" or "conflictual" are difficult to define operationally and have different connotations for clinicians from various perspectives, these symbols are useful in clinical practice. Since relationship patterns can be quite complex, it is often useful to represent them on a separate genogram. Illustrating the relationships of the Freud family is a chancy business. Figure 5 presents some of the possible relationship patterns that the available background information on the family suggests to us. Among the many complications at this level of genogram construction are the following problems: (a) depicting how relationships change over time; (b) depicting the changing patterns of over- and underfunctioning in a family; (c) depicting relationships which are seen differently from the perspective of different family members; (d) depicting ambivalent relationships, such as hostile-dependent relationships, or those in which a child continually seeks approval from a distant parent. One must be satisfied to illustrate only the grossest level of relationship to help the clinician keep key family patterns in mind.

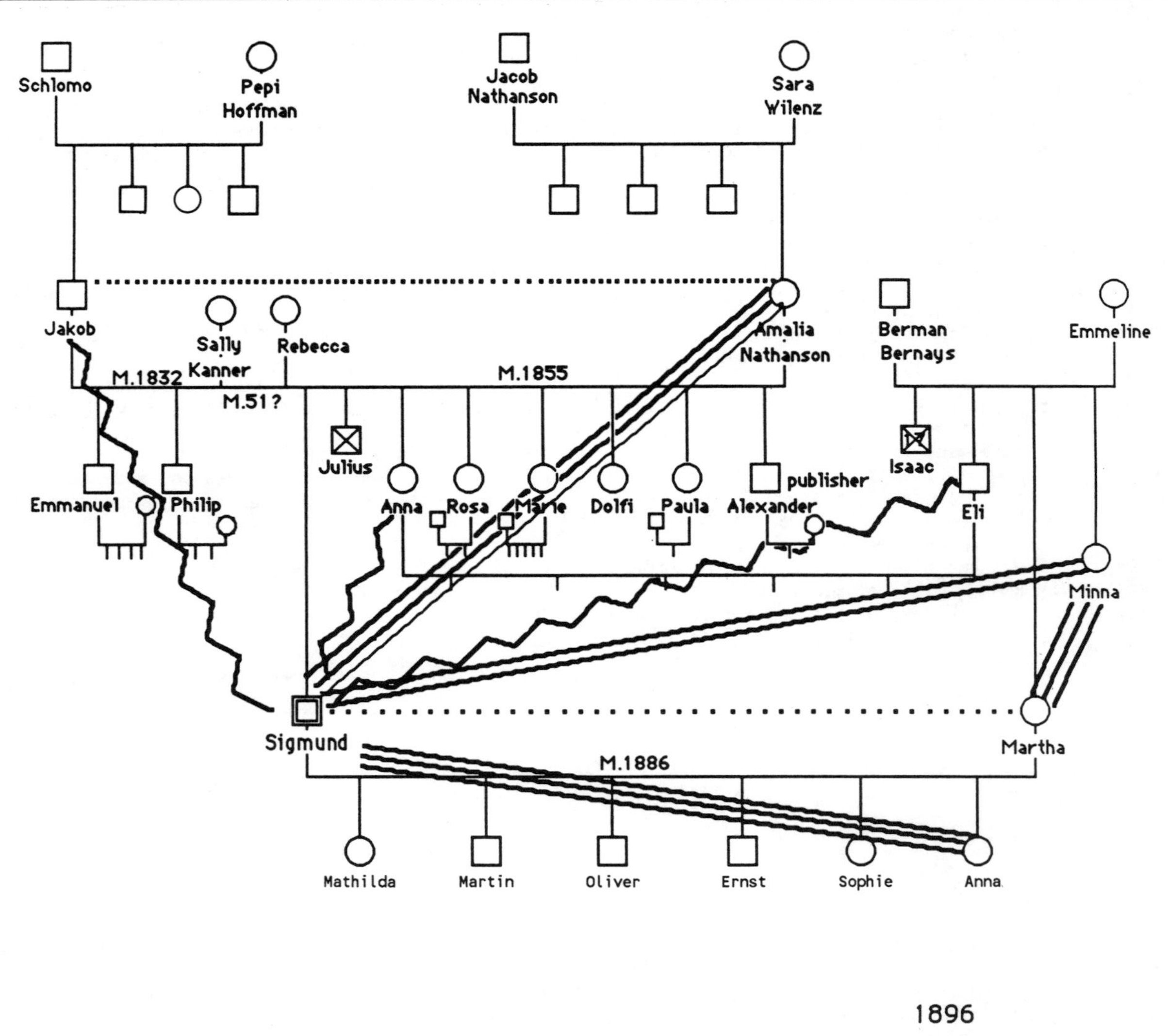

Figure 5. Freud family relationships.

Complex Genograms. The Freud family is relatively simple to map. Even here, however, the cross-marriages between the Freud and Bernays family pose a challenge for depicting the tangled web of relationships. In modern families with multiple marriages and divorces and shifting family membership, drawing the genogram and including all the relevant information can become very complex indeed (see McGoldrick & Gerson, 1985). Since genograms can become very complex, there is no set of rules that will cover all contingencies. Generally, the focal point of a genogram is the Index Person, and details about others are shown only as they relate to this person. The complexity of the genogram will thus depend on the depth and breadth of the information included. Genograms are necessarily schematic and cannot detail all the vicissitudes of a family's history. For example, it would be unlikely that the following would appear on the typical Freud genogram: (a) Sigmund did not attend his sister Anna's wedding; (b) Sigmund did not attend his mother's funeral and sent his daughter, Anna, as the "family representative"; (c) Minna's fiancé, Ignaz Schonberg, was Sigmund's patient and friend; (d) Sigmund was his daughter Anna's analyst; and (e) Minna's bedroom in the Freud household was located behind the master bedroom, with no exit except through the latter room.

INTERPRETING GENOGRAMS

Since the genogram has developed primarily out of the family systems theory of Murray Bowen (1978), the conceptual framework for analyzing genogram patterns has been based on his ideas. What follows is for the most part derived from Bowen's work. We use six categories for interpreting genograms: family structure, life cycle fit, pattern repetition across generations, life events and family functioning, relational patterns and triangles, and family balance and imbalance.

FAMILY STRUCTURE

The family structure as mapped on a genogram includes household composition, sibling constellation, and other unusual family configurations. Where one fits in the family structure can influence one's functioning, relational patterns, and the type of family formed for the next generation. Examining sibling constellation and other elements of family structure mapped on genogram allows one to hypothesize about personality characteristics and relational patterns.

The lines and figures on a genogram provide a lot of information about a family's basic structure. The bare genogram of the Freud family in Figure 6 (p. 212) illustrates this point. From this skeletal genogram alone, the clinician can generate a number of hypotheses.

Household Composition. One glance at the structure of the genogram usually reveals the family's composition; that is, whether the family is intact, a single-parent household, a remarried family, a three-generational household, or a household including extended family members.

The first thing evident on the Freud genogram is that Jakob had three wives; Sigmund came from a remarried family. Such a structure always raises questions about the connections between the different parts of the family. For example, how well did Jakob's children from his first marriage relate to their stepmother, and did the children from each marriage get along well with each other? Similarly, what did it mean for Jakob that Sigmund was his third son, and for Amalia, that he was her first? In terms of the household composition in the next generation, we note the presence of Martha's unmarried sister, Minna. This should alert the clinician to the possible impact of an extended family member living in the household, particularly Minna's relationship with her sister and brother-in-law and her possible position as a "second mother." Minna lived in the household from 1895. Did this create triangles with Sigmund and his wife, or with the children, over who was the preferred mother figure? Also, we know about at least one nanny. What role did servants or nursemaids play in the family relationships?

Sibling Constellation. The importance of birth position, sex, and number of years in age from other siblings has long been discussed in the literature, although there has not always been agreement on the role sibling constellation plays in development (Adler, 1958; Bank & Kahn, 1982; Ernst & Angst, 1983; Forer, 1976; Sutton-Smith & Rosenberg, 1970; Toman, 1976). Many factors come into play that influence the role of sibling

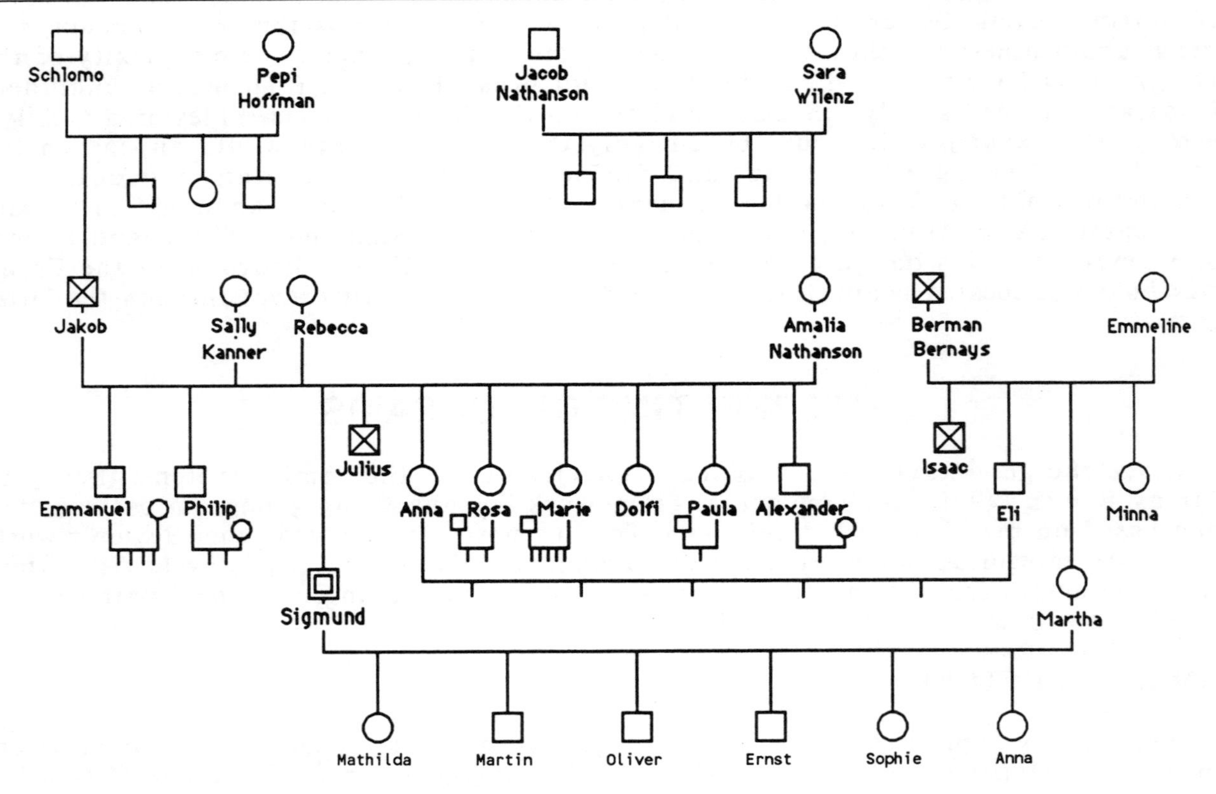

Figure 6. Freud family - bare genogram.

patterns, such as the timing of the child's birth in the family's history, special characteristics of a child, a family's "program" for each child, and parental biases regarding sex differences. In addition, ethnic groups vary in the role that sibling position plays in the family. Equally important, sibling patterns are undergoing significant changes, primarily because of different child-bearing and child-rearing patterns that have followed the increased availability of birth control, the women's movement, the entry of more women into the work force, and changing family structures. These factors all complicate our understanding of sibling patterns in a family. Nevertheless, we will venture some hypotheses about typical sibling patterns which are especially evident when mapped on a genogram. These hypotheses derive primarily from the work of Walter Toman (1976).

Sibling position can have particular relevance for one's emotional position in a family and future relations with a spouse and children. For example, an oldest child is more likely to be over-responsible, conscientious, and parental, while the youngest is more likely to be childlike and carefree. The oldest and youngest children often hold special positions in a family.

Sigmund was the oldest of his mother's 7 surviving children, followed by 5 sisters, and finally a brother 10 years later. We know that Sigmund held a special position in his family. He had a very intense relationship with his mother, who always referred to him as her "Golden Sigi." By all accounts, he was the center of the household. In addition to being the oldest, he was also the only son (after the second son died) for many years. The preference for sons over daughters shown in the Freud family has been characteristic of virtually all cultures. It is evidenced clearly in the family story that when Freud's sister, Anna, wanted to play the piano her mother bought one, but immediately got rid of it when Sigmund complained that the noise bothered him, and the sisters never had any further piano training. Sigmund's special position is further shown by the family having given him the privilege of naming his younger brother, Alexander, born when Sigmund was 10 years old.

Sigmund was the third son of his father, who had been married twice before. This may have made Sigmund even more important to his mother as the first child of her family with Jakob. Sigmund had two brothers who were a generation older than he. It is interesting that for the first 3 years of life Sigmund was raised almost as a younger brother to his nephew, John, who was a year or so older than he. Freud has commented on the importance of this relationship: "Until the end of my third year we (Sigmund and John) had been inseparable; we had loved each other and fought each other and...this childish relationship has determined all my later feelings in intercourse with persons my own age" (Jones, 1953, p. 8).

The oldest will sometimes feel resentment towards the later born, feeling threatened or displaced by the new arrival. These feelings can linger into adulthood. Sigmund's relationship with his sister, Anna, seems never to have been very close, and they were alienated as adults. From a very early age, he may have seen her as an intrusion and she may have resented his special position and privileges in the family. As will be discussed later, she was born at a difficult time for Sigmund and the family, which may have exacerbated his feelings against her.

The youngest may also have a special position in the family, that of the "baby," but may sometimes take on the role of caretaker as the parents age. This seems to be the case with Sigmund and his youngest daughter, Anna. Throughout his life, they were very close (she, rather than his wife, took care of him when he was ill), and she alone among the children never married, devoted herself to her father, and chose to carry on his life work.

The importance of sibling position will often appear in marital choices. It appears that those who repeat their sibling relationship in their marriage have a greater likelihood of complementarity and marital stability. Interestingly, in the Freud and Bernays families, the oldest brother married the next oldest sister in the other family, and in both cases the men appear to have dominated the relationship (a characteristic obviously reinforced by the culture).

Unusual Family Configurations. Sometimes there are unusual family configurations on the genogram that will suggest further exploration. As mentioned previously, there were cross-marriages in the Freud and Bernays families where brother and sister married sister and brother. This appears as an unusual configuration on the genogram and raises questions about how the couples formed and how the two families responded to the marriages. Further exploration reveals some negativity between these two family branches, which will be discussed in more detail later.

LIFE CYCLE FIT

The genogram is scanned for the family's life-cycle stage (see Carter & McGoldrick, 1980), because this suggests the tasks a family will be dealing with at any moment in its history. Most importantly, we look for discrepancies in age or life-cycle stage of family members and transitions that occur "off time," the most traumatic being untimely deaths.

In terms of life cycle fit, what is immediately apparent on the genogram (see Figure 2) is the discrepancy in age between Sigmund's father and mother. Jakob was 20 years older than Amalia, and his oldest son from his first marriage was older than his young wife, suggesting possible conflicts or at least uncomfortable feelings between the sons and the new wife. Jakob's older son had a son even before Sigmund was born, so that both Amalia and her daughter-in-law were having children during the same period. Although the sons reportedly emigrated to London for economic reasons, it is interesting to observe that the emigration occurred only a few years after their father's new marriage and the beginning of the new family.

The Freud and Bernays families had their share of untimely deaths. Both Sigmund and Martha had experienced the death of a young sibling and Minna's fiancé died, leaving her unmarried for the rest of her life. Much later, in 1930, Sigmund wrote of the death of his 4-year-old grandson: "I have spent some of the blackest days of my life in sorrowing about the child. At last I have taken hold of myself and can think of him quietly and talk of him without tears. But the comforts of reason have done nothing to help; the only consolation for me is that at my age I would not have seen much of him" (quoted in Clark, 1980, p. 441). He appeared to go into a depression for at least 3 years.

His strong reaction seems to be due partly to his own diagnosis of cancer coinciding with the untimely death of a favorite grandchild. In a later section, we will discuss further the impact of death on family functioning.

PATTERN REPETITION ACROSS GENERATIONS

Families repeat themselves. What happens to one generation will often repeat itself in the next; the same issues tend to be played out from generation to generation, though the actual behavior may take a variety of forms. Bowen (1978) terms this the multi-generational transmission of family patterns. The hypothesis is that relationship patterns in previous generations could provide implicit models for family functioning in the next generation. On the genogram we look for patterns of functioning, relationships, and structure continuing or alternating from one generation to the next.

We know very little about pattern repetition in the Freud family. We do know that Sigmund's paternal grandfather, Schlomo, who died a few months before Sigmund was born and for whom he was named, was a rabbi (Clark, 1980, p. 110). Sigmund, as a professor, perhaps followed in his footsteps - some would argue as a teacher of a new religion, psychoanalysis. It is possible that the calling to teach skipped a generation. Also interesting was the pattern of one child in each generation taking responsibility for the care of the elderly parents. Quite common in Vienna of that time, this would often be a daughter who never married, but devoted her young life to her parents. In the Freud family, this role was filled by Dolfi among Sigmund's siblings, and by Anna among his children, who also followed in his footsteps by becoming an analyst.

LIFE EVENTS AND FAMILY FUNCTIONING

We take a systemic view of the "coincidence" of events. Concurrent events in different parts of a family are not viewed simply as random happenings; rather, they are seen as often systemically interconnected. In addition, critical events are more likely to occur at some times than at others, especially at the nodal points of life cycle transition in a family's history. Symptoms tend to cluster around such transitions in the family's life cycle, when family members face the task of reorganizing their relations with one another to go on to the next phase. It is helpful to track changes in a family's long-term functioning as they relate to critical family life events and transitions. We examine the genogram carefully for the coincidences of life events; the impact of life changes, transitions, and traumas; anniversary reactions; and the role of social, economic, and political events.

In the Freud family, there were certain critical periods during which a series of important family events occurred. These are highlighted in Figure 7 (p. 215). The first critical period occurred around Sigmund's birth. In 1855, his father, Jakob, married Amalia Nathanson. Seven months later, Jakob's father died. Three months after this, Sigmund was born. A year later, Julius was born, but he died after 8 months. Then, after another 2 years, Jakob's two oldest sons moved to England, and Jakob and his family moved from Freiberg probably to Leipzig. And finally, a year later, Jakob moved his family again to Vienna. One can speculate about the impact of the two deaths (Jakob's father and the infant son, Julius) on the family and its relation to the chain of events that followed. Perhaps Jakob's move was partly a decision to leave a place where much misfortune had recently been experienced. In any event, Sigmund was born during a difficult time for the family and seemed especially valued as a result.

A second critical period occurred from 1895 to 1896. Sigmund's favorite child, Anna, was born on December 3, 1895. The following year, his sister-in-law, Minna, moved into the household, and on December 23 of that year Sigmund's father died, a loss which Sigmund said was the most significant and upsetting in the life of a man. Not surprisingly, he went into a depression during this period and began his famous self-analysis. It is interesting that Anna, who like her father was born at a difficult point in her family's history, was the only one to become an analyst.

It is important to note that both critical periods occurred at transitional points in the Freud family life cycle. The first occurred around a marriage (Jakob's third) and the second around the birth of the last child. In clinical practice, we find that families are more vulnerable to change around transitional points in the family life cycle. Thus, we

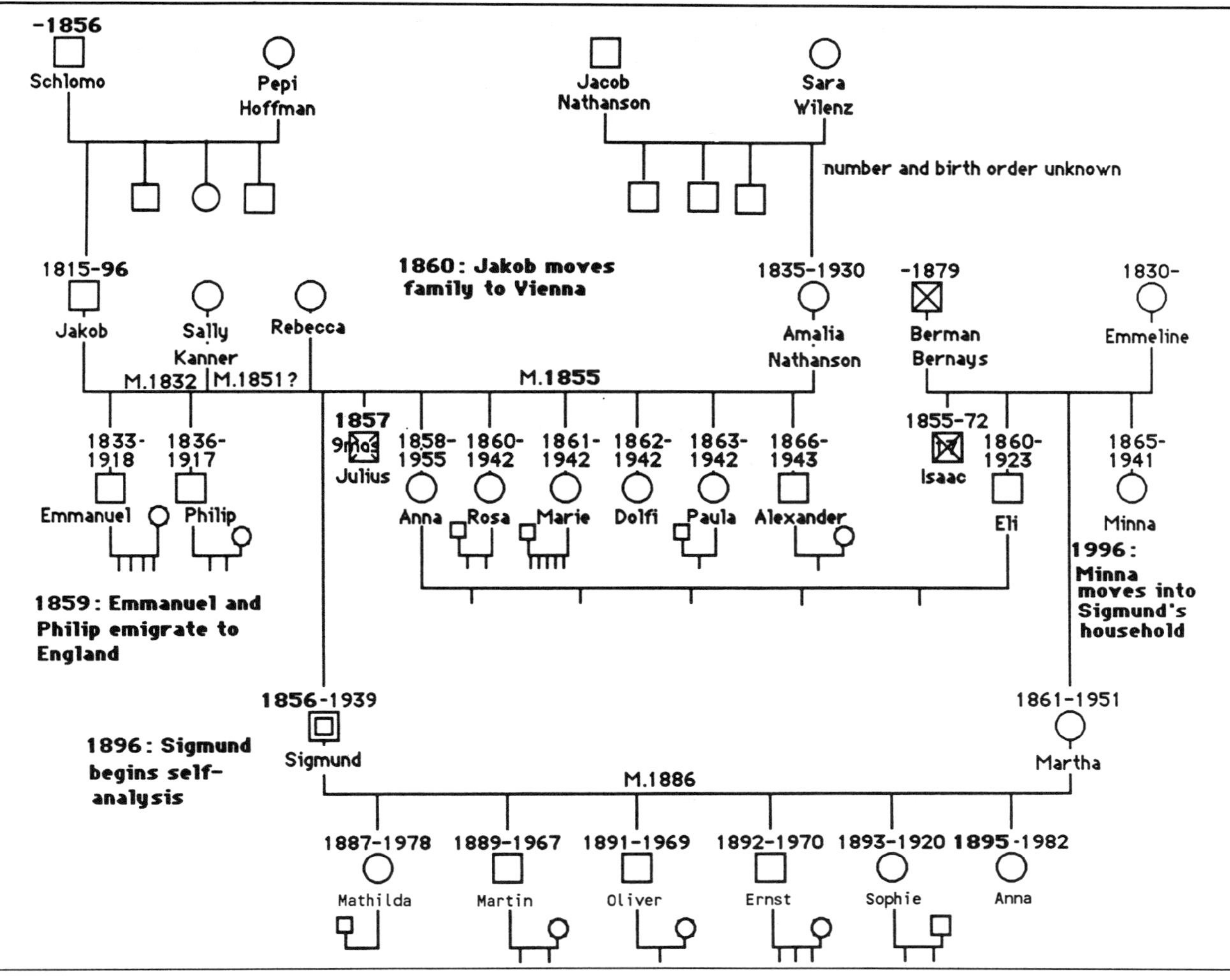

Figure 7. Freud family - critical periods.

pay particular attention to these nodal points when examining genograms for coincidences of family events or changes in family functioning.

Some deaths have more impact on a family than others. Particularly traumatic are untimely deaths such as the early death of Sigmund's brother, Julius. Another example was the death of Sigmund's 4-year-old grandson, which was mentioned previously.

RELATIONAL PATTERNS AND TRIANGLES

While it is beyond the scope of this contribution to cover the theoretical complexities that underlie the interpretation of relational patterns on the genogram, we will discuss briefly the concept of triangles in understanding family relationships. A triangle is a set of three relationships in which the functioning of each dyad is dependent on and affects the other two. The formation of triangles in a family involves two people bringing (triangling) a third into their relationship, which usually lessens the difficulties in the initial dyad. Two family members, for example, may join in helping a third, who is labeled "victim," or gang up against a third, who is labeled "villain." It is the collusion of the two in relation to the third that defines a triangle (Bowen, 1978).

There are many different types of triangles, including parent/child triangles, couple triangles, in-law triangles, triangles in divorced and remarried families, triangles in families with foster and adopted children, multigenerational triangles, and triangles with people outside the family. (For further discussion of each type of triangle, see McGoldrick & Gerson, 1985.) A family can have a number of different triangles, each triangle being part of an interlocking network.

We will focus on two triangles in the Freud family. The first is the triangle involving Jakob Freud, his third wife, and Jakob's sons from his previous marriage, Philip and Emmanuel (see Figure 8). This is an example of a remarried family triangle. In this type of triangle, there are predictable patterns: Often, the children from the previous marriage will resent the new parent, experiencing him or her as an intruder and an imperfect replacement for the idealized other parent. On the other hand, the new parent may find it difficult to find a comfortable role in the family and may see the children from the old marriage as preventing the clear establishment of a new family with the spouse. Since there is no direct information, we can only speculate on the situation in the Freud family shortly before and after Sigmund's birth. Amalia had married a man twice her age who had two previous wives and two sons. The distance between the families was exaggerated by the fact that the sons were approximately her own age. It is likely that she was feeling some tension regarding their presence, even though one had already married and moved out. The sons were probably having their own difficulties adjusting to this very young stepmother who was so eager to have her own family, beginning with Sigmund. Jakob, no doubt, was caught in the middle. It is not surprising that within a few years, both sons had emigrated to England, particularly after economic stresses (business failure) were added to the possible family stresses.

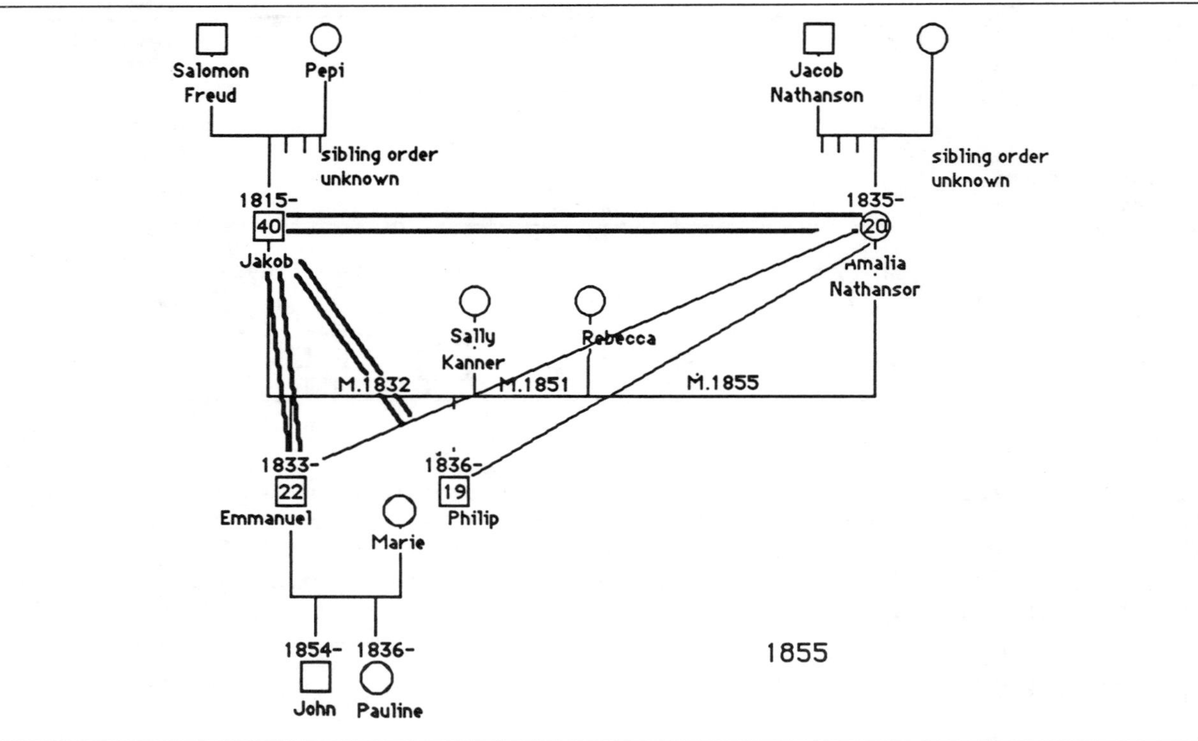

Figure 8. Freud family - remarried family triangles.

A second triangle involves Sigmund, his wife, Martha, and her nuclear family, the Bernays (see Figure 9, p. 217). Actually, this triangle began even before they were married. During their long courtship Sigmund wrote to Martha: "From now on you are but a guest in your family...For has it not been laid down since time immemorial that the woman shall leave father and mother and follow the man she had chosen?" (letter in E. L. Freud, 1960, p. 23). Sigmund particularly resented his mother-in-law who moved her family, including Martha, from Vienna during the period they were engaged and before they could marry, due to a lack of money. Sigmund also did not get along well with his brother-in-law, Eli, although they had been friends before Sigmund met Martha. Eli married Sigmund's sister, Anna, in 1883. Sigmund did not attend the wedding, or even mention the event in his letters to Martha, although he was writing her almost daily. Perhaps Sigmund especially resented their marriage when his being able to marry seemed so far away. Sigmund's negative feelings toward his sister and brother-in-law seemed to

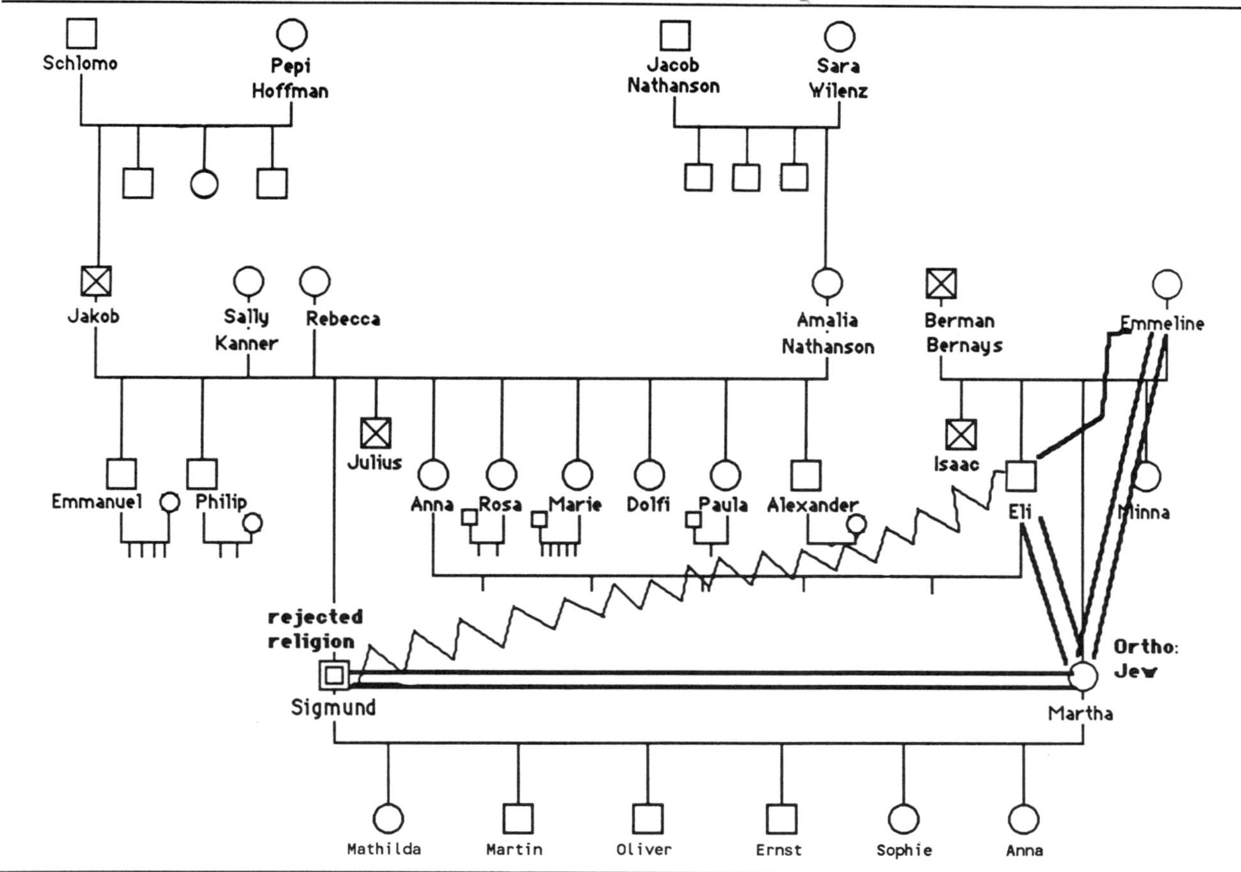

Figure 9. Freud family - in-law triangles.

intensify when they emigrated to New York and the less educated Eli became very wealthy, while the highly educated Sigmund struggled for survival. On the other hand, Martha's sister, Minna, was not only accepted by Sigmund, particularly after she became part of the Freud household, but even became more of a confidante and traveling companion for Sigmund than his wife. We know very little about Martha's attitude toward her husband's relationship with her sister.

FAMILY BALANCE AND IMBALANCE

Balance and imbalance speak to the functional whole of a family system. Contrasting characteristics are usually present in the same family. In well-functioning families, such characteristics usually balance one another out. Patterns of balance and imbalance can best be seen by looking for contrasts and characteristics that stand out. The clinician then wonders how these contrasts and idiosyncrasies fit together into a functional whole. For example, if one person is doing poorly in a family in which everyone else is doing well, the question immediately arises as to what role the dysfunction may play in the family. Such balances and imbalances may be seen in the areas of family structure, roles, level of functioning, and resources.

In the Freud family, one thing that immediately stands out in Sigmund's generation is that he was the only male for almost 10 years, until Alexander was born. Given the high value placed on males in his family and the loss of a brother at very early age, this imbalance in gender probably led to high expectations being placed on him. In terms of sex roles, there was the typical role imbalance of that era; Sigmund earned the living and was the family authority while Martha ran the house, organizing everything to meet her husband's needs. Such a strict dichotomy seen in a more modern family would immediately raise the possibility of marital stresses due to such rigid sex-role typing. There was also a contrast in religious observance in Sigmund's and Martha's families. While both were Jewish, Martha came from an Orthodox family while Sigmund's family seemed to be more assimilated. In fact, Martha remained an Orthodox Jew throughout her life, despite Sigmund's rejection of religion. Again, seeing such contrasts on the genogram should lead the clinician to further explore how the imbalance is handled by the family system.

THE FUTURE OF THE GENOGRAM

Using the Freud family, we have demonstrated the basic principles for interpretation of the genogram. We believe that inferences based on the genogram can be very useful in generating hypotheses for understanding the family. These hypotheses allow the clinician to better engage with the family, unblock systemic and emotional impasses, clarify family patterns, and reframe and detoxify family issues. The uses of the genogram in clinical practice are as varied as are the ways of doing family therapy.

However, we believe the value of the genogram has just begun to be tapped. Our work in this area is a first step in the effort to standardize the genogram and explicate the principles underlying its use. The genogram has yet to be tested as a scientific instrument: Its reliability and validity have not been demonstrated and much work is yet to be done to empirically show its clinical utility.

One of the most exciting possibilities of the genogram is its potential for further research on family patterns. Since so many clinicians routinely collect family information with genograms, there is a vast pool of family data just waiting to be tapped. What is needed is a way to gather together all this information so it will be available for research. We believe that the computerization of the genogram may be a solution.

Gerson has developed a computer program for generating genograms on the Apple II and Macintosh computers. Although still in a rudimentary stage of development, the program can already draw genograms based on family information entered into the computer. The computer solves many of the space and design problems that can make drawing and revising genograms so tedious. In addition, the computer creates an electronic database for family information. The next step is to pool the data into a large computer which can begin to analyze the complex family patterns seen across families.

In sum, we believe that development of the genogram as both a clinical and research instrument has just begun. We hope our efforts to describe and explain the principles of the genogram will promote further growth in its use and development.

Randy Gerson, PhD, is currently on the staff of the Atlanta Institute for Family Studies, where he does training in family therapy and maintains his private practice. Prior to his present position, he was on the faculty of the Family Institute of Westchester. His training is in clinical psychology and family therapy and he has published a book and other articles on family assessment. Other interests include the use of computers in family therapy training and the investigation of the systemic histories of the families of famous personalities. Dr. Gerson may be contacted at 61 8th Street, Atlanta, GA 30327.

Monica McGoldrick, MSW, is currently Associate Professor and Director of Family Training, Psychiatry Department and CMHC of UMDNJ-Rutgers Medical School, Piscataway, New Jersey, and also works at Family Institute of Westchester. Her books include *Genograms in Family Assessment, Ethnicity and Family Therapy,* and *The Family Life Cycle: A Framework for Family Therapy.* She is an Advisory Editor of *Family Process, JMFT,* and several other major family journals and is on the Board of the American Family Therapy Association. She was formerly Secretary of the American Orthopsychiatric Association. Other areas of interest include women's issues, death and the family, and family therapy with one person. Ms. McGoldrick can be contacted at Family Training Unit UMDNJ, CMHC, Piscataway, NJ 08854.

RESOURCES

Adler, A. (1958). *What Life Should Mean to You?* New York: Capricorn Books.

Bank, S. P., & Kahn, M. D. (1982). *The Sibling Bond.* New York: Basic Books.

Bowen, M. (1978). *Family Therapy in Clinical Practice.* New York: Jason Aronson.

Bradt, J. (1980). *The Family Diagram.* Washington, DC: Groome Center, 5225 Loughboro Road.

Carter, E. A., & McGoldrick, M. (1976). Family therapy with one person and the family therapist's own family. In P. J. Guerin (Ed.), *Family Therapy* (pp. 193-219). New York: Gardner.

Carter, E. A., & McGoldrick, M. (1980). *The Family Life Cycle: A Framework for Family Therapy.* New York: Gardner.

Engel, G. (1975). The death of a twin: Mourning and anniversary reactions: Fragments of 10 years of self-analysis. *International Journal of Psychoanalysis, 56,* 23-40.

Ernst, C., & Angst, J. (1983). *Birth Order: Its Influence on Personality.* New York: Springer Verlag.

Forer, L. (1976). *The Birth Order Factor.* New York: Simon & Schuster.

Gerson, R. (1980, April 8). *A Computer-Assisted Family Genogram and Family Chronology Service.* Presentation on genograms at the annual meeting of the American Orthopsychiatric Association, Boston, MA.

Guerin, P. J. (Ed.). (1976). *Family Therapy.* New York: Gardner.

Guerin, P. J., & Pendagast, E. G. (1976). Evaluation of family system and genogram. In P. J. Guerin (Ed.), *Family Therapy* (pp. 450-464). New York: Gardner.

Hadley, T., Jacob, T., Miliones, J., Caplan, J., & Spitz, D. (1974). The relationship between family developmental crises and the appearance of symptoms in a family member. *Family Process, 13,* 207-214.

Hartman, A. (1978). Diagramatic assessment of family relationships. *Social Casework, 59,* 465-476.

Holmes, T. H., & Masuda, M. (1974). Life change and illness susceptibility. In B. S. Dohrenwend & B. Dohrenwend (Eds.), *Stressful Life Events: Their Nature and Effects* (pp. 45-72). New York: John Wiley & Sons.

Jolly, W. M., Froom, J., & Rosen, M. G. (1980). The genogram. *Journal of Family Practice, 10,* 251-255.

Lieberman, S. (1979). *Transgenerational Family Therapy.* London: Croom Helm.

McGoldrick, M. (1980). Problems with family genograms. *American Journal of Family Therapy, 7,* 74-76.

McGoldrick, M., & Gerson, R. (1985). *Genograms in Family Assessment.* New York: W. W. Norton.

McGoldrick, M., Rohrbaugh, M., Weiss, H., Tomm, K., & Gerson, R. (1983, April 8). *Genograms: Applications in Family Therapy, Family Medicine, and Research.* Presentation at the annual meeting of the American Orthopsychiatric Association, Boston, MA.

Medalie, J. H. (1978). *Family Medicine: Principles and Applications.* Baltimore: Williams & Wilkins.

Milhorn, H. T. (1981). The genogram: A structured approach to the family history. *Journal of the Mississippi State Medical Association, 22,* 250-252.

Mullins, M. C., & Christie-Seely, J. (1984). Collecting and recording family data - the genogram. In J. Christie-Seely (Ed.), *Working with the Family in Primary Care* (pp. 179-191). New York: Praeger.

Pendagast, E. G., & Sherman, C. O. (1977). A guide to the genogram. *The Family, 5,* 3-14.

Rakel, R. E. (1977). *Principles of Family Medicine.* Philadelphia: W. B. Saunders.

Rogers, J., & Durkin, M. (1984). The family history: The utility of a semi-structured interview. *Family Systems Medicine, 2,* 176-187.

Sproul, M. S., & Gallagher, R. M. (1982). The genogram as an aid to crisis intervention. *Journal of Family Practice, 14,* 959-960.

Starkey, P. J. (1981). Genograms: A guide to understanding one's own family system. *Perspectives in Psychiatric Care, 19,* 164-173.

Stolorow, R. D., & Atwood, G. E. (1979). *Faces in a Cloud: Subjectivity in Personality Theory.* New York: Jason Aronson.

Sutton-Smith, B., & Rosenberg, B. G. (1970). *The Sibling*. New York: Holt, Rinehart & Winston.

Toman, W. (1976). *Family Constellation* (3rd ed.). New York: Springer.

Wachtel, E. F. (1982). The family psychic over three generations: The genogram revisited. *Journal of Marital and Family Therapy, 8*, 335-343.

Woolf, V. V. (1983). Family network systems in transgenerational psychotherapy: The theory, advantages and expanded applications of genograms. *Family Therapy, 10*, 119-137.

Wright, L. M., & Leahey, M. (1984). *Nurses and Families: A Guide to Family Assessment and Intervention*. Philadelphia: F. A. Davis.

BIOGRAPHICAL/FREUD FAMILY

Interviews with Hella Bernays and Edward Bernays, niece and nephew of Freud.

Bank, S., & Kahn, M. D. (1980-1981). Freudian siblings. *Psychoanalytic Review, 67*, 493-504.

Bernays, Anna Freud. (1940, November). My brother Sigmund Freud. *The American Mercury*, pp. 336-337, 340.

Bernays, E. L. (1965). *Biography of an Idea*. New York: Simon & Schuster.

Clark, C. W. (1980). *Freud: The Man and the Cause*. London: Jonathan Cape and Weidenfeld & Nicolson.

Eissler, K. R. (1978). *Sigmund Freud: His Life in Pictures and Words*. New York: Helen and Kurt Wolff Books, Harcourt Brace Jovanovich.

Engelman, E. (1976). *Berggasse 19*. New York: Basic Books.

Freeman, L., & Strean, H. S. (1981). *Freud and Women*. New York: Frederick Ungar Publishing Co.

Freud, E. L. (1960). *Letters of Sigmund Freud*. New York: McGraw-Hill.

Freud, M. (1958). *Sigmund Freud: Man and Father*. New York: Vanguard.

Freud Lowenstein, S. (1980). Book review: Freud und sein vater. *Family Process, 19*, 2.

Fromm, E. (1959). *Sigmund Freud's Mission*. New York: Grove.

Glicklhorn, R. (1969, January). The Freiberg period of the Freud family. *Journal of the History of Medicine, 24*, 37-43.

Jones, E. (1953, 1956, 1957). *The Life and Work of Sigmund Freud* (3 Volumes). New York: Basic Books.

Krull, M. (1986). *Freud and His Father*. New York: W. W. Norton.

Mannoni, O. (1968, 1971). *Freud*. New York: Vintage.

Natenberg, M. (1955). *The Case History of Sigmund Freud: A Psycho-Biography*. Chicago: Regent House.

Roazen, P. (1975). *Freud and His Followers*. New York: Alfred A. Knopf.

Wallechinsky, D., & Wallace, I. (1975). *The People's Almanac*. Garden City, NY: Doubleday.

TREATING CLIENTS WHO HAVE AIDS*

John C. Gonsiorek

> "sunt lacrimae rerum, et mentem
> mortalia tangunt" - *Aeneid*, I, 461-2

Most of the media coverage and a significant proportion of research funding for acquired immune deficiency syndrome (AIDS) have been focused on medical aspects of this lethal disease. Many clients with AIDS or AIDS-related illnesses report that their psychological and social needs are often given inadequate attention. Health care personnel are just beginning to recognize that attending to the psychosocial needs of persons with AIDS is an integral and crucial part of basic medical care for these populations. This contribution will outline the psychological and social factors affecting individuals with AIDS and related illnesses, and suggest some therapeutic strategies for counseling and psychotherapy with these individuals.

BASIC INFORMATION ABOUT AIDS

AIDS has been known to exist in the United States since 1979. There are indications that this disease has existed for a somewhat longer period of time in central Africa, perhaps since the 1960s. AIDS is an illness in which an individual's immune system becomes seriously compromised and deteriorates to the point that the body cannot adequately defend against many malignancies and infectious agents. Typically, an individual with AIDS succumbs to these. The most common, accounting for over 80% of cases, are Kaposi's sarcoma (KS) and Pneumocystis carinii pneumonia (PCP), although individuals with the syndrome are susceptible to a wide variety of other opportunistic illnesses. As of early April, 1986, the Center for Disease Control (CDC) reported over 19,000 cases of AIDS in the United States, and it is believed that the number of new cases is doubling every 6 to 12 months.

It is generally believed that a recently isolated retrovirus, termed HTLV3 (Popovic et al., 1984) causes AIDS. This "single agent" model of AIDS postulates that the HTLV3 virus weakens the immune system, rendering the body defenseless against opportunistic infections. Although there remain a number of unresolved questions about the HTLV3 virus (Laurence, 1985), the ways in which this virus affects the body are becoming increasingly well understood. Another etiologic model of AIDS, the "immunologic overload" theory (Sonnabend, Witkin, & Purtilo, 1984), hypothesizes that multiple assaults upon the immune system by repeated exposure to various pathogens, drug abuse, and maladaptive health and lifestyle habits overwhelm the immune system and create a permanent state of immune suppression. Although the second viewpoint appears to be a minority one, the state of data about AIDS is such that no reasonable theory can be discarded.

*The author would like to thank a number of people whose detailed criticism was very helpful: N. Douglas Elwood, MA, Park Place Clinic, Minneapolis; John Heefner, MD, Metropolitan Clinic of Counseling, Minneapolis; Hanan Rosenstein, MD, Minneapolis; and Scott Strickland, MD, St. Louis Park Medical Center, St. Louis Park, MN. I would also like to express my appreciation to B and K, a friend and client respectively, who have been extraordinarily helpful in my understanding the experience of having AIDS.

Martin and Vance (1984) have suggested an interactive model combining the first two. According to their model, "exposure to an AIDS agent will lead to clinically significant symptomatology only under conditions of host vulnerability" (p. 1306). Although most of the media attention and research efforts have been concerned with single agent models, Martin and Vance emphasize that in many medical conditions, "exposure to a pathogenic agent is a necessary, but rarely sufficient condition to induce frank expression of disease symptomatology...few diseases involve agents that have 100% attack rate" (p. 1305). Martin and Vance present a well argued methodological analysis of AIDS research. The important point for this discussion is that their critique suggests much of the theorizing and research concerning AIDS has serious flaws.

The CDC reports that approximately 51% of the individuals diagnosed with AIDS have died from it. Current understanding of the illness suggests that most, if not all, individuals with the diagnosis will die of its related infections or malignancies. However, it is also important to note the geographical concentration of AIDS cases. One-third of all cases in the United States are in the metropolitan New York City area, and approximately 10% each in San Francisco and Los Angeles. To understand what this means, consider the following. It is estimated that 1% of the gay men in San Francisco have already died of AIDS and another 2-3% have the diagnosis. It is estimated that approximately 70% of gay males in San Francisco have been infected with the HTLV3 virus (see discussion below for the differences between HTLV3 infection and AIDS). The cumulative effects of illness, death, and grief resulting from AIDS have been overwhelming in certain communities in the United States.

It is important to note that 73% of AIDS cases are homosexual or bisexual men, 17% are intravenous drug users, and 3% are transfusion recipients. However, there is a peculiarity in the CDC figures cited above: Heterosexual intravenous drug users are counted in the drug user category, but homosexual or bisexual male drug users are counted in the homosexual or bisexual category. Data from New York City, which tallies intravenous drug users separately regardless of sexual orientation, suggest that intravenous drug use runs a close second to sexual orientation as a risk factor. There is at least one state, New Jersey, where intravenous drug users account for as many cases as homosexual or bisexual men. Nonetheless, it is clear that homosexual and bisexual men have been the hardest hit by the AIDS epidemic.

If one looks back upon recent epidemics, such as the polio epidemics of the 1940s and 1950s and the swine flu scare of the mid-1970s, it is clear that the validity of even conservative pronouncements from respected authorities has not been impressive. The social and political climate concerning AIDS in the United States places enormous pressure upon researchers and medical personnel to provide information and reduce ambiguity quickly. This, in addition to standard methodological problems that beset research, produces a situation conducive to the exercise of bad judgment and premature conclusions concerning research and clinical findings. Both the individual with AIDS and the therapist must cope with an uncomfortable amount of ambiguity concerning even the most basic information about the disease.

THE SOCIAL CONTEXT OF HOMOSEXUALITY

Despite recent attitudinal changes in some segments of the United States population, most individuals have been socialized with the implicit or explicit belief that homosexuality is in some way criminal, sinful, inferior, or second class. Individuals who eventually become homosexual or bisexual are exposed to the same homophobic set of attitudes, manifested in gay and bisexual individuals as internalized homophobia (see Gonsiorek, 1984; Malyon, 1982). Because it is generally believed that sexual transmission of the virus, combined with a large number of sexual partners in some segments of the gay male community, is the reason for the high incidence of AIDS in gay and bisexual men, the AIDS epidemic reinforces this stereotypical and prejudicial view of sexual expression between men as dangerous and damaging. The pervasiveness of this stereotype can be seen in the illogical method of data reporting concerning gay and bisexual males versus intravenous drug users utilized by the CDC. As has been noted (Coates, Temoshok, & Mandel, 1984; Mandel, 1983; and Martin & Vance, 1984), these biases have not only crept into the media coverage of AIDS, but into basic medical research. AIDS has rapidly assumed a position as a metaphor, for both high risk populations and the society in general. This metaphorical conceptualization of AIDS will doubtless prove as mystifying and dehumanizing as comparable metaphorical understandings of tuberculosis and cancer have been (see Sontag, 1978). This social context of oppression of homosexuality will directly affect the relationship between a gay client and a health care provider (Gonsiorek, 1980).

THE SOCIAL AND PSYCHOLOGICAL IMPACT OF AIDS

CLIENT CONCERNS

In recent years a number of articles have paved the way toward understanding the psychosocial aspects of AIDS (Cassens, 1985; Coates et al., 1984; Joseph et al., 1984; Malyon & Pinka, 1983; Mandel, 1983; Mandel et al., 1985; Morin & Batchelor, 1984; Morin, Charles, & Malyon, 1984). Before describing specific social and psychological issues, however, it is important to describe the different kinds of AIDS-related conditions because the social and psychological issues vary somewhat between them.

First, there are individuals who have received a formal diagnosis of AIDS. The CDC publishes a detailed set of diagnostic criteria for AIDS. The prognosis for this group is very poor. Most people who have received the diagnosis have died. No one has fully recovered from AIDS, and the current belief is that barring any major treatment advances, most if not all individuals with this diagnosis will die of one of its opportunistic illnesses. Typically this diagnosis is the culmination of a long period of illness, fatigue, and numerous medical problems. Often the diagnosis is a confirmation of the person's worst fears; typically the individual has known for sometime that he is quite sick, although on occasion, the illness and diagnosis do come on quite suddenly.

AIDS Related Complex (ARC) is an AIDS-related condition. Individuals with ARC have clinical and laboratory evidence of a compromised immune system, can have a variety of medical symptoms ranging from mild to debilitating, and occasionally have certain infections that are not sufficient to warrant a diagnosis of AIDS. Current thinking is that somewhere between 5% and 20% of individuals with ARC will eventually develop AIDS. Because these data are based on only a few years of study, this prediction can only be made for approximately 4 to 5 years. After that period, the prognosis of ARC individuals is unknown.

Next there are individuals who have positive results on tests for HTLV3 antibodies. These individuals may not be symptomatic; if they have significant symptoms, they are usually classified in the ARC group. Current prognostic understanding is that approximately 10% of individuals who are positive for HTLV3 antibodies will develop AIDS, but again this prediction can only be made for roughly 4 to 5 years. Some seropositive individuals have had no awareness of any infection or even knowledge that they were being tested for HTLV3. Although some may seek out such testing, many individuals donating blood or sperm, applying for insurance policies, or being administered other medical evaluations were given the test for HTLV3 antibodies without their knowledge, so this information may come as a surprise.

There are others, sometimes called the worried well, who show no sign of illness and have not been tested as positive for HTLV3 antibodies, but who are intensely preoccupied with the fear of getting AIDS. This group includes individuals who may not know their test status, but may also include those who know they have tested negative, or who cognitively understand that their risk is low, but who are nevertheless preoccupied with the fear of getting AIDS.

There are some noteworthy differences between these groups. Persons with a formal diagnosis of AIDS have the least amount of ambiguity. Some persons with AIDS, who have gone through a prolonged period of having a diagnosis of ARC, report a sense of relief about finally knowing where they stand. Individuals with ARC may be every bit as ill on a day-to-day basis as individuals with AIDS, but are in the most ambiguous situation. Not surprisingly, some researchers report that individuals with ARC have greater degrees of psychological distress, yet have less attention paid to their psychosocial needs than individuals with AIDS (see Mandel et al., 1985).

Finally, two other groups should be mentioned. Individuals with AIDS or an AIDS-related illness who are not gay or bisexual men suffer the same turmoil. They are also sometimes faced with discrimination and prejudice they have never before encountered because it is presumed they are really gay or bisexual. In most places, the majority of persons with AIDS *are* gay or bisexual, and services are oriented for this population, so other individuals may feel left out or neglected. Those that come to mind most easily in this regard are hemophiliacs who have acquired AIDS through blood transfusions. In addition, family and friends of persons with AIDS may experience very high levels of distress yet, because they are not themselves ill, may be perceived and perceive themselves to be in no need of assistance.

Many of the psychological processes experienced by people facing death and dying are common in individuals with AIDS-related illness (Kubler-Ross, 1969). Mandel et al. (1985) report that in studies comparing AIDS patients with other groups receiving terminal diagnoses, the psychological reactions were comparable. In addition to all the psychological dynamics stemming from the death and dying process, there is another set of psychological factors and social problems. The metaphor I use to conceptualize this situation is of a hurricane within a hurricane, a whirlwind of social processes surrounding an individual experiencing a storm of internal psychological processes.

EXTERNAL CONCERNS

Typically the information that an individual has AIDS elicits powerful reactions from that person's environment. These reactions are frequently so disruptive that they become a major source of stress. The following describes some of the major sources of external stress, but is by no means exhaustive.

The reactions of friends and acquaintances are usually intense, but may also be ambivalent. Not only may the friends and acquaintances worry about the loss of their friend and begin handling their grief in a variety of ways, but they themselves may be members of a high-risk group. Their friend's diagnosis of AIDS may abruptly present them with the reality of their own vulnerability. In regions where AIDS has not yet had a major impact, many individuals in the gay community may still be attempting to deny that the epidemic can happen in their locale. The response of such people may be to continue their denial by withdrawing from their friend or acquaintance with AIDS. In areas that have been very hard hit by AIDS, persons may be weary and exhausted from the endless suffering and death, and may be unwilling or unable to bear the emotional strain of yet another friend becoming ill and dying. Friends or acquaintances who are uninformed may have unrealistic fears of casual contagion which may exacerbate their withdrawal. At a time when the person with AIDS may be most in need of the support and comfort of friends and acquaintances, support may be ambivalent, or inconsistent.

Another external source of stress can be the biological family of the person with AIDS. If a gay or bisexual man has already informed his family about his sexual orientation, any lingering discomfort the family may have about the sexual orientation may surface. Some families who had seemed adjusted to a member's homosexuality have become homophobic in response to the news that the person has AIDS, or to the AIDS epidemic itself even when their family member remains healthy. For an individual who has not told his family about his sexual orientation, this diagnosis presents a very painful dilemma. If he tells his family about both his sexual orientation and the diagnosis, it may be too much for a family to deal with, and he risks losing support when it is most needed. If he does not tell the family, not only is family support unavailable, but he will be going through his own grieving process with some very crucial issues unresolved. Telling the family about AIDS and not about the sexual orientation is usually not an option, as sexual orientation is likely to be the first question the family asks. There is a macabre but telling AIDS joke that illustrates this point: "What is the hardest thing about having AIDS? Trying to convince your mother that you are Haitian."

Another external factor is discrimination. In addition to the various kinds of discrimination in employment, housing, access to services, credit, and so on that gay men frequently face, the AIDS epidemic has created a new and specific wave of discrimination which is larger than the issue of sexual orientation itself. A recent issue of the newsletter of the American Civil Liberties Union (Stoddard, 1985) had as its lead story the civil liberties violations occurring as a result of the AIDS crisis. It is important to note that some of this discrimination occurs in an unusually intrusive fashion. Not only are people with AIDS denied housing, fired from jobs, dropped from certain insurance coverages, denied access to service, and so on, but there have been situations where individuals have been screened for the AIDS virus without their knowledge or consent and then discriminated against. For example, some insurance companies, employers, or blood banks have screened individual donors for the HTLV3 virus and then used the positive test result as a basis for discrimination.

Financial loss represents another area of external stress. Individuals may lose their jobs or be unable to work fully. They may lose their insurance coverage and see their financial resources rapidly eroded by the cost of their medical care. Average cost of treatment for one AIDS patient may vary from $50,000 to $100,000, but there have been situations where the cost of medical care exceeded $1,000,000, depending on the kinds of opportunistic illnesses the person had and the types of treatments attempted.

It should also be noted that the clinical course of AIDS can vary dramatically; therefore, people with AIDS, like people with other variable illnesses such as lupus or multiple sclerosis, may have a very difficult time with disability policies. For most employers and insurance companies, the concept of disability is a static one where an individual is or is not able to work in certain ways or a certain percentage of the time. This concept of disability does not apply to illnesses that, in their natural course, wax and wane. Persons with AIDS may find their insurance carriers, employers, and even family and friends insensitive or suspicious about their degree of disability, as they may appear extremely ill one day and fine and fully functioning a few days later. Out of financial necessity, a sense of identity derived from work, or other reasons, a person with AIDS may elect to stay working as long as possible. If the employer does not know the medical situation, there may be considerable intolerance for the person's erratic work schedule due to the fluctuations of the illness. If the employer does know the person's medical status, there may be pressure from other employees or from management itself to remove the person with AIDS from the job, either out of a mistaken fear of contagion, outright discrimination, or simply blind fear. Systems such as Social Security, various state programs, and various private insurance disability programs are often complicated to deal with, have considerable delays, or, in a variety of ways, may be unsympathetic to the special circumstances of the person with AIDS.

Publicity about AIDS may constitute another external stress. Media coverage is often sensationalistic and distorted, and at times overtly antigay. Probably the most common problem is excessive mystification or misinformation from the media. Two examples follow. The media sometimes refer to ARC as pre-AIDS, which suggests that all ARC patients will eventually develop AIDS. The prognosis of ARC patients is not entirely understood, and what is known to date suggests that only a minority will develop AIDS.

Another case involves reporting of the pediatric incidence of AIDS. For the most part, the origin of pediatric cases of AIDS is well understood. These are children who have either received blood transfusions, frequently because of hemophilia, or they have been born to mothers who have AIDS. Yet, in the media discussion of pediatric cases, there is rarely an explanation given, feeding into fear and mystification which frequently also turns into antigay sentiment. The pediatric cases also present another area of ambivalence for many gay men. On the one hand it is a relief to see the nation taking AIDS seriously as a result of pediatric cases, but it is also a bitter and grim reminder of the second-class status of gay men in the United States, that a relatively small number of pediatric cases has aroused more concern, sympathy, and concrete support than the deaths of thousands of gay men.

The medical restrictions necessitated by AIDS are also a considerable source of stress, particularly because it is not entirely understood what measures should be taken. Depending on the opinion and education of one's physician, a person with AIDS may be told to avoid everything from pets, to people with colds, to fresh produce, or to continue life as normal. It can be a frustrating and overwhelming experience for previously healthy individuals to deal with the bureaucracy of the medical system and insurance companies. Health care personnel may be phobic, because of the fear of AIDS, antihomosexual sentiment, or both, or may be insensitive or uninformed about the special needs of AIDS patients. There have been numerous reports of unconscionable lapses in basic care provided to AIDS patients, particularly inpatients, and especially those who are indigent.

Finally, as experiments with drug treatments for AIDS begin, persons with AIDS will face another set of external stresses regarding medical options. Most of the drugs being prepared for experimental treatment of AIDS have serious and debilitating side effects, and some of them are powerfully immune-altering. In the near future, many AIDS patients will be faced with the decision of whether to take an immune-altering drug while parts of their immune system are still intact, running the risk of further impairing their immune system, or to wait until their immune system is overwhelmed to take such a medication, when it may be too late for effective treatment. Even in the best of circumstances, it is very difficult for a consumer of health care services to sort through the pros and cons of experimental treatments, particularly when the cost-benefit analysis may be a life or death matter. Quality of life issues often affect these decisions, and health care personnel, particularly physicians, are often poorly trained to help patients evaluate such concerns.

PSYCHOLOGICAL REACTIONS

Approximately 70% of the AIDS cases in the United States occur among individuals 40 and younger, and 68% of the cases among individuals between the ages of 20 and 40. By and large, this is an age group which has not come to terms with its mortality and which has not had the experience of seeing peers grow old and die. This is also an age group where men tend to be externally focused on careers and success, and less prone to introspection and consideration of existential issues. In a sense, AIDS primarily strikes an age group which is developmentally unprepared to deal with issues of death, dying, and grief. Further, most people have age peers as their friends and acquaintances, and persons with AIDS may find that their support group is equally ill equipped to deal with these issues.

Because of internalized homophobia or, in some cases, other aspects of personality structure, some persons receiving a diagnosis of AIDS or an AIDS-related illness have responded with self and other destructive behaviors. These may include abuse of alcohol or drugs, putting oneself or others at medical risk, not complying with medical regimens, and so on. A therapist working with such individuals should be sensitized to the possibility that they may be acting out internalized homophobia by punishing themselves or other gay men.

Another psychological issue is the loss of sexuality. For persons with AIDS or AIDS-related illnesses who remain sexually active, safer sex procedures are crucial for preventing the spread of the illness and protecting themselves against re-exposure to HTLV3. For persons who are not HTLV3 infected, the safer sex procedures may literally spell the difference between life and death. However, safer sex procedures which essentially prohibit the exchange of bodily fluids, especially semen, are quite restrictive. The sexual activities an individual engages in often have complex psychological meaning. A clinician must be sensitive to the fact that choosing safer sex procedures is not like a Chinese food menu where a person simply selects from column A because column B is too dangerous. The loss of preferred modes of sexual expression is a deep and profound loss; persons who have shifted to safer sex procedures and away from riskier activities may experience it as such.

Loss of control is another pervasive psychological issue. As mentioned above, AIDS tends to strike an age group of males who value the exercise of control over the world. Almost every aspect of the life of a person with AIDS becomes out of control. It is hard to imagine a situation where more things have the potential to unpredictably go awry than one in which an incurable and fatal illness, which comes on suddenly in the prime of life, is paired with considerable social stigma. The medical system may give confusing double messages to persons with AIDS. On the one hand, they may be encouraged to actively monitor their physical status and to take control of a variety of areas of their lives, such as diet, exercise, and other preventive measures. At the same time, they may be expected to dutifully accept the vicissitudes of the health care system.

Another kind of psychological loss rarely discussed is the loss of touch, separate from the loss of sexuality. Many persons with AIDS complain that physical affection is virtually absent from their lives because of isolation, fear of contagion by others, or their own fear of being contagious or contracting an infection. The losses of touch and sexuality hit especially hard for the gay male community. The freedom to be openly affectionate and comfortably sexual with another man has been difficult to achieve both socially and personally. The self-imposed suppression of these areas often has profound psychological meaning for individuals who only a decade ago may have risked life and limb to win the right to such expression.

Because of changes in their bodies, persons with AIDS or AIDS-related illnesses may view themselves as diseased, dirty, or lethal. These feelings may be separate from or intertwined with internalized homophobia. This is not merely a psychological phenomenon. Persons with this range of illnesses may undergo both subtle and obvious changes in their bodies. As with the loss of control issue, persons with AIDS may be given a confusing double message by the medical system about an appropriate level of somatic concern. On the one hand, the person may be encouraged to monitor his body for even the most subtle changes, yet may be met with annoyance when he regularly reports these minor changes, especially as some of the symptoms may be quite variable or ephemeral in nature. For example, many persons with AIDS report changes in their skin tone, texture, coloring, and "feel." Yet these events may not be easily observed by another. What one physician may view as hypochondriacal preoccupation, another may view as responsible self-care. As persons with AIDS frequently have several physicians who specialize in the various ailments they endure, they may get very different messages in this area. Some persons with AIDS may become extremely ill, nearly die of an infection, and then entirely recover from that particular infection, while others may get a different sort of malignancy that produces bruises, disfigurement, and overt scarring, which may never be cured. Therefore, the body image concerns that a given person has may not only differ from those of another person with AIDS, but may change over time.

A person with AIDS is undergoing at least two very different physical processes. The immune system is under attack from the HTLV3 virus, and there is increasing evidence that central nervous system tissue is also under attack by this virus (Holland & Tross, 1985). Neurologic and neuropsychological impairment can range from mild, short-term memory problems to gross dementia. The early manifestations of this neuropsychological impairment may include motor and coordination impairment, difficulty in concentrating, changes in affect, short-term memory problems, and others. These are again variable and often ephemeral symptoms, and persons with AIDS and their clinicians may have difficulty determining whether such symptoms are signs of early neuropsychological impairment, anxiety or depression, an opportunistic infection, or somatic overconcern. Although a neuropsychological assessment can often be helpful in tracking this impairment at its middle and later stages, it is often less useful for detecting subtle impairment in its early stages. Neuropsychological impairment in AIDS is much more frequent than was earlier thought, and clinicians should keep informed of new developments in this area.

Symptoms of anxiety and depression are quite common in individuals with AIDS or AIDS-related illnesses. Mandel et al. (1985) reported that a number of factors predict a more adaptive adjustment to the illness. These include making concrete changes in one's lifestyle to optimize quality of life and health, sharing one's medical status and information about one's health with others, mobilizing one's support system, and not blaming oneself for the illness. They also found that patients with ARC appeared to have higher degrees of psychological distress than patients with AIDS. Given the added ambiguity of ARC, this situation may not be surprising. An immobilizing depression or anxiety state may not only be painful to the person with AIDS, but may interfere with the ability to engage in more adaptive responses to the illness.

SUGGESTIONS FOR CLINICAL WORK WITH AIDS PATIENTS

Given the variability of the medical course, the external social stressors, and the psychological meaning of the illness for the person, the therapeutic strategy may need to vary as a consequence of prominent issues for a particular AIDS client.

MANAGING CLINICAL SYMPTOMS

Crisis management issues are usually paramount immediately after the illness is recognized, although they can occur at any time in working with a patient having AIDS.

Frequently the maladaptive reactions of the external world are as much a problem for the person with AIDS as the illness itself and internal psychological events. Helping the client with AIDS to make concrete goal-oriented improvements in daily life to reduce the stress, particularly from external events, is very important. Because so many events may be impinging on the person at one time, helping the client prioritize and choose which things to tackle and which to temporarily, or perhaps permanently, avoid, is an important task. This crisis-oriented focus can reduce the psychological distress of the client and help him regain some sense of control.

It is important to manage symptoms of anxiety and depression to prevent a client from becoming immobilized, withdrawn, and overwhelmed. However, it is also important to do so in a way that respects the grieving process. The therapist must often walk a fine line between allowing the grieving process to emerge versus allowing the patient to become immobilized by depression, thereby setting in motion a new series of stressful events. Psychiatric evaluation and use of medication may be an important tool in managing debilitating levels of depression and anxiety.

The clinician should keep a sharp watch for overt or subtle behavior that is destructive to oneself and others. These may be manifestations of internalized homophobia or reflections of other personality factors. For example, though it may be useful for a client to take a critical and questioning attitude toward the medical regimens offered, continued noncompliance with reasonable medical requests may be self-destructive. Refusing to contain the spread of the virus through safer sex practices, if the client does remain sexually active, may be a manifestation of hostility directed toward other gay men.

Often after an initial crisis period, the client may begin to reinstate control in some areas of life, such as dealing with friends and family, restoring a support system, and handling the health-care system assertively. This is frequently accompanied by some degree of denial about death. As the illness progresses in an overt way medically, this constructive denial will break down. The grieving process will resume more openly. Existential issues of meaning may emerge, and the client will face the tasks of closure with friends, lovers, and family, and external preparations for death such as wills, wishes about terminal medical treatment, and so on.

Mandel et al. (1985) make a very important point about denial. They suggest there is no such thing as false hope, that hopelessness is deadly. Retaining a sense of hope may be one of the most important therapeutic tasks. Clinicians may do a disservice to clients by depriving them of this under the guise of breaking through denial about their prognosis. I would suggest that if a person's reality testing about his illness is intact, as evidenced by compliance with reasonable medical regimes, awareness of risks about being infected and being infectious, and appropriate attending to external stressors, then whatever sense of hope he may have about his future, even if it flies in the face of the current grim prognosis, is productive and therapeutic. Hope may become destructive denial only when it leads to these realities being ignored or distorted.

Much of the time, therapy with persons having AIDS consists of exploring various psychological issues, attempting to clarify but not directing the process. The clinician working with AIDS clients will likely have to manage shifts in therapeutic style from a crisis management, goal-oriented approach during periods of high stress, to more indirect, reflective approaches during periods of processing grief or other psychological events. In any case, it is important not to contribute further to the loss of control experienced by many persons having AIDS. It is important to be goal-directed with the unmanageable aspects of life, but not too interventionist concerning the person's emotional state. When at all possible, the clinician should attempt to empower the person. The therapist should be attentive to cues that the constructive denial is breaking down. A client may very gingerly test a therapist's - and his own - willingness to face death. If the therapist is unwilling, the client may also back away. The therapist may need to *gently* take the initiative in this area.

I cannot emphasize enough that no psychotherapeutic treatment of a person with AIDS is complete until that individual is connected with a support group including others sharing the condition and status. Groups provide opportunities that individual therapy can never reproduce, such as support from one's peers, reality testing, generation of new options for coping, and a sense of friendship and understanding that a physically healthy therapist is simply unlikely to offer. Initially, many persons with AIDS are reluctant to attend such groups and offer a great deal of resistance to doing so, some of which may be rooted in their denial about their illness, but some of which may be realistic concerns about privacy and confidentiality. In general, I would suggest that a person with AIDS be guided towards such groups by the individual therapist in a consistent but not abrupt or demanding manner.

MANAGING THERAPIST ISSUES

It should go without saying that clinicians who are homophobic or uncertain of their attitudes about homosexuality should first address these issues before working with clients who have AIDS or AIDS-related illnesses. Gonsiorek (1980, 1984) and Morin and Charles (1983) discuss these concerns. Therapists who have not worked through their own resolution of death and dying will have a a difficult time, also. Therapists working with AIDS clients must be willing to work with the client until death.

The clinician working with AIDS victims must keep responsibly informed about the rapidly changing medical developments of this disease, both to guide treatment planning and to model an active stance for the client. Fears of contagion and insensitivity to the changing pace of therapy with such clients may be indications that misinformation or countertransference issues need to be addressed. Fear of death, concern with one's own mortality, grief, and loss will all be issues for clinicians. The only certain thing is that the clinician is likely to be intensely uncomfortable at times. Most therapeutic endeavors operate on an assumption that the client's options will expand as therapy continues. Clients with AIDS, as with other terminal illnesses, operate in a context of shrinking options, which can be stressful for therapists not experienced in working with dying clients.

Clinicians will have to be exquisitely sensitive to issues of confidentiality, realizing that a single careless case note that comes to the attention of an insurance carrier, employer, and so on, may mean loss of employment, housing, or insurance coverage for the patient. This is clearly a situation where carelessness on the part of the clinician may unnecessarily contribute to the external stress of the client.

All therapists, but especially gay therapists, will have to be cautious about enmeshment with clients having AIDS-related conditions. It can be exceptionally painful for a therapist who has helped a client weather coming-out issues, to work again with the same client struggling to come to terms with his HTLV3 infection.

The clinician may have to periodically serve as advocate for the client in a variety of situations. The most common of these is in dealing with other aspects of the health care system. Mental health professionals are probably the best trained of health care professionals to deal with the psychological issues raised by AIDS. In particular, they may be more experienced than some physicians in processing decisions about treatment options. It may often be necessary to have joint meetings with other health care staff or to take a more active role than is typical in therapy in dealing with the client's support system. Examples may include family sessions, couples sessions, sessions where a roommate or friends may be present, and so on.

Finally, it is important for the therapist to obtain regular support and consultation so that issues are not "dumped" on the client by the therapist. There is every indication that the AIDS epidemic will be significantly worse in the near future. I would recommend that each clinician monitor his or her own stress level and make deliberate decisions about how many clients with AIDS can reasonably be managed at any point in time.

John C. Gonsiorek, PhD, is currently Director of Psychological Services at Twin Cities Therapy Clinic in Minneapolis, and is a Clinical Assistant Professor of Psychology at the University of Minnesota. He received his PhD in clinical psychology from the University of Minnesota in 1978. He has published a variety of articles, and edited two books on mental health issues pertaining to sexual orientation and identity, as well as other topics. Dr. Gonsiorek may be contacted at Physicians & Surgeons Building #506, 63 S. 9th Street, Minneapolis, MN 55402.

RESOURCES

CITED REFERENCES

Cassens, B. (1985). Social consequences of the Acquired Immunodeficiency Syndrome. *Annals of Internal Medicine, 103,* 768-771.

Coates, T., Temoshok, L., & Mandel, J. (1984). Psychosocial research is essential to understanding and treating AIDS. *American Psychologist, 39,* 1309-1313.

Fisher, K. (1983, July). Stress: The unseen killer in AIDS. *APA Monitor,* pp. 20-21.

Gonsiorek, J. (1980). What health care professionals need to know about gay men and lesbians. In M. Jospe, J. Nieberding, & B. Cohen (Eds.), *Psychological Factors in Health Care* (pp. 297-311). Lexington, MA: D. C. Health.

Gonsiorek, J. (1984). Psychotherapeutic issues with gay and lesbian clients. In P. A. Keller & L. G. Ritt, *Innovations in Clinical Practice: A Source Book* (Vol. 3, pp. 69-84). Sarasota, FL: Professional Resource Exchange, Inc.

Holland, J., & Tross, S. (1985). The psychosocial and neuropsychiatric sequelae of Acquired Immune Deficiency Syndrome and Related Disorders. *Annals of Internal Medicine, 103,* 760-764.

Joseph, J., Emmons, C., Kessler, R., Wortman, C., O'Brien, K., Hocker, W., & Schaefer, C. (1984). Coping with the threat of AIDS: An approach to psychosocial assessment. *American Psychologist, 39,* 1297-1302.

Kubler-Ross, E. (1969). *On Death and Dying.* London: MacMillan.

Laurence, J. (1985). The immune system in AIDS. *Scientific American, 253,* 6, 84-93.

Malyon, A. (1982). Psychotherapeutic implications of internalized homophobia in gay men. In J. Gonsiorek (Ed.), *Homosexuality and Psychotherapy: A Practitioner's Handbook of Affirmative Models* (pp. 59-68). NY: Haworth Press.

Malyon, A., & Pinka, A. (1983). Acquired Immune Deficiency Syndrome: A challenge to psychology. *The Professional Psychologist, 7*(4), 1-11. (Available from California Psychological Association)

Mandel, J. (1983). *Biopsychosocial Aspects of the Acquired Immune Deficiency Syndrome.* Paper presented at American Psychological Association Convention, Anaheim, CA.

Mandel, J., Moulton, J., Temoshok, L., & Woods, W. (1985, September). *Overview of Treatment Issues in Working with Persons with AIDS and ARC.* Paper presented at a conference on AIDS: Policy, Administrative and Clinical Issues of Mental Health, San Francisco, CA.

Martin, J., & Vance, C. (1984). Behavioral and psychosocial factors in AIDS: Methodological and substantive issues. *American Psychologist, 39,* 1309-1314.

Morin, S., & Charles, K. (1983). Heterosexual bias in psychotherapy. In J. Murray & P. Abramson (Eds.), *Bias in Psychotherapy.* NY: Praeger.

Morin, S., Charles, K., & Malyon, A. (1984). The psychological impact of AIDS on gay men. *American Psychologist, 39,* 1288-1293.

Nichols, S. (1985). Psychosocial reactions of persons with Acquired Immune Deficiency Syndrome. *Annals of Internal Medicine, 103,* 765-767.

Nieberding, J. (1983). *Role of the Health Psychologist Working with AIDS Patients.* Paper presented at American Psychological Association Convention, Los Angeles, CA.

Popovic, M., Sarngadharan, M., Read, E., & Gallo, R. (1984). Detection, isolation, and continuous production of cytopathic retroviruses (HTLV-III) from patients with AIDS and pre-AIDS. *Science, 224,* 497-500.

Sonnabend, J., Witkin, S., & Purtilo, D. (1984). AIDS: An explanation for its occurrence among homosexual men. In P. Ma & D. Armstrong (Eds.), *Acquired Immune Deficiency Syndrome and Infections of Homosexual Men.* NY: York Medical Books.

Sontag, S. (1978). *Illness as Metaphor.* NY: Farrar, Straus & Giroux.

Stoddard, T. (1985). The AIDS crisis. *Civil Liberties, 355,* 1, 3.

ASSOCIATIONS

The following organizations have a long history of working with clients having AIDS-related illnesses, and have produced a variety of materials on this topic.

Gay Men's Health Crisis, Box 274, 132 W. 24th Street, New York, NY 10011.
Shanti Project, 890 Hayes Street, San Francisco, CA 94117.
Pacific Center AIDS Project, P.O. Box 908, Berkeley, CA 94701.

INTRODUCTION TO SECTION II: PRACTICE MANAGEMENT AND PROFESSIONAL DEVELOPMENT

This section of *Innovations* includes contributions that deal with practice management and professional development. Successful practice management requires careful consideration of many important issues. In fact, these issues change almost from month to month as new mechanisms for service delivery are introduced. Many believe that the entire face of service delivery will change dramatically over the next several years.

Four clinicians describe their private practices in this section. Each practice is unique in a number of ways, and these authors should provide the reader with an interesting perspective on the diversity of psychological practice.

Next, an attorney describes how the clinician can use small claims court for collections. The collection of fees is a difficult and sensitive issue for most clinicians. Hussey discusses, in very practical terms, how to effectively use small claims court, including suggestions on several important pitfalls.

Meek provides a brief discussion of "client snatching." She addresses some of the delicate issues involved when a client already in treatment decides to seek a new therapist. This is an area of confusion for many practitioners, and her discussion skillfully addresses some of the concerns.

Frankel offers a very important contribution on changes in the health care delivery system. As a psychologist who has been on the forefront of changes within California, Frankel has some interesting perspectives on the impact of new health care delivery mechanisms in mental health. The contribution includes specific suggestions for practitioners who are considering involvement in one of the newer forms of service delivery.

Finally, Meek provides a brief discussion of how to use an answering machine in a clinical practice. Many practitioners work in small, solo practices which cannot afford full-time clerical support. She contrasts the advantages of an answering service with those of an answering machine, which she has found effective in her own practice. Her anecdotal experiences will be of interest to anyone who uses or is considering the use of an answering machine.

THE PRIVATE PRACTICE
OF PSYCHOLOGY:
FOUR VARIATIONS

Herbert J. Freudenberger, Mark H. Lewin,
Carroll L. Meek, and Lawrence G. Ritt

During one of the editorial "brainstorming" sessions for this volume, discussion was focused on topics that might be helpful to clinicians considering independent practice. As the discussion progressed, we began to generate questions that potential independent practitioners might ask colleagues who were already functioning in the private sector. How do you select a community for your practice? How do you decide on a location for your office within your chosen community? How do you design a functional office? What *is* a functional office? What are relevant issues to consider in shaping your physical space to fit your professional needs? How do you furnish an office? What are the relationships between a practitioner's personality, clinical orientation, client needs, and office design? How do you plan for future growth? How do you manage a practice? Are there common mistakes that practitioners make in establishing a private practice?

When we considered possible formats for answering some of these questions, the best method seemed to be to invite several psychologists with different types of independent practices to discuss these issues in an informal and personalized fashion. The only structure we provided was to ask that they address some of the questions we had generated during our initial editorial conference. This contribution is a compilation of their responses.

Our contributors are:

Herbert J. Freudenberger. Dr. Freudenberger has maintained a psychoanalytic practice in the New York metropolitan area for the past 30 years. He is a Fellow of the American Psychological Association and author of several books and articles, including the recent bestselling *Women's Burnout* from Penguin Books. He may be contacted at 18 East 87th Street, New York, NY 10128.

Mark H. Lewin. Dr. Lewin is a full-time practitioner in Rochester, New York. He also writes and lectures extensively on professional issues including the management aspects of public and private practice. He is a Diplomate in Clinical Psychology, ABPP, and serves on a number of boards of trustees, helping to expand the use of behavioral science knowledge and technology in the community. Dr. Lewin can be contacted at the Upstate Psychological Service Center, 756 East Main Street, Rochester, NY 14605.

Carroll L. Meek. Dr. Meek is currently in independent practice as a counseling psychologist in Pullman, Washington. For many years prior to opening her practice, she was a psychologist in Counseling Services at Washington State University. She has contributed several articles to the *Innovations* series as well as other publications. Dr. Meek may be contacted at The Professional Mall, S. E. 1205 Professional Mall Boulevard, Pullman, WA 99163.

Lawrence G. Ritt. Dr. Ritt is in private practice in Sarasota, Florida. He is also the Publisher of the Professional Resource Exchange, Inc. He is immediate Past President of the Florida Psychological Association. He holds a doctoral degree in clinical psychology. Dr. Ritt can be contacted at the Professional Resource Exchange, 635 S. Orange Avenue, Suite 4, Sarasota, FL 33577.

HERBERT J. FREUDENBERGER

I have been in psychoanalytic practice for 30 years. When I began to practice in 1956, I was located at 890 Park Avenue, New York City. Why there? Because it was available and the rent was reasonable. I wanted to remain in New York City because I believed that the metropolitan area would offer the widest range of patients and problems.

It was a correct assumption. New York offered me the ability to meet with many colleagues and to complete my psychoanalytic training at the National Psychological Association for Psychoanalysis with Dr. Theodore Reik. I also hoped that the presence of many colleges and universities would afford me the opportunity to teach at one of them and, happily, this proved to be so. I taught, on a full and part-time basis, undergraduate and graduate psychology courses. This also gave me the public exposure I needed, so that my first set of patients were predominantly students or their family and friends. New York also offered me the possibility of becoming active in professional organizations. I served a number of years on the board of the New York Society of Clinical Psychologists, and was elected its President on two separate occasions.

As the years marched on, my interests shifted to the drug abusing population. I helped start the first Free Clinic in New York City for "hippie" LSD and amphetamine abusers, and created the health component of the first Hispanic drug therapeutic community. This ultimately led to my seeing, in practice, many Hispanic men and women, the staffs of alcohol and drug programs, and the graduates of these programs.

My work in practice as well as "on the street" was most exciting and growth provoking. It made me re-evaluate my fee structure and some of my treatment approaches. Consequently, I partially shifted and retrained myself in group therapy and became one of the first practitioners to work with the chemical abuser in independent practice. A portion (about 25%) of my practice is working with this group of chemical abusers. The major changes that have taken place over the years are the drug of choice of this group of patients, and my ability to innovate treatment techniques.

Working with the varied populations, attempting new approaches, led ultimately to my developing the concept of burnout, and to writing the first article, in 1973, on this, now most prevalent concept. Two books have since been produced on this subject.

About 8 years ago, I moved my office to 18 East 87th Street. I had become a bit wiser by now because I bought the space and now own a cooperative office. I gutted the entire space. My individual office is approximately 19 feet by 24 feet. It is artificially separated by couch-chairs and overhead lighting, thus allowing me to shift my therapeutic location from the private part of the space to the group area as the working day evolves. This gives me the opportunity to function in different capacities during the therapeutic day. I believe that this ability to shift my sitting space and to work with a different therapeutic modality has also enabled me to maintain a creativity and a joy of work and living.

I designed the waiting room, which is approximately 10 feet by 16 feet and has a working fireplace, to appear as a living room. There are comfortable couches available; an octave table stands in the corner and is used by many of my patients to write their thoughts pre- or post-session. A fully equipped kitchen can provide coffee. Next to the kitchen is an area for a part-time male secretary who handles my books and typing and does so much to make my life more comfortable and productive.

My office reiterates the atmosphere of a living room. Only a desk in the corner hints at the possibility that this is an office. Having grown up in Europe in a wonderful home, until Hitler changed it all, "gemutlichkeit" and "willkomen" were major bywords of my family. I suspect it is what I had hoped to create in my living room/office space.

My diplomas and awards are inconspicuously displayed. The room has more than ample seating. The couch-chairs are all movable, so that when I conduct a seminar, workshop, or large group marathon sessions, I can comfortably sit 20-25 people.

In my office I have three exits and entrances. This is to allow anonymity for individuals and colleagues from other cities who do not wish to have it known that they are in therapy.

I work with my colleague, Dr. Penny Russianoff, who is located cross-town from me. We sometimes share couple-patients and have conducted workshops and seminars together for the past 12 years. This has allowed us both to learn and to "spell" each other during the course of a class seminar or extended group. A percentage of my referrals are from former or present patients. Another group is referred by physicians - a cardiologist, internist, pharmacologist/psychiatrist and dermatologist. These referrals, as well as those that I receive through my men's and women's burnout publications, are generally persons under stress. Some individuals self-refer as a result of my public TV, lecture, or radio appearances.

I work with a team of accountants, and legal and financial advisors, and have developed a personal pension plan system that I and others follow and administer during the course of a year.

We have separate storage materials for our records and have successfully cataloged the numerous newspaper, magazine, radio, and TV coverages that I have been fortunate enough to obtain through my publications on burnout, anxiety, impaired professionals, and chemical abusers.

My office is furnished with a mixture of antiques and modern art, a reflection of who I am as a person. Therapy is difficult enough without making the therapeutic environment appear uninviting or unpleasant. The highest compliment that a new or old patient can convey is to comment that they felt welcome and relatively comfortable in the waiting room during their initial visit. Oh yes, we also try to have fresh plants and flowers present in the waiting room.

Most of my clients are between the ages of 20 to 60. They are about equally divided between men and women. My groups pretty much exemplify the gestalt of New York City. You might find a successful attorney, physician, or stockbroker sitting with an alcoholic, a police officer, teacher, nurse, middle management executive, dentist, a call girl, a pimp, a salesperson, a secretary, vice president of a bank, hospital administrator, restaurant owner, or computer specialist - just to name a few.

I could not complete my thoughts about my work without commenting about the importance of my fine wife of 23 years and my three young adult children - one of whom is training to become a psychologist.

In all the years of practice I have seldom regretted my choice of profession. I have given and also believe have received much, have grown and matured. In many ways there has been more than an equal exchange with the many men and women patients who I have been privileged to work with during these 30 years.

MARK H. LEWIN

THE SETTING

"This I beheld or dreamed it in a dream." So starts "Opportunity" by Edward Roland Sill, a poem that I first learned in fifth grade. The lines resurfaced in my mind in April of 1975 when I walked into a poorly kept building just east of downtown Rochester's "inner loop." The previous owners had permitted the building to drift into neglect while their business moved similarly. Their mortgage had been foreclosed just as I was planning to expand my solo practice. The building had been an elegant private home at the turn of the century. Stained glass windows, deep beamed ceilings, warm woods, large rooms with oversized carved pocket doors, five fireplaces, and plenty of space all graced the facility. The location was good, and there was a parking area on the property. In addition, four city buses stopped within a few steps of the building. This permitted servicing of the less affluent segments of the population as well as middle class and organizational clients that I had targeted.

I fell in love with the building despite broken ceilings, dismantled central heating, an unsafe porch, and its marginal neighborhood. The Eastman Dental School, one block east of the building, was planning to move as was a city school district administration building. A cultural district was being planned for the area just to the west; no one knew what the impact of that would be on the surrounding areas.

I rushed in where angels fear to tread. Fortunately, the intervening 10 years have been good to the neighborhood. A church has remained; The Eastman Dental School has been transformed into a center for light, high technology industry; a neighborhood group has encouraged the rehabilitation of the houses north of us; the school building has been transformed into housing and commercial spaces; and the surrounding areas of the city are being rejuvenated. A major hospital is less than a mile south of us and professional offices are scattered through the area.

Our building is three stories plus a basement, which we have renovated and renamed the "lower level." We use it to house our outplacement and career management service. This lower level has four offices, a library, a large common area for meetings and general "rapping," and its own bathroom.

Our main reception area is on the first floor. A secretary-receptionist is situated in this area, along with our current files, photocopying machine, and other office equipment. We keep current issues of magazines on display: *Natural History, New York Magazine, Life, Psychology Today, Business Week, Inc., Readers Digest, Family Circle*, and *Working Woman* are available, as are a few books. A special selection for children is in another magazine rack. Several clients have spontaneously made favorable comments about the selection and up-to-date quality of our offerings.

Beyond the reception area are two large offices, a room for our office manager, a testing room, a bathroom, and storage closets. At the rear of the building is a conference room in which we hold staff meetings, group sessions, and team building meetings. We also hold business breakfasts and luncheons there. It is a private setting where confidentiality is no problem, as it can be in restaurants. In addition, it saves us time - we do not have to travel back and forth from restaurants. The clients and gatekeepers who meet in the conference room experience our organization as stronger because we have the space to host them.

The second level has two sections. One is a suite of two offices, plus storage space and a bathroom. The other section is rented out as a two-bedroom apartment. It can easily be converted into four offices when the need arises. The third floor is also rented out. One part is a lovely studio apartment that would make an ideal conference area; we have run workshops and held meetings there in the past. The final one-bedroom apartment on the third floor will probably remain rented so that there will always be someone in the building.

Rochester, a metropolitan area of 600,000 people in western New York, is a fine city with a history of progressively approaching the delivery of psychological and health care services. The Eastman Kodak Company and Xerox Corporation are its two major employers. Bausch and Lomb, Sybron Corporation, and General Motors' Delco and Rochester Products Divisions, as well as many tool and die, printing, and high tech companies play a major role in the community. The population in general is at a high socio-economic and educational level. Eight colleges and universities are in the area, as is a major medical center, Strong Memorial Hospital. Four health maintenance organizations actively vie for participants. We are a healthy, happy group of citizens who complain about (but secretly take pride in and exaggerate) the frozen assets of our snow-belt heritage.

My practice has evolved from a solo enterprise to a group of seven. It started out as one clinical psychologist serving the community, making his own appointments, typing his reports, emptying his own wastebasket, and doing his own planning. It was (and remains) my deep belief that psychology has more to offer than merely "seeing clients" in the traditional clinical mode. I began using my clinical psychological skills in industrial and in community organization settings; I also discovered a need for vocational and career planning within the context of exploring client needs. I was having fun, sensing professional challenge, and feeling that I was contributing to the community. But I was also overworked. What to do?

PLANNING AND MANAGING SERVICES

I developed a business plan for expanding in a systematic way. An outline of the business plan can be found on pages 59-61 of my 1978 book. My first colleague was an industrial psychologist, my second a clinical psychologist. In the past 8 years, after assessing changes in the community and its needs, and because of the increasing competitive pressures of the HMOs, our model has changed. The HMOs now draw large numbers of people who used to seek psychological services on the open market, but who are not "locked in" to the services provided "for free" by their HMO. We still offer individual, marriage, and family psychotherapy, neuropsychological evaluations, and evaluations of families involved in custody disputes, but we are changing our emphasis. Our major source of clinical referrals is now attorneys. This was the result of a systematic effort to educate them to the ways we can help them help their clients. We made the effort because of our prediction that medical referrals would be greatly reduced by the change in health care delivery planned for Rochester. The prediction was accurate and our plan has been successful.

Career planning and outplacement services have become a major source of our income and service delivery. We have hired a full-time career counselor. A psychologist begins the process with a comprehensive psychological evaluation that focuses on the individual's intellectual efficiency, motivation and personality characteristics, social skills and insight, administrative-managerial-organizational abilities, and vocational-career interests. The career counselor, in conjunction with the psychologist, then helps the client develop and implement a career plan.

Organization development, team building, strategic planning, conflict management, morale surveys, pre-hire and pre-promotion evaluations, manager training and development, and other human resources management services are also an integral part of our offerings.

We, as psychologists, are not fully prepared to meet all of the needs of our organizational client. We, therefore, decided to seek the services of a business consultant with whom we could work comfortably and well. We found such a professional. He joined us, and both we (the psychologists) and he have noted the synergistic benefits to our clients (and to us) of the integration of our insights and services.

Our newest division is being developed to help our clients meet their training needs. Training involves teaching and leads to behavior change. That is the work of psychology. We have designed programs to teach managers how to manage more effectively; workers and managers how to monitor and improve the quality of their work; and business people how to plan and organize their business and personal lives. We will also develop training "packages" and products. This can reduce our sole dependence on the fee for service practice that we have enjoyed but in which we develop no real "equity."

LESSONS LEARNED

What have we all learned in 18 years of practice? First, the practice of psychology can be fun. It can support a pleasant lifestyle, and most importantly it can make meaningful contributions to the community. Second, planning and awareness of community trends can help develop a thriving practice and avoid "unexpected" problems and competitive pressures. Third, there can be real advantages to taking a broad view of the ways in which psychological insights can serve the community. A diverse array of individual and organizational clients can benefit from our interventions. Psychology is only one of the behavioral sciences; we have learned that we can enhance the quality of our services by joining forces with other specialists whose skills are compatible with ours - even if we sometimes overlap. Fourth, psychology is a science, but the practice of psychology is both a profession and a business. We succeed when we meet our clients' needs and serve them well. Our practice thrives on management and careful planning.

CARROLL L. MEEK

TYPE OF PRACTICE

I work alone in a small independent practice. I have no receptionist or bookkeeper and no "live" answering service (I use a telephone answering machine - see "Guidelines for Using an Answering Machine in Your Practice," pages 271-276). I even clean my own office. I employ an accountant to deal with the submission of tax forms. I pay a psychiatrist for consultation twice a month concerning medical difficulties and problem patients. I have several colleagues that I contact when I am bored or desire collegial contact.

COMMUNITY DESCRIPTION

My practice is in Pullman, Washington, a community with 26,000 people - a figure that includes 16,000 Washington State University (WSU) students. Pullman is 9 miles from Moscow, Idaho, a community with 17,000 people including 8,000 University of Idaho students. Both universities provide counseling services to students free of charge.

The university settings provide an academic atmosphere and, typical residents are likely to be highly educated. Both communities are classified as rural, with the second-highest business (next to the universities) probably being farming. There are many smaller nearby communities which draw individuals into my practice.

LOCATION OF OFFICE

My office is located approximately one-half mile from WSU and Memorial Hospital, which also houses WSU's Student Health Center. The Professional Mall is an office complex with medical prestige and familiarity to those who reside in our area. The Mall is composed of three buildings that form an upside-down "U" shape and are fronted by a large, green lawn with flowering trees. There is adequate parking and handicapped persons' access. My office is in an alcove between a Social Security office and a pharmacy. It has bathrooms nearby, a very small waiting area, and a drinking fountain. Although the space I rent does not include the "waiting area," I was given permission to install two small chairs outside my office door. In addition to the offices in my building, the other two buildings contain dentists, physicians, a financial management firm, and an insurance agency.

Because of the type of traffic, and because I am situated close to the parking lot, my office sign is seen by many individuals everyday. My sign, at the outside door, says:

> Carroll L. Meek, PhD
> Counseling Psychologist
> Licensed
> National Register of Health
>   Service Providers in Psychology
> Counseling and Consultation
> (Individual, Couple, Child, and
>   Adolescent Therapy)

Individuals see this sign when walking by, and it "registers." I always ask people how they got my name and many have mentioned that they saw my sign on the way to an appointment with another professional in the Mall.

The area is a quiet one which is heavily utilized by medical patients. Most individuals know about it and it is easy to find, even if people are not already familiar with it. I have been renting this space for 4 years. It has been perfect for my needs. Patients have been impressed with its accessibility and decor, and university professors who teach psychology and human services classes have even requested permission to bring their students to the office to see my private practice setting.

DESCRIPTION OF PRACTICE

Because I worked at WSU's Counseling Services for 13 years, my reputation and name were already known. My practice was, therefore, already somewhat established even though I did not see private patients while I was employed at the university. My practice is much more varied than I expected it would be. I consult with community leaders, professionals, many university faculty, and blue-collar workers. I see teenagers, university students, and children. I treat individuals, couples, and families; occasionally I make house calls. I have a difficult practice, but it is highly rewarding and challenging. People want to read about their diagnoses and request detailed and technical information about their treatment. This need for scientific information is partly because of their educated status, but also because I encourage their active involvement in treatment.

I have "word-of-mouth" referrals, some from physicians, counseling centers, and other therapists. I receive many self-referrals from my listing in the yellow pages. Although I feel sorry for individuals who have to "pluck a name out of a hat" like that, many people do.

OFFICE LAYOUT

The room I occupy is only 14 by 18 square feet. I divided the room by placing bookcases at a right angle from the door. The room, divided as it is, creates a small office area on one side, where I have a small refrigerator, coffee maker, desk, typewriter and work table, two extra straight-backed chairs, file cabinet, telephone answering machine, and so on. On the therapy side, I have two easy chairs, a 200-year-old crusader chair, a rocking chair, a leather sofa, end tables with table lamps, floor lamp, and a lateral file (see Figure 1).

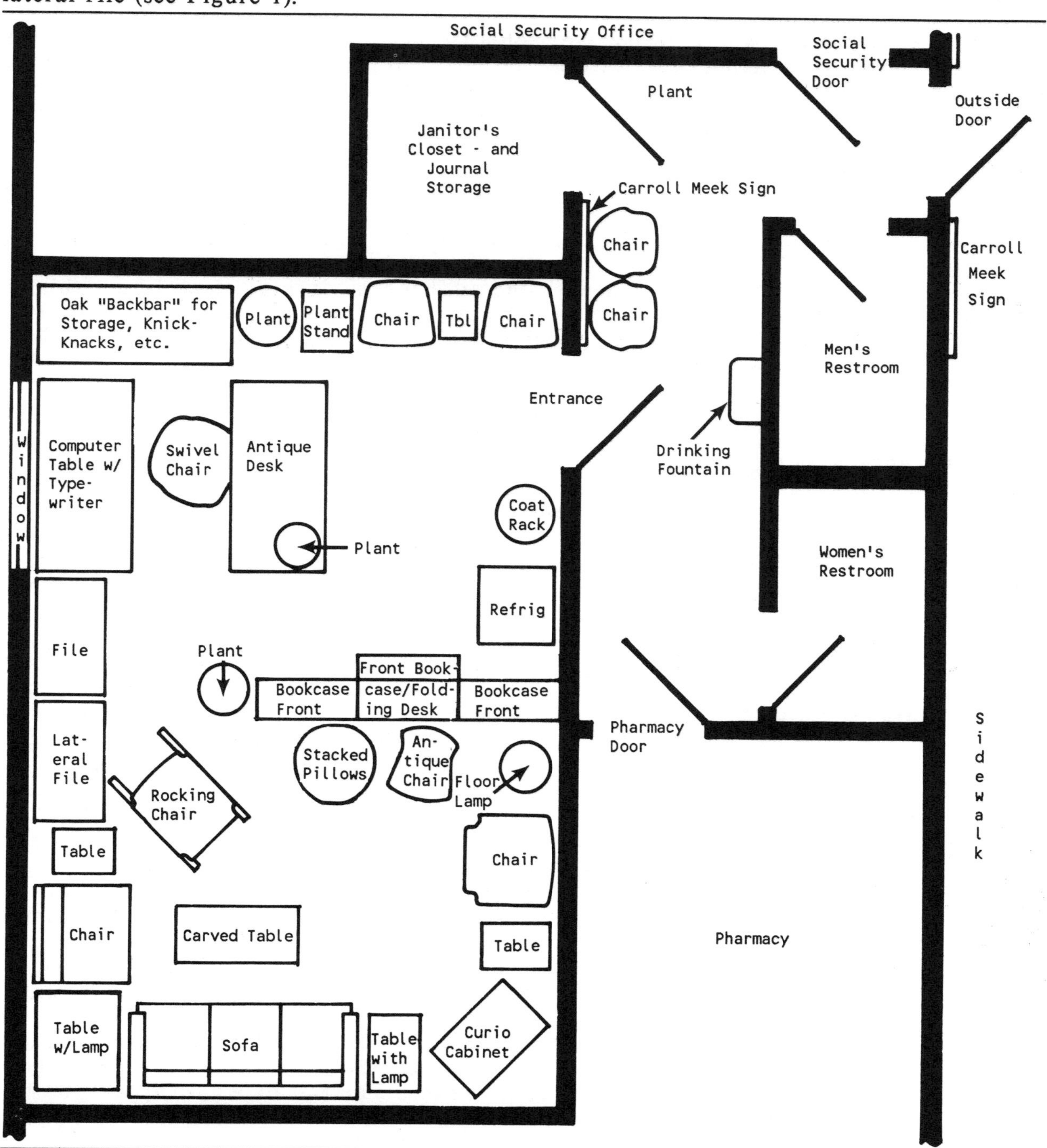

Figure 1. Drawing courtesy of Aachen Designers, Gainesville, FL.

The smallness of the counseling area seems to provide security to individuals and many people have spontaneously commented that it is most comfortable and relaxing to be in an area like mine. I see deeply distressed individuals go instinctively to the innermost chair. The chair many initially pick is also the one most likely to be the furthest from mine (the rocking chair). As they develop more trust, they change chairs, often with the explanation, "I want to get a different view." They may move closer to me until as therapy proceeds they are sitting in the chair closest to mine. I have seen this sequence of chair changes so many times that I view it as a sign of progress in therapy. I have also seated comfortably, although cozily, as many as seven people in the therapy area.

OFFICE DECOR

When people see my *Office Policy Statement* (Meek & Editors, 1985) out of context, they often feel that it is too businesslike or harsh. The down-to-business aspect of my *Statement* is tempered by the office atmosphere I have attempted to provide. I have learned in the 4 years of my practice that the first impression people receive is not by my *Statement*, anyway. First impressions are formed by what people encounter when they initially enter my small office.

Because I took a year's leave of absence from WSU to see if I could establish, and would like working in a private practice, I knew that if my effort were to be successful, I would need to furnish an office that looked like it had been there for a long time. This meant decorating it with sturdy furnishings, expensive accents, and so on. Therefore, I chose solid Danish oak furniture. I also added antiques to the office, mixing old and new.

The office took a medieval turn with the addition of an old, black "gun cabinet" someone made 50 years ago, and with some persuasion, the antique dealer turned it into a curio cabinet to which I added a leaded-glass castle, some porcelain music boxes, some unicorns, a jumping jack, and a few vases. The curio cabinet was the turning point which made one look around for the "missing suit of armor." The castle-like decor, therefore, happened by accident. The office, from the beginning, took on a long-established impression which has served me well.

When I look at my office atmosphere in retrospect, I find that I have more than unconsciously provided people with a statement of myself. When people first walk through the door, they are making decisions about whether they think I am going to be able to help them.

One 16-year-old whose treatment would have been paid for by Social and Health Services if she would agree to pursue therapy at the local clinic, decided she would pay for my services out of her own part-time job instead. I tried to persuade her to at least try every therapist at the local clinic so she would not have to sacrifice her hard-earned wages. She was terribly patient with my efforts at persuasion until she finally blurted out, "Carroll! Have you seen *their* offices?" Atmosphere is important to 16 year olds!

People are first greeted by my 10-year-old receptionist - a very seasoned Maltese dog who has worked with me since she was a puppy. Having worked with WSU students for several years and in my private practice for 4 years, she is a bit reserved. She escorts people to their seats (literally) and takes her place on the couch and sleeps until the next therapy hour. Sometimes individuals express regret that she is not a lap dog, but she isn't, and children and adults respond readily to the explanation that she is basically shy and does not require or like a lot of attention. When the bell on the outside door rings for the next appointment, however, she is right there, looking for her next "customer." People seeing a dog at the Professional Mall come looking for her owner - I sometimes think *she* generates referrals, but does not get credit. Teenage and college students have reported to their parents, "Hey! I couldn't believe it! She has a *dog* in her office!" Parents hearing that know their offspring have started therapy. How many kids, reporting home, say *anything* about their first therapy session?

The second impression is formed by my 15-year-old philodendron and other vining plants, which have enveloped one-third of my office ceiling and one-fourth of the office walls. I suppose the third impression is formed by me. The rest of what captures notice seems to be idiosyncratic as far as individual preferences and tastes are concerned. Plants seem to be very important to most people. I usually keep one semi-sick plant in the office along with the healthy ones; when people inquire about it, I tell them that because it got the same treatment as all the rest, I have to assume it is not trying hard enough.

I also have an antique reproduction, inlaid-wood chiming clock. I have no idea how I ever managed to do therapy for 16 years without a chiming clock. The half-hour chime tells the person that he or she has utilized half the session, and for many it gets them moving much more quickly than they were in the first half.

The walls of my office are decorated with paintings and photographs of various castles. There are tapestries I have made myself, and they provide the opportunity for my patients to see that *anything* can be accomplished with patience and sustained effort.

One set of parents wanted an "unusual" therapist, because they did not feel that previous therapy had been successful in establishing a relationship with their 15-year-old suicidal son. The referral source said, "Have we got a therapist for you!" The first session left the boy running home excitedly to tell his parents about the office and the dog. "I'll tell you," he said, "she's a witch." When I asked him whether he thought I was a *good* witch or a *bad* witch, he only smiled, but he brought many of his friends by my office (I supposed they were there to help him decide).

Therapists need to provide intentional statements about who they are. They generally do it, unwittingly, anyway. A sterile, white office where individuals peer around looking for nurses with syringes does not provide an atmosphere for openness and candor; it also convinces people that they may be "beyond help." Many people come to me because they feel they do not fit in; seeing me and my office convinces them that idiosyncrasy is okay, it just needs to be channeled into appropriate outlets.

I have had colleagues ask me whether all the debris in my office provides too much stimulation or too many diversions to work fully in therapy. I have never had that happen. When comments are made about various things in my office, I use them to the maximum as therapy tools. I find that even off-hand comments generally mean something.

OFFICE FUNCTION

I hang a sign outside my office door which says, "I am in conference, please do not disturb. If you have an appointment, please ring the bell at the time of your appointment." I work afternoons and evenings. I serve coffee, tea, and hot chocolate (with marshmallows).

Although my office is well insulated from sounds inside and outside, I installed a radio speaker underneath one of the chairs outside my office door. This makes it virtually *impossible* for a "listening ear" to hear anything inside my office. People have asked me if I am lonely because I work alone. I worked in institutional settings for 16 years! I have not missed it and contrary to popular opinion it is virtually *impossible* for a *therapist* to work alone! In addition, I pay a supervisor for two sessions per month. My husband is a psychiatrist and I also have several friends who are experts in their respective fields. When I need additional contact, the phone is right there and a luncheon engagement is only 24 hours away.

LAWRENCE G. RITT

In 1970, I moved to Sarasota, Florida and assumed the directorship of a new community mental health clinic. Sarasota is located on the Gulf of Mexico approximately 60 miles south of Tampa. Over the past 16 years, I have witnessed this county's emergence from a small, undeveloped "artist's colony" community of approximately 60,000 into a sprawling, multifaceted area with a population of just under 250,000. Sarasota County is the 17th fastest growing metropolitan area in the country. It also has the second highest per capita income in Florida; a major factor in understanding the proliferation of amenities that contribute to the quality of life of the area (outstanding restaurants, a symphony orchestra, museums, three equity theatres, specialty shopping areas, etc.). Major industries include tourism, home construction, light manufacturing, and agriculture. Although there are many retirees in the area, there is also a large and viable business and professional community spanning all age groups.

My professional activities as clinic director included a pleasant mix of direct client services, teaching, consultation, program development, and administration. The clinic had an entrepreneurial spirit; our talented, imaginative, and energetic staff was creatively building a new program to meet identified community needs. However, it became obvious after 4 years that our clinical-entrepeneurial orientation needed to be supplemented by greater emphasis on management and administration. I resigned as director in 1974 after deciding that I wasn't interested in changing roles to meet the program's emergent needs. I briefly considered a clinical academic position, but decided to "take the plunge" and become an independent practitioner, instead.

When I entered independent practice in 1974, there were two other psychologists, four psychiatrists, and two clinical social workers in private practice. That number has now increased to approximately 75 full and part-time practitioners.

I opened my first office across the hall from one of the other psychologists and we made arrangements to share a part-time secretary and answering service. Our building was located three blocks from the public hospital on the town's main artery (appropriately called Tamiami Trail to signify the fact that it runs from Tampa to Miami). Our two story building had an open courtyard with an immense palm tree in the center. The other tenants included a group practice of pediatricians, several dentists, and a real estate management firm. I leased a 400 square foot office consisting of two rooms; a 12' x 12' open space that served as a secretarial area/waiting room and a large inner office. I purchased a new teak desk with lots of little cubbyholes and drawers. Several weekends of garage sales led to the acquisition of a desk chair, end tables, table lamps, and a couple of comfortable side chairs. My desk was placed against a wall where I could use it for testing, telephone calls, and paperwork but where it would not intrude into the living room style seating arrangement that I prefer when working with psychotherapy clients and families.

In 1976, all the fronds fell off the palm tree (leaving a huge, dead phallic symbol in our courtyard), and all of the professional tenants abandoned the building as it became obvious that the landlord did not intend to provide adequate maintenance. I moved into a new building in the downtown area. That location was chosen based on a careful examination of where my clients lived and worked.

My second office was located in a delightful Spanish-style stucco building with iron gates, a bricked courtyard, an abundance of tropical greenery, and perfect architectural scale. I rented 650 square feet of unfinished space. Modifying that space to meet my needs was great fun! My landlord, Ron Spector, is a marvelous fellow who implemented all of my ideas perfectly. The finished office consisted of an irregularly shaped waiting room, a separate secretarial area with a window to the waiting area, a short hall with a hospitality area (coffee, tea, cold drinks, and water), a small testing/play room, and a large (12' x 22') inner office.

I spend more time at my office than at home and have discovered that both I and my clients are most relaxed and productive when we work in a truly comfortable, quiet, and private setting. Responding to that discovery, I devoted a great deal of attention to all of the construction and furnishing details of my second office.

All interior walls were built to double thickness with sound-absorbing wallboard, air-conditioning ductwork was designed to totally baffle noise transmission, and oversized solid wood doors were installed and weather stripped throughout the space. With my office door closed, neither I nor my clients had any concerns about our conversations being overheard and there were no external distractions (except for occasional bird sounds emanating through the courtyard window).

The office color scheme consisted of earth tones. Dark plush carpeting and light grained wallpaper were installed throughout the space. One wall in my inner office was diagonally paneled in rough-grained natural cedar. I kept my teak desk and supplemented it with a 10 foot teak wall unit of cabinets and bookshelves. I bought a comfortable, plush recliner/rocker; distraught clients routinely seem to find the gentle rocking motion of this chair to be highly soothing. I added three incredibly comfortable (and indestructible) Knoll chairs and arranged them in a separate triangular seating arrangement with two simple square end tables; I used this area for marital and family therapy, depositions, and conferences (pulling in additional chairs from other rooms as needed). I indulged myself by buying an ergonomic desk chair. Although my clients often comment that my "straightback" chair looks less comfortable than theirs, the truth is that I can sit for hours in this chair in absolute comfort. Finishing touches included some of my favorite paintings, photographs, sculpture, and lots of tropical green plants in floor containers and hanging pots.

In 1979, I reluctantly decided it was time to leave my marvelous second office. That decision was based on an increasingly difficult parking situation (as several restaurants opened on our block) and the need for more space to accommodate the newly-formed publishing company that produces this series. When I notified my favorite landlord of my decision, he informed me that he was building a new complex about six blocks away that would have ample parking and would be architecturally quite similar to the building I was vacating. Within a week, I had signed on as his first tenant and began to recreate my old office in his new building.

Based on the premise that "if it works, don't fix it," the waiting room, testing/play room, hospitality area, and inner office in my current (third) office are almost identical to my second office. We also used exactly the same soundproofing features, carpeting, wallpaper, and cedar paneling. I did rent an additional 400 square feet to allow for a second psychologist's office and increased storage and filing space in the secretarial area. A door in the secretarial area connects my office to the office suite that houses the publishing company staff.

As I look back over the 12 year course of my career as an independent practitioner, I realize that I have been following a notably circular path. More specifically, I find that I have returned to many of the same activities that I abandoned when I entered private practice in 1974.

When I first entered practice, I was almost exclusively office and hospital based. I conducted three to six psychological evaluations a week. The balance of my time was spent in individual, marital, and family therapy. Initially, my referrals came primarily from the nonpsychiatric medical community, local schools, attorneys, and the other contacts I had made during my tenure at the mental health clinic. Although I still receive referrals from those sources, I now find that approximately 30% of my referrals come from former clients.

With the passage of time, a definite office ambience has evolved. I want my clients to be comfortable and relaxed in the office. Instead of couches and loveseats, I chose individual chairs for the waiting room. I didn't want a seating arrangement that imposed intimacy with total strangers. All of my magazines are current and include *People*, *Time*, *U.S. News and World Report*, *Architectural Digest*, *Smithsonian*, *Town and Country*, and *Psychology Today*. I keep a plastic crate of small games, books, and magazines for children. An FM radio is set to a classical station. Clients and their families are invited to help themselves to coffee, tea, and cold drinks. The waiting room also contains an acrylic "Take One" display of useful client handouts including pamphlets explaining our office policies (Keller & Ritt, 1982), psychological services (Florida Psychological Association, 1985), and psychotherapy (Lacks, Stolz, & Levine, 1983).

I have a full-time secretary who answers the phone, attends to the needs of waiting clients, types, handles bookkeeping and fee collections, interacts with insurance companies, scores standardized tests, and makes appointments for old clients. I speak with all new referrals on the telephone prior to setting their first appointment. These telephone contacts provide me with an opportunity to answer questions, alleviate client concerns, insure that the referral is appropriate, discuss fees and office policies, identify information the client may want to obtain before our first session (e.g., records from prior therapists), refer to other health care providers when indicated, and generally set the stage for our first face-to-face contact. I routinely respond to all phone calls daily. If it is obvious that I won't be free until late, my secretary invites both clients and referral sources to leave numbers where they can be reached in the evening.

As a general policy, I ask psychotherapy clients to pay their fees at the end of each session. When clients feel their insurance will pay all or a portion of the charges, my secretary requests their consent to call the carrier to prescreen coverage, current deductibles, and policy limitations. Once those issues are clarified, I will accept insurance assignment. Clients seem to appreciate my willingness and desire to discuss fees in an open and straightforward manner. I also feel these discussions set a precedent for openness and honesty regarding other therapeutic issues.

I routinely see some clients on a *pro bono* basis. My willingness to see occasional clients without charge is not an altogether altruistic decision. In my opinion, professionals gain a great deal of community respect when they accept indigent referrals from judges, physicians, and agencies.

I cannot remember how I ran my office prior to the advent of microcomputers. My letters and reports sometimes go through six or more revisions; however, my word-processing secretary has little difficulty accommodating my periodic perfection. I also have a computer discretely hidden inside the teak cabinets in my office. I use this terminal for typing progress notes, quick memos, and maintaining an online "to do" list. We also use our computers for test scoring and interpretation, database and literature searches, and telecommunicating with other psychologists on electronic bulletin boards.

In discussing the joys of my practice, I would be remiss if I didn't mention Terry Proeger, the psychologist who has been sharing my office space since 1980. I can't imagine a more satisfactory collegial arrangement than the relationship we share. My respect for his professional expertise allows me to relax when I'm on vacation or otherwise unavailable to my clients. I know Terry can handle any crisis they experience during my absence. Our regular case conferences almost always lead to insights that enable us to better serve our clients. There is also great comfort in knowing we are available to assist each other with difficult clinical, professional, and ethical issues.

Although I still enjoy providing "traditional" diagnostic and treatment services and spend approximately 50% of my time in such endeavors, I discovered early in my private practice career that I yearned for more diversity. I enjoy the challenges of forensic work and increasingly accept referrals for evaluations and consultations related to criminal and civil cases. I also do frequent custody evaluations and mediation for local judges. Working with a large national Employee Assistance Program has provided an opportunity to do the type of crisis intervention work that was so stimulating at the mental health clinic.

When I first left the clinic, I found myself periodically grieving over the loss of opportunities to use my skills as a community psychologist. Then it occurred to me that such opportunities were not lost; I had simply misplaced them! With a little effort, I have been able to establish a wide range of training and consultative relationships. I serve as a case, program, and community systems consultant to a children's mental health program. I also have ongoing and regularly scheduled consultative relationships with a local rehabilitation/work adjustment facility, a substance abuse program, and offer training, consultative, and EAP-type services to our fire department and paramedics. In addition, I provide weekly supervision to a recently graduated clinical psychologist.

In closing, I want to note that I have served as a member of the Executive Council of the Florida Psychological Association since 1979. I mention this fact only because I want to stress the important role I feel my colleagues on the Council have played in my professional development. They freely share their expertise and are outstanding models for developing new roles and skills. Their feedback and critique of my work products have proven invaluable. In addition, I thoroughly enjoy their company.

RESOURCES

Florida Psychological Association. (1985). *What Is Psychology: A Guide to Psychological Services*. Tallahassee, FL: Florida Psychological Association.

Keller, P. A., & Ritt, L. G. (1982). Fee information. In P. A. Keller & L. G. Ritt (Eds.), *Innovations in Clinical Practice: A Source Book* (Vol. 1, p. 381). Sarasota, FL: Professional Resource Exchange, Inc.

Lacks, P., Stolz, J., & Levine, J. (1983). A guide to psychotherapy. In P. A. Keller & L. G. Ritt (Eds.), *Innovations in Clinical Practice: A Source Book* (Vol. 2, pp. 443-446). Sarasota, FL: Professional Resource Exchange, Inc.

Lewin, M. H. (1978). *Establishing and Maintaining a Successful Professional Practice*. Rochester, NY: Professional Development Institute.

Meek, C. L., & Editors. (1985). A collection of office forms. In P. A. Keller & L. G. Ritt (Eds.), *Innovations in Clinical Practice: A Source Book* (Vol. 4, pp. 345-360). Sarasota, FL: Professional Resource Exchange, Inc.

HOW TO USE SMALL CLAIMS COURT FOR COLLECTIONS

William R. Hussey

How many patients do you bill periodically without really expecting any payment? You are probably tempted to write these off as bad debts, but perhaps some inner sense of justice prompts you to want to find a way to bring these nonpaying patients to justice. After all, they agreed to purchase your services, your time, and your professional advice, and now they verge on getting all that for nothing. It just is not right.

The purpose of this contribution is to describe the small claims court alternative to abandoning these claims, and educate you to its use. But why bother? Can you justify the effort, and the expense of your time? Can you succeed? If you win in court, what are the chances you will collect? Wouldn't your time perhaps be better spent in refining your list of patients to weed out those who appear to be poor payment risks? Is trying to collect old bills through small claims court really worth it?

My answer is: Yes, generally it is worth it, but only if you make it work for you. You can, with a little experience, streamline your small claims court collection work so that it takes a minimum of your time. Also, you can establish or enhance your reputation in the community as someone who stands up for what you believe in, someone who cannot readily be taken advantage of.

Patients of professionals do not pay for a variety of reasons. It is probably easier to get away with not paying a professional than with not paying almost any other creditor. If people do not pay their phone bill, telephone service is cut off. If they do not pay their electric bill, their electricity is cut off. If they do not pay a charge account bill promptly, credit is cut off, and a bad credit report goes into a central credit reporting agency. However, if they do not pay a professional, usually nothing happens. So, even with well-intentioned people, professionals become the last to be paid, because there is no pressure to pay them. The small claims court process can provide that pressure.

PREPARATION

One of the first things you should do is gear your office procedures to anticipate the nonpaying patient. This is not negative thinking; it is simply being realistic. Obviously, every effort should be made to collect for services when they are rendered. However, there are many occasions when on-the-spot payment is impossible or impractical. Questions of insurance coverage may be present, the patient may be in need of immediate service but not then equipped with cash or check to pay for it, services may be rendered away from the office, or a variety of other situations may occur to inhibit immediate payment.

It is relatively easy to establish office procedures to track patients and payments. However, the need to keep critical information about patient visits confidential must always take precedence over such procedures. Any clinician who enters this type of collection process must consider carefully the requirements of professional ethics and statutes regarding patient privilege. Still, within those limitations, the data you collect at intake may provide a useful trail to contact a patient who has moved and failed to pay your bill. To what extent you permit your office staff to use these intake data to make discreet inquiries of various sources about the whereabouts of a nonpaying patient must remain your personal decision.

You can, however, readily establish payment sources by making a photocopy of every check that comes through the office. It is a simple procedure to gather all payment checks that come in during the course of a day, or whatever time period elapses between deposits, and line the checks up on a photocopy machine before sending them to the bank for deposit. Those checks will reveal the account number and the name of the bank your patient is then dealing with. Later, if you are trying to collect a small claims court judgment you have obtained against this patient, any check photocopies will disclose a bank account that may still be open and can be garnished. Also, a telephone call to a bank suggesting that you have a check from a certain patient in the amount of, say, $150, and identifying the account, will often elicit from the bank whether there are funds in the account at that moment to cover such a check.

Promptness also tends to pay off. Many surveys have been conducted showing a steep rise in nonpayment of bills as they age. Such studies have shown that uncollectability of accounts may go from 10% after 30 days to 40% after 60 days to 80% after 90 days. I do not vouch for the accuracy of those percentages, but only for their representation of the sharp decrease in collectability as time passes. You can help your patients as well as yourself by not allowing large bills to build to a point where they may be unmanageable.

SMALL CLAIMS COURT OVERVIEW

The small claims court is at the bottom of the court system. Although the name "small claims court" is probably the most common, the court also can be found under the guise of justice court, municipal court, common pleas court, court of summary procedure, and other names. For uniformity, we will continue to refer to it as "small claims court." Sometimes a small claims court will be a division of another court, providing for prompt and summary handling of certain defined claims.

In all cases, the court will define the monetary limits of what it considers to be a small claim. These can run from a low of $300 up to highs of several thousand. It is vital that you make sure that any claim you present to the court is within the monetary limits of your jurisdiction's small claims court. Otherwise, you will not be able to use the relatively simple and easy procedures of a small claims court, and will probably require the services of an attorney to lead you through the thicket of required procedures if you are thrust into a higher court. This, of course, is another incentive to prompt action, before the amount of the bill exceeds the limits of the small claims court.

Small claims courts generally like to be thought of as "people's" courts, a place where the average citizen can come to get disputes resolved quickly and informally. Yet, most of the judges in these courts recognize that their courts are often used as collection facilities by loan companies, charge account creditors, and professionals. Also, most of the judges who sit on the small claims court bench were previously practicing lawyers, and came to the court steeped in the formal rules and procedures of the higher courts. Some have difficulty letting go of those procedures, and will require more formality than would seem to be the intent of the court. Therefore, at the outset, it is usually a good idea to sit in on a session or two of a small claims court to watch different judges, if your community has more than one handling small claims, so that you get a feeling for the manner in which the court operates, and the degree of strictness followed by each judge. This should not be an extensive research project, but something to which you might devote several hours before plunging into the unfamiliar courtroom arena.

The definition of a small claim is determined by your state's law delineating the jurisdiction of a small claims court. Generally, small claims courts are not geared to require a defendant to do something, as opposed to ordering a defendant to pay something. Suits in small claims courts are almost invariably for money. The amount of money sought must be within the maximum jurisdictional limits of the court. These days, $1,500, $2,000, and $2,500, are common ceilings. Filing fees will often vary depending upon the amount of the claim, with the charge for a $300 claim less than for a $500 claim, which in turn would be less than a $1,000 claim, and so forth.

USING A SMALL CLAIMS COURT

All courts, even those handling small claims, have a set of rules that they follow. You will need to know them. Also, most small claims courts have certain forms that they require you to use.

One of the first things you should do, after sitting in on a few hearings, is visit the office of the court clerk handling small claims and get copies of all the forms required and procedures used, plus a copy of the rules of procedure for the court. The clerk's office may not have available extra copies of those rules, but a clerk can probably tell you where you can get a copy. Most law libraries will have a set of these rules, and most courthouses have a law library. Public libraries will also sometimes have them, and if you cannot immediately get a copy of the rules, you can at least find out the name and address of the publisher of the books containing them, and call or write to the publisher to get a copy.

You will generally use your time and the court process more economically and efficiently if you gather a group of claims together and start them all at one time. The court clerk will usually try to accommodate you by setting all your cases for hearing on the same day, and at or near the same time, and may even give you some discretion as to the day and time, so as to coincide best with your work schedule. Although initially you should file the claims in person so that you become familiar with the way in which they are handled and set up, after you have done this a few times in person, you can probably arrange to get the claims filed by mail, and have the court clerks do most of the administrative work for you.

PREPARING A CLAIM

Although there is a certain art to pleading a case well, that is much more important in courts at a higher level than small claims. What you need essentially is a short, straightforward statement, setting forth what you believe you are entitled to and why.

Since courts have long been used to collect unpaid bills and accounts, two general principles of law have evolved which you should learn and use. The most important is called "account stated." This applies when you have sent out by mail to someone who owes you money a statement showing the status of that person's account with you, specifying the amount of money claimed and what it is for. If your delinquent patient does not raise any objection within a reasonable period of time following receipt of this invoice, it then becomes an "account stated." This substantially simplifies the proof needed to establish your basic claim: you simply show the court a copy of the statement you sent, and testify as to how and when you sent it to the patient, who made no objection to it, and therefore the money is owed. When you get into court, that is all you have to prove. The burden then shifts to defendants to offer proof as to why the bill should not be paid, if in fact they have, or think they have, any defenses. But they have the burden of proving those defenses, and you do not have to negate them. I believe you will find that this procedure is the one you will use most often.

Related to this, but less likely to apply with a professional, is the legal principle called "open account." Although similar to the "account stated" procedure, an open account refers to the extension of a general line of credit to someone, where goods or services are furnished and bills rendered on a continuing basis, and progress payments are made at regular intervals. Businesses often use this for a continuing customer, a supplier, or a manufacturer under a long-term contract. Although it is unusual for a professional to extend a continuing line of credit, because it is possible I have mentioned it here.

GETTING THE DEFENDANT INTO COURT

Absolutely vital to the successful prosecution of any small claims court case is getting the defendant under the jurisdiction of the court. In fact, if a defendant does not answer and a judgment is entered in your favor by default, the only available basis for challenging that judgment is that the court did not properly obtain jurisdiction. Therefore, you must follow precisely the requirements of serving process on the defendant so that the court obtains jurisdiction, and can render a judgment that will be binding and enforceable.

As a general rule, the defendant must be served personally with a copy of your claim and a "summons" either to appear in court or to answer your claim within a certain period. If the summons and your claim are personally served on the defendant by a person authorized by law to do so, the court then acquires jurisdiction, and can make rulings affecting the defendant. Therefore, personal service of a summons and claim on a defendant is something you should always strive for.

Lawmakers recognize that people will often attempt to evade having a summons and claim served on them, will move, conceal their whereabouts, or otherwise become very difficult if not impossible to locate. Laws have therefore been enacted that allow a certain latitude in serving a claim on a defendant. Usually a little more latitude is allowed with small claims cases than with others, because the claim is small by nature, and if the attempted service on or notice to the defendant does not actually reach him or her, any judgment against the defendant still will not be as serious a matter as it would be if there were a much more substantial claim.

Therefore, many small claims courts allow a summons and claim to be served on a defendant by certified or registered mail. Although this procedure may be more convenient and less expensive than getting personal service through a deputy sheriff or someone similar, there is a certain risk of insufficient service, because you need to have a signed return receipt showing that the papers were received. Since certified or registered mail deliveries are usually attempted during the day, a household where everyone works will have no one home to receive the mail delivery and sign for it. In those cases, a small notice form is left in the mailbox, requesting the addressee to come to the post office to pick up the mail and sign for it. If the addressee suspects that you or anyone else may be attempting to collect money, he or she may simply refuse to go to the post office and pick up the letter, and after a time it will be returned to the sender with the notice "unclaimed." This is *not* effective service. On the other hand, if delivery is attempted on someone at the defendant's address who refuses to accept the court's papers, and the return receipt is marked "refused," courts will often accept that as valid service.

Whenever a defendant fails to appear in court at a scheduled time, the judge usually looks immediately in the court's file for written proof that the defendant was properly served with the claim and summons. If service was not proper, the judge will tell you to go back and try again. Of course, if that happens on all or most of the claims you have scheduled before the court on any given date and time, your trip to the courthouse that day will be wasted. Thus, if you have 15 claims all scheduled at one time, insufficient service on five of them probably will not make much difference, so service by registered or certified mail might be worth the cost saving. On the other hand, if you have only one or two claims to bring before the court, and you do not have good service of process on those defendants, you may find yourself eating a distasteful chunk of wasted time.

What kind of service of process is acceptable in your small claims court is something that the clerk's office generally will know and be able to acquaint you with. Questions such as the validity of registered or certified mail, whether mail can be accepted by a family member other than the defendant, and whether refused mail has been effectively served, may need to be researched by you or by a lawyer. Since laws differ from state to state, you will need to check on the laws where you practice.

Locating a disappearing debtor can often present a real challenge. Here is where some of the original information you obtained on a new patient, as discussed previously, can pay off, by allowing someone in your office to track down a debtor through phone calls to employers or relatives of the debtor. Again, the sooner you bring your claim after concluding that the patient is reluctant to pay, the fresher the trail will be and the better chance you will have of locating him or her.

PREPARING FOR TRIAL

Some small claims courts have a pre-trial procedure, which is, in effect, a mandatory initial meeting. Here the judge will review the case, see if there is any possibility of settlement, try to determine how long the trial of the case will take, and then set a trial date. If your state law or local rules authorize such a procedure, you will find it can be very effective in resolving claims at that pre-trial meeting. So, whenever you can, use the pre-trial conference to attempt settlement, or to eliminate much time and effort in trial preparation that might otherwise be required without it.

Always come to a pre-trial conference armed with knowledge of your claim and the documents which you will need to prove it. If you are willing to compromise, consider in advance the extent to which you will compromise on each claim. If your court allows progress payments on judgments, compute in advance what you believe are the minimum installment payment amounts and maximum payment period you want.

If you are using the "account stated" procedure, you should bring to the pre-trial conference copies of the bills you sent out, data on the date each bill was sent, whether or not any response was obtained, and how you verified that the address that the bills went to was a valid address for the defendant.

Generally, you will *not* need to bring witnesses to the pre-trial conference, but you should know whether any witnesses will be needed, and if any are, be prepared to provide their names and addresses to the court and your opponent.

Despite the court's apparent reliance on written documents filed with the court, the evidence you must use to prove your case still comes from live witnesses. Even when a document is introduced into evidence, it must be introduced through a live witness who can prove what the document is, where it came from, who it went to, and its purpose. Therefore, although you might think it ought to be acceptable simply to mail in to the court a copy of an unpaid bill, the court will require you to produce either yourself or another person in your office who can testify to the validity of the bill and when and where it has been sent.

Throughout this narrative I have continually referred to "you" as the professional who owns the practice, performed the services, and rendered the bill. However, many of you will have office managers or billing clerks who handle most of the billing for you, and may well know more about it than you do. Can they come to court and testify, and if they do, would you also have to come? The answer to those questions, like so many others, is: "It depends." If you are suing on an account stated, and your court follows a pre-trial conference procedure, the billing clerk in your office who verifies addresses and handles mailing of statements could certainly appear at any pre-trial conference, if you have given that person settlement authority and general authorization to act as your agent in collection matters.

If you have incorporated into a professional association or professional corporation, anyone you send to court should be an officer of the corporation. If your corporation is owned entirely by you, and you hold all the offices, you should probably make the person who goes to court for you an assistant secretary or assistant treasurer, because as a general rule only corporate officers have authority to act for a corporation and will be acceptable to the court.

If the amount of your fee or the necessity for or quality of the services you have rendered is challenged by a defendant, then you will have to appear personally to provide testimony as to the reasonableness of the charges and necessity for the services. You might also need to have another professional provide expert testimony as to the reasonableness of the charges and the necessity for the services. Although that is nearly always required in higher level courts, it is often dispensed with in small claims court. It is, again, simply a possible requirement, and you should verify the procedure followed in your area.

If you do need to provide live testimony from a witness other than either you or someone in your office, you should *always* have a subpoena served on each witness you will need, even if the witness is a friend of yours. There are several reasons for this. A subpoena carries with it the power of the court to enforce it. No one likes to take time off to come to court, and many employers are very reluctant to let their employees have time off to come to court as witnesses, yet when the employee has a subpoena, neither the employee nor the employer has any real choice in the matter. Also, witnesses subpoenaed to come to court generally have a shade more believability than those who come voluntarily. These witnesses are perceived as testifying not because they want to do a favor for the person presenting their testimony, but because they have something valuable to say and have been required to come, putting aside other things that day they might rather be doing. If a witness is subpoenaed and does not appear at the required time and place, you will then have grounds for a continuance that you will not have if the witness is supposed to show up voluntarily, and does not.

Subpoenas are issued by the court clerk. They are often served by a local deputy sheriff or a licensed process server. Licensed process servers will usually be listed in the yellow pages, often under private investigators, if not found under the "process server" heading.

Subpoenas may also require a witness to bring something, such as records or documents or any other tangible thing that the witness has in his or her possession or has control over, and which you need to present in your case. A subpoena requiring a witness both to appear and to bring something is commonly called a "subpoena duces tecum," and courts sometimes use different forms for a subpoena duces tecum than for a simple subpoena to appear, so check your court's forms.

If your court does not have a pre-trial procedure, you will need to come to the initial hearing fully prepared to present your case with testimony and documents. Some courts that do not use a pre-trial procedure still permit the plaintiff to obtain an automatic continuance if the defendant comes to the initial hearing without filing any kind of written pleading in advance indicating what his or her defenses are. However, until you are sure of the procedure your small claims court follows, it will usually pay you to be prepared to go to trial at any such initial hearing, unless instructions on any of the court documents tell you otherwise.

The final word on this subject is a warning to read carefully all court documents. The court will assume that you have read its documents, that you understand what is in them, and that you are prepared to follow their instructions. There are few things as embarrassing as having a judge inform you in front of everyone in the courtroom that the question you asked, or the procedure you claim ignorance of, appears as instructions in the court's documents, and you simply failed to read them. For a trained professional, this is particularly embarrassing. If you find any written instruction from the court that you do not understand, ask someone in the clerk's office to explain it to you.

HANDLING COUNTERCLAIMS

A counterclaim is what its name implies: a claim that goes counter to your claim; a claim back against you. Counterclaims are generally divided into mandatory and permissive. A mandatory counterclaim is one arising out of the same transaction or occurrence as the main claim, and must be made in the same proceeding, or it is considered to be abandoned. A permissive counterclaim is a claim a defendant has back against the plaintiff which does not arise out of the same transaction or occurrence, and may be brought as part of this same case or not, at the defendant's choice.

The counterclaim a professional most often will encounter is one for malpractice (professional negligence) arising out of the same services for which the professional is making the claim against the defendant. Many lawyers use the principle that the best defense is a good offense. More often than not, if you are confronted with a counterclaim, a lawyer will be representing the defendant. If you receive a counterclaim for professional negligence, notify your insurance carrier immediately and demand that the insurer defend you for this counterclaim. Although technically you can still handle the collection portion of your claim by yourself, I would urge you to arrange to have the lawyer hired by your malpractice insurer handle the entire case for you.

Malpractice is increasingly the subject of new state laws which set guidelines and limitations on malpractice suits. Unless you are personally involved in promoting the enactment of such laws, you will probably not be familiar with their many ramifications, and should rely upon your malpractice insurer and its attorneys to determine whether the defendant's malpractice claim will be permissible. Also, a malpractice claim generally will not be within the jurisdictional limits of a small claims court, and will need to be transferred to a higher level court.

Although you may occasionally see a full-blown malpractice counterclaim, it is more likely that you will encounter a discontented patient whose real complaint is that he or she does not think you did anything to help the presenting problem and so does not want to pay you. Courts may allow such a counterclaim to preserve the court's image as a people's court, responsive to an individual's claims. However, any claim that challenges the competency of you or the services you have rendered must be based upon and proved by the testimony of another expert in the same field. A defendant making a counterclaim asserting dissatisfaction with your services should have that claim dismissed at the end of his or her case if he or she has not presented expert testimony to prove that your care and treatment fell below the standard of care for those in your specialty field in your community.

If a counterclaim of any kind is made against you, I would also urge you to have a court reporter present at trial. Judges are often elected, and thus are particularly sensitive to the concerns and feelings of the citizens coming before them. Rather than risking the wrath of a resident who may feel squelched if the judge does not permit an extensive monologue about dissatisfaction with your services, the judge may well allow a full airing of grievances and complaints. Although you would certainly rather not have to listen to this recital (probably having heard it already), no problem would arise unless the judge also accepted the claim without appropriate proof. If that happens, you may wind up on the wrong end of the judgment, or lose your case when you really should not have, and your only recourse then is appeal. Appellate judges have difficulty reviewing a case unless there is a record of the proceedings and testimony. Therefore, whenever you anticipate the possibility of an appeal, you should spend the money for a court reporter to take down the proceedings, even if you never have them transcribed. The cost typically will not exceed $100, and more likely will range from $40 to $60.

Although a dissatisfied patient's claim of professional negligence must be proved by expert testimony, and the standard of care is the standard set by your profession, such a claim is not one you want to confront regularly. So, as a guideline in deciding whether or not to sue for an unpaid bill, you might want to think twice about suing if you were uncomfortable with the services rendered or the procedure you followed in caring for the patient.

PRE-TRIAL PROCEDURES

The pre-trial conference was touched upon earlier, and will be reviewed briefly here. The court's goal is to settle the case if at all possible, and to get it ready for trial if it cannot be settled. The court documents usually will outline the procedure to follow and the material to bring to a pre-trial conference, and that procedure should be followed exactly. You should also bring your calendar and appointment book so that you can work with the court in setting a trial time that will interrupt your schedule as little as possible.

Higher courts have a number of procedures which allow each side to discover information about the other side's case. In small claims court such procedures are very limited, but one usually allowed is the taking of depositions. This is the sworn testimony of a witness taken in advance of trial and used at trial under certain circumstances spelled out in the rules, such as when a witness (deponent) is out of the area, and in some cases, when an expert witness is used. Also, many small claims courts have procedures which allow you to require your opponent to give you documents in his or her possession that you need to prove your case.

The extent to which your small claims court allows the use of these and other pre-trial preparation and investigation procedures (called pre-trial discovery) will be found in your court's rules, which provides another reason to obtain a copy of those rules before you venture into the small claims courtroom.

TRIAL

Trials have taken place in an almost infinite number of forms over the period of recorded history. In any form, they constitute a "trial" to the participants even though our procedures have civilized the process compared to the trials by fire and by ordeal of ancient times. Despite the preparation that goes into getting ready, the unexpected still occurs, and dealing with it is challenging.

A lot of people become frustrated because the small claims court does not work the way they think it ought to. Many think a small claims trial is like appearing before a marriage counselor or an arbitrator. They believe that all they should have to do is come in and tell their story, then let the other side give their version, and the arbitrator (judge) will decide who is right. Some small claims courts still work that way, but most do not. And they do not because, although much of the formality of the higher courts is relaxed, most judges are reluctant to let go of the trial procedural rules completely.

Judges usually will require direct examination, and probably will allow cross-examination, of witnesses. Cross-examination tests the witness's memory, opportunity and ability to observe, knowledge of the subject matter, and possible bias or prejudice. It is in the cross-examination of witnesses that most lay people who use small claims court get mixed up, and consequently fail to use one of the most effective means available for searching out truth.

The small claims trial agenda commonly mirrors the procedure followed in the higher courts, but simply takes less time because the subject matter (the claim) is usually simple and limited. Although many small claims judges bypass an opening statement and ask you to begin presenting your testimony immediately, it is usually a good idea to be prepared with a very brief opening statement that outlines the nature of the case and what you intend to prove. You may have outlined this at a pre-trial conference, but between the conference and the time of your trial, the judge may have handled hundreds of other cases, and probably will not remember yours. Therefore, be prepared with a brief (about 1 minute) outline of your case. However, if the judge orders you to skip it, do not try to override this decision simply because you have prepared an opening statement and want to give it. Instead, call your first witness (which may be yourself).

The case proceeds as follows: The claimant (you) presents the claim through one or more witnesses. After each witness the defendant has an opportunity to cross-examine that witness about the testimony he or she has given, or the documents offered into evidence. Next, the defendant presents any defenses he or she may have through his or her own testimony or the testimony of any other witnesses. You have the right to cross-examine the defendant and any defense witnesses about their testimony or documents. If the defendant has any counterclaim, that counterclaim is presented next as if it were a new claim. You have the right, first, to cross-examine any witnesses the defendant presents in support of the counterclaim. After the defendant is finished presenting proof on the counterclaim, you can then present your defenses to the counterclaim through your testimony or the testimony of any other witnesses you might have. The defendant then has the right to cross-examine your witnesses.

As a practical matter, the lines between these sections of the trial often fade or disappear, for testimony will overlap, and by the time each of you has finished the first round of witnesses, all the available evidence may have been presented.

If, at the conclusion of your case, the defendant believes you have not presented sufficient evidence to prove your claim, he or she may move to dismiss it; likewise, at the conclusion of the defendant's defense, or at the conclusion of the defendant's counterclaim, you may move to dismiss any of the defenses or the counterclaim on the basis that the defendant did not present sufficient evidence to support the defense or the counterclaim. However, in most small claims courts, you will not need to make a motion to dismiss; the judge will generally do it if either you or your opponent has not presented enough proof to sustain any claim or defense.

When each side is finished, the court may give each of you a minute or two to comment on the evidence and what you believe it has proved. Again, small claims judges often bypass this to speed things along, especially if the issues to be decided are uncomplicated.

Some of the defenses you might be confronted with, which are referred to as affirmative defenses because the defendant must prove them, are such things as payment, compromise and settlement, waiver of the right to make the claim, and the statute of limitations or laches (i.e., you waited too long to bring the claim).

The greatest difficulty most people have in small claims court is learning when and how to ask questions. Everybody has a story to tell and is impatient to tell it. When they should be asking questions of their opponent or a witness, they instead keep trying to testify and argue, to present their side of the case. If you are the only witness for your case, obviously you cannot ask yourself questions, but will simply present your claim in narrative fashion to the judge. On the other hand, if you present any witnesses to the court, you should direct questions to those witnesses that are general in nature, such as where, when, what, how, and why.

To get a document into evidence through a witness, ask if the witness can identify the document. If the answer is yes, ask the witness then to identify what the document is by description, date, purpose, origin, and how it came into the witness's possession or knowledge. After it has been identified, hand it to the judge and say, "I offer this into evidence." The judge will then mark it as an exhibit and enter it into the court record.

Most courts' rules allow photocopies. This has largely done away with the old, so-called "best evidence" rule, which required you to put an original document into evidence, unless for some reason you could not, and then you had to explain why. (Contrary to the belief entertained by many, the "best evidence" rule does not refer to a quality or hierarchy of proof, such as giving documents more credibility than live testimony.)

Your proof for a claim based upon an account stated might go something like this: You or your bookkeeper would have at hand a carbon copy or photocopy of one or several bills sent to the defendant. If you were present and offering the testimony of your bookkeeper, you would do it in question and answer form. But if you or your bookkeeper were testifying alone, you would simply identify the documents as bills sent to the defendant and indicate that they bear the dates that the bills were mailed to the defendant, that the defendant never objected to the bill, that none of the bills came back to you as being undeliverable, and perhaps that you called the defendant's residence and verified that the address you used was correct.

If the defendant did not raise any objection to the bill when it was sent to him or her, that is all you have to do. A defendant's claim that "I haven't got the money to pay you now," is not a valid objection to the bill. An account stated can only be defeated by proof that the defendant never got it or is not the person who owes the bill, or that the bill is not owed for some reason.

If you are confronted with a written defense before trial that claims some or all of the services were not rendered, you may then need to produce an appointment book to verify that the defendant had an appointment on the date you claim, and you can testify that in fact you rendered the services then. This is something that your bookkeeper could not do. Your professional opinion that the services were necessary and that the price was reasonable is generally sufficient, and can only be overcome by testimony from another expert saying that the services were not necessary or the amount charged is unreasonable.

JUDGMENT

Sometimes a judge will give his or her final judgment in a contested case at the end of the hearing. More often, especially in recent years, judges have been delaying their decisions until everybody leaves the courtroom, for sometimes emotions run high in small claims court cases, especially if the claim has been hotly contested.

The court's ruling will be given in the form of a document entitled, "Judgment," or "Final Judgment," and represents the final determination by the court as to who wins, and if you do, how much money will be awarded. The judgment will also include costs that are taxable against your opponent under the laws of your state. Generally, the filing fee, the cost of serving the claim and the summons on the defendant, the cost of certified mail if that is used, the fee paid to each witness who testified at trial, and the cost of subpoenaing each witness, will all be taxed against the losing party. If you are claiming unpaid bills of $300, and have court costs of $75, your total judgment would be for $375 if you win.

A final judgment in small claims court is entered in the *court* records, but is not recorded in the *public* records unless you pay an additional sum to accomplish that. You should always do so, and spend whatever money is necessary to have a certified copy of the judgment recorded in the public records. When recorded, it will remain a valid lien against a judgment debtor's property for up to 20 years. It will appear on the debtor's credit record until paid or discharged in bankruptcy. In most areas, recording a certified copy of the judgment can be accomplished for $10 or less, and the cost gets added to your judgment.

Judgments earn interest at whatever rate your state law sets. Most states have modernized their judgment interest statutes so that judgments now earn from 8% to 12% per year, simple interest.

If a defendant does not appear when required for a pre-trial conference or scheduled trial, a judgment will be entered in your favor by default. Still, you may have to provide some minimum evidence if the judge questions whether you are entitled to receive the amount you are seeking.

Collecting a judgment is often very difficult, and some state's laws make it tougher than others. The court will not collect your judgment for you, but has procedures which will assist you. Costs incurred in collecting are added to your judgment.

Execution is a term often thought of only in relation to the ultimate penalty for criminal activity. However, its much more common use refers to a procedure for collecting on a judgment. A writ of execution, obtained from the court, entitles you to have a deputy sheriff seize and sell property owned by a defendant against whom you have a judgment (henceforth referred to as the "judgment debtor"), to satisfy the judgment. This sounds like a simple process, but it becomes complicated when a judgment debtor's property is subject to a lien which equals or exceeds the value of the property (such as an auto loan balance in excess of a car's value).

Sheriffs sometimes get into trouble if a deputy executes on the wrong property. So, the sheriff will want you to put up an execution bond of one and a quarter to two and a half times the amount of the money you are after, indemnifying him or her if the deputy makes a mistake that infringes upon someone else's rights. You have to be very specific in identifying the property you want the sheriff to execute on, so you must find out precisely what property the judgment debtor owns. Checking on motor vehicles is usually relatively easy, because the Department of Motor Vehicles in most states has very accurate and up-to-date records of the ownership of cars and trucks. But checking on other property can be much more difficult.

Generally, you must first attempt execution before you can use other means to collect a judgment. However, most sheriffs recognize the problems associated with execution, so they accommodate by making a demand for payment at the defendant's residence, then return the writ unsatisfied if they do not collect anything (and they usually don't). That satisfies the law requiring an attempt at execution.

A much more promising source is garnishing the judgment debtor's bank account. You can garnish the account and have the bank pay you the money directly. That sounds like a great idea, but how do you find out the defendant's bank? Well, if you kept copies of any checks received from the judgment debtor at the time any payment was made, then you know both the bank and the account number the judgment debtor was then using. He or she may have changed banks, but if not, that account may be your pot of gold.

You may also use what is called "discovery in aid of execution," which is designed to force the judgment debtor to disclose his or her assets, what form they are in, and where they are located. One method is to send out written questions, called interrogatories. The court will compel answers if the judgment debtor ignores you. Interrogatories involve only mailing expense and the time it takes to prepare them, but they seldom yield useful information because people quickly learn to provide evasive answers. An oral deposition, also allowed but more expensive, is much more effective. Usually you will only need to pay for the court reporter's attendance time, which should average about

$50. (Ordering the deposition transcribed by the court reporter raises the cost substantially, but is seldom necessary.)

Wage garnishments have been severely limited in recent years by federal law, and are not nearly as effective as they once were. If the judgment debtor is the head of a family, other exemptions may be available as well.

Judgment debtors often ask to pay in installments, which most courts allow and sometimes even encourage. Interest keeps running during the installment term, unless the court rules otherwise. This may be a good solution, for it provides a steady income to you, and puts the judgment pay-off in the realm of reality for a working person who is having a tough time making ends meet.

CONCLUSION

All this may sound terribly complicated and not really worth the time, trouble, and effort. Yet, as you begin doing it, you will find that the process can be streamlined, and will become repetitive.

As time goes on, you will find that some claims are worth pursuing while others are not, and you will learn the difference. You will certainly also find that the small claims collection process becomes more effective the more efficient you make it, as you bundle claims together to get them all heard at the same time.

I hope this has helped you, and wish you every success in your collection efforts.

William R. Hussey, Esquire, currently maintains a general law practice with his son in Fort Lauderdale, Florida. Prior to opening his Florida practice in 1970, he was an attorney in Michigan and, for approximately 9 years, worked in radio, television, and direct mail advertising. After obtaining his law degree in 1962, much of his time was involved in handling collection cases for insurance companies. Mr. Hussey may be contacted at 1540 E. Commercial Boulevard, Fort Lauderdale, FL 33334-5793.

CLIENT SNATCHING:
A DEFENSE

Carroll L. Meek

Soon after beginning my independent practice, "therapist shoppers" began to appear in my office. I was unprepared. I did not want to be accused of "client snatching" (Ewing, 1983) by my peers in the interest of seeing to it that my business did not fail.

The first time it happened, the client did not mention that, "Oh, by the way, I have been seeing therapist X for the past 8 years," until the end of the session! Was I, now, a "client snatcher?" I told the client that I needed to confer with X to determine the suitability of changing therapists. The client graciously consented. To my utter amazement, X said, "I really think she has received all she can from me; it would do her a world of good to see another therapist. I think you would be good for her."

The second time it happened, the client told me she had been in therapy with Y and had been totally put off by something that had happened during one of the sessions. Once again, I was unprepared. I told her she needed to go back to her previous therapist and tell Y that she wanted to begin therapy with someone else. She also agreed! I think that request of mine cost her $40 or $45!

The third time, I tried my tactic as mentioned for therapist Y, and the client looked at me and said, "Carroll, I don't know if I am going to like you, yet! Why should I have to terminate with Z and burn my bridges before I know that you are going to suit me any better?"

That did it! I decided to reread the *Ethical Principles of Psychologists* (American Psychological Association, 1981a). The standards emphasize that serving the rights of consumers is more important than anything else, and require referrals to be made to agencies and other people when they are more appropriate to deliver services to clients.

Acceptable medical practice encourages second opinions. Some third-party payors require them. Insurance companies are requiring, more and more, second opinions before costly medical procedures can be obtained. Because psychotherapy can certainly be a costly procedure, third-party payors may soon require second opinions for the necessity of psychotherapy, as well.

In my *Office Policy Statement*, I have the following statement:

If you have any questions or any concerns about your course of contact with me, please discuss these issues with me. In signing this contract, you are agreeing that should you have *any* dissatisfaction or concern about your treatment, or should you wish to contract with another psychologist or a psychiatrist for services, you will do your best to indicate that you are making the change and *why* you wish the change to be made. If you are unhappy with your services here and need help finding additional or alternate assistance, I will do my best to help you locate a more suitable referral or therapy resource. (Meek & Editors, 1985, p. 349)

Although many people have asked questions about the course of therapy and/or their diagnoses, no one has elected to talk directly with me about their intention to locate another therapist. There is an opportunity on my *Evaluation of Service* form to specify "I am in therapy with someone else." Some have indicated that they are in therapy with someone else. These people may have changed for financial reasons or may have moved, but some may also have decided that another therapist would be more useful to them, decided to try it without burning their bridges with me, and chose to pursue therapy elsewhere.

Clients who seek alternate forms of therapeutic assistance are telling us something. I believe their efforts to find a person who better relates to them should be reinforced and condoned. No one has ever snatched a client from me who did not serve him or her better.

Competition is a source of strength to a profession and it provides clues for self-evaluation. I know my colleagues well enough not to harbor *any* illusions that I am better at all things than they are. I know some of them possess personalities and techniques which suit different people better.

What we are talking about, then, is not client snatching, but client retention - that is retaining those who need and can profit from your services. Therapists can do a great deal to retain their own clients. Focusing on the ones that "got snatched" offers an irresistible temptation to blame someone else for one's own shortcomings, rather than taking responsibility for it oneself. Clients who "got snatched" provide a great deal of information about "what might have gone wrong."

There are several other points which need to be considered which may directly or indirectly relate to the matter of client retention, and which will help practitioners avoid complaints from others about having their clients "snatched."

1. *Keep your clients appraised of your continuing desire to provide the best possible service to them.* Incorporate a statement in an *Introduction to Therapy* (Meek & Editors, 1985) handout indicating that you welcome feedback from them regarding what is or is not helpful as therapy proceeds. Informing clients that you will be asking them for periodic evaluation also lets them know that what they think of you and your work with them is an ongoing process and will continue to be important to you.

2. *Get to know your colleagues' skills and areas of expertise.* You are less likely to be accused of "client snatching" if your colleagues know you as well, including your ethical standards. If you ultimately treat their clients, your colleagues will have to assume there were good reasons for it. Knowing your colleagues also opens the door for consultation when you have a puzzling professional concern.

3. *Refer to other therapists regardless of whether your own schedule is full.* Referrals to other therapists indicate that you are interested in maintaining good relationships with them. In addition, they are less likely to accuse you of continuing your business at their "expense," or of being greedy.

4. *Establish good working relationships with your clients' personal physicians.* Some physicians are quite adept in ascertaining whether psychotropic medications are likely to be helpful to your clients. They are also willing to help with your concerns about side effects which clients may have mentioned to you, but may not have mentioned to them. They, therefore, stand to profit from working with you as well. They will help you rule out physiological bases for difficulties encountered by clients. It is important to avoid the temptation to assume that aches and pains are due to stress or other psychological factors without continuing to rule out physical causes or other treatment needs. When physicians profit from working with you, they become excellent referral resources as well.

5. *If there is a psychiatrist in your area who is willing to consult with you on a fee-per-hour basis, this may provide you and your clients many dividends.* An arrangement made by you to contract for help from another professional in medically related areas of expertise in which you are less well-prepared, will lend credibility to your work if someone ever has a major complaint about you. In addition, your psychiatric consultant may occasionally consent to provide an evaluation of an amorphous client (i.e., one who is not demonstrating good progress; one who is presenting a diagnostic dilemma; one who is dubious concerning the appropriate course of treatment; one who is having difficulties finding the proper medication through a personal physician; or one whose personal physician may want an additional opinion).

If a consultation session is necessary for one of your clients, this arrangement clarifies the expectations of all parties. The implied statement made by the process is that this person is a medical or psychiatric *consultant*; the purpose is not to seek a therapist to suit the client better. Validation by the consultant regarding the appropriateness of treatment also instills confidence that everyone is proceeding properly, and lets the client know that you are doing everything in your power to insure adequacy of treatment.

The best protection against encroaching therapists and client attrition is to be the best therapist possible. If not, then expectations for client retention are not going to be met.

Carroll L. Meek, PhD, is currently in independent practice as a counseling psychologist. Prior to her four year old private practice, she was a psychologist in Counseling Services at Washington State University, Pullman, Washington for 13 years. She received her PhD from the University of Idaho, Moscow, Idaho in 1972. In addition to her work at Washington State, she was a counselor at the University of Idaho's Counseling Center for 1 year and was counselor and head resident at the University of Wisconsin-Oshkosh for 2 years. Dr. Meek may be contacted at The Professional Mall, S. E. 1205 Professional Mall Boulevard, Pullman, WA 99163.

RESOURCES

American Psychological Association. (1981, June). Ethical principles of psychologists. *American Psychologist, 36,* 633-639. (a)

American Psychological Association. (1981, June). Specialty guidelines for the delivery of services by clinical psychologists. *American Psychologist, 36,* 640-651. (b)

American Psychological Association. (1981, June). Specialty guidelines for the delivery of services by counseling psychologists. *American Psychologist, 36,* 652-663. (c)

Ewing, E. P. (1983). Ethical issues in clinical practice. In P. A. Keller & L. G. Ritt (Eds.), *Innovations in Clinical Practice: A Source Book* (Vol. 2, pp. 399-410). Sarasota, FL: Professional Resource Exchange, Inc.

Meek, C. L., & Editors. (1985). A collection of office forms. In P. A. Keller & L. G. Ritt (Eds.), *Innovations in Clinical Practice: A Source Book* (Vol. 4, pp. 345-360). Sarasota, FL: Professional Resource Exchange, Inc.

CHANGES IN HEALTH CARE DELIVERY: A GUIDE FOR THE INDEPENDENT PRACTITIONER

A. Steven Frankel

PROFESSIONALS, GOVERNMENT, AND BUSINESS

When I was an adolescent, I played poker with two close friends on an ongoing basis. It was a wild game: Even at nickel-dime-quarter stakes, one of us usually got taken for a bundle (too often me), and another made out like a bandit (too often one of my friends). When I mentioned anything about my losses to my parents, I heard, "Someone always gets it in the neck when you play three-handed poker."

Currently, government, business, and professionals are playing "three-handed poker" with the health care system. Their conflicting goals necessitate a change in that system.

BACKGROUND: ESCALATING HEALTH CARE COSTS

For some years, practitioners and practice agencies, including hospitals (hereafter called "providers"), have been on the up side of the three-handed poker game that has been played by providers, government, and business. Health care costs in recent years have escalated at rates that far exceed inflation, and providers and provider groups have done quite well. However, if you were the one who had to pay for care that can cost up to $600 per day for room and board plus up to $300 per day for professional fees and another $100 for ancillary charges, and if you had to pay these costs for a year or so per patient, and if you were financially responsible for an increasing number of people each year who needed these services, you would probably be quite concerned.

There are many reasons, some quite logical, for the escalation of health care costs. Although mental health costs have constituted only a small portion of escalating health care costs, they too are caught up in one of the most fundamental shifts in the human service delivery system in the history of this country. Health care costs, which amount to approximately 10% of the Gross National Product (GNP) of this nation, have gotten so high that the government and businesses who pay the bills have simply decided they cannot continue to do so. Realistically, there will simply not be enough money available to pay these costs.

THE LEGISLATIVE RESPONSE: CALIFORNIA AND THE FEDERAL GOVERNMENT

While concerns about health care costs have not been a recent problem in this country, they became so serious that in 1982 the California Legislature passed two laws that began to change the way health care is delivered and paid for. State Assemblyman Robinson's bills (AB799 and 3480), which were intended to address an ineffective and inefficient state health care system called Medi-Cal (Medicaid in states other than California), provided for businesses and insurance companies to negotiate fees with providers. Thus, the private sector and the government, which had been footing the bills for health care at ever increasing "reasonable and customary rates," were now able to establish fee schedules for various health care services and were able to shift some of the costs of health care back to the insureds by increasing deductibles, paying percentages of fees, and even capping or limiting the absolute amount of dollars available for certain types of services (e.g., providing for a $50,000 lifetime mental health benefit). Additionally, these laws provided for "third party payors" to contract directly with providers for discounted services, and to provide incentives for their insureds to utilize these discounted services.

The federal government's Medicare program moved to payment for services based on Diagnostic Related Groups (DRGs). Various disorders, regardless of their clinical relationship to each other, were paid for at the same rate because they fell into the same DRG. Thus, for example, an acute schizophrenic episode might qualify for 4 days worth of hospitalization, just as an appendectomy would.

PREDICTIONS THAT HAVE COME TRUE

In 1982, I wrote an article describing the above changes, and predicted that the future would see health care being delivered in any of the following ways: comprehensive pre-paid health care plans (HMOs); discounted fee-for-service provider groups (PPOs and IPAs); the "traditional" fee-for-service model, in which insureds choose their own providers and pay some portion of the fee left unpaid by insurance ("co-payment"); and perhaps an "executive" type of insurance policy, in which people pay high premiums for the comfort of knowing that the policy will pay 100% of the costs of services of any licensed provider. Other forms of health care delivery were predicted, limited only by the "creativity and political and financial savvy of providers and insurers" (Frankel, 1982, p. 29).

"SPITTING INTO THE WIND":
THE RESPONSE FROM PROFESSIONALS

THE CALIFORNIA EXPERIENCE

In California, as across the nation, providers began to realize that these legislative changes spelled three kinds of trouble. First, the autonomy of the professions to set fees for their services - a hallmark of an independent profession - would be compromised. Professionals would be shifted from the status of co-equal players in the "three-handed poker game" to that of mere laborers. Second, with cost-control measures of all kinds being instituted by third party payors, providers could not count on being able to stay in business as accustomed. They would now have to learn to be business people in addition to losing their identities as professionals. Third, providers feared for the quality of health care that they would be able to provide, especially in the areas of diagnostic testing, length of hospital stay (associated with thoroughness of care), and use of expensive treatment techniques. Professionals saw that they (and perhaps their patients) were about to "get it in the neck."

Almost instantaneously, professional societies and their political and legislative lobbying divisions went into action. Attorneys were hired, lobbyists engaged, funds solicited, new action groups created, and even interdisciplinary cooperation emerged to deal with the common enemy. The California Medical Association, in its Medical Executives' Memo of July 6, 1982, stated that:

> preliminary analysis of AB3480...reveals significant conflicts with other insurance code provisions and with other state laws...There have been numerous court decisions holding that insurance companies cannot contract with physicians to provide medical services. The Medical Practices Act (in California) also prohibits such arrangements. The new language in AB3480 was hastily enacted, reflecting the legislature's last-minute budget frenzy, by-passing usual hearings and opportunities for public participation...Legal counsel...concludes that implementa-

tion of these AB3480 provisions in the manner envisioned by the insurance industry will require additional legislation.

Provider organizations hoped that a strong and well-financed attack in the legislative and judicial arena would make the new laws unimplementable, and that other solutions less repugnant to provider groups could be sought. Wrong again!

PROFESSIONAL GROUPS AS DOMINOES

I suppose that my own experience as chair person of the "Strike Force," as we called the action group of the California State Psychological Association's (CSPA) Division of Clinical and Professional Psychology, is a good example of what happened to all such groups. First, I confess that my involvement with professional organizations is fundamentally self-serving, in that I like to be able to climb a tree, see what is coming, and be in a position to deal with it before it hurts me. When I climbed this particular tree, I looked off into the distance and I saw them coming. They were big, they were burly, they were mean, hungry, and not in a mood to talk. They knew that they had an enormous amount of power and they were right. Worst of all, they were coming my way. I did what any reasonable human would do. I climbed down from the tree, warned everybody about what I had seen, and ran in the other direction (forming a Preferred Provider Organization or PPO, with another psychologist and three psychiatrists).

The first mission of the Strike Force (now independent of CSPA and called the California Association of Psychology Providers - CAPP) was to hire legal counsel to begin to fight these laws in the courts. To date, CAPP's greatest contribution has been to successfully sue the State of California's Department of Health Services to assure that psychologists cannot be discriminated against in terms of their status and privileges in hospitals. The importance of this is that membership on hospital staffs increases the chances of being included in one of the many PPOs that are springing up. Our efforts thus changed from figuring out how to "beat" them to figuring out how to join them. Professional groups across the nation have followed suit.

THE "BUSINESSIZATION" OF HEALTH CARE

While the major worry of professional groups in America has been "socialized" health care, what we have seen in the past 4 years might be considered "businessized" health care. In this form of health care, a few huge health care delivery organizations compete to offer a broad variety of health care products to consumers. Business principles are applied to all aspects of health care delivery to make health care an enterprise that provides the greatest good for the greatest number at costs that are bearable and nonescalating - all while the business makes a profit. To accomplish such a task, the business community has brought its own concepts to health care, along with other changes that must be made to support the implementation of these concepts.

Hospitals have been purchased in record numbers by competing chains. Health care products such as supplementary health insurance for the aged and short-stay programs for substance abuse, eating disorders, stress management, and depression are marketed. Outreach programs for assessing blood pressure, emergency care centers, ambulatory surgery centers, imaging centers (e.g., CAT scans), weight-control programs, and a myriad of similar services are marketed to self-insured corporations, insurance companies, and businesses, as well as to the public. Hospital ownership corporations are providing brand names in the health care market that represents 10% of our GNP. One company provides free artificial heart implant procedures, generating enormous publicity with each procedure. Insurance companies are being purchased by hospital ownership corporations so that these companies can now cover all of the bases of service provision, including capturing large numbers of people who will use the companies' services.

COST CONTAINMENT: THE PRINCIPLE AND SOME EXAMPLES

One of the most important lessons to be learned from the business sector is that one cannot pay out more money than one takes in. If more money must be paid out than is taken in and survival is important, there are two alternatives: either find ways to increase monies entering the system (e.g., raise prices) or decrease expenditures. Since increases in costs are what (supposedly) started all of these problems, cost containment is the concept that is most relevant to economic survival. Examples of cost containment efforts include (a) pre-treatment authorization, which requires prior approval of charges by a representative of the insuring organization; (b) requirement of a second opinion to pay surgery charges; and (c) utilization review of available data and budgetary pressures to determine the necessity for a particular test, treatment, or treatment location. If those reviewing the treatment do not agree that it is medically necessary, they may recommend against paying for it. When the services have already been provided, either because the provider felt them necessary or because the provider was not familiar with such cost containment methods, the provider may not be paid at all. This places the burden of payment on the patient. In cases where the patient cannot pay, the provider has worked for free. This process is called "shifting the risk to the provider." Providers do not like it, as a rule.

Such programs have saved insuring organizations a great deal of money, and thus are very much in favor in the insurance industry at this time. These cost containment procedures should not, however, be confused with "quality assurance" or "quality control," procedures designed to make sure that the quality of care is maintained at a high level. Unfortunately, confusion between these two concepts abounds in the industry.

CONTRACTS

Part of the "businessization" of health care concerns redefining the relationships between providers and payors. These relationships are defined in contracts.

Fee-for-Service Contracts. Until recently, providers have primarily been paid via a fee-for-service relationship with the patient and the patient's insurance company. A fee is assigned to each service as it is provided, and the insurance company agrees, via contract with the patient, to reimburse for "reasonable and customary" charges for services.

Capitated Contracts. The capitated contract asks a provider to determine the amount of services that a particular patient group will consume in a year. Health Maintenance Organizations (HMOs) have been using this model for some time. The monies necessary to provide the agreed-upon amount of services are paid by the insurer to the provider group at the beginning of the contract year, and that is all the money the provider can get. If the provider has estimated accurately, there will be at least enough money to pay for required services. If the provider has overestimated utilization, there will be money left at the end of the year (profit), perhaps to be divided among the individual providers. However, if the provider has underestimated utilization, the services will have to be provided anyway, at a financial loss. Capitated contracts are much like playing the commodity market - both up-side and down-side risks can be substantial. Making these kinds of predictions is a highly sophisticated area of business, and it is not always done successfully (witness the number of HMO groups that have sprung up and died away in recent years). It should be approached with great caution and much consultation!

EAPs - THE MOST POPULAR PEOPLE IN THE NATION

In their efforts to contain costs without risking quality of care, many organizations have developed Employee Assistance Programs (EAPs). These are often in-house entities staffed by professionals (e.g., nurses, social workers, marriage/family counselors, etc.), which have the responsibility for coordinating the human service needs of the insureds so they do not overutilize services. EAP directors often set up in-house programs designed to reduce utilization of certain services. For example, they may offer stress-reduction programs to employees to reduce the need for individual employees to obtain these services privately (and presumably more expensively). EAP staff often provide psychological counseling to employees before referring them to independent professionals. In this way, they are "gate keepers" of utilization. Because they sit at the hub of so many referrals, they are very popular among professionals, who clamor for opportunities to take them to lunch, dinner, or anywhere else - just to get on the referral list.

Companies with so few employees that an in-house EAP program cannot be economically justified may contract with independent EAP organizations. Such organizations provide services to many companies, and are springing up like wildfire. Functioning of two private model EAPs is discussed in earlier volumes of the *Innovations* series (McInroy & Howard, 1984; Vehlow & Kropp, 1982). People who work for such organizations are also popular with enterprising professionals.

EAPs, whether in-house or contracted, can in turn contract with providers for services. Fee-for-service arrangements are more popular than capitated contracts. In California, any organization wishing to engage in a capitated contract with an EAP organization must be licensed under the Knox/Keene Act - legislation designed to insure that a contracting provider group is reputable and will be in business for some time. Gaining registration under this act is an extraordinarily tedious process, requiring specialized legal assistance - for a considerable amount of money.

TROUBLE IN PARADISE: EVEN BUSINESSMEN MAKE MISTAKES

While it looks like the businessization of health care is well under way, all is not well. Some of the largest and most well-capitalized health care companies have not been as thoughtful as they might. While they were busy acquiring hospitals and insurance companies, they may have not paid enough attention to the fact that both governmental and private sector cost containment programs were being implemented with a vengeance. Hospital beds were going empty, sometimes because procedures were not being authorized as medically necessary, other times because outpatient centers, ambulatory surgery centers, and other such programs were offering the same procedures that used to be performed in hospitals. Sometimes, between DRGs, utilization review, and technological advances, beds were empty because patients were discharged very quickly.

Medical/surgical hospital bed occupancy rates have dropped drastically. Some hospital ownership companies have noticed that psychiatric beds are a bit less empty than medical/surgery beds, and are converting medical/surgery beds to psychiatric beds as quickly as possible. This is likely to have consequences for psychiatric hospitals, draining off some of the patients who would otherwise be filling those beds. It is now clear that hospital ownership may not be as financially rewarding as it was thought to be, and stock prices of some of these companies have fallen. The lesson to be learned is that no one has a corner on the market of knowledge about health care delivery. We need a great deal more thought, information, and collaboration between the three hands at our poker game, because everyone may get it in the neck if we don't.

In summary, the businessization of health care seeks to use market forces to control costs. A competitive environment is being created. Professionals who expect to flourish economically must either bring some resources into the system by working more hours (hourly fees will be capped by payors), or develop cost containment procedures of their own. Professionals, especially those who have been in independent practice for some time, may have priced themselves out of the new market, and this group is most likely to be affected (and very upset) about changes in the delivery system. They often point to traditional concerns about professionals who advertise, professionals who hire other professionals, and so on, as examples of the terrible things that are happening in health care. While these concerns are at times quite reasonable, the reality of the times remains. This is not a time to be paralyzed with shock and dismay. It is a time to think and to act.

"ACRONYMOUS" DEBATES: RESPONSES
FROM THE PROFESSIONAL COMMUNITY

In response to the developments in health care delivery, professionals have developed a variety of cost-conscious vehicles that can exist with or without the large health care corporations (although, as specific groups do well, they seem to be developing relationships with the large corporations). Some of these vehicles have actually been around for some time, while others are newer. Virtually all are known by their initials.

HMOs

An HMO is a Health Maintenance Organization, a pre-paid health care organization that meets certain federal criteria, and that includes both providers and facilities for service provision. Registered with the federal government, HMOs are required by federal law to include mental health care in their contracts, but the extent of such coverage is not required to be very thorough. For that reason, many HMOs prefer to limit mental health programs to their insureds. Some refer cases to independent providers after screening, while others have an in-house mental health staff. Providers in HMOs are sometimes eligible to become partners, but often this status is available only to physicians. Psychologists and other mental health professionals are often employees of such organizations. In HMOs, the gate keepers of specialist services (such as those of mental health professionals) must agree that such services are medically necessary before a patient is seen by a specialist. This is done to control costs, often by a "utilization review" committee, and many times without input by a member of the very specialty group that could offer the most informed opinion about need. Federal law requires companies with more than 25 employees that offer health care benefits to offer a registered HMO as one alternative health care plan. Data suggest that employees find HMOs attractive. Enrollment is generally rising and new HMOs are developing with increasing frequency.

PPOs AND IPAs

When a group of providers, usually with facilities such as hospitals or clinics, bands together to offer discounted services in the hopes of gaining a higher volume of business, the resulting organization is called a Preferred Provider Organization (PPO). Such an organization seeks primarily to provide fee-for-service contracts at reduced rates with businesses and groups of insureds. At times, rather than reduced rates, a PPO will agree to intensive utilization review as a way to contain costs. PPOs, therefore, have some flexibility. A PPO can offer fee-for-service contracts with some groups, while offering to provide pre-paid or capitated contracts with others (in California, such PPOs are required to register under the Knox/Keene Act, as mentioned above).

The Independent Practitioner Association (IPA) is a kind of PPO - often a group of practitioners who band together to offer services, but who may not have a facility as part of their organization. It has the same kind of flexibility as any other PPO in offering health care services.

Unlike most HMOs, providers can join more than one PPO and IPA. HMO employees typically work at the HMO site and provide services to patients of that HMO only. In a PPO or IPA, the professional typically works out of his or her own office. As with HMOs, laws vary from state to state concerning the role that psychologists and other mental health professionals play in PPOs and IPAs. Some states (e.g., California) require that the services of psychologists be included by PPOs that offer mental health services "whenever possible" - whatever that means.

HMOs and PPOs or IPAs can be single purpose health care plans; for example, one dealing with mental health only. Such a plan could offer pre-paid or discounted fee-for-service mental health services. These might include acute care psychiatric hospitalization, outpatient and day patient programs, and outreach and specialty (e.g., eating disorder, stress management) programming. One mental health PPO is described by Bindman and Hefele (1985).

HMOs and PPOs can also be organized in several ways, and can form any of a variety of relationships with other entities, depending on state and federal law. For example, in California the law provides for multidisciplinary corporations. In such corporations, physicians, psychologists, social workers, and marriage and family counselors can all hold shares of stock in the same corporation. Interdisciplinary corporations can provide the services of all of their component parts and can act as corporate entities in terms of business activities.

Further, provider groups like HMOs and PPOs or IPAs can enter joint ventures with other provider groups or health care service organizations (e.g., hospital corporations) to form new entities for health care delivery. For instance, a joint venture between a mental health PPO and a hospital ownership corporation might lead to a hospital in which profits are shared with providers. (Profit sharing has been more common in general health care than in mental health, especially among nonphysician mental health professionals.) Such business concepts are limited only by law, energy, and imagination.

"CAVEAT EMPTOR": THINGS TO CONSIDER BEFORE JOINING A PPO OR IPA

Michele Licht is an attorney who has been involved with the psychology profession for some years. She has prepared a list of concerns that all practitioners should address with any PPO or IPA before agreeing to participate as a provider. Her list of concerns includes:*

1. Organizational Form of the PPO.

   PPOs will be structured and organized in a variety of ways but most commonly they will be sponsored by an insurance company, provider group or entrepreneurial group.
   You should be concerned with the financial viability of the PPO, its potential for maintaining an adequate subscriber pool, its reputation, and other basic organizational traits.

2. Covered Services.

   It is recommended that you request the PPO to provide you with a standard provider contract. Specifically, you will want to be aware of what benefits and exclusions the PPO will provide for psychological services and any deductibles or co-payments which may be required. Knowing this information can help you avoid future problems, and can also be useful in assisting a client/patient in understanding available benefits.

3. Provider Compensation Schedule.

   Read the Provider Contract carefully to understand how you will be reimbursed for your services and what limitations, if any, will be placed on your reimbursement. If there is a payment schedule, *MAKE SURE YOU UNDERSTAND IT*. Most Provider Contracts will ask you to accept a discount of your usual fee or of the usual or customary fee in your area as determined by the PPO.
   You should also read the Provider Contract to determine whether you may bill the subscriber directly for non-covered services. Some PPO Provider Contracts require that the provider accept PPO reimbursement as payment in full and restrict *ANY* direct billing of subscribers, even for non-covered services.
   In addition, you should check the contract to see whether the PPO is required to pay you within a specified number of days.

---

*The material contained here is summarized from "P.P.O.s: Everything You've Always Wanted to Know But Were Afraid to Ask" by M. Licht, 1984, <u>The Professional Psychologist</u>, <u>6</u>, pp. 27-29. Included by permission of the author and publisher.

4. Buy-In Fee.

   Many PPOs require that providers make a one-time payment to the PPO for the privilege of being a participating provider and being listed in a directory of plan providers. If there is a buy-in fee, you should carefully analyze the PPO's stability and its ability to maintain an adequate patient pool, versus your investment in it.

5. Risk of Loss.

   Some PPO contracts require that providers share in the risk of loss. For example, the PPO may withhold a percent of the provider's payment for a year. If the PPO has had a good year, it may give the provider back the amount withheld plus a share in the profits. If the PPO does not do well, the provider may be asked to take the withheld amount as a loss.

6. Utilization Review.

   Make sure you understand exactly how the PPO's utilization review process will function. If there is a panel set up to review psychological services, what is the make-up of that panel? How frequently will reviews be conducted? Will there be an appeal process established and if so, what standards will be used in the review? On what basis may reviews be initiated?

7. Referral Arrangements.

   Some PPO contracts require that their providers only refer patients to other PPO participating providers. Therefore, you may wish to review the list of other participating providers before signing on.

8. Provider Directory.

   Some PPO contracts require that you permit your name and address to be given to PPO subscribers. This may include listing in a directory of PPO participating providers. This would most likely be to your advantage as a referral source. You may, however, want to request that the PPO give you an opportunity to review any materials using your name before they are distributed, to avoid the potential for ethical problems.

9. "Hold Harmless" Clauses.

   Some PPOs require that the provider carry all malpractice risks and hold the PPO completely harmless. This presents serious problems for providers. For example, if treatment is terminated prematurely because of a PPO determination, the PPO should share in any liability. However, a hold harmless clause would make the provider *SOLELY LIABLE*, even though the PPO made the determination. Moreover, many liability policies exclude contractually assumed liability. Thus you may not be covered at all under any policy carried by the PPO.

10. Professional Insurance Policy.

    Review your own professional insurance policy to make certain that there are no exclusions which may apply to your contracting with the PPO.

11. Contract Hospitals.

    Find out which hospitals will be available for admission of PPO subscribers. Most PPOs limit admissions to hospitals which have contracted with the PPO.

If you do not have privileges at the contracting hospitals, find out what arrangements will be made if a patient of yours requires hospitalization.

12. Continuity of Care.

Read the Provider Contract to determine what provision is made for continuing treatment of subscribers who are under active treatment if and when the subscriber contract is terminated. (Licht, 1984, pp. 27-28)

CONCLUSIONS

There is no doubt that a revolution in health care delivery is upon us. There is also no doubt that many of the new delivery mechanisms and organizations that have emerged and continue to emerge will disappear over time, while others will flourish. At this time, professionals must find alternative vehicles for the provision of their services - vehicles that are cost-effective as well as high in quality. The shift in the nature of health care delivery raises new questions about the nature of ethics and professionalism, and these questions also must be addressed.

A. Steven Frankel, PhD, is a past Director of Clinical Training at U.S.C., where he is an Adjunct Associate Professor of Psychology. An ABPP Diplomate in Clinical Psychology, he serves on the Board of Family and Child Therapeutic Services in Torrance, and has a private practice in the Palos Verdes area. He has been a consultant to Brotman Memorial Medical Center in Culver City, and remains the consulting psychologist at Del Amo Hospital in Torrance, where he bases his inpatient practice and research. Dr. Frankel may be contacted at 24520 Hawthorne Boulevard, Suite 110, Torrance, CA 90505.

RESOURCES

Bindman, A. J., & Hefele, T. J. (1985). Preferred provider organizations. In P. A. Keller & L. G. Ritt (Eds.), *Innovations in Clinical Practice: A Source Book* (Vol. 4, pp. 203-214). Sarasota, FL: Professional Resource Exchange, Inc.

Frankel, A. S. (1982). Preferred providers, platitudes and panic: Standards of practice and the insurance industry. *Professional Psychologist, 6*, 27-30.

Licht, M. (1984). P.P.O.s: Everything you've always wanted to know but were afraid to ask. *Professional Psychologist, 8*, 27-29.

McInroy, J. D., & Howard, S. G. (1984). Developing an employee assistance program within a clinical practice. In P. A. Keller & L. G. Ritt (Eds.), *Innovations in Clinical Practice: A Source Book* (Vol. 3, pp. 353-364). Sarasota, FL: Professional Resource Exchange, Inc.

Vehlow, Jr., C. M., & Kropp, C. L. (1982). Developing employee assistance programs. In P. A. Keller & L. G. Ritt (Eds.), *Innovations in Clinical Practice: A Source Book* (Vol. 1, pp. 334-342). Sarasota, FL: Professional Resource Exchange, Inc.

GUIDELINES FOR USING AN ANSWERING MACHINE IN YOUR PRACTICE

Carroll L. Meek

I recently taught an intensive week-long graduate course entitled, "The Ins and Outs of Establishing a Private Practice." As with most graduate courses, I learned more than I expected and ultimately pondered many issues raised by the members of the group. The class was small, and half were already self-employed in an independent psychotherapy practice. Two-thirds of them were most interested in discussing the advantages and difficulties inherent in a telephone answering machine system of taking calls, versus hiring an answering service (an agency in which calls from many businesses are taken when the business is either closed or personnel are unable to answer) or employing a receptionist.

YOUR OWN RECEPTIONIST

Although I had a faculty position waiting for me after having taken a year's leave of absence from my university, I knew that I wanted to make my private practice successful. Having been employed in institutions for 16 years, I was already familiar with the difficulties in keeping secretarial personnel happy. I knew that I was not an adept supervisor - individuals harbored jealousies and I found that it was easy for classified staff to take advantage of me. I was tired of the diversions created by office intrigue. The expense involved (wages, insurance, workers' compensation, social security, retirement, etc.) was a formidable consideration. Finally, I wanted to enter a private practice without another mouth to feed, in case I had to return later to the faculty position I held at the university.

Because our rural area (Pullman, Washington/Moscow, Idaho) is quite small and people have tended to live here for long periods of time, it seems that everybody knows everybody. Before I opened my business, I knew that many people in our communities drove to Spokane, Washington (80 miles away) to insure their anonymity when seeking psychological services.

I wanted to be in charge of my own schedule and whether I accepted someone into therapy. I wanted to do my own typing and bookkeeping, and to be the main spokesperson for my business: fees, practices, and so on. What, then, would I have paid my receptionist to do? I could not think of a thing, so I automatically dismissed this alternative as a possibility. The individuals in practice in my class had receptionists and were feeling the pressure of providing for them, as well as earning their own income. I do not know whether they worried about confidentiality problems, but I would have. Taking time to train a receptionist was also something I did not want to do. Others, as well as my own experience, told me that secretary-receptionists would want an occasional afternoon off, sick leave, and/or vacation pay. Since independent practitioners do not receive the same compensation, paying someone while not working seemed ludicrous to me. Colleagues had mentioned that their employees quickly became used to birthday parties, teas, or an occasional lunch on the boss, not to mention National Secretary's Week.

A PROFESSIONAL "LIVE ANSWERING SERVICE"

I have a colleague who has hired an answering service. She believes it offers a personal touch. I have called her office when she has switched the lever which transfers her calls to the answering service. The conversation goes something like this: "Hello, Dr. X's office." "Could I speak to Dr. X, please?" "Dr. X is in conference right now" (this answering service is probably across town; the only information the service has is that Dr. X has flipped the switch). "Would you like me to have her return your call?" "Well, no; could you tell me when she will be free and I will call her back then?" "No, I don't know when she will be available. Would you like to leave your name and number?" Now, if I am a caller wishing to maintain my anonymity, I have to give this stranger my name and number. I may even wrongly assume that this is Dr. X's receptionist, sitting right outside Dr. X's door. If pressed, the answering service will have to admit that they answer phones for many businesses in the area. This admission is likely to occur if the caller says, "Would you have her call me as soon as she is free? It's *very* important." "Well, she usually calls several times a day to obtain her messages; that's all I can tell you."

My typewriter repair representative has such an answering service. It has taken me a good 5 years to learn that all she wants to know is the typewriter model, what I think is wrong with it, my name, and my telephone number. That is it! She is not prepared to tell me how much it is going to cost, when the repairman is going to call me back, where he is at the present time, or anything else.

THE ANSWERING MACHINE

To be perfectly honest, I really only considered an answering machine. I knew there was a likelihood I would lose business because of it, but having a job waiting in the wings allowed me to care a little less about lost business. Besides, when confronted with an answering machine myself, I found that I was perfectly capable of uttering the words, when I really wanted the person to contact me. Having called individuals who wanted to contact me, many, many times before I *finally* got an answer, has permitted me to breathe a sigh of relief for my own answering machine. At least people do not have to wait for more than one ring before the phone is answered, and my recorded message is delivered.

RECORDING MESSAGES

I use three cassette tapes. The first is used when I am in conference; individuals then know immediately that I am in my office. It says:

Hello. This is Carroll Meek. Because I am in conference right now, I am unable to answer the phone. If you would like me to call you, please leave your name and telephone number and I will get back to you as soon as I can. If you choose to leave a message, please wait for the tone. Thank you very much for calling.

The second cassette is used when I am at home. Because I work afternoons and evenings, individuals become accustomed to calling me in the mornings to make appointments. Otherwise, they are confronted with the frustration of trying to get through to me at the office when I am in conference, hour after hour, or back to back. This cassette says:

Hello. This is Carroll Meek. I am not at this number right now. You may (in case I am in transit) reach me at (208) 882-3343. If you choose to leave a message, instead, please give me your name and telephone number and I will call you as soon as I can. If you choose to leave a message, please wait for the tone. Thank you very much for calling.

I purposely decided not to indicate that the number on the second cassette was my home telephone number, because new callers are hesitant to call a professional at home when inquiring about services or wanting to make an appointment. Old callers know it is my home telephone number and that I utilize mornings to schedule appointments. Because my *Office Policy Statement* (Meek & Editors, 1985) informs people that they may feel free to call for help at my home telephone number (and that they will be charged therapy time for it), they feel very free to do so.

I do not change the first two cassettes until the tape wears out. The third cassette is utilized when I am on vacations or out of town. I also use the third cassette for days I choose not to come to the office. The tape is changed as the situation warrants. Examples of messages are:

Hello. This is Carroll Meek. I will not be back in the office until ___(date)___. You may leave your name and telephone number and I will get back to you as soon as I return to the office on ___(date)___. If you choose to leave a message, please wait for the tone. Thank you very much for calling.

Hello. This is Carroll Meek. I will not be in today. If you would like to call me at (208) 882-3343, please feel free to do so. If you choose to leave a message, instead, please give me your name and telephone number and I will call you on ___(day)___. If you decide to leave a message, please wait for the tone. Thank you very much for calling.

The tapes, themselves, have a label where you can assign a title. It saves time and inconvenience if you write the content of the tape on the label (i.e., "in conference," "at home," and "vacation"). Also, because the tapes have a tendency to wear out quickly, I found it useful to write the date of first usage on the tape. If it wears out before 3 months, label it "defective," and take it back to the store where purchased. Because the tapes seem to be the weakest link in recording devices, it may be useful for you to purchase several. Some tapes are defective at the very outset. When using a new tape for recording clients' messages, make a call to yourself and deliver a message to be certain that the new tape will actually record it. Once, when I was ill for 3 days, I had a complete tape with no messages; I could hear that there were voices on it, but could not hear the message. This was the most frustrating disappointment my machine has provided.

There are a few helpful tips concerning how to record messages. First, the message should be planned to include all of the necessary details. Tell callers what information they should leave for you. It is also important to mention the recording tone which is the caller's cue to start talking. If the end of your message can be timed to end just before the tone, results are usually best.

I once did an interview with a radio announcer for one of our local stations. He told me that if you have a smile on your face and a lilt in your voice, individuals are more likely to listen to what you have to say. I have heeded his advice in making my recorded messages. It is important to sound cheerful, confident, and pleasant without being supercilious, condescending, or stumbling. I have listened to telephone recordings which sound frankly depressed and/or arrogant. In learning to record your messages, several trials may be necessary before you have one that you are comfortable with and that delivers your message in the manner you intend. I have found it helpful to keep cards in my file with the text written on them, so that I can read it directly; it gives me one less thing to focus on. After recording your message, it is important to listen to it a couple of times, and if you are not pleased with your effort, try again until you are completely satisfied. You may also want to check your own recorded message every week or so, because when a tape starts wearing out (they do so very frequently) your voice starts sounding mushy and a little sluggish. You will find that your patients will be very helpful in telling you about this if it occurs without your notice.

PATIENTS' REACTIONS

When people are in therapy in my office, they have an opportunity to see, firsthand, that messages left on the phone are not heard by those inside the office. When someone calls, the phone rings once and the answering machine clicks on. There is a little whirring which is not very loud, and the machine clicks off when the caller hangs up.

Many people do not realize that they may turn the machine barely on (no volume at all), and the message is still received on the recording, even though the volume is technically off. I used to unplug the telephone during conferences so that people could be spared the one ring. However, I found that after my patient left and I had listened to my messages, I went merrily on my way without remembering to plug the phone back in, so even with the answering machine off (I was, after all, available), no calls could come through. I decided that people could endure the one ring, and I would not have to be troubled with one more thing to remember. Although the machine is only 3 to 8 feet away from any of us during a session, it is quiet enough that it creates no disruption. I do call attention to the machine for first-time clients, however, because once during a session, my client looked at the red light on the machine and politely inquired, "Are we being recorded?"

Some people refuse to leave messages and choose, instead, to keep calling until I can answer personally. They might say, "I'm the one who has been calling. I can't leave a message on that thing." When I inquire more directly, they indicate that the major problems are that they don't know how they sound (I tell them, normal, just like they were speaking to me directly) and that they do not know how to hang up on a machine. I tell them to just say "Bye," and hang up. The machine automatically hangs itself up when no further sound is forthcoming. I also tell individuals that I offer desensitization to phone answering machines at absolutely no charge. All they have to do is call once per day for five days and leave a message. If individuals are basically shy, I tell them to just say, "Bob called" (or whoever they are), and I will recognize the voice and will know to return the call. Besides, after a conversation like this, I already know the "Bob" who is phone-answering-machine phobic and will know exactly who to call.

I also use the recorded message as a way for patients to keep me up to date on their progress and physician consultations (between sessions), and/or changes in medication(s). I request that people leave messages of this nature between therapy appointments, and they are apt to do so.

I have had many people express appreciation regarding my answering machine, once they get used to it. They can track my whereabouts just by the cassette I have in the machine at the time. Sometimes I have had people leave urgent messages on my machine on weekends. I have chastised them severely and have indicated that I do not listen to my messages until I go to the office on Monday afternoons. My answering machine has a beeper that permits me to call my office and obtain my messages on weekends, but it is a toll-charge call between my Moscow home and Pullman office. Also, if I forget to push the "stop" button, the machine tape continues to roll after I have hung up and within 30 minutes after my call, there is no tape available for others wishing to leave messages. I have found it easier to train people to listen to the tape, which tells them what to do. The two times during the 3 years of my practice when people left urgent weekend messages on my machine, coincidentally happened to be on the two Saturdays I went to the office to tidy up, do reports, or do other homework. So, I guess someone is looking out for me *and* my patients. After getting a scolding about the risky nature of trying to catch me in my office on Saturdays, individuals are much less likely to do it again, without calling me at home first.

I have had some humorous experiences with that machine, but only one which was extremely aggravating. This concerned several days of useless and obscene messages from some youngsters. Fortunately, the behavior stopped and has not recurred.

The humorous experiences are much more frequent. Because the phone rings once when the answering machine is on, I discovered that if I was sitting at my desk and the phone rang, I had a tendency to answer it on the first ring. I soon figured out that when I answered on the first ring, answering-machine phobics hung up assuming that they had obtained my recording again. I now wait for two or three rings before picking up the phone, so that people know I am live and not the recording. I also say, "Hello," since "This is Carroll Meek" indicates a recorded message.

I have had people pursue appointments because, after hearing the recording, they decided that they "liked my voice," and (before ever talking to me directly) that they wanted to enter therapy. One woman wanting a female therapist, and noting the masculine spelling of my name, was relieved that I was female when she heard my recording. Also, individuals can cancel their appointments any time up to the time of their appointment, so the telephone answering machine makes this possible any time, day or night.

Once I answered the phone and a very hesitant, reluctant voice said, "You! It's you! I didn't want to talk to you! I just wanted to leave a message!" I indicated that we could hang up, I could turn the machine on, and he could deliver his message. He said, "No, I may as well talk to you!" People know that they can fill me in and leave messages (between appointments) and that they will not be charged for recorded messages.

I have also had people call to "just hear my voice," which has seemed to be reassuring to those in crisis. Knowing that I am just a phone call away seems to be therapeutically helpful.

People have appreciated the added confidentiality involved because I work alone, with no live answering service or receptionist. Although it takes a little training to use my service and track my steps, it is generally appreciated. Individuals have spontaneously commented that they get quick answers when calling me and know how to track me down based on the cassette I have in the machine at the time. There is no doubt that my answering machine is a personal service, and individuals have expressed appreciation for it.

Also, I give people an evaluation questionnaire (Meek & Editors, 1985) once a year. The answering machine has *never* been mentioned as an inconvenience, a nuisance, or an office practice that anyone would recommend be changed.

EQUIPMENT CONSIDERATIONS

In selecting your answering machine, there are several features to consider. First, like many modern electronic devices, answering machines may break down. Can you have the equipment quickly repaired by your dealer or a local repair center? Does your dealer have a loaner for emergencies? If the answer to either question is no, you should consider the need for a backup machine in the event yours fails.

Other issues have to do with system features. Will you want to check messages while you are away from the office? This requires a pocket-size remote device which allows you to call in and retrieve messages. For the most part this is a straightforward process, which is available at a reasonable price. Some machines can even be directed to change messages from other locations. Is this a feature you want? Is it practical? Keep in mind that effective messages require some careful planning.

Last, all machines are not the same in terms of their ability to answer, to terminate messages, and so on. First, consider whether you can control the number of rings before the machine answers. Some machines will answer without a ring to disturb your session. My machine has a dial which regulates the number of rings before the machine answers the phone. Once, I unwittingly changed the dial, so that the phone rang a number of times before the machine answered. Callers, knowing that I set my machine on one ring, decided the machine was not on at all and hung up. I have now taped the dial in the correct position.

Second, if you have a small office, the noise a machine makes is no small consideration. Before buying, listen to the machine in action; imagine how it will sound if it interrupts your session several times. Finally, make sure the machine is easy to operate. Most modern answering machines are, but play with it to see if the controls make sense. Record a message and see how it sounds. Find out if you can return it if you are not comfortable with it in your office.

Part of making an answering machine work is finding one with which you are comfortable and which has the features you want. The best advice is to buy where you can try the machine, where you can return it if you desire, and where same-day repair service is available.

Carroll L. Meek, PhD, is currently in independent practice as a counseling psychologist. Prior to her 4 year old private practice, she was a psychologist in Counseling Services at Washington State University, Pullman, Washington for 13 years. She received her PhD from the University of Idaho, Moscow, Idaho in 1972. In addition to her work at Washington State, she was a counselor at the University of Idaho's Counseling Center for 1 year and was counselor and head resident at the University of Wisconsin-Oshkosh for 2 years. Dr. Meek may be contacted at The Professional Mall, S. E. 1205 Professional Mall Boulevard, Pullman, WA 99163.

RESOURCES

Meek, C. L., & Editors. (1985). A collection of office forms. In P. A. Keller & L. G. Ritt (Eds.), *Innovations in Clinical Practice: A Source Book* (Vol. 4, pp. 345-360). Sarasota, FL: Professional Resource Exchange, Inc.

INTRODUCTION TO SECTION III: ASSESSMENT INSTRUMENTS AND OFFICE FORMS

This section of *Innovations* includes a variety of instruments, checklists, and forms for practitioners to use in collecting and organizing information. It reflects the goal of our series to responsibly share useful materials.

Although some of the materials included here have been formally developed and normed, others were designed for informal application and should not be used as formal instruments. We have included them because we feel they can be used effectively by practitioners to collect information from their clients. The value of forms and instruments depends upon appropriate application by clinicians who use them. It is important to emphasize that they are not necessarily designed to generate the types of inferences often associated with more formalized tests with a long history of use. Readers should recognize potential as well as stated limitations of these materials and use them in accord with accepted ethical principles of psychologists.

Given the limitations noted above, we have attempted to insure that the materials which follow include sufficient information to allow readers to evaluate their appropriate application. Certain basic information and instructions have been included with each contribution and, when necessary, the Resource section contains references to more detailed information. Readers who wish to use such material are advised to obtain the additional resources. If there is a desire to use the material for research purposes, most authors would appreciate being contacted so that information may be shared.

Faiver has prepared a revised version of the Mental Status Examination which was included in the first volume of the *Innovations* series. Many readers have reported that this is a useful format for the Mental Status Examination. Faiver's revision makes the form consistent with the *DSM-III*, which was introduced after the first volume appeared, and also provides some elements of a client history that are not routinely included in the Mental Status Examination.

Beckham's Coping Strategies Scales for Depressed Patients is an instrument that some readers may find useful in their assessment and treatment of individuals who are depressed. It has potential value in identifying the coping strategies that work for individual patients. The data obtained from this instrument may lead to specific discussions in therapy and give the clinician some idea of how to build on a client's unique strengths.

The Social Adjustment Self-Report Questionnaire, contributed by Weissman, evaluates basic areas of a client's social functioning. It is presented in a straightforward format that the client can complete himself or herself. This instrument has been used in a wide variety of research settings and frequently has been applied with depressed clients. Its potential applications include pre- and post-measures of clients who are receiving therapeutic interventions designed to improve their social functioning.

The final instrument in this section is the Strain Questionnaire developed by Lefebvre and Sandford. This questionnaire examines various factors which are commonly related to stress. Its use grows from work in behavioral medicine settings where there is often a need to help clients reduce their levels of stress.

Readers are encouraged to submit materials from their clinical offices or research for consideration in future volumes. Information about preparing contributions may be obtained by writing to the Senior Editor at the Professional Resource Exchange, Inc.

THE MENTAL STATUS EXAMINATION-REVISED

Christopher M. Faiver

Crary and Johnson's (1982) "Structured Mental Status Examination" has been an invaluable resource in my practice and teaching because of its descriptive and methodological design. The form which follows expands the Crary and Johnson instrument to include other information, including elements of history, which may be helpful to the clinician.

The present form follows the same general format and uses the same method of recording (the reader may wish to refer to Johnson, Snibbe, and Evans' text on *Basic Psychopathology* [1975, 1981] for a detailed discussion of this format). This form includes new individual items in two of Crary and Johnson's five major categories and adds two new sections and an expansion of the former instrument's diagnostic section. The following is a breakdown of modifications:

CATEGORY	ITEM ADDITIONS
BEHAVIOR	Social-Interpersonal Functioning
	Sleeping Habits
	Eating Habits
	Substance Ab(use)
THINKING	Impaired Concentration
	Retardation
	Suicidal Plans
	Homicidal Plans
	Guilt

NEW SECTIONS

Previous Mental Health Contacts
Treatment Plan

REVISED SECTION

Diagnostic Impression (*DSM-III*)

Crary and Johnson note that the structure and systematization of their instrument contribute to a flow from mental status observation to diagnostic inferences and treatment planning. My revision of their form incorporates and adds to their observations, but also takes into consideration the patient's previous mental health contacts, including medications, from which a diagnostic impression is drawn. Also, the revised structural flow concludes with a brief, but systematic treatment plan.

Following from Crary and Johnson's (1982) instructions, "a check should be placed in the column labeled *not present* even if no evidence of a problem is observed. If the abnormality is minimally present or occurs only occasionally, a check is placed in the second column labeled *slight or occasional*. If the abnormality is more pronounced in severity or frequency, a check is placed in the third column labeled *marked or repeated*. A distinction is made between current abnormalities and those experienced in the past. The notation 'HX' is placed in either of the last two columns to signify an abnormality not currently reported but which is described as occurring in the past. The notation 'ND' is used in the first column to indicate if a determination was not attempted during the examination or could not be inferred from the observations. Space is also available at the end of each section for qualification of recorded marks. The final item on the form is space for a diagnosis followed by a listing of the mental status examination which led to the diagnosis" (page 227).

MENTAL STATUS EXAMINATION-REVISED*

CLIENT'S NAME________________________________ OBSERVER'S NAME________________________________

NOTATION SYMBOLS ✔ = Determination made   HX = <u>History</u> = Described but not demonstrated
                  ND = <u>No Data</u> and cannot be inferred

		Not Present	Slight or Occas.	Marked or Repeated
Appearance	1. physically unkempt, unclean................			
	2. clothing disheveled, dirty.................			
	3. clothing atypical, unusual, bizarre........			
	4. unusual physical characteristics...........			

Comments Re Appearance:

			Not Present	Slight or Occas.	Marked or Repeated
Behavior	Posture	5. slumped.....................................			
		6. rigid, tense...............................			
		7. atypical, inappropriate....................			
	Facial Expression Suggests	8. anxiety, fear, apprehension................			
		9. depression, sadness........................			
		10. anger, hostility...........................			
		11. decreased variability of expression........			
		12. bizarreness, inappropriate.................			
	General Body Movements	13. accelerated, increased speed...............			
		14. decreased, slowed..........................			
		15. atypical, peculiar, inappropriateness.....			
		16. restlessness, fidgety......................			
	Amplitude and Quality of Speech	17. increased, loud............................			
		18. decreased, slowed..........................			
		19. atypical quality, slurring, stammer........			
	Counselor - Client Relationship	20. domineering................................			
		21. submissive, overly compliant...............			
		22. provocative................................			
		23. suspicious.................................			
		24. uncooperative..............................			

*The present form is a revision from <u>Innovations in Clinical Practice: A Source Book</u> (Vol. 1, pp. 229-230) by W. G. Crary and C. W. Johnson, 1982, Sarasota, FL: Professional Resource Exchange, Inc. Also from <u>Basic Psychopathology: A Programmed Text</u> (pp. 227-230) by C. W. Johnson, J. R. Snibbe, and L. A. Evans, 1975, New York: Spectrum Publications, Inc. Also from <u>Basic Psychopathology: A Programmed Text</u> by C. W. Johnson, J. R. Snibbe, and L. A. Evans, 1981, Jamaica, NY: SP Medical & Scientific Books. Copyright © 1981 by the SP Medical & Scientific Books. Reprinted by permission. The revised form incorporates elements of history not included in the original form.

			Not Present	Slight or Occas.	Marked or Repeated
Behavior (Cont'd)	Social Interpersonal Functioning	25. impaired....................................			
	Sleeping Habits	26. increased....................................			
		27. decreased....................................			
	Eating Habits	28. overeating....................................			
		29. anorexic....................................			
	Substance (ab)use	30. alcohol (ab)use............................			
		31. other drugs ( ) (ab)use..			

Comments Re Behavior:

		Not Present	Slight or Occas.	Marked or Repeated
Feeling (Affect and Mood)	32. inappropriate to thought content...........			
	33. increased lability of affect...............			
	predominant mood is:			
	34. blunted, absent, unvarying.................			
	35. euphoric....................................			
	36. anger, hostility............................			
	37. fear, anxiety, apprehension.................			
	38. depression, sadness........................			

Comments Re Feeling:

		Not Present	Slight or Occas.	Marked or Repeated
Perception	39. illusions....................................			
	40. auditory hallucinations.....................			
	41. visual hallucinations.......................			
	42. other types of hallucinations..............			

Comments Re Perception:

			Not Present	Slight or Occas.	Marked or Repeated
Thinking	Intellectual Functioning	43. impaired level of consciousness............			
		44. impaired attention span....................			
		45. impaired abstract thinking.................			

			Not Present	Slight or Occas.	Marked or Repeated
Thinking (Cont'd)	Intellectual Functioning (Cont'd)	46. impaired calculation ability...............			
		47. impaired intelligence......................			
		48. impaired concentration.....................			
		49. retardation................................			
	Orientation	50. disoriented to person......................			
		51. disoriented to place.......................			
		52. disoriented to time........................			
	Insight	53. difficulty in acknowledging the presence of psychological problems.....................			
		54. mostly blames others or circumstances for problems...................................			
	Judgment	55. impaired ability to manage daily living activities.................................			
		56. impaired ability to make reasonable life decisions.................................			
	Memory	57. impaired immediate recall..................			
		58. impaired recent memory.....................			
		59. impaired remote memory.....................			
	Thought Content	60. obsessions.................................			
		61. compulsions................................			
		62. phobias....................................			
		63. derealization...depersonalization..........			
		64. suicidal ideation..........................			
		65. suicidal plans.............................			
		66. homicidal ideation.........................			
		67. homicidal plans............................			
		68. delusions..................................			
		69. ideas of reference.........................			
		70. ideas of influence.........................			
		71. guilt......................................			
	Stream of Thought (as manifested by speech)	72. associational disturbance..................			
		73. thought flow decreased, slowed.............			
		74. thought flow increased.....................			

Comments Re Thinking:

Previous Mental Health Contacts	outpatient - describe............	
	inpatient - describe.............	
	medication - list................	

Comments Re Previous Contacts:

	Axis	Code #	Diagnosis	✔ if Primary
Diagnostic Impression (DSM-III)	I			
	II			
	III			
	IV			
	V			
	as manifested by the following MSE item(s):			

Comments Re Diagnosis:

		Objectives:	Methods:
Plan	Treatment	1.	1.
		2.	2.
		3.	3.
		4.	4.
		5.	5.
	Frequency of Contacts		Expected Date of Achievement
	Review	Date:	
	Modifications	Date:	

Comments Re Plan:

Christopher M. Faiver, PhD, is presently Assistant Professor of Counseling at Youngstown State University in Youngstown, Ohio, and maintains a private practice in psychology with PsyCare, Inc., of Warren, Ohio. Prior to his present position, he was associated with Trumbull County Mental Health Center and Rebecca Williams Community House, both of Warren, Ohio. An Ohio licensed psychologist, he is listed in the National Register of Health Service Providers in Psychology and serves as an adjunct staff member at several local hospitals. He received his doctorate in Educational Psychology (counseling specialty) at Case Western Reserve University. Dr. Faiver may be contacted c/o the Department of Counseling, Youngstown State University, Youngstown, OH 44555.

RESOURCES

Crary, W. G., & Johnson, C. W. (1982). Introduction to the Mental Status Examination. In P. A. Keller & L. G. Ritt (Eds.), *Innovations in Clinical Practice: A Source Book* (Vol. 1, pp. 227-230). Sarasota, FL: Professional Resource Exchange, Inc.

Johnson, C. W., Snibbe, J. R., & Evans, L. A. (1975). *Basic Psychopathology: A Programmed Text.* New York: Spectrum Publications.

Johnson, C. W., Snibbe, J. R., & Evans, L. A. (1981). *Basic Psychopathology: A Programmed Text* (2nd ed.). Jamaica, NY: SP Medical & Scientific Books.

THE COPING STRATEGIES SCALES FOR DEPRESSED PATIENTS

E. Edward Beckham

Depression is one of the problems most commonly encountered by mental health professionals. Current psychological theories generally imply that depression can result from a failure to cope with stressful circumstances through the use of cognitive or behavioral coping mechanisms. A variety of kinds of coping mechanisms in depression have been investigated, including activity and work, self-care and maintenance, pharmacological alternatives, help and comfort seeking (Rippere, 1977), and emotional and informational support seeking (Coyne, Alwin, & Lazarus, 1981). (For a complete discussion of the literature, see Billings & Moos, 1985.) Some sex differences have been found. Funabiki, Bologna, Pepping, and FitzGerald (1980), for example, found that women coped with depression more often than did men by talking with close friends and by overeating. Men, on the other hand, were more likely to become involved in activities. Doerfler and Richards (1981) found that women who developed new interpersonal relationships were more likely to get over their depression than women who did not.

The Coping Strategies Scales (COSTS) (Beckham & Adams, 1984) were designed to measure a wide range of behaviors and thoughts that might occur in persons attempting to cope with depression. Behaviors included in the COSTS were not necessarily designed to reflect healthy strategies as conceptualized by mental health professionals. Instead, they were meant to reflect the widest possible range of individual responses. Second, the COSTS were designed to reflect recent coping attempts rather than how persons might cope in general or under hypothetical situations. Third, the scales were designed to reflect whether a person felt better, worse, or the same after coping behaviors were performed.

QUESTIONNAIRE DEVELOPMENT

Items for the COSTS were drawn from the empirical literature on how people cope with depression (e.g., Rippere, 1977). They were also taken from literature on how people cope with physical disability and illness (e.g., Bulman & Wortman, 1977), and how people deal with death and grief (e.g., Chodoff, Freedman, & Hamburg, 1964). Finally, items were taken from the general literature on coping and adaptation (e.g., White, 1974) and from books on the treatment of depression which give psychotherapeutic advice on coping with such symptoms (e.g., Beck et al., 1979).

Items taken from the above sources formed a pool of 143 items. Ten categories of coping behavior that were inclusive of the total items in the pool were rationally defined. These categories and their definitions are shown in Table 1 on the next page. The pool of 143 items was given to 8 members of the faculty of the Department of Psychiatry and Behavioral Sciences at the University of Oklahoma Health Sciences Center for assignment to one of the 10 categories. Items were retained if at least 6 out of 8 raters agreed on scale assignment. This criterion was met by 108 items. A total of 34 additional items were then generated and submitted to 5 of the original 8 clinicians. Items for which there was 80% agreement on scale placement (face validity) were retained.

TABLE 1: COPING STRATEGIES

---

1. BLAME - Looking for the person who caused one's problems, whether it be oneself or someone else.

2. EMOTIONAL EXPRESSION - Venting anger, anxiety, despondency, and so on.

3. EMOTIONAL CONTAINMENT - Holding feelings in or hiding feelings from others, including but not limited to anger, depression, or anxiety.

4. SOCIAL SUPPORT/DEPENDENCY - Looking to friends, relatives, or professionals to listen to one's problems or to help with one's problems.

5. RELIGIOUS SUPPORT - Looking to scriptures, to God, or to some religious institution for help with one's problems.

6. PHILOSOPHICAL/COGNITIVE RESTRUCTURING - Thinking about one's problems in a new way that makes them less threatening or more tolerable.

7. GENERAL ACTIVITY - Doing something physically or mentally that is unrelated to one's problems - neither specifically trying to solve them nor avoid them.

8. AVOIDANCE/DENIAL - Avoiding thinking about one's problems; avoiding talking about one's problems; or avoiding doing something which would remind one of them.

9. PROBLEM SOLVING - Gathering information about one's problems, thinking about possible solutions, deciding upon a course of action, or carrying out a course of action.

10. PASSIVITY - Having thoughts about one's problems that neither attempt to resolve nor to avoid them, but rather to accept or dwell on them.

Items were then given to subjects either in psychotherapy or entering psychotherapy who had a primary diagnosis of nonpsychotic depression, or who were being treated for another disorder such as anxiety, but where their therapist judged depression to be a significant part of their problem. In order to have as representative a sample as possible, subjects were drawn from a psychiatric outpatient clinic, an inpatient hospital psychiatric ward, private practice, and a day hospital. Patients included low income individuals as well as those of middle and high income. There were 53 males and 47 females, ages 18 to 71 years old. The average Beck Depression Inventory (BDI) score of the sample was 21.0. The COSTS were administered to these subjects, and the scales were then correlationally refined. Items that did have a correlation of at least $r = .25$ with their assigned scale, or that did not correlate more highly with their assigned scale than one of the other scales, were dropped. Internal reliabilities of the 10 scales were moderate to high - ranging from .62 to .86. In a replication study of 64 additional patients, the original alpha internal reliability coefficients were essentially confirmed.

Several of the scales were expected to relate to depression, and this was confirmed. Scale 1 (Blame) correlated $r = +.31$ (p < .001) with the BDI. Levels of General Activity were correlated $r = -.34$ (p < .001) with the BDI, and Passivity increased as depression increased ($r = +.26$; p < .001). It was also found that persons became more expressive of emotions as their depression increased ($r = +.22$; p < .01). Not all scales, however, had significant correlations with the BDI, indicating that the COSTS measure more than the general level of depression or dysphoria.

In filling out the COSTS, subjects indicated whether they felt better, worse, or the same after performing a particular behavior or having a particular thought. This allowed for the gathering of information about which types of behaviors and cognitions were helpful or harmful. Items which were frequently reported to have made subjects feel better included taking steps to overcome their problems, helping others, trying to focus on the good things in their lives, being with friends, trying to do things which they typically enjoyed, doing something constructive, seeking out information that would help them resolve their problems, and talking to friends about their problems. Behaviors and cognitions which were frequently reported to make them feel worse included keeping their feelings bottled up inside, worrying about their problems a lot, being very emotional, thinking about their problems over and over again, holding in feelings, blaming themselves for problems, and preventing themselves from crying.

It is interesting that seeking information to help resolve problems was often rated as making persons feel better, while thinking about problems over and over again was frequently rated as making persons feel worse. It appears from the above items that those behaviors which take an active mental or physical stance toward overcoming depression are likely to make persons feel better, while those which lead to a passive stance tend to make persons feel worse.

SUGGESTIONS FOR FUTURE RESEARCH

While there has been no test-retest reliability study for the COSTS, the high levels of internal reliability are suggestive of good scale stability over time, although test-retest reliability studies still must be done. Further validation studies of the COSTS are needed to establish their relationship to other measures of coping and to observer-rated measures of coping. Another promising avenue of validation research would be to contrast the coping styles of persons with two different personality styles, such as histrionic and compulsive types of personalities. Finally, research is needed to test the psychometric properties of a simplified response format (i.e., "yes," the person has done the behavior in the last 2 weeks versus "no," they have not).

SUGGESTIONS FOR USE OF
THE COSTS IN CLINICAL PRACTICE

Norms are provided in this article for the COSTS for a mixed sample of depressed inpatients and outpatients. Through the use of these norms, the clinician can judge what types of coping skills a particular patient is using most and which he or she is using least. While more research is needed, it would seem likely that a "healthy" coping profile would include moderate levels of emotional expression, emotional containment, and social support seeking. High levels of problem solving and cognitive restructuring are likely to be adaptive unless they reflect an obsessive tendency. High levels of passivity or avoidance should alert the clinician that the client is probably not facing up to his or her problems. Because these scales are designed to measure behaviors more than attitudes, results can be fed back to patients with the idea that they can change their behavior. Scale scores are not meant to represent long-term, enduring character traits, but rather behaviors which can be changed in the near future. Readers are also reminded that scores should be interpreted with caution because this is an instrument that requires further study before it is fully developed.

The clinician may also find it helpful to examine the efficiency of the patient's coping, that is, the degree to which the person is feeling better as a result of his or her various coping attempts. Clients may benefit from reviewing with the therapist the things they are doing which make them feel better and those which make them feel worse.

One problem the clinician may encounter with these scales is difficulty in scoring. The scales were originally designed to be scored by having answers entered numerically into a computer. Some clinicians may still wish to do this with a personal computer and the author will be glad to provide an SAS scoring routine free of charge. Nevertheless, hand scoring can be done using the information provided in Table 2 on the next page.

TABLE 2: SCORING INFORMATION

Each item is scored one (1) when a subject checks that he or she did it and felt better, did it and felt worse, or did it and felt the same. Each item is scored zero (0) when the subject indicates that he or she has not done it in the past 2 weeks.

```
Scale  1:  9, 25, 27, 43, 63, 67, 74, 91, 106, 117
Scale  2:  8, 12, 19, 58, 61, 99, 111, 122, 127
Scale  3:  7, 29, 49, 65, 75, 79, 101, 113, 119, 133, 135, 139
Scale  4:  3, 26, 32, 36, 37, 44, 45, 52, 73, 77, 82, 83, 92, 123, 136
Scale  5:  28, 33, 69, 70, 94, 107, 108, 116, 120, 131
Scale  6:  10, 16, 24, 57, 64, 66, 71, 80, 85, 86, 87, 95, 100, 103, 104, 114, 118, 130, 137, 142
Scale  7:  1, 14, 18, 30, 31, 39, 42, 46, 55, 62, 72, 78, 93, 109, 110, 115, 125, 126, 129, 132, 134,
           138, 140, 141
Scale  8:  5, 13, 17, 20, 48, 50, 51, 76, 88, 96, 105
Scale  9:  6, 11, 22, 40, 41, 53, 56, 60, 81, 89, 124
Scale 10:  4, 15, 34, 38, 47, 54, 68, 90, 97, 128
```

Composite Scale (Emotional Expression, Social Support Seeking):
```
          3, 8, 9, 12, 19, 20, 25, 26, 27, 32, 35, 36, 37, 38, 40, 43, 44, 45, 47, 52, 58, 61, 63, 67,
          77, 82, 85, 91, 92, 99, 100, 106, 111, 112, 117, 122, 127, 136
```

Composite Scale (Emotional Containment, Passivity):
```
          5, 6, 7, 29, 34, 49, 54, 65, 68, 75, 79, 88, 90, 101, 113, 119, 128, 133, 135, 137, 139
```

Composite Scale (Individual Coping Activity and Cognitive Restructuring):
```
          1, 11, 13, 14, 18, 30, 31, 39, 42, 46, 48, 50, 55, 62, 70, 71, 72, 78, 80, 83, 84, 86, 87,
          89, 93, 94, 95, 98, 102, 104, 105, 110, 114, 115, 116, 123, 125, 126, 129, 132, 134, 138,
          140, 141, 142
```

Norms are for mildly to severely depressed patients

T-Score Values (M = Mean, SD = Standard Deviation)

```
Scale  1:  M =  5.06, SD = 2.60
Scale  2:  M =  5.57, SD = 2.38
Scale  3:  M =  9.36, SD = 2.78
Scale  4:  M =  7.75, SD = 3.97
Scale  5:  M =   4.4, SD = 3.21
Scale  6:  M = 12.60, SD = 4.44
Scale  7:  M = 12.68, SD = 4.59
Scale  8:  M =  8.04, SD = 2.51
Scale  9:  M =  7.81, SD = 2.10
Scale 10:  M =  6.88, SD - 1.95
```

Composite Scale (Emotional Expression, Social Support Seeking):
```
          M = 20.73, SD = 8.16
```

Composite Scale (Emotional Containment, Passivity):
```
          M = 14.55, SD =  4.5
```

Composite Scale (Individual Coping Activity and Cognitive Restructuring):
```
          M = 25.6, SD = 8.09
```

Name_______________________________
Age________________________Sex_______________________
Date____
Therapist____

COPING STRATEGIES SCALES (COSTS)

The purpose of this questionnaire is to find out how people deal with feeling "depressed" or "down." On the following pages are activities which you may have done in the <u>last 2 weeks</u>. After each activity indicate whether, as a result of it, you felt:

      1. better   2. worse   3. the same

or, if you did not do the activity, check

      4. did not do it

In the <u>last 2 weeks</u>, have you:	As a result, did you feel			I did not do it in the last 2 weeks
	better	worse	the same	
1. read a lot?	( )	( )	( )	( )
2. watched a lot of TV?	( )	( )	( )	( )
3. talked with friends or relatives about your problems?	( )	( )	( )	( )
4. tried to accept your problems?	( )	( )	( )	( )
5. told yourself that you don't have any problems?	( )	( )	( )	( )
6. tried to resolve your problems in the way you have handled past problems?	( )	( )	( )	( )
7. hidden your feelings from others?	( )	( )	( )	( )
8. been very emotional compared to your usual self?	( )	( )	( )	( )
9. hated someone for causing your current problems?	( )	( )	( )	( )
10. tried to find some meaning in your difficult situation?	( )	( )	( )	( )
11. taken steps to overcome your problem?	( )	( )	( )	( )
12. let one or more people know how irritated you are with them?	( )	( )	( )	( )
13. tried to get away from the things that remind you of your problems?	( )	( )	( )	( )
14. listened to music?	( )	( )	( )	( )
15. decided to accept your problems?	( )	( )	( )	( )
16. told yourself that your problems are small compared to those some people have?	( )	( )	( )	( )
17. tried not to worry about your problems?	( )	( )	( )	( )

In the <u>last 2 weeks</u>, have you:	As a result, did you feel			I did not do it in the last 2 weeks
	better	worse	the same	
18. tried to do things which you typically enjoy?	( )	( )	( )	( )
19. expressed anger at your spouse or someone close to you?	( )	( )	( )	( )
20. stayed away from other people?	( )	( )	( )	( )
21. drunk alcohol or used drugs to help reduce your feelings of depression?	( )	( )	( )	( )
22. sought out information (before today) that would help you resolve your problems?	( )	( )	( )	( )
23. done something wild, reckless, or illegal?	( )	( )	( )	( )
24. decided that something good can come from your situation?	( )	( )	( )	( )
25. blamed others for your problems?	( )	( )	( )	( )
26. followed the advice of others to resolve your problems (not advice received today)?	( )	( )	( )	( )
27. blamed yourself for your problems?	( )	( )	( )	( )
28. tried to bargain with God or a Supreme Power to help you overcome your problems?	( )	( )	( )	( )
29. decided not to let others see how you are feeling?	( )	( )	( )	( )
30. exercised?	( )	( )	( )	( )
31. gone for a drive?	( )	( )	( )	( )
32. found yourself often asking others for help?	( )	( )	( )	( )
33. tried to live a better life according to your religious beliefs?	( )	( )	( )	( )
34. given up?	( )	( )	( )	( )
35. gone over your problems in your mind over and over again?	( )	( )	( )	( )
36. done things to get the attention of others?	( )	( )	( )	( )
37. asked others for help (not including coming to a mental health professional today)?	( )	( )	( )	( )
38. thought about your problems a lot?	( )	( )	( )	( )
39. been involved in recreation or pleasurable activities?	( )	( )	( )	( )
40. made a major change in your lifestyle - gotten a divorce, changed jobs, and so on?	( )	( )	( )	( )
41. read books on self-help for depression?	( )	( )	( )	( )
42. bought some new things for yourself?	( )	( )	( )	( )

In the <u>last 2 weeks</u>, have you:	As a result, did you feel			I did not do it in the last 2 weeks
	better	worse	the same	
43. decided that your problems have been caused by other people?	( )	( )	( )	( )
44. talked to a friend about your problems?	( )	( )	( )	( )
45. done little about your problems, hoping that others would help you?	( )	( )	( )	( )
46. done housework (cleaning, polishing, straightening)?	( )	( )	( )	( )
47. worried about your problems a lot?	( )	( )	( )	( )
48. tried to keep your mind off things that are upsetting you?	( )	( )	( )	( )
49. expressed little emotion to others in the past week?	( )	( )	( )	( )
50. tried to distract yourself from your troubles?	( )	( )	( )	( )
51. avoided thinking about your problems?	( )	( )	( )	( )
52. complained to friends and relatives about your problems?	( )	( )	( )	( )
53. made plans to overcome your problems (besides coming to a mental health professional today)?	( )	( )	( )	( )
54. tried to take what comes without letting it bother you and without complaining?	( )	( )	( )	( )
55. done something creative or artistic?	( )	( )	( )	( )
56. thought about ways to overcome your problems?	( )	( )	( )	( )
57. reminded yourself that you have dealt with unpleasant situations before?	( )	( )	( )	( )
58. expressed anger that others were not making adequate efforts to help you?	( )	( )	( )	( )
59. told yourself that other people have problems like yours?	( )	( )	( )	( )
60. carefully weighed the pros and cons of different alternatives to solving your problems?	( )	( )	( )	( )
61. told others that you were depressed or emotionally upset?	( )	( )	( )	( )
62. become more involved in life and taken on more responsibilities?	( )	( )	( )	( )
63. thought a lot about who is responsible for your problems (besides yourself)?	( )	( )	( )	( )
64. told yourself that other people have dealt with problems such as yours?	( )	( )	( )	( )
65. tried not to bother other people with how you felt?	( )	( )	( )	( )

In the <u>last 2 weeks</u>, have you:	As a result, did you feel			I did not do it in the last 2 weeks
	better	worse	the same	
66. been less demanding in what you require of yourself?	( )	( )	( )	( )
67. thought a lot about how you have brought your problems on yourself?	( )	( )	( )	( )
68. decided to wait and see how things turn out rather than making an effort to change them?	( )	( )	( )	( )
69. read the Scriptures?	( )	( )	( )	( )
70. become more active in your church or synagogue?	( )	( )	( )	( )
71. tried to look at your situation philosophically?	( )	( )	( )	( )
72. gone to movies?	( )	( )	( )	( )
73. let others take care of you?	( )	( )	( )	( )
74. decided that your current problems are a punishment for past actions?	( )	( )	( )	( )
75. masked your true feelings when with others?	( )	( )	( )	( )
76. tried to think positively and ignore the negative in your life?	( )	( )	( )	( )
77. sought sympathy from others?	( )	( )	( )	( )
78. gone shopping?	( )	( )	( )	( )
79. felt angry but held it in?	( )	( )	( )	( )
80. tried to focus on the good things in your life?	( )	( )	( )	( )
81. asserted yourself and taken positive action on problems that are getting you down?	( )	( )	( )	( )
82. sought reassurance and moral support from others?	( )	( )	( )	( )
83. talked with people who have had problems similar to yours?	( )	( )	( )	( )
84. told jokes?	( )	( )	( )	( )
85. told yourself you could not have prevented the troubles you experienced?	( )	( )	( )	( )
86. thought about your accomplishments, your strengths, and/or your abilities?	( )	( )	( )	( )
87. told yourself that some good for others can come out of your misfortune?	( )	( )	( )	( )
88. tried not to think about the bad aspects of your situation?	( )	( )	( )	( )
89. taken steps to improve your problems?	( )	( )	( )	( )

In the <u>last 2 weeks</u>, have you:	As a result, did you feel			I did not do it in the last 2 weeks
	better	worse	the same	
90. resigned yourself to your problems?	( )	( )	( )	( )
91. thought about how your problems have been caused by other people?	( )	( )	( )	( )
92. let others tell you how to get better (not including a mental health professional you may have seen today)?	( )	( )	( )	( )
93. become more active than usual?	( )	( )	( )	( )
94. turned your life over to God?	( )	( )	( )	( )
95. decided that there is a purpose behind your adversity?	( )	( )	( )	( )
96. avoided people that remind you of your problems?	( )	( )	( )	( )
97. accepted the fact that you are a sick person?	( )	( )	( )	( )
98. read humorous articles, stories, and so forth?	( )	( )	( )	( )
99. let others see how you really feel?	( )	( )	( )	( )
100. decided that you can grow and learn through your suffering?	( )	( )	( )	( )
101. prevented yourself from crying?	( )	( )	( )	( )
102. made humorous comments or wise cracks?	( )	( )	( )	( )
103. told yourself that other people have problems like your own?	( )	( )	( )	( )
104. looked for how you can learn something out of your bad situation?	( )	( )	( )	( )
105. avoided unpleasant situations?	( )	( )	( )	( )
106. gotten angry at God?	( )	( )	( )	( )
107. tried to follow God's will for you?	( )	( )	( )	( )
108. asked for God's guidance?	( )	( )	( )	( )
109. worked overtime?	( )	( )	( )	( )
110. become more sexually active?	( )	( )	( )	( )
111. let others see how bad you feel?	( )	( )	( )	( )
112. decided you deserve what you are experiencing?	( )	( )	( )	( )
113. kept your feelings bottled up inside?	( )	( )	( )	( )
114. told yourself that it is normal to feel depressed or anxious sometimes?	( )	( )	( )	( )
115. eaten more than usual?	( )	( )	( )	( )
116. become more religious?	( )	( )	( )	( )

In the <u>last 2 weeks</u>, have you:	As a result, did you feel			I did not do it in the last 2 weeks
	better	worse	the same	
117. decided that you deserve what you are experiencing?	( )	( )	( )	( )
118. decided that your depression or misfortune is not due to anything in particular, but is just a result of chance?	( )	( )	( )	( )
119. tried to act as if you were not upset?	( )	( )	( )	( )
120. asked someone to pray for you?	( )	( )	( )	( )
121. slept more than usual?	( )	( )	( )	( )
122. cried in the presence of someone else?	( )	( )	( )	( )
123. been with friends?	( )	( )	( )	( )
124. tried to figure out why you feel depressed?	( )	( )	( )	( )
125. gone for a walk?	( )	( )	( )	( )
126. tried to keep busy with things to do?	( )	( )	( )	( )
127. cried when by yourself?	( )	( )	( )	( )
128. decided to wait and see if your problem will resolve itself?	( )	( )	( )	( )
129. done something constructive?	( )	( )	( )	( )
130. lowered your expectations of yourself?	( )	( )	( )	( )
131. prayed for help?	( )	( )	( )	( )
132. gone out?	( )	( )	( )	( )
133. hid your irritation with others?	( )	( )	( )	( )
134. engaged in active recreation (tennis, skiing, etc.)?	( )	( )	( )	( )
135. held in your feelings?	( )	( )	( )	( )
136. depended on your family or friends more than usual?	( )	( )	( )	( )
137. told yourself that your problems will pass?	( )	( )	( )	( )
138. immersed yourself in your work or housework?	( )	( )	( )	( )
139. tried to act as if you weren't feeling bad?	( )	( )	( )	( )
140. helped others?	( )	( )	( )	( )
141. played with children or watched them playing?	( )	( )	( )	( )
142. told yourself that your problems are only a small part of your life?	( )	( )	( )	( )

E. Edward Beckham, PhD, is currently an Assistant Professor in the Department of Psychiatry and Behavioral Sciences at the University of Oklahoma Health Sciences Center in Oklahoma City where he is working on the NIMH Treatment of Depression Collaborative Research Program. He also works in the Inpatient Mental Health Unit of Oklahoma Memorial Hospital. He received his PhD in clinical psychology from Texas Tech in 1980. His publications include *Handbook of Depression: Treatment, Assessment, and Research*, published in 1985, which he co-edited. Research interests focus on the role of cognitions in the etiology and treatment of depression. Dr. Beckham may be contacted at the Department of Psychiatry and Behavioral Sciences, OU Health Sciences Center, P. O. Box 26901, Oklahoma City, OK 73190.

RESOURCES

Beck, A. T., Rush, A. J., Shaw, B. F., & Emery, G. (1979). *Cognitive Therapy of Depression.* New York: Guilford Press.

Beckham, E. E., & Adams, R. L. (1984). Coping behavior in depression: Report on a new scale. *Behavior Research and Therapy, 22,* 71-75.

Billings, A. G., & Moos, R. H. (1985). Psychosocial stressors, coping and depression. In E. E. Beckham & W. R. Leber (Eds.), *Handbook of Depression: Treatment, Assessment, and Research* (pp. 940-974). Homewood, IL: Dorsey Press.

Bulman, R. J., & Wortman, C. B. (1977). Attributions of blame and coping in the "real world": Severe accident victims react to their lot. *Journal of Personality and Social Psychology, 35,* 351-363.

Chodoff, P., Freedman, S. B., & Hamburg, D. (1964). Stress, defenses, and coping behavior: Observations in parents of children with malignant disease. *American Journal of Psychiatry, 120,* 743-749.

Coyne, J. C., Alwin, C., & Lazarus, R. S. (1981). Depression and coping in stressful episodes. *Journal of Abnormal Psychology, 90,* 439-447.

Doerfler, L. A., & Richards, C. S. (1981). Self-initiated attempts to cope with depression. *Cognitive Therapy and Research, 5,* 367-371.

Funabiki, D., Bologna, N. C., Pepping, M., & FitzGerald, K. C. (1980). Revisiting sex differences in the expression of depression. *Journal of Abnormal Psychology, 89,* 194-202.

Rippere, V. (1977). Some cognitive dimensions of antidepressive behavior. *Behavior Research and Therapy, 15,* 185-191.

White, R. W. (1974). Strategies of adaptation, an attempt at systematic description. In G. V. Coelho, D. A. Hamburg, & J. E. Adams (Eds.), *Coping and Adaptation* (pp. 47-68). New York: Basic Books.

THE SOCIAL ADJUSTMENT SELF-REPORT QUESTIONNAIRE

Myrna M. Weissman

Social adjustment, including the way in which a person fills various social roles, is an important consideration in assessing the functioning of individuals who seek help for mental health problems. The scale described in this contribution was designed to provide an efficient self-report measure of social functioning in several different role areas. Data obtained from a variety of populations support its use.

DEVELOPMENT

The Social Adjustment Self-Report Questionnaire (SAS-SR) is derived from the Social Adjustment Scale (SAS). SAS, which was developed and normed on depressed outpatients, is presented in an interview format described elsewhere (Weissman & Paykel, 1974). It has subsequently been used with other groups of psychiatric patients. More detailed information about SAS is available from the author at the address provided in the biography.

Data regarding reliability and validity of the SAS-SR are discussed in Weissman and Bothwell (1976). Comparisons between an interview rating of social adjustment and self-report using the scale ranged from $r = .40$ (family unit) to $r = .76$ (marital) on individual scales. The overall agreement between the two methods was .72.

The current version of SAS-SR contains 54 questions that measure a respondent's role performance over the past 2 weeks in the following areas: (a) work outside the home, (b) work at home, (c) work as a student, (d) social and leisure, (e) extended family, (f) marital, (g) parental, (h) family unit, and (i) economic. Responses can be used to compute scores for each role area and an overall adjustment score.

The SAS-SR has a number of potential applications with various psychiatric populations or community groups. Data available from previous studies (Weissman et al., 1978) provide normative comparisons which may be of use to clinicians and researchers. The scale can be used in mental health settings as a screening instrument or for determining base line functioning and subsequent changes among patients receiving treatment. Several recent articles that illustrate the use of the scale in research are included in the Resource section.

ADMINISTRATION AND SCORING

The SAS-SR is a paper-and-pencil test completed by the subject. In cases where the subject is illiterate, or unable to complete the questions for any other reason, items may be taken by a relative or significant other. Someone familiar with the instrument should be available to instruct the subject about the format, answer questions, and check for completeness.

Two scores are obtained:

1. An *overall adjustment score* is based on a sum of all items, divided by the number actually scored. Only one of the three work areas listed below is used to compute the overall score.
2. A *role area mean score* is based on a sum of the items in a role area, divided by the number of the items actually scored in that area.

Scores of 8, indicating that an item did not apply to a particular subject, are treated as missing data.

The following role areas are scored:

Item Number	Role Area
1-6*	Work Outside Home
7-12*	Work at Home
13-18*	Work as a Student
19-29	Social and Leisure
30-37	Extended Family
38-46	Marital
47-50	Parental
51-53	Family Unit
54	Economic

***Note:** Only one work area is used to compute the overall adjustment score.

NORMATIVE DATA

Normative data are available on a sample of 774 subjects. Table 1 on the next page contains social adjustment role means and overall adjustment by sex and by sample totals in four populations.

Details regarding the collection of the normative data are available in Weissman et al. (1978). Two primary populations are represented: a community sample of 482 subjects and a psychiatric outpatient sample of 292 subjects. The clinical symptom groups in Table 1 were identified on the basis of clinician ratings and administration of several symptom scales described in Weissman et al. (1978).

When making interpretations regarding scores, the user is reminded to take the subject's base line of functioning into consideration. For example, certain individuals who have chronically functioned at a relatively low level socially may appear to be doing poorly following treatment, when they have actually improved in comparison to their previous level.

TABLE 1: SOCIAL ADJUSTMENT ROLE MEANS AND OVERALL ADJUSTMENT BY SEX AND THE TOTAL SAMPLE IN THE FOUR POPULATIONS*[a]

Populations	Social Adjustment Role Means																		Overall Adjustment		
	Work			Social and leisure			Extended family			Marital			Parental			Family unit					
	N	M	SD	N	M	SD	N	M	SD	N	M	SD	N	M	SD	N	M	SD	N	M	SD
Community sample																					
Male	127	1.26	.31	205	1.83	.51	201	1.33	.31	170	1.72	.46	101	1.35	.41	194	1.35	.51	205	1.56	.32
Female	272	1.46	.50	277	1.83	.53	274	1.34	.35	191	1.77	.49	175	1.43	.43	270	1.54	.62	277	1.61	.34
Total	399	1.40	.46	482	1.83[b]	.52	475	1.34	.33	361	1.75	.48	276	1.40	.42	464	1.46	.58	482	1.59	.33
p-Value		<.001			NS			NS			NS			NS			<.001			NS	
Acute depressives																					
Male	23	2.57	.77	36	2.91	.70	36	2.13	.67	22	2.42	.45	18	2.38	.73	29	2.68	.75	36	2.56	.44
Female	149	2.47	.74	155	2.83	.65	155	2.15	.69	93	2.46	.58	101	2.25	.82	140	2.86	.91	155	2.53	.46
Total	172	2.48	.75	191	2.85	.66	191	2.15	.69	115	2.45	.55	119	2.27	.81	169	2.83	.89	191	2.53	.46
p-Value		NS			NS			NS			NS			NS			<.01			NS	
Alcoholics																					
Male	9	1.62	.67	35	2.44	.82	35	1.91	.62	15	2.02	.62	9	1.67	.57	27	2.24	1.13	35	2.17	.65
Female	17	1.93	.55	19	2.59	.72	17	2.23	.66	7	2.19	.67	8	1.88	.65	18	2.82	1.07	19	2.36	.50
Total	26	1.82	.62	54	2.50	.79	52	2.02	.65	22	2.07	.64	17	1.77	.62	45	2.46	1.14	54	2.23	.61
p-Value		NS			NS			NS			NS			NS			NS			NS	
Schizophrenics																					
Male	4	1.25	.19	12	2.51	.74	12	1.53	.32	3	1.85	.21	2	1.63	.13	5	1.87	.81	12	1.99	.47
Female	35	1.66	.78	35	2.37	.77	35	1.66	.79	19	1.98	.75	18	1.61	.67	29	1.85	1.02	35	1.95	.66
Total	39	1.62	.75	47	2.40	.76	47	1.63	.70	22	1.97	.70	20	1.61	.64	34	1.85	.99	47	1.96	.62
p-Value		NS			NS			NS			NS			NS			NS			NS	

[a]Ns vary because the subject did not have the role and assessment, therefore, was not applicable.
[b]NS, not significant.

*From "Social Adjustment by Self-Report in a Community Sample and in Psychiatric Outpatients" by M. M. Weissman, B. A. Prusoff, W. D. Thompson, P. S. Harding, and J. K. Meyers, 1978, Journal of Nervous and Mental Disease, 166(5), p. 322. Copyright © 1978 by Williams & Wilkins Co. Reprinted by permission.

SOCIAL ADJUSTMENT SELF-REPORT QUESTIONNAIRE

We are interested in finding out how you have been doing in the last *2 weeks*. We would like you to answer some questions about your work, spare time, and your family life. There are no right or wrong answers to these questions. Check the answers that best describe how you have been in the last *2 weeks*.

WORK OUTSIDE THE HOME

Please check the situation that best describes you.

I am 1 ___ a worker for pay. 4 ___ retired.
      2 ___ a housewife.   5 ___ unemployed.
      3 ___ a student.

Do you usually work for pay more than 15 hours per week?

      1 ___ Yes   2 ___ No

Did you work any hours for pay in the last 2 weeks?

      1 ___ Yes   2 ___ No

Check the answer that best describes how you have been in the last 2 weeks.

1. How many days did you miss from work in the last 2 weeks?

    1 ___ No days missed.
    2 ___ One day.
    3 ___ I missed about half the time.
    4 ___ Missed more than half the time but did make at least one day.
    5 ___ I did not work any days.
    8 ___ On vacation all of the last 2 weeks.

If you have not worked any days in the last 2 weeks, go on to Question 7.

2. Have you been able to do your work in the last 2 weeks?

    1 ___ I did my work very well.
    2 ___ I did my work well but had some minor problems.
    3 ___ I needed help with work and did not do well about half the time.
    4 ___ I did my work poorly most of the time.
    5 ___ I did my work poorly all the time.

3. Have you been ashamed of how you do your work in the last 2 weeks?

    1 ___ I never felt ashamed.
    2 ___ Once or twice I felt a little ashamed.
    3 ___ About half the time I felt ashamed.
    4 ___ I felt ashamed most of the time.
    5 ___ I felt ashamed all the time.

4. Have you had any arguments with people at work in the last 2 weeks?

    1 ___ I had no arguments and got along very well.
    2 ___ I usually got along well but had minor arguments.
    3 ___ I had more than one argument.
    4 ___ I had many arguments.
    5 ___ I was constantly in arguments.

5. Have you felt upset, worried, or uncomfortable while doing your work during the last 2 weeks?

    1 ___ I never felt upset.
    2 ___ Once or twice I felt upset.
    3 ___ Half the time I felt upset.
    4 ___ I felt upset most of the time.
    5 ___ I felt upset all of the time.

6. Have you found your work interesting these last 2 weeks?

    1 ___ My work was almost always interesting.
    2 ___ Once or twice my work was not interesting.
    3 ___ Half the time my work was uninteresting.
    4 ___ Most of the time my work was uninteresting.
    5 ___ My work was always uninteresting.

WORK AT HOME

Housewives answer Questions 7-12. Otherwise, go on to Question 13.

7. How many days did you do some housework during the last 2 weeks?

    1 ___ Every day
    2 ___ I did the housework almost every day.
    3 ___ I did the housework about half the time.
    4 ___ I usually did not do the housework.
    5 ___ I was completely unable to do housework.
    8 ___ I was away from home all of the last 2 weeks.

8. During the last 2 weeks, have you kept up with your housework? This includes cooking, cleaning, laundry, grocery shopping, and errands.

    1 ___ I did my work very well.
    2 ___ I did my work well but had some minor problems.
    3 ___ I needed help with my work and did not do it well about half the time.
    4 ___ I did my work poorly most of the time.
    5 ___ I did my work poorly all of the time.

9. Have you been ashamed of how you did your housework during the last 2 weeks?

    1 ___ I never felt ashamed.
    2 ___ Once or twice I felt a little ashamed.
    3 ___ About half the time I felt ashamed.
    4 ___ I felt ashamed most of the time.
    5 ___ I felt ashamed all the time.

10. Have you had any arguments with salespeople, tradesmen, or neighbors in the last 2 weeks?

    1 ___ I had no arguments and got along very well.
    2 ___ I usually got along well, but had minor arguments.

   3 ___ I had more than one argument.
   4 ___ I had many arguments.
   5 ___ I was constantly in arguments.

11. Have you felt upset while doing your housework during the last 2 weeks?

   1 ___ I never felt upset.
   2 ___ Once or twice I felt upset.
   3 ___ Half the time I felt upset.
   4 ___ I felt upset most of the time.
   5 ___ I felt upset all of the time.

12. Have you found your housework interesting these last 2 weeks?

   1 ___ My work was almost always interesting.
   2 ___ Once or twice my work was not interesting.
   3 ___ Half the time my work was uninteresting.
   4 ___ Most of the time my work was uninteresting.
   5 ___ My work was always uninteresting.

FOR STUDENTS

Answer Questions 13-18 if you go to school half time or more. Otherwise, go on to Question 19.

What best describes your school program? (Choose one)

   1 ___ Full time.
   2 ___ 3/4 time.
   3 ___ Half time.

Check the answer that best describes how you have been the last 2 weeks.

13. How many days of classes did you miss in the last 2 weeks?

   1 ___ No days missed.
   2 ___ A few days missed.
   3 ___ I missed about half the time.
   4 ___ Missed more than half the time but did make at least one day.
   5 ___ I did not go to classes at all.
   8 ___ I was on vacation all of the last 2 weeks.

14. Have you been able to keep up with your class work in the last 2 weeks?

   1 ___ I did my work very well.
   2 ___ I did my work well but had minor problems.
   3 ___ I needed help with my work and did not do well about half the time.
   4 ___ I did my work poorly most of the time.
   5 ___ I did my work poorly all the time.

15. During the last 2 weeks, have you been ashamed of how you do your school work?

   1 ___ I never felt ashamed.
   2 ___ Once or twice I felt ashamed.
   3 ___ About half the time I felt ashamed.
   4 ___ I felt ashamed most of the time.
   5 ___ I felt ashamed all of the time.

16. Have you had any arguments with people at school in the last 2 weeks?

   1 ___ I had no arguments and got along very well.
   2 ___ I usually got along well but had minor arguments.
   3 ___ I had more than one argument.
   4 ___ I had many arguments.
   5 ___ I was constantly in arguments.
   8 ___ Not applicable; I did not attend school.

17. Have you felt upset at school during the last 2 weeks?

   1 ___ I never felt upset.
   2 ___ Once or twice I felt upset.
   3 ___ Half the time I felt upset.
   4 ___ I felt upset most of the time.
   5 ___ I felt upset all of the time.
   8 ___ Not applicable; I did not attend school.

18. Have you found your school work interesting these last 2 weeks?

   1 ___ My work was almost always interesting.
   2 ___ Once or twice my work was not interesting.
   3 ___ Half the time my work was uninteresting.
   4 ___ Most of the time my work was uninteresting.
   5 ___ My work was always uninteresting.

SPARE TIME

Everyone answer Questions 19-27.

Check the answer that best describes how you have been in the last 2 weeks.

19. How many friends have you seen or spoken to on the telephone in the last 2 weeks?

   1 ___ Nine or more friends.
   2 ___ Five to eight friends.
   3 ___ Two to four friends.
   4 ___ One friend.
   5 ___ No friends.

20. Have you been able to talk about your feelings and problems with at least one friend during the last 2 weeks?

   1 ___ I can always talk about my innermost feelings.
   2 ___ I usually can talk about my feelings.
   3 ___ About half the time I felt able to talk about my feelings.
   4 ___ I usually was not able to talk about my feelings.
   5 ___ I was never able to talk about my feelings.
   8 ___ Not applicable; I have no friends.

21. How many times in the last 2 weeks have you gone out socially with other people? For example, visited friends, gone to movies, bowling, church, restaurants, invited friends to your home?

   1 ___ More than three times.
   2 ___ Three times.
   3 ___ Twice.
   4 ___ Once.
   5 ___ None.

22. How much time have you spent on hobbies or spare time interests during the last 2 weeks?

For example, bowling, sewing, gardening, sports, reading?

1 ___ I spent most of my spare time on hobbies almost every day.
2 ___ I spent some spare time on hobbies some of the days.
3 ___ I spent a little spare time on hobbies.
4 ___ I usually did not spend any time on hobbies but did watch TV.
5 ___ I did not spend any spare time on hobbies or watching TV.

23. Have you had open arguments with your friends in the last 2 weeks?

1 ___ I had no arguments and got along very well.
2 ___ I usually got along well but had minor arguments.
3 ___ I had more than one argument.
4 ___ I had many arguments.
5 ___ I was constantly in arguments.
8 ___ Not applicable; I have no friends.

24. If your feelings were hurt or offended by a friend during the last 2 weeks, how badly did you take it?

1 ___ It did not affect me or it did not happen.
2 ___ I got over it in a few hours.
3 ___ I got over it in a few days.
4 ___ I got over it in a week.
5 ___ It will take me months to recover.
8 ___ Not applicable; I have no friends.

25. Have you felt shy or uncomfortable with people in the last 2 weeks?

1 ___ I always felt comfortable.
2 ___ Sometimes I felt uncomfortable but could relax after a while.
3 ___ About half the time I felt uncomfortable.
4 ___ I usually felt uncomfortable.
5 ___ I always felt uncomfortable.
8 ___ Not applicable; I was never with people.

26. Have you felt lonely and wished for more friends during the last 2 weeks?

1 ___ I have not felt lonely.
2 ___ I have felt lonely a few times.
3 ___ About half the time I felt lonely.
4 ___ I usually felt lonely.
5 ___ I always felt lonely and wished for more friends.

27. Have you felt bored in your spare time during the last 2 weeks?

1 ___ I never felt bored.
2 ___ I usually did not feel bored.
3 ___ About half the time I felt bored.
4 ___ Most of the time I felt bored.
5 ___ I was constantly bored.

Are you a single, separated, or divorced person not living with a person of opposite sex; please answer below.

1 ___ YES, answer Questions 28 and 29.
2 ___ NO, go to Question 30.

28. How many times have you been with a date these last 2 weeks?

1 ___ More than three times.
2 ___ Three times.
3 ___ Twice.
4 ___ Once.
5 ___ Never.

29. Have you been interested in dating during the last 2 weeks? If you have not dated, would you have liked to?

1 ___ I was always interested in dating.
2 ___ Most of the time I was interested.
3 ___ About half of the time I was interested.
4 ___ Most of the time I was not interested.
5 ___ I was completely uninterested.

FAMILY

Answer Questions 30-37 about your parents, brothers, sisters, in-laws, and children not living at home.

Have you been in contact with any of them in the last 2 weeks?

1 ___ YES, answer Questions 30-37.
2 ___ NO, go to Question 36.

30. Have you had open arguments with your relatives in the last 2 weeks?

1 ___ We always got along very well.
2 ___ We usually got along very well but had some minor arguments.
3 ___ I had more than one argument with at least one relative.
4 ___ I had many arguments.
5 ___ I was constantly in arguments.

31. Have you been able to talk about your feelings and problems with at least one of your relatives in the last 2 weeks?

1 ___ I can always talk about my feelings with at least one relative.
2 ___ I usually can talk about my feelings.
3 ___ About half the time I felt able to talk about my feelings.
4 ___ I usually was not able to talk about my feelings.
5 ___ I was never able to talk about my feelings.

32. Have you avoided contacts with your relatives these last 2 weeks?

1 ___ I have contacted relatives regularly.
2 ___ I have contacted a relative at least once.
3 ___ I have waited for my relatives to contact me.
4 ___ I avoided my relatives, but they contacted me.
5 ___ I have no contacts with any relatives.

33. Did you depend on your relatives for help, advice, money, or friendship during the last 2 weeks?

1 ___ I never need to depend on them.
2 ___ I usually did not need to depend on them.

3 ___ About half the time I needed to depend
        on them.
4 ___ Most of the time I depend on them.
5 ___ I depend completely on them.

34. Have you wanted to do the opposite of what
    your relatives wanted in order to make them
    angry during the last 2 weeks?

    1 ___ I never wanted to oppose them.
    2 ___ Once or twice I wanted to oppose them.
    3 ___ About half the time I wanted to oppose
        them.
    4 ___ Most of the time I wanted to oppose
        them.
    5 ___ I always opposed them.

35. Have you been worried about things happening
    to your relatives without good reason in the
    last 2 weeks?

    1 ___ I have not worried without reason.
    2 ___ Once or twice I worried.
    3 ___ About half the time I worried.
    4 ___ Most of the time I worried.
    5 ___ I have worried the entire time.
    8 ___ Not applicable; my relatives are no
        longer living.

EVERYONE answer Questions 36 and 37, even if your
relatives are not living.

36. During the last 2 weeks, have you been think-
    ing that you have let any of your relatives
    down or have been unfair to them at any time?

    1 ___ I did not feel that I let them down
        at all.
    2 ___ I usually did not feel that I let them
        down.
    3 ___ About half the time I felt that I let
        them down.
    4 ___ Most of the time I have felt that I let
        them down.
    5 ___ I always felt that I let them down.

37. During the last 2 weeks, have you been think-
    ing that any of your relatives have let you
    down or have been unfair to you at any time?

    1 ___ I never felt that they let me down.
    2 ___ I felt that they usually did not let
        me down.
    3 ___ About half the time I felt they let
        me down.
    4 ___ I usually have felt that they let me
        down.
    5 ___ I am very bitter that they let me down.

Are you living with your spouse or have you been
living with a person of the opposite sex in a
permanent relationship?

    1 ___ YES, please answer Questions 38-46.
    2 ___ NO, go to Question 47.

38. Have you had open arguments with your partner
    in the last 2 weeks?

    1 ___ We had no arguments and we got along
        well.
    2 ___ We usually got along well but had
        minor arguments.
    3 ___ We had more than one argument.

4 ___ We had many arguments.
5 ___ We were constantly in arguments.

39. Have you been able to talk about your feelings
    and problems with your partner during the last
    2 weeks?

    1 ___ I could always talk freely about my
        feelings.
    2 ___ I usually could talk about my feelings.
    3 ___ About half the time I felt able to talk
        about my feelings.
    4 ___ I usually was not able to talk about my
        feelings.
    5 ___ I was never able to talk about my
        feelings.

40. Have you been demanding to have your own way
    at home during the last 2 weeks?

    1 ___ I have not insisted on always having
        my own way.
    2 ___ I usually have not insisted on having
        my own way.
    3 ___ About half the time I insisted on having
        my own way.
    4 ___ I usually insisted on having my own way.
    5 ___ I always insisted on having my own way.

41. Have you been bossed around by your partner
    these last 2 weeks?

    1 ___ Almost never.
    2 ___ Once in a while.
    3 ___ About half the time.
    4 ___ Most of the time.
    5 ___ Always.

42. How much have you felt dependent on your
    partner these last 2 weeks?

    1 ___ I was independent.
    2 ___ I was usually independent.
    3 ___ I was somewhat dependent.
    4 ___ I was usually dependent.
    5 ___ I depended on my partner for everything.

43. How have you felt about your partner during
    the last 2 weeks?

    1 ___ I always felt affection.
    2 ___ I usually felt affection.
    3 ___ About half the time I felt dislike
        and half the time affection.
    4 ___ I usually felt dislike.
    5 ___ I always felt dislike.

44. How many times have you and your partner
    had intercourse?

    1 ___ More than twice a week.
    2 ___ Once or twice a week.
    3 ___ Once every 2 weeks.
    4 ___ Less than once every 2 weeks but at
        least once in the last month.
    5 ___ Not at all in a month or longer.

45. Have you had any problems during intercourse,
    such as pain these last 2 weeks?

    1 ___ None.
    2 ___ Once or twice.
    3 ___ About half the time.
    4 ___ Most of the time.

5 ___ Always.
8 ___ Not applicable; no intercourse in the last 2 weeks.

46. How have you felt about intercourse during the last 2 weeks?

    1 ___ I always enjoyed it.
    2 ___ I usually enjoyed it.
    3 ___ About half the time I did and half the time I did not enjoy it.
    4 ___ I usually did not enjoy it.
    5 ___ I never enjoyed it.

CHILDREN

Have you had unmarried children, stepchildren, or foster children living at home during the last 2 weeks?

    1 ___ YES, answer Questions 47-50.
    2 ___ NO, go to Question 51.

47. Have you been interested in what your children are doing - school, play, or hobbies during the last 2 weeks?

    1 ___ I was always interested and actively involved.
    2 ___ I usually was interested and involved.
    3 ___ About half the time interested and half the time not interested.
    4 ___ I usually was disinterested.
    5 ___ I was always disinterested.

48. Have you been able to talk and listen to your children during the last 2 weeks? Include only children over the age of 2.

    1 ___ I always was able to communicate with them.
    2 ___ I usually was able to communicate with them.
    3 ___ About half the time I could communicate.
    4 ___ I usually was not able to communicate.
    5 ___ I was completely unable to communicate.
    8 ___ Not applicable; no children over the age of 2.

49. How have you been getting along with the children during the last 2 weeks?

    1 ___ I had no arguments and got along very well.
    2 ___ I usually got along well but had minor arguments.
    3 ___ I had more than one argument.
    4 ___ I had many arguments.
    5 ___ I was constantly in arguments.

50. How have you felt toward your children these last 2 weeks?

    1 ___ I always felt affection.
    2 ___ I mostly felt affection.
    3 ___ About half the time I felt affection.

4 ___ Most of the time I did not feel affection.
5 ___ I never felt affection toward them.

FAMILY UNIT

Have you ever been married, ever lived with a person of the opposite sex, or ever had children? Please check.

    1 ___ YES, please answer Questions 51-53.
    2 ___ NO, go to Question 54.

51. Have you worried about your partner or any of your children without any reason during the last 2 weeks, even if you are not living together now?

    1 ___ I never worried.
    2 ___ Once or twice I worried.
    3 ___ About half the time I worried.
    4 ___ Most of the time I worried.
    5 ___ I always worried.
    8 ___ Not applicable; partner and children not living.

52. During the last 2 weeks have you been thinking that you have let down your partner or any of your children at any time?

    1 ___ I did not feel I let them down at all.
    2 ___ I usually did not feel that I let them down.
    3 ___ About half the time I felt I let them down.
    4 ___ Most of the time I have felt that I let them down.
    5 ___ I let them down completely.

53. During the last 2 weeks, have you been thinking that your partner or any of your children have let you down at any time?

    1 ___ I never felt that they let me down.
    2 ___ I felt they usually did not let me down.
    3 ___ About half the time I felt they let me down.
    4 ___ I usually felt they let me down.
    5 ___ I feel bitter that they have let me down.

FINANCIAL

EVERYONE please answer Question 54.

54. Have you had enough money to take care of your own and your family's financial needs during the last 2 weeks?

    1 ___ I had enough money for needs.
    2 ___ I usually had enough money with minor problems.
    3 ___ About half the time I did not have enough money but did not have to borrow money.
    4 ___ I usually did not have enough money and had to borrow from others.
    5 ___ I had great financial difficulty.

Myrna M. Weissman, PhD, is currently a Professor of Psychiatry and Epidemiology at Yale University School of Medicine, and Director of the Depression Research Unit of Connecticut Mental Health Center. She has also been a Visiting Senior Scholar at the Institute of Medicine, National Academy of Sciences in Washington, DC. She received her doctorate from Yale University in 1974. Her specialty area is in psychiatric epidemiology and she has received a number of awards for her work in this area. Her current research is on the epidemiology of psychiatric disorders in the community, and the treatment and the genetics of affective disorders. Dr. Weissman may be contacted at Yale University School of Medicine, Depression Research Unit, 350 Congress Avenue, New Haven, CT 06519.

RESOURCES

Chevron, E. S., & Rounsaville, B. J. (1983). Evaluating the clinical skills of psychotherapists: A comparison of techniques. *Archives of General Psychiatry, 40,* 1129-1132.

Norman, D. K., & Herzog, D. B. (1984). Persistent social maladjustment in bulimia: A one-year follow-up. *American Journal of Psychiatry, 141,* 444-446.

Richman, J. (1984). Sex differences in social adjustment: Effects of sex role socialization and role stress. *Journal of Nervous and Mental Disease, 172,* 539-545.

Rounsaville, B. J., Sholomskas, D., & Prusoff, B. A. (1980). Chronic mood disorders in depressed outpatients: Diagnosis and response to pharmacotherapy. *Journal of Affective Disorders, 2,* 73-88.

Weissman, M. M., & Bothwell, S. (1976). Assessment of social adjustment by patient self report. *Archives of General Psychiatry, 33,* 1111-1115.

Weissman, M. M., & Paykel, E. S. (1974). *The depressed woman: A study of social relationships.* Chicago: University of Chicago Press.

Weissman, M. M., Prusoff, B. A., Thompson, W. D., Harding, P. S., & Meyers, J. K. (1978). Social adjustment by self-report in a community sample and in psychiatric outpatients. *Journal of Nervous and Mental Disease, 166,* 317-326.

THE STRAIN QUESTIONNAIRE

R. Craig Lefebvre and Sandra L. Sandford

The Strain Questionnaire (SQ) (Lefebvre & Sandford, 1984) was developed to measure strain (stress) as a syndrome of physical, behavioral, and cognitive symptoms that are elicited, to varying degrees, by environmental demands upon an individual. Several self-report measures assess stress stimuli or the process of transaction between the person and his or her environment (i.e., coping scales). The few instruments that purport to evaluate the response of stress have either emphasized only the somatic aspects of the response or have been couched in the context of an affective state such as depression or anxiety. Despite an extensive history of research in this area, little effort has been expended toward the development of a self-report instrument that measures the everyday manifestations of the stress response (cf. Selye, 1976, pp. 174-177). These manifestations include physical, behavioral, and cognitive signs. Such an oversight has three important implications for the clinician:

1. The impact of behavioral and cognitive symptoms on levels of reported stress cannot be assessed.
2. The possible interactive, or causal, relationships between these three response systems cannot be delineated.
3. No possibility exists for the identification of idiosyncratic stress syndromes that might then dictate specific intervention techniques.

From this perspective, the assessment of all modalities of the stress (here referred to as strain) response is important to clinical diagnosis and prescription. Although studies are still necessary to further validate various aspects of the SQ, it appears to be a valid and reliable measure of strain in both cross-sectional and longitudinal studies (Lefebvre & Sandford, 1984, 1985). It also has potential as a screening tool to identify those persons most likely to benefit from specific stress management techniques.

DEVELOPMENT

An item pool of 48 physical, behavioral, and cognitive signs of strain were generated by reference to Selye (1976) and Lefebvre and Lawlis (1979). Four clinical psychology doctoral-level interns with experience in treating stress disorders were asked to sort the items into either physical, behavioral, or cognitive categories. Inter-rater reliability of these sorts ranged from $r = .88$ to $r = 1.00$.

All 48 items were included in the SQ. Individuals were instructed to "circle the letter which most closely corresponds to how often *in the past week* you have experienced or felt each of the items listed." Responses were recorded as A = never, B = rarely, C = sometimes, D = frequently, and E = constantly. These responses were subsequently transposed to numerical equivalents (A = 1, E = 5) for statistical analyses. In subsequent work, these adjectives have been anchored with the descriptors A = never (0 days/week), B = rarely (1-2 days/week), C = sometimes (3-4 days/week), D = frequently (5-6 days/week), E = constantly (7 days/week).

RELIABILITY OF SCORES

Estimates of internal consistency for each subscale - physical, behavioral, and cognitive - and the total SQ were computed by use of the Spearman-Brown split-half reliability and Cronbach alpha statistics. In addition, test-retest correlations were obtained from a subsample of 68 graduate business students who completed another SQ 4 weeks after the first administration.

The data shown in Table 1 indicate moderately high internal consistency of the SQ and the component scales, and, given the fluid nature of strain, good stability over a 1 month time period.

TABLE 1: RELIABILITY OF THE SQ AND ITS SUBSCALES

Scale	Split-Half	Alpha	Test-Retest
SQ	.88	.94	.79
Physical	.87	.92	.75
Behavioral	.62	.71	.77
Cognitive	.86	.86	.73

NORMS

Normative data for the SQ, shown in Table 2, were obtained on 285 males and 127 females ($N = 412$) who had a mean age of 33 years (range 17-58 years). This group consisted of 38 elementary and secondary education teachers and 45 insurance agents who were enrolled in stress management classes; 110 naval engineers and 119 graduate business students who completed it as part of a battery of instruments assessing health-related behaviors and attitudes; and 100 undergraduate students who also took it as part of a battery of questionnaires.

TABLE 2: NORMS FOR THE SQ AND ITS SUBSCALES

Scale	Mean	SD	Range	Maximum
SQ	86	25	48-189	240
Physical	50	16	28-116	140
Behavioral	22	6	12-44	60
Cognitive	14	5	8-37	40

SCORING

The SQ is composed of three scales as enumerated earlier: physical, behavioral, and cognitive. Scoring procedures are based on these scales plus the full SQ score. The left-hand column of the SQ contains the 28 physical signs of strain ("backaches" to "pre-menstrual tension or missed cycles"). They are followed in the right-hand column by 12 behavioral items ("spent more time alone" to "accident proneness"), and eight cognitive signs of strain ("believe the world is against you" to "think things can't get any worse"). Each scale score is calculated by summing the individual symptom ratings within the scale.

In a factor analysis of the SQ, Lefebvre and Sandford (1985) identified 11 orthogonal factors. Items loading on each of these factors are shown in Table 3 on the next page.

APPLICATION

Before considering the application of the SQ in clinical practice, several cautionary notes are warranted. First, the SQ has not been standardized on clinical populations

---

TABLE 3:   SQ ITEM LOADINGS ON DERIVED FACTORS (IN DESCENDING ORDER OF IMPORTANCE)

Factor 1:   Cognitive 1 behavior strain
             Items: 42, 45, 44, 48, 29, 41, 43, 46, 30, 31, 32, 35

Factor 2:   Vague physical complaints
             Items: 4, 5, 16, 14, 2, 3, 6, 13, 18

Factor 3:   Gastrointestinal complaints
             Items: 9, 10, 8, 33, 11, 32

Factor 4:   Chronic muscle tension and sleep disturbance
             Items: 17, 26, 34, 19, 7, 47, 18, 46

Factor 5:   Cephalic activity
             Items: 21, 22, 19, 20, 36

Factor 6:   Back problems/accident proneness
             Items: 1, 2, 27, 40

Factor 7:   Perspiration
             Items: 23, 24, 20

Factor 8:   Menstrual complaints
             Items: 28, 14

Factor 9:   Cardiopulmonary activity
             Items: 12, 13, 25, 15

Factor 10:   Substance abuse
             Items: 37, 39

Factor 11:   Prescription drug use
             Items: 38

---

presenting with stress complaints. Thus, any generalizations to this group must be made with the caveat that they are derived from nonclinical samples. Second, no studies are yet complete which demonstrate the sensitivity of the SQ to reductions in strain. Lefebvre & Sandford (1984) have demonstrated, however, its predictiveness for increases in levels of strain and depression. And finally, its prognostic utility in clinical settings has yet to be tested.

In interpreting the SQ, one must first look at the SQ to determine if the overall strain level is high. For research purposes, the mean has been used to determine "High" versus "Low" strain. Clinically, persons who are at least one standard deviation above the mean on the SQ can be expected to be experiencing significant strain.

After inspecting the SQ total score, each subscale score should be reviewed following the same criteria as outlined above. The total SQ score, and each of the component scales, should then be compared to obtain a profile of strain reactivity. For instance, a person with a score of SQ = 95, physical = 70, behavioral = 15, and cognitive = 10, would have only a slight elevation in total strain, yet a significant elevation in physical signs of strain.

The determination of divergent scale scores, as depicted in the last example, would be reflected in the clinical intervention. Persons high in physical signs of strain would most likely benefit from both exercise prescription and relaxation techniques. Individuals high in behavioral symptoms should be instructed in the use of behavior management skills to remedy these problems. People with many cognitive signs of strain can be targeted for cognitive restructuring techniques such as rational-emotive therapy. Until a firm empirical base is established for these recommendations, however, these techniques should not be used exclusively for these specific strain responses. Rather, the target techniques should serve as a focal strategy in treatment planning, but certainly not be the only one.

Some clinicians may also want to take advantage of the factor scores to further refine their intervention efforts. Of particular relevance to stress management are the physical factors that emerge from the SQ, which can be differentially addressed by progressive muscle relaxation methods and autogenic training. Progressive relaxation methods appear best suited for individuals expressing physical strain through (a) chronic muscle tension and sleep disturbance, (b) cephalic activity, and (c) back problems. Autogenic training would be more appropriate for individuals reporting strain as (a) gastrointestinal complaints, (b) perspiration, (c) menstrual complaints, and (d) cardio-pulmonary activity.

The Strain Questionnaire should be viewed as both a diagnostic and evaluation instrument. Obviously, people will respond with different types of strain symptoms both across situations and across time. The SQ can be used to evaluate progress in managing stress symptoms over the course of individual or group therapy. Its use as an evaluation tool within the context of stress management seminars not only educates participants to the everyday signs of strain, but also allows them to focus their efforts on learning the stress reduction methods that may be most beneficial to their unique situation. The use of an instrument such as the SQ may lead to more individually tailored approaches to stress management which avoid trying to fit everyone to the clinician's favorite technique.

STRAIN QUESTIONNAIRE*

Please read the following list and circle the letter that most closely corresponds to how often *in the past week* you have experienced or felt each of the items listed.

A = Not at all   B = 1 or 2 days   C = 3 or 4 days   D = 5 or 6 days   E = Everyday

1. backaches	A B C D E	29. spent more time alone A B C D E
2. muscle soreness	A B C D E	30. irritability A B C D E
3. numbness or tingling in body	A B C D E	31. impulsive behavior A B C D E
4. heaviness in arms or legs	A B C D E	32. easily startled A B C D E
5. weakness in body parts	A B C D E	33. stuttering/other speech
6. tense muscles	A B C D E	dysfluencies A B C D E
7. pain in neck	A B C D E	34. insomnia A B C D E
8. nausea or upset stomach	A B C D E	35. inability to sit still A B C D E
9. diarrhea or indigestion	A B C D E	36. smoking A B C D E
10. tight stomach	A B C D E	37. use of recreational drugs A B C D E
11. loss of or excessive appetite	A B C D E	38. use of prescription drugs A B C D E
12. pain in heart or chest	A B C D E	39. use of alcohol A B C D E
13. shortness of breath	A B C D E	40. accident proneness A B C D E
14. faintness, dizziness	A B C D E	41. believe the world is
15. racing heart	A B C D E	against you A B C D E
16. light headedness	A B C D E	42. feeling out of control A B C D E
17. headaches	A B C D E	43. urge to cry or run
18. hot or cold spells	A B C D E	away and hide A B C D E
19. lump in throat	A B C D E	44. feeling of unreality A B C D E
20. dryness of throat and mouth	A B C D E	45. feeling that you are no good A B C D E
21. teeth grinding	A B C D E	46. inability to concentrate A B C D E
22. trembling or nervous tics	A B C D E	47. nightmares A B C D E
23. sweating	A B C D E	48. think things can't get
24. sweaty hands	A B C D E	any worse A B C D E
25. itching	A B C D E	
26. cold or warm hands	A B C D E	
27. frequent need to urinate	A B C D E	
28. pre-menstrual tension or		
missed cycles	A B C D E	

R. Craig Lefebvre, PhD, is currently the Intervention Unit Coordinator of The Pawtucket Heart Health Program. He is also an Assistant Professor (research) of Community Health at Brown University, and an Adjunct Assistant Professor of Psychology at the University of Rhode Island. His degree is in clinical psychology, and he has held post-doctoral fellowships at the University of Virginia and the University of Pittsburgh. He has published extensively in the field of behavioral medicine, with particular interests including cardiovascular disease prevention and community-based approaches to health promotion. Dr. Lefebvre may be contacted at The Pawtucket Heart Health Program, The Memorial Hospital, Prospect Street, Pawtucket, RI 02860.

Sandra L. Sandford is currently completing her graduate studies in clinical psychology at the University of Pittsburgh. Her interests include moderators of life stressors, and neuropsychological and neurophysiological sequalae of hepatic diseases. Ms. Sandford may be contacted at Department of Psychology, University of Pittsburgh, Pittsburgh, PA 15231.

RESOURCES

Lefebvre, R. C., & Lawlis, C. F. (1979). A rational approach to medical disorders. *Rational Living, 14,* 17-22.

Lefebvre, R. C., & Sandford, S. L. (1984). *The Modulation of Stress: Analysis of Effects in a High-Risk Psychosocial Context.* Paper presented at the annual meeting of the Society of Behavioral Medicine, Philadelphia, PA.

Lefebvre, R. C., & Sandford, S. L. (1985). A multi-modal questionnaire for stress. *Journal of Human Stress, 11,* 69-75.

Selye, H. (1976). *The Stress of Life* (rev. ed.). New York: McGraw-Hill.

INTRODUCTION TO SECTION IV: COMMUNITY INTERVENTIONS

Although the primary focus in the *Innovations* series is on clinical interventions, we have included this section because of our firm belief that practitioners often select relatively narrow roles that may limit their potential influence on the community. Mental health professionals are in an excellent position to address a diversity of problems that are sometimes overlooked by traditional practitioners. In Volume 5 we have included three examples of potential clinician involvement outside the consulting room. By selecting these, we hope to stimulate thinking about strategies for influencing a larger number of people than might be served through psychotherapy.

In the first contribution, Scogin and Beutler provide guidelines for the psychological screening of law enforcement candidates. Mental health professionals have played a growing role in law enforcement programs over the years. The selection of law enforcement candidates has become an important issue in many communities. These authors provide an up-to-date review of appropriate assessment techniques for this purpose. They also provide guidelines for avoiding common pitfalls when psychologists become involved in screening.

Everly's contribution introduces a relatively new role for mental health professionals: occupational health psychology. He illustrates how consultants can become involved with the enhancement of physically and mentally healthy behaviors in the work place. His stepwise approach is based on a comprehensive understanding of needs in the work place.

Finally, in the third contribution to this section Dangel and Blevins offer a brief clinician's guide to selecting parent training programs. Over the past decade an increasing number of mental health professionals have become involved in offering parent training programs. At the same time there has been a steady increase in the diversity of programs which are available for this purpose. These authors suggest issues which clinicians should consider in selecting training programs and provide a short overview of several of the more popular programs.

PSYCHOLOGICAL SCREENING OF LAW ENFORCEMENT CANDIDATES

Forrest Scogin and Larry E. Beutler

The purpose of this contribution is to offer readers an overview of practices in psychological screening of law enforcement candidates. It is primarily designed for practitioners who are interested in establishing a consultative relationship with a law enforcement agency; however, practitioners already involved in psychological screening may find the contents a useful review. The following topics are covered in varying depth: the history of psychological screening of law enforcement candidates, the ethical contours of psychological consultation to law enforcement agencies, the purposes of psychological screening, the instruments and techniques widely used, the research evidence in support of the practice, and finally, a proposed assessment battery. Although our focus is on pre-employment screening, psychological evaluations are also used in promotion and retention decisions. The use of psychological screening by law enforcement agencies is increasing, so opportunities to contract with agencies for provision of this service may be available to more clinicians. It is our hope that this contribution will assist readers in mastery of this relatively new, challenging, and potentially rewarding professional activity.

HISTORY

In 1967, the President's Commission on Law Enforcement issued its report detailing abuse and unprofessional behavior on the part of law enforcement personnel. One of the recommendations of the commission was the use of psychological screening of law enforcement candidates. In 1973, the National Advisory Commission on Criminal Justice Standards also recommended psychological examination as part of the selection process for law enforcement candidates. Recommendations of this sort legitimized police psychology and opened many doors for practitioners interested in law enforcement consultation. Though the tasks of the law enforcement consultant or full-time police psychologist may be varied (Fitzhugh, 1983), the primary duty is and will probably remain psychological assessment of officer candidates. The practice of law enforcement psychological screening is still in its infancy, however, and the research and recommendations presented here reflect this state of affairs. The imprecise nature of our assessment practices makes it necessary that clinicians be aware of ethical and legal parameters in law enforcement screening. The following section presents an overview of these issues.

ETHICAL AND LEGAL ISSUES

The sharp increase in the use of psychological screening in law enforcement agencies in the past decade has led to concerns about ethical and legal standards in this field (Inwald, 1985a). The Equal Employment Opportunity Commission (EEOC) requires that hiring practices be unbiased and that selection procedures be validated. Superimposed on these requirements is the concern of many law enforcement agencies about vicarious liability. The case of *Bonsignore v. City of New York* demonstrates the risks of vicarious liability. In this case, a department was held negligent for not having conducted a psychological evaluation of an officer who subsequently shot and disabled his wife and killed himself. Thus, law enforcement agencies are caught in the dilemma of leaving themselves open for litigation whether or not they utilize psychological testing. Increasing numbers of agencies appear to be choosing the option of pre-employment psychological screening.

Practitioners who are interested or involved in psychological assessment of law enforcement candidates should be aware of the implications of denying a position to an individual based on psychological screening. Inwald (1985b) has proposed a set of guidelines for conducting pre-employment psychological screening. The guidelines are summarized here.*

1. Pre-employment psychological test results should be used as one component of the overall selection process. Psychological recommendations should not be used as the sole criterion for a hire/no hire decision.
2. A comprehensive rationale and definition of the psychological screening program's goals should be provided to the law enforcement agency. This should be developed in conjunction with administrators and guided by an appraisal of agency needs as well as the abilities of mental health specialists.
3. A rating system should be developed that provides for more than a "yes" or "no" determination of psychological suitability.
4. Both formal and informal training efforts should be made to clarify goals and psychological testing procedures for administrators.
5. Before conducting their own clinical assessments of candidates, practitioners should familiarize themselves with the specific field of psychological testing for law enforcement officers.
6. A psychological "job analysis" should be obtained by interviewing departmental personnel and/or taking survey information regarding those psychological attributes considered most important for effective officer behavior.
7. A comprehensive test battery of written psychological instruments should be administered to candidates, with the results available to psychological staff before follow-up interviews are conducted.
8. Written tests should be validated for use with law enforcement officer candidates, and the tests should be normed by sex and race. In smaller departments, data comparing populations and job requirements can be developed to support the transferability of validation studies from larger agencies.
9. Specific cutoff scores should be avoided unless such scores have been cross-validated in research studies in the agency where they will be used.
10. Written tests should be pilot tested before being adopted into a final psychological screening battery.
11. Written instruments should contain well-defined, preferably behavioral, scales and should avoid the need for largely subjective interpretation.
12. "One-on-one" follow-up interviews for all candidates should be held to properly verify written tests results and to gather additional relevant information before a final evaluative report is made.
13. A standardized, behaviorally oriented interview format should be employed, with all psychological material, including background data and test results, evaluated by interviewers in advance.
14. Core questions in the interview, including those which allow for open-ended follow-up questions, should be periodically reviewed and possibly edited so that practitioners can increase their probability of collecting the most relevant information in a limited time period.
15. While a clinical assessment of overall emotional adjustment may be made, clinical diagnoses or psychiatric labeling of candidates should be avoided when the goal is to identify those individuals whose emotional adjustment difficulties may adversely affect specific job performance.

---

*The guidelines are summarized here with permission from "Proposed Guidelines for Conducting Pre-Employment Psychological Screening Programs" by R. E. Inwald, March 18, 1985, *Crime Control Digest*, *19*, pp. 3-6. Copyright © by Washington Crime News Services.

16. Written job-related psychological reports should be prepared for each candidate tested, avoiding psychological jargon and "hospital language."
17. Administrators directly involved in making hiring decisions should be provided with full written reports and the information necessary for easy interpretation of all documents.
18. Psychologists should retain their professional consultant status, rather than performing selection tasks more appropriate for personnel officers (such as making final hiring decisions).
19. Validation efforts should be made to tie final "suitability" ratings to behavioral criteria measures (e.g., terminations, disciplinary infractions, excessive absenteeism, lateness and/or supervisory ratings, etc.).
20. If possible, base line data on critical criteria measures (such as rates of serious incidents, negative reports, etc.) should be collected for future comparisons before a psychological testing program is implemented.
21. Clear disclaimers should be made so that reports evaluating current emotional stability or suitability for a job in law enforcement will not be deemed valid after a specific period of time (such as 6 or 8 months).
22. Pre-employment test results should be used only for making pre-employment hiring decisions and doing follow-up research where individual officer identities are protected.
23. Provisions should be made for the security of all testing materials, either on or off agency premises.
24. If candidates will be denied employment based on psychological testing results, they should be allowed an opportunity to appeal negative decisions.
25. Only licensed psychologists or mental health professionals, trained and experienced in psychological test interpretation and assessment techniques, should be retained to conduct psychological screening for law enforcement agencies.
26. When mail order or computerized tests are employed, a mental health professional should be given the primary responsibility for interpreting and verifying individual results.
27. If a decision based even in part on psychological results is challenged, providers of the psychological testing services should be prepared to defend their procedures, conclusions, and recommendations.

The most important of these guidelines include the following: (a) psychological evaluation should be only one component of the selection process; (b) practitioners should become acquainted with the field of psychological screening of law enforcement candidates; (c) only licensed or certified psychologists or similarly qualified professionals should be involved in psychological screening of law enforcement candidates; and (d) practitioners should be prepared to defend their assessment practices and selection recommendations. All of these factors have a major bearing on who conducts psychological screening, the techniques used in the screening process, the type of recommendations made, and the influence these recommendations have on the final hiring decision.

PURPOSES OF EVALUATION

Two fundamentally different approaches are proposed for the use of psychological screening. One of these emanates from a base in clinical psychology and operates from three fundamental assumptions: (a) personality variables are continuing, individual characteristics that predispose one's ability to adjust to job demands; (b) disturbances of personality can occur both in terms of coping style (the individual uses an inefficient method of coping with difficulties) and coping adequacy (the individual has low stress tolerance generally); and (c) these enduring personality characteristics, more than a given task or environment, determine performance within a department.

A second approach to psychological screening emphasizes the role of the officer system and the organizational structure. This approach derives from a personnel model of fitting person to task and is also based upon three fundamental assumptions: (a) various tasks require variations in skill level, tolerances, and interests; (b) the fit of the task to the person's aptitude, more than any continuing and enduring personality traits, is likely to determine the quality of job performance; and (c) a task analysis of the particular job and environment is required to predict a desired effect.

Operating from a clinical perspective, psychologists evaluate a candidate's emotional well-being, flexibility, intellectual capacity, and available social resources through which stress might be discharged or managed (e.g., Beutler et al., 1985). The primary goal of such a psychological screening is to eliminate from consideration those candidates who have serious personality disorders, are unable to adjust to a diverse environment, and do not have available sufficient social support systems to assist them in monitoring behavior and discharging anxiety. This approach assumes that there is a core of common experiences within any given law enforcement agency and a corollary core of requisite skills. This approach also assumes that these skills are by and large emotional in nature and reflect one's flexibility. The assumption is made that the ability to perform any individual task is less important than the ability to adapt to a changing environment. Interpersonal relationships, more than aptitudes for specific activities, are seen as the determinants of job adjustment and success.

This model of psychological assessment clearly comes from a background in psychopathology. In contrast, the personnel approach to psychological screening assumes that individual tasks rather than general skills will determine the best fit and the maximal achievement. This approach comes more from a human engineering viewpoint. It attempts to assess human aptitudes and strengths in concert with the demands of specific and individualized tasks. The distinction of this viewpoint from the clinical one can be seen in the type of decisions and recommendations made. From a clinical perspective, one makes a general decision about whether or not a particular applicant is suitable to the job of police officer. From the second viewpoint, applicants are judged as suitable for a particular task within the scope of the police officer's job. A general statement is less likely to be rendered about the person's overall suitability for the role of police officer (e.g., Burkhart, 1980). The strength of the personnel model is in its ability to match particular individuals to specifically needed skills. It confronts difficulties, however, when applied to small departments in which officers must do a variety of tasks and specialization is not feasible.

Ideally, some combination of these two approaches may be recommended. Within such a comprehensive model, the most apparent and primary question may well be the candidate's initial and subsequent mental health, although the match of the candidates' strengths and weaknesses to a particular job or task may also become appropriate. The ensuing recommendations and discussions are based on the assumptions of the clinical model of law enforcement psychological screening.

The psychological assessment of a law enforcement candidate should be comprehensive and designed to address several questions, the most apparent being the candidate's mental health. More specifically, is there evidence in the assessment of a formal psychiatric disorder? This task is familiar to mental health practitioners trained in psychodiagnostic evaluation. Ruling out psychiatric disorders, however, is probably the least important function of pre-employment psychological screening. Few frankly psychotic, clinically depressed, or outright sociopathic individuals present themselves as law enforcement candidates. On the other hand, many law enforcement candidates do present with features of clinical disturbances. The task of the consultant is to ascertain the extent to which these features will interfere with effective professional behavior, which in turn is determined by the demands of the particular position.

A practitioner may choose to assess and include in a report many additional areas of functioning beyond traditional diagnostic considerations. Some areas pertinent to law enforcement work include a candidate's stress tolerance and capacity to perform under stressful conditions, general intellectual ability, likely employment stability, potential for alcohol and drug abuse, relations with authority figures and peers, and ability to be appropriately assertive. Assessment of additional topics may be useful, based upon consultation with agency administrators and analyses of the jobs that candidates will assume.

The written report of the psychological screening takes a different form than the traditional psychodiagnostic report. We recommend that summary "probability of risk" statements be made for each of the domains of functioning mentioned earlier. For example, a summary statement for employment stability might read, "This candidate presents acceptable risk in the area of job stability," or "This candidate presents moderate risk in the area of job stability." A final, overall statement of risk can be worded similarly. Unless the candidate presents obviously unconventional or inappropriate characteristics, recommendations to hire or not hire on the basis of psychological assessment should be made only as probability statements. Rather than mere subterfuge, such a reporting style reflects the accuracy of our assessment techniques and predictions.

When preparing reports, practitioners should avoid mental health jargon in favor of terminology more readily assimilated by the law enforcement administrator. Similarly, diagnostic impressions or treatment recommendations are not particularly useful or pertinent, even though evidence from the assessment may suggest one or both. Brevity is also appreciated by "bottom-line" oriented law enforcement administrators.

INSTRUMENTS AND TECHNIQUES

Deciding which among the many assessment techniques is best suited for psychological screening of law enforcement candidates is a difficult task. Murphy (1972) surveyed 203 police agencies and found that 36 different types of psychological screening procedures, ranging from the well-known Minnesota Multiphasic Personality Inventory (MMPI) to the not-so-well-known Self-Prepared Psychological Test, were in use. Clearly, no consensus existed in the Murphy (1972) survey, and it is doubtful that the situation has changed dramatically to date. Selection of assessment techniques is determined by several factors, including analysis of factors presumably related to effective job performance, time and budget constraints, and practitioner familiarity and training.

Successful pre-employment screening requires that practitioners be familiar with the agency to which they consult. This can be accomplished through conversation with administrators regarding optimal job performance and desired officer characteristics. Practitioners must also familiarize themselves with the day-to-day job demands of the positions for which they will screen candidates. Interviewing officers already on the job and accompanying officers through several shifts of work can prove invaluable in developing a feel for job demands. Any attempt to screen candidates without such preliminary fact finding is ill-advised.

As stated earlier, psychological assessments of law enforcement candidates should be comprehensive. If at all possible, the assessment should include a clinical interview. The purpose of the interview in a law enforcement psychological screening is different from that of a traditional diagnostic interview. Nonetheless, the practitioner should be alert to signs of psychopathology, particularly personality disorders. Law enforcement work seems to attract a number of individuals who exhibit high authoritarianism or excessive thrill seeking behavior, characteristics which are detrimental to law enforcement work. A set of standard interview questions is recommended to insure comparability of assessment data. If it is possible to conduct the assessment in two sessions, the practitioner may use the results of the objective measures to guide the clinical interview. Deviant responses to the paper-and-pencil measures should be corroborated through the clinical interview. Questions about potentially damaging aspects of a candidate's behavior need be carefully worded; for example, the question, "How much do you usually drink when you have something to drink?" is more likely to elicit useful information than the question, "Do you drink alcohol?"

In addition to a clinical interview, we recommend a paper-and-pencil assessment of personality in screening law enforcement candidates. The MMPI is the most frequently used instrument of this sort (Murphy, 1972). However, the MMPI should never be used as the sole measure of psychological functioning, nor should a candidate be denied employment solely on the basis of deviant responses to the MMPI. Understandably, most candidates approach the MMPI somewhat guardedly. If the validity of the results is questionable, discussion of response style with the candidate and readministration is an option that the authors have used.

Several studies have examined the utility of the MMPI in predicting officer performance. Saxe and Reiser (1976) found that MMPI scores differentiated officers who continued from those who separated from the Los Angeles Police Department. However, these authors also note that both groups fall within "normal" ranges on the scale, thus limiting the utility of the MMPI in predicting subsequent officer performance. Beutler et al. (1985) found significant associations between several individual MMPI and composite scale scores and officer performance. For example, these investigators found significant positive correlations between candidate MMPI Depression scale scores and subsequent supervisor rated technical proficiency. The danger of using one instrument in screening is demonstrated by a similar significant positive correlation between Depression scale scores and grievances lodged against the officers by citizens. Perhaps the most useful empirical finding of this study is the significant positive correlation between candidate's mean MMPI scale elevation and subsequent officer suspensions. Thus, the MMPI appears to possess some predictive validity. Unfortunately, establishment of cutoff scores with adequate sensitivity and specificity has not been achieved.

Some consultants have questioned the use of the MMPI for screening law enforcement candidates. The most common criticism is that although the MMPI was developed for use with clinical populations, law enforcement screening usually involves assessing nonpathological populations. An instrument that can be used in lieu of or in conjunction with the MMPI is the Inwald Personality Inventory (IPI; Inwald, Knatz, & Shusman, 1982). The IPI is a 310 true-false item instrument which yields 26 separate scales, designed specifically for assessment of law enforcement officers. Four content areas are included in the IPI, designed to measure validity, "acting out," internalized conflict, and interpersonal conflict. Inwald and her colleagues have published several studies reporting the predictive validity of the IPI (Inwald & Shusman, 1984; Shusman, Inwald, & Landa, 1984). The IPI appears to be gaining popularity among police psychology practitioners, though many will probably continue to use the MMPI due to familiarity and convenience.

Other paper-and-pencil personality inventories used by law enforcement consultants include the California Psychological Inventory (CPI), the 16 Personality Factors Questionnaire (16 PF), and the Eysenck Personality Inventory (EPI). Because these inventories have not been evaluated as extensively as the MMPI and the IPI, practitioners interested in using them may wish to consider small-scale validation studies within their own agencies.

In addition to a measure of general personality functioning, many practitioners include an assessment of specific psychiatric symptomatology in their screenings. The Symptom Checklist (SCL-90; Derogatis, Rickels, & Rock, 1976) is a 90-item instrument widely used by mental health practitioners and researchers. This instrument is useful for assessing the level of distress and stress tolerance among law enforcement candidates.

General intellectual functioning should also be assessed. Often, agencies will have required candidates to pass a civil service type examination prior to psychological screening. Nonetheless, a brief screening of intelligence provides useful information. We have used the Shipley Institute of Living Scale (Shipley, 1940) for this purpose. The measures of verbal intelligence and abstraction provide indices of relative cognitive strengths and weaknesses. Below or well above average scores on intelligence scales merit attention; well below average scores bring into question the candidate's ability to handle the intellectual demands of law enforcement work, but well above average intelligence may lead to dissatisfaction with the duties of law enforcement or difficulties in adjustment to law enforcement administrative practices.

The candidate's ability to get along with the public, peers, and authority figures is an essential component of effective law enforcement performance, and thus merits assessment. Data from the clinical interview and the paper-and-pencil personality measure will provide some information on this dimension of functioning. We have found inclusion of a specific instrument to assess interpersonal style a useful component of an assessment battery. The Fundamental Interpersonal Relations Orientation Scale (FIRO; Schutz, 1958) assesses three normally occurring interpersonal needs: inclusion, affection, and control. Each of these needs is further divided into willingness to be receptive to that need in others and to the desire to express that need towards others. Scores on this instrument can aid in prediction of an individual's interpersonal functioning. For example, Beutler et al. (1985) found significant positive correlations between candidates' expressed affection scores and supervisors' subsequent ratings of their interpersonal ability as officers. Wanted control, on the other hand, was negatively correlated with rated interpersonal ability.

Many other instruments have been or could be used in psychological screening of law enforcement candidates. Unfortunately, little research has been done that examines the predictive validity of many of these psychological screening techniques. A review of existing studies follows.

RESEARCH ON PSYCHOLOGICAL SCREENING OF LAW ENFORCEMENT CANDIDATES

The primary test of the utility of psychological screening of law enforcement candidates is predictive validity. That is, do individuals judged more likely to do poorly in law enforcement work on the basis of psychological evaluation indeed perform more poorly? Establishing the predictive validity of psychological screening techniques is an exceedingly difficult task. Burkhart (1980) and Inwald (1985a) have discussed at length the inherent difficulties in establishing predictive validity. For example, the establishment of relevant criteria by which to judge success is problematic. Ratings by supervisors appear to be biased in many cases (Beutler et al., 1985; Fitzhugh, 1983). Also, many behaviors that are blatantly inappropriate, such as abuse of deadly force, rarely occur. Another major impediment is the necessity of eliminating from candidacy those individuals who perform poorly on the psychological evaluation. It is ethically and legally questionable to allow apparently psychologically unfit candidates to assume law enforcement positions. From a research validation perspective, however, eliminating individuals with poor scores or performance restricts the range and limits the establishment of predictive validity. Although these difficulties are not insurmountable, they have limited the number of effective predictive validity studies.

Spielberger, Spaulding, Jolley, and Ward (1979) examined the validity of a number of personality and demographic variables in predicting officer performance. These researchers established as their criterion the success or failure of the officer at 1 year of service. Success was defined as satisfactory performance or rehirability, whereas failure was defined as unrehirability or failing to pass the police academy. The CPI discriminated between successes and failures, with successes more likely to have high scores. Four demographic or biographical items also distinguished the two groups: Successful officers were more likely to report (a) participation in high school athletics, (b) fewer family moves, (c) less need for job encouragement, and (d) higher needs for achievement and societal contributions.

Saxe and Reiser (1976) compared the MMPI scores of a group of successful police applicants to the scores of a group of applicants who passed the psychological screening but later separated from the department. Although statistically significant, the differences in the two groups' scores are quite small, and inspection of the group profiles reveals little configural variation. Nonetheless, as Saxe and Reiser (1976) conclude, "the significant statistical differences between the groups may reveal specific attributes which relate to success on the job" (p. 424).

Inwald and her colleagues have conducted several predictive validity studies on personality and psychological functioning measures. Shusman et al. (1984) compared the validity of the MMPI and the IPI in predicting correction officer job performance. Success and failure were categorized in a fashion similar to that employed by Saxe and Reiser (1976). If still on the job after 1 year, one was a success; if terminated, one was a failure. Shusman et al., using discriminate function analysis, found that the IPI correctly predicted 73% of the retained-terminated officers, while the MMPI correctly identified 63%. In terms of actual job performance, as indicated by absenteeism, lateness, and disciplinary interviews, the IPI and MMPI were almost identical in their discriminatory power, with correct identification in the 50% to 60% range. These results suggest that the IPI and MMPI are viable instruments for the assessment of law enforcement candidates, but that the use of a single instrument or technique is unlikely to yield data of sufficient breadth to predict the multifaceted behavior demanded in law enforcement work.

Beutler et al. (1985) examined the predictive validity of a battery of psychological assessment techniques. Three police departments were included in the study: a university police department, a community college police department, and an inner-city police department. Officers were assessed on several psychological instruments, including the MMPI, the EPI, the FIRO-B, the Shipley Institute of Living Scale, the SCL-90, and the Bender-Gestalt (Bender, 1938). Variables to be predicted included supervisory ratings of interpersonal ability and technical proficiency, and personnel record documentation of vehicular reprimands, force reprimands, participation in continuing education, commendations, grievances, suspensions, and referrals to counseling. Psychological assessment variables were significantly associated with the supervisory ratings of interpersonal ability and technical proficiency. Psychological evaluation data were also significantly associated with the personnel record variables. The ability of any one of the instruments used alone in this study to predict officer performance, however, was quite poor. Nonetheless, taken collectively, the results of psychological assessment techniques designed to tap varied facets of functioning accurately predicted much of officers' subsequent professional behavior. Despite the overall predictive power of the battery used in this study, commendations and participation in continuing education, two positive indices, were not predicted by psychological assessment data. As stated earlier, our ability to predict job performance at present seems to be in the area of negative performance. We can screen out those who are likely to do poorly, but we cannot predict who will be exemplary officers.

RECOMMENDED PROCEDURES

The procedures to be followed in conducting psychological screening of law enforcement candidates will vary depending upon the department one serves. Fitzhugh (1983) provides useful suggestions for establishing and maintaining consultation with law enforcement agencies. We bypass contractual considerations involved in psychological screening and move to procedures to be implemented with candidates.

It is recommended that informed consent be obtained from all candidates prior to psychological assessment. The consent form may include statements delimiting confidentiality, the purposes of the evaluation, and the possible use of assessment data in research. The assessment itself should include both paper-and-pencil measures and an in-depth clinical interview. Where feasible, the written instruments should be completed by the candidate in an initial sitting, and the results of these measures should be used to guide the practitioner in the conduct of the subsequent interview.

When the assessment is completed, a written report should be prepared. The report should identify strengths and weaknesses of the candidate relevant to the performance of the particular job that he or she seeks. Diagnostic labels should be avoided, as should outright recommendations to hire or not hire. Probability statements for each of the identified areas of officer performance are recommended instead. A sample report outline is provided on page 326.

Decisions about who shall have access to the psychological screening report should be made in consultation with agency administrators. The period of time for which the assessment results are considered to be valid should also be made clear. Six months to a year is a reasonable time frame. Finally, candidates should be given feedback on the results of their psychological assessment, whether or not they are subsequently hired.

PROPOSED COMPONENTS OF A
PSYCHOLOGICAL SCREENING BATTERY
FOR LAW ENFORCEMENT CANDIDATES

Following are proposed components of a screening battery for law enforcement candidates. Recommendations for specific instruments are made, with the choice of instrument at the discretion of the individual practitioner.

1. *Background Information* - Information regarding history of the candidate's family, education, marital experience, employment, and drug and alcohol use, arrests, and so forth. A form used by the authors is presented on pages 327-328.

2. *Personality Inventory* - A measure of the candidate's general personality style and functioning, including current distress level, interpersonal style, energy level, suspiciousness, and sociopathy. The MMPI and the IPI appear to be the instruments of choice on this dimension, though some practitioners may prefer the CPI, EPI, of 16 PF.

3. *Intellectual Functioning* - A brief assessment of intellectual functioning is recommended. A full-blown intellectual assessment is not recommended due to time constraints. A selected subtest or two of the Wechsler Adult Intelligence Scale-Revised (Wechsler, 1981), such as Vocabulary or Information, may be used. The Shipley Institute of Living Scale is another brief instrument that assesses intelligence.

4. *Symptomatic Distress Level* - A measure of the candidate's specific symptomatology, such as the presence of phobias, interpersonal sensitivity, somatization, psychoticism, hostility, or anxiety. The SCL-90 appears to be the instrument of choice in this assessment.

5. *Interpersonal Style* - This area of functioning may be adequately assessed by the MMPI or IPI, but we recommend additional assessment of this most important component of effective law enforcement behavior. The FIRO-B has been used by the authors to assess a candidate's expressed and wanted control, inclusion, and affection.

6. *Clinical Interview* - This most important component of the assessment may include inquiries related to the results of the written assessments as well as standard interview questions.

SUMMARY

Psychological screening of law enforcement candidates is a challenging task. Practitioners trained to assess in clinic and hospital settings are asked to apply their expertise to a nonpathological group and to make difficult predictions. Despite its complexity, the importance of accurate screening cannot be overemphasized. Law enforcement personnel are given a badge and a gun, two devices easily abused. The consequences of inaccurate or nonexistent assessment can, therefore, be extremely detrimental. Unfortunately, our assessment practices are not precise. We have presented research that suggests that psychological evaluation data can predict, albeit not powerfully, the future performance of law enforcement candidates. Dedication on the part of psychologists to validate screening procedures will continue to open the doors of law enforcement agencies to psychological expertise. Accurate screening of law enforcement candidates should be a goal of both police and psychologists as well as a societal necessity.

LAW ENFORCEMENT CANDIDATE EVALUATION

NAME: DATE:

AGE: REFERRANT:

REASON FOR REFERRAL:

ASSESSMENT TECHNIQUES:

BACKGROUND AND PROBABLE JOB STABILITY:

COGNITIVE FUNCTIONING AND JUDGMENT:

INTERPERSONAL AND PEER RELATIONSHIPS:

AUTHORITY RELATIONSHIPS AND LEADERSHIP:

SUMMARY:

BACKGROUND INFORMATION

Name____

Sex________________ Age________________ Last grade of school completed____________________________

Highest diploma or degree earned____

Are you currently married?___________________________ How long?_______________________________

How many times have you been married?____

How many children do you have?____

How many times have you and your spouse separated?____

Are you now separated?___________________________ What's the worst thing about your marriage?________________

____

What is your current employment?____

Position?____

How long have you been employed in your current job?____

Since high school, how many full-time jobs have you held?____

What were they and for how long?

    1. ____

    2. ____

    3. ____

    4. ____

    5. ____

    6. ____

    7. ____

    8. ____

    9. ____

    10. ____

Have you ever been fired from a job?___________________________ Explain______________________________

____

How many times have you been charged with a legal violation (exclude traffic offenses)?___________________

What were the charges and approximate dates?

    1. ____

    2. ____

    3. ____

    4. ____

    5. ____

How many traffic violations have you received in the past 3 years?_______________________________

    For what?____

Where did you grow up?____

What did your father do?____

What did your mother do?____

How many different houses did you live in before you turned 16?_______________________________

Were your parents ever divorced?______________________ Why?_________________________________

____

Who did you live with?____

Did either of your parents have a drinking problem?____

How many times was your mother married?____

How many times was your father married?____

Have you ever been in the armed forces?____

Which branch?____

When discharged?______________________ What type?____

What type of disciplinary action did you receive?____

Highest rank obtained?____

Are you taking any medications?______________________ What?_________________________________

What have you been hospitalized for?

    1. ____ Date_______________________________

    2. ____ Date_______________________________

    3. ____ Date_______________________________

How did you do in school?____

What kind of trouble did you get in as a kid?____

____

Why do you want to be a law enforcement officer?____

____

____

____

Forrest Scogin, PhD, is currently Assistant Professor of Psychology at the University of Alabama in Tuscaloosa. Prior to his present position, he was a Post-Doctoral Fellow at the University of Arizona in Tucson. His training is in clinical psychology and his other interests include clinical geropsychology and psychotherapy research. Dr. Scogin may be contacted at the Department of Psychology, University of Alabama, University, AL 35486.

Larry E. Beutler, PhD, is currently Professor of Psychiatry and Psychology, Chief of Clinical Psychology Programs, and Director of Clinical Research within the Department of Psychiatry at the University of Arizona. Dr. Beutler has been a consultant to the Texas Department of Corrections, Houston Police Department, University of Arizona Police Department, South Tucson Police Department, and Pima College Police Department. He is also Associate Editor of the *Journal of Consulting and Clinical Psychology* and serves on the review boards of numerous professional journals. He received his training in clinical psychology from the University of Nebraska-Lincoln and served on the faculties of Duke University Medical School, Stephen F. Austin State University, and Baylor College of Medicine prior to assuming his current position. He has published approximately 200 articles and papers and is the author or co-author of four books. Dr. Beutler can be contacted at the Department of Psychiatry, University of Arizona College of Medicine, Tucson, AZ 85724.

RESOURCES

Bender, L. (1938). *A Visual Motor Gestalt Test and Its Clinical Use* (Research Monograph No. 3). New York: American Orthopsychiatric Association.

Beutler, L. E., Storm, A. Kirkish, P., Scogin, F., & Gaines, J. A. (1985). Parameters in the prediction of police officer performance. *Professional Psychology, 16,* 324-335.

Bonsignore v. City of New York. (1981, September 14). 78-0240, in *New York Law Journal.*

Burkhart, B. R. (1980). Conceptual issues in the development of police selection procedures. *Professional Psychology, 11,* 121-129.

Derogatis, L. R., Rickels, K., & Rock, A. F. (1976). The SCL-90 and the MMPI: A step in the validation of a new self-report scale. *British Journal of Psychiatry, 128,* 280-289.

Fitzhugh, W. P. (1983). New roles in consultation with police. In P. A. Keller & L. G. Ritt (Eds.), *Innovations in Clinical Practice: A Source Book* (Vol. 3, pp. 371-387). Sarasota, FL: Professional Resource Exchange, Inc.

Inwald, R. E. (1985). Administrative, legal, and ethical practices in the psychological testing of law enforcement officers. *Journal of Criminal Justice, 13,* 367-372. (a)

Inwald, R. E. (1985). Proposed guidelines for conducting pre-employment psychological screening programs. *Crime Control Digest, 19,* 1-6. (b)

Inwald, R., Knatz, H., & Shusman, E. (1982). *The Inwald Personality Inventory Manual.* New York: Hilson.

Inwald, R. E., & Shusman, E. J. (1984). Personality and performance sex differences of law enforcement officer recruits. *Journal of Police Science and Administration, 12,* 339-347.

Murphy, J. J. (1972). Current practices in the use of psychological testing by police agencies. *Journal of Criminal Law, Criminology and Police Science, 63,* 570-576.

Saxe, S. J., & Reiser, M. (1976). A comparison of three police applicant groups using the MMPI. *Journal of Police Science and Administration, 4,* 419-425.

Schutz, W. C. (1958). *The Interpersonal Underworld.* Palo Alto, CA: Science and Behavior Books.

Shipley, W. C. (1940). A self-administered scale for measuring intellectual impairment and deterioration. *Journal of Psychology, 9,* 371-377.

Shusman, E. J., Inwald, R. E., & Landa, B. (1984). Correction officer job performance as predicted by the IPI and MMPI: A validation and cross-validation study. *Criminal Justice and Behavior, 11,* 309-329.

Spielberger, C. D., Spaulding, H. C., Jolley, M. T., & Ward, J. C. (1979). Selection of effective law enforcement officers: The Florida Police Standards Project. In C. D.

Spielberger (Ed.), *Police Selection and Evaluation: Issues and Techniques* (pp. 231-251). New York: Praeger.

Wechsler, D. (1981). *Wechsler Adult Intelligence Scale-Revised: Manual.* New York: Psychological Corporation.

INSTRUMENTS

Fundamental Interpersonal Relations Orientation - Behavior (FIRO-B). A brief inventory measuring six dimensions of behavior toward others, which can be administered in about 20 minutes. Available from Consulting Psychologist Press, Inc., 577 College Avenue, P. O. Box 11636, Palo Alto, CA 94306. Phone: (415) 857-1444.

Inwald Personality Inventory (IPI). Available from Hilson Research, Inc., 119-19 83rd Avenue, Kew Gardens, NY 11415.

Shipley Institute of Living Scale. A brief test assessing vocabulary and abstract thinking which can be administered in about 20 minutes. Available from Western Psychological Services, 12031 Wilshire Boulevard, Los Angeles, CA 90025. Phone: (213) 478-2061.

Symptom Checklist-90-Revised (SCL-90-R). A 90-item, self-report, symptom checklist which can be administered in about 15 minutes. Available from Clinical Psychometric Research, 1228 Wine Spring Lane, Towson, MD 21204. Phone: (301) 321-6165.

AN INTRODUCTION TO OCCUPATIONAL HEALTH PSYCHOLOGY

George S. Everly, Jr.

> "Even the most cost-conscious society should recognize that
> money spent on human capital is the single most important
> investing it can make." - *Newsweek*, October 18, 1982

The American culture has entered a new age - the "Age of Health Promotion." In this age, prevention is considered as important as treatment, and lifestyle and health-related behavior patterns are viewed as the quintessential points of intervention for affecting human health status. The work place, where most adults spend at least one-third of their lives, is considered by many as an ideal setting within which to promote health through programs designed to affect lifestyle and health behavior. In this contribution I provide a brief rationale for the development of behavioral technologies for health promotion, examine the current status of occupational health psychology, propose one such intervention model, and finally, make some recommendations for the training of occupational health psychologists.

A RATIONALE FOR OCCUPATIONAL HEALTH PSYCHOLOGY

Before developing a rationale for the existence of occupational health psychology programs, it seems useful to introduce the reader to the concept of occupational health psychology itself. Occupational health psychology is a specialized field of application of the larger discipline of health psychology (Division 39 of the American Psychological Association). Briefly stated, health psychology is dedicated to the application of psychological theories, principles, and practices to the prevention, diagnosis, treatment, and rehabilitation of physical disease and dysfunction. Occupational health psychology, then, is the practice of health psychology relating to, or in the context of, the occupational milieu.

There is much to support the existence of health psychology in general, and more specifically, occupational health psychology. Table 1 on the next page demonstrates that lifestyle is the single most important factor contributing to the 10 leading causes of death prior to age 75. Public health scholar Lawrence Green argues that lifestyle/behavior is the main determinant of human health in the United States. He states:

> Behavior influences health directly through preventative health behavior and lifestyle in general. The environment is behaviorally influenced through social action and through peoples' exposure of themselves to the environmental risks. The effect of medical care on health depends on illness behavior and sick-role behavior, the appropriate utilization of services, and the effective following of medical regimens. (Green, 1981, p. 20)

TABLE 1: ESTIMATED CONTRIBUTION FOR FOUR FACTORS TO THE 10 LEADING CAUSES OF DEATH, AGES 1 TO 75 (EXPRESSED IN PERCENT)

Causes of Death	Factors			
	Lifestyle/ Behavior	Environment	Biology	Medical Care
Heart Disease	54	9	25	12
Cancer	37	24	29	10
Motor Vehicle Accidents	69	18	1	12
Other Accidents	51	31	4	14
Stroke	50	22	21	7
Homicide	63	35	2	0
Suicide	60	35	2	3
Cirrhosis	70	9	18	3
Influenza/Pneumonia	23	20	39	18
Diabetes	34	0	60	6
All 10 Causes Combined	51	20	19	10

From <u>Ten Leading Causes of Death in the United States</u> by the U.S. Center for Disease Control, 1980, Washington, DC: USDHHS.

According to Stephen Weiss (1985):

> Since 1900, we have seen an increase of 20 years in the lifespan of the average American. However, a close inspection of these figures reveals that the major changes have taken place during the childhood years, the result of immunization, penicillin, and other pharmacologic discoveries to combat the acute infectious diseases. For the 45-year old male, however, the increase in life span since 1900 has amounted to only about three years. Thus, the progress toward ameliorating the effects of the chronic degenerative disease has left much to be desired. (p. x)

Table 1 illustrates that the leading cause of the chronic degenerative diseases described by Weiss is lifestyle. John Knowles (1977) offers a cogent summary by stating "... over 99% of us are born healthy and suffer premature death and disability only as a result of personal misbehavior and environmental conditions" (p. 58).

Thus we see a rationale for attending to lifestyle as an important determinant of health status. Furthermore, by virtue of education and training, no discipline is better prepared to help change behavior than professional psychology.

Why employ the occupational environment as a vehicle for addressing issues of health-related behavior/lifestyle? Consider the following:

1. This country's health care costs are estimated to exceed $300 billion, and the cost is increasing by about 10% to 12% each year. Furthermore, American corporations will pay over 25% of these costs - an amount roughly equivalent to 10% of their operating budgets (American Institute of Certified Public Accountants, 1981).
2. Alcoholism increases employee absenteeism by 2.5 times and increases the accident rate by 3 to 5 times (National Chamber Foundation, 1978).
3. Smoking two packs of cigarettes a day doubles the absenteeism rate among such smokers (National Chamber Foundation, 1978).
4. Smoking is thought to contribute to 325,000 premature deaths each year. The cost of recruiting replacements for executives lost to heart disease alone is estimated to be $700 million per year (Goldberg, 1978).
5. Finally, according to the National Chamber Foundation Report (1978):

> The workplace may be a setting particularly well-suited to effective and widespread health promotion programs. Through the programs, business can help employees and their families achieve and maintain better health. The programs have the potential to benefit not only the individual participants, but also the sponsoring company. (p. ix)

In summary, it is clear that employers have a vested interest in the health status and health-related behavior of their employees. Business and industry pay over 25% of this nation's health care costs. Furthermore, most corporations' health insurance premiums are "experience rated," that is, the more claims filed, the higher the subsequent insurance premium. Obviously, greater corporation operating costs lower profits. Employees will spend one-third of their lives in the work place. For many, it is the hub of their social existence; it can be the hub of their quest for health as well (see Cohen, 1985).

CURRENT STATUS OF
OCCUPATIONAL HEALTH PSYCHOLOGY

Apparently, as a response to the statistics cited in the previous section, promotion of occupational health has become increasingly prevalent. The beginning of the current thrust can be traced back to the mid 1970s. It was then that several large corporations began serious occupational health promotion initiatives. Today, companies such as Kimberly-Clark, IBM, Control Data, and Johnson & Johnson lead the field in sophisticated health promotion programs. It has been estimated that as many as 1500 companies currently have such programs in operation (Weiss, 1985).

Corporate programs come in diverse forms. A traditional program might have the following elements:

1. Before entering any form of intervention program, employees are usually screened (although this function can be free-standing, not necessarily in preface to intervention programs). Health screening might include a behavioral health risk appraisal, general medical examination, blood analysis, treadmill EKG, vision and audiometry examinations, and perhaps a readiness-for-physical-exercise evaluation. Depending on the scope of the program, psychological status may be assessed, as well.
2. After the screening is complete, employees are usually counseled concerning the findings. Specific recommendations about personal health promotion are then made by a health educator or counselor.
3. Following the health and risk factor counseling session, employees may be referred to health resources in the community, or they may take advantage of in-house health promotion programs. Typical programs include: (a) smoking cessation, (b) stress management, (c) physical exercise/aerobics, (d) weight control, (e) cardiovascular hypertension screening and management, (f) accident prevention (especially back injury prevention), (g) nutrition education, and (h) psychological services. Psychological services may or may not be part of the traditional health promotion effort.

The above may be referred to as a traditional "modular" intervention approach. Everly and Feldman (1985) reviewed such an approach to health promotion at the work site. In their review the structure and effectiveness of various programs and modules was examined. They discovered a variety of approaches with varying rates of participation and success. They concluded that multidimensional interventions, regardless of the target problem, appear to have the greatest potential for lasting success, as opposed to unidimensional modular formulations.

It is important to consider the financial impact of such programs upon the corporation's balance sheet. In other words, are these programs cost effective? Historically, there seemed to be an implicit assumption that a favorable financial return on health promotion efforts would naturally be forthcoming. Or, if financial justification for such programs could not be demonstrated, such efforts seemed justifiable from a humanitarian perspective. The harsh reality may be that if interest rates skyrocket again, or if corporate resources diminish, health promotion efforts at the work site may be endangered. Useful reviews of the financial aspects of health promotion can be found in studies by Spencer (1984), Hollander, Lengermann, and DeMuth (1985), and Smith, Haight, and Everly (1986).

Some preliminary data on program effectiveness exist and are encouraging: In 1979, a survey of 34 companies that had established physical fitness programs revealed that 60% of these programs were estimated to yield a return greater than the costs of the program (Olive & Kirkpatrick, 1982). Companies such as Equitable Life Assurance, Campbell Soup, and New York Telephone have offered dollar estimations of return-on-investment. Some estimates are as high as 6 to 1 return on dollars invested (Berry, 1981). Others claimed such benefits decreased turnover, lowered medical utilization, decreased absenteeism, increased productivity, and improved public image. These claims are clearly preliminary and, to a degree, speculative. Currently there is a dearth of reliable cost benefit data on the utility of such programs. Nor have major changes in absenteeism, productivity, and morale been reliably demonstrated. Part of the difficulty in generating such data is the traditional "modular" approach to program development. In the next section, an alternative approach to program development is described.

A "SYSTEMS CONSULTATION" APPROACH TO OCCUPATIONAL HEALTH PSYCHOLOGY

Traditionally, corporate management has defined the health-behavior problems to be served by narrow-focus programs, such as smoking cessation and stress management programs. Such modular approaches have typically assumed that (a) health-related behavior is unidimensional, and therefore is most responsive to pre-packaged, narrowly defined, unidimensional interventions; (b) modular unitary focus interventions are unidimensional; (c) corporate managers have correctly assessed employees' needs; (d) corporate managers have correctly identified the appropriate form of intervention to meet their needs; (e) corporate managers are capable of effectively communicating their needs and expectations to the individual(s) responsible for health promotion program development; and (f) managers' expectations for success are reasonable and congruent with current capabilities and resources (adapted from Schein, 1969). These are dangerously unreliable assumptions.

Many corporate managers simply do not understand what health promotion is, or how it can be achieved. Furthermore, they seldom appreciate the costs associated with such efforts or how they can accurately measure success. To remedy these problems, a different approach to the development of occupational health psychology programs was created. This approach will be referred to as a "systems consultation" model.

The fundamental goal in the development of the systems consultation model was to create a model for program development that would be sensitive to the environment, needs, and expectations of differing organizations and their respective managements. In achieving such a goal, it is clear that managerial satisfaction with behavioral outcome, as well as cost effectiveness, can be maximized.

The systems consultation model is based on a model of organizational development activities known as process consultation. As used in the present context, it refers to the collaborative efforts of the health promotion team and corporate management to achieve the desired health promotion outcome. In this model, those responsible for health promotion program development, whether external consultants or salaried corporate staff, assume the role of health behavior consultants to corporate management and policy makers. The steps in the systems consultation model are described below.

STEP 1

The individual(s) responsible for the development of the occupational health promotion initiative meet with management personnel to identify (a) perceived needs associated with employee health-related behavior; (b) implicit expectations for outcome; and (c) explicit goals for the health promotion program.

This process, in its ideal form, is a collaborative exchange. The four most common generic goals associated with occupational health promotion efforts are (a) increased employee satisfaction; (b) decreased employee morbidity; (c) decreased health-related costs; and (d) increased productivity.

STEP 2

Perform a microanalysis of the respective constituents of each respective goal.

1. To increase employee satisfaction, it is necessary to determine, from the employees, the relative degree of *desirability* that work site health promotion programs would have and specifically what types of programs they would *utilize*.
2. It is important to identify the most common causes of employee morbidity that are amenable to behavioral alteration.
3. It is critically important to identify the *actual* sources of health-care dollar expenditure, rather than simply to make assumptions based upon national, community, or industry averages.
4. The *actual* sources of productivity erosion that may be amenable to health-related behavioral intervention must be identified. The most common variables in this category are absenteeism and turnover.

STEP 3

Formulate the outcome variables that will be used to assess the relative success of the intervention. The formulation of these variables depends upon the preceding microanalysis and goal identification. Appropriate measurement techniques must be used. Satisfaction questionnaires and program utilization statistics may be employed to assess employee satisfaction. Health records and medical utilization reports may be used to assess employee morbidity. Various financial models and insurance fees may be used to assess health-related cost as an outcome variable. See Smith et al. (1986) for a review of this issue. Finally, absenteeism, turnover, or general unit productivity statistics may be used to assess productivity as an outcome variable.

STEP 4

Design and implement a health promotion program specifically based upon the preceding steps. Community resources, external consultants, and in-house personnel and programs represent potential resources.

STEP 5

Conduct assessment of outcome variables using the methods generated in Step 3.

STEP 6

This final phase of the systems consultation model provides the opportunity to return to any of the previous five phases or to continue with longitudinal follow-up.

The systems consultation model of occupational health behavior program development is graphically summarized in Table 2 (p. 336). This model is designed to be flexible and dynamic enough to meet the idiosyncratic needs of each organization in which it is employed. Such an approach maximizes goal attainment as well as cost effectiveness. The systems consultation model is based upon collaboration between health professionals and management personnel to best meet the needs of the organization.

In the final sections of this contribution, the professional preparation of the occupational health psychologist will be discussed.

A CASE EXAMPLE

The author was asked to create a stress management program for a large entertainment and tourist-oriented business concern. Employees typically worked four or five 12-hour shifts a week, and it was not uncommon for management personnel to work 60 to 100 hours a week. Top management was well aware of the excessive stress placed

---

**TABLE 2:   THE "SYSTEMS CONSULTATION" MODEL OF OCCUPATIONAL
HEALTH PROMOTION PROGRAM DEVELOPMENT**

```
Step 1 - Collaborative Consultation for Goal Formation
Step 2 - Microanalysis of Goal Constituency
Step 3 - Formulation of Outcome Measurements
Step 4 - Program Design and Implementation
Step 5 - Assessment
Step 6 - Reformulation or Follow-Up
```

---

upon its employees and wanted to provide some corporate-sponsored support. A simplistic and naïve remedy to this problem would be to shorten working hours or hire more employees. However, it was considered highly desirable to be employed by this corporation, where front line employees who dealt directly with customers could easily earn $50,000 to $80,000 per year with only a high school education. Management personnel could earn over $100,000 per year. Much of the stress upon these workers was a self-driven desire to achieve; the long hours and stressful conditions were considered part of the job and endemic to the industry.

STEP 1

I met with top-level management to discuss the nature of the problem and to solicit from them any pre-conceived notions of how the problem could be dealt with. Management informed me that "stress" was the problem, although they were not sure what that meant operationally. They knew that their employees were prime candidates for "burn out" and that the job placed significant pressures on their employees' home lives. Similarly, many employees were showing signs of stress-related diseases. It was decided that decreased employee morbidity would be the outcome variable for the health promotion intervention.

STEP 2

The next step was to determine what types of morbidity should constitute the goal. General health complaints would serve as the major constituent. Implicit in such a decision was the recognition that excessive stress could play a contributing role in a host of physical and psychiatric complaints.

STEP 3

Having accepted general health as the variable in need of improvement, the next step was to formulate outcome measures. We decided to use professional health care utilization as our outcome measure. Previous health-care utilization data were available from this self-insured company. Such data were retrospectively used to establish a 2-year pre-intervention base line.

STEP 4

The next step was to meet individually with each of 42 department heads to gather historical and background information. On-site observation was also utilized. On the basis of the previous steps, a two-stage intervention was designed and implemented. In the initial stage, a series of information-oriented seminars provided each employee with a several hour introduction to the nature of stress and potential remedies. In the second stage, an in-house employee assistance program was developed. Community resources were also mobilized in the effort.

STEP 5

The 1-year outcome data are now being collected and analyzed.

STEP 6

On the basis of the initial outcome data, alterations of the existing program will be considered.

TRAINING THE OCCUPATIONAL HEALTH PSYCHOLOGIST

The traditionally trained psychologist is simply not prepared to function effectively in the occupational health promotion environment. Typically, counseling or clinical psychologists are best prepared to enter this field, yet their training typically needs augmentation.

My experience suggests that the professional best suited for work in this arena is a hybrid. These individuals will have been trained in (a) counseling or clinical psychology, (b) business administration or industrial psychology, (c) medical physiology, and (d) public health or health education. Careful analysis of the occupational health promotion environment reveals that promoting behavior health at the work site represents a blending of these four professions. Thus, occupational health psychology may represent a post-doctoral specialty. At the present time, I know of no such formalized training programs. Rather, the interested student must prepare him or herself to enter this field through a conscious blending of these respective disciplines. Once accomplished, however, such professionals may represent a formidable professional resource both to private and public sectors.

SUMMARY AND RECOMMENDATIONS

In the year 1900, the leading causes of death in the United States were the infectious diseases. In the 1980s, the leading causes of death are the chronic degenerative diseases. In the early 1900s, our approach to the amelioration of such diseases was based upon the "one germ - one disease" model promulgated by Pasteur. While appropriate then, it no longer seems reasonable to attack the chronic degenerative diseases of the 1980s with this reductionistic, mechanistic mentality. Yet it may be argued that using the traditional modular approach to health promotion is analogous to using the "one germ - one disease" approach to amelioration of disease. Both systems typically see a unitary problem and a unitary solution, unclouded by the realities of inter-relationships and synergy. This contribution has provided the reader with a brief rationale for occupational health psychology and has briefly described a dynamic and flexible systems consultation model of occupational health promotion.

I have further argued that the professional best suited to provide and develop occupational health promotion activities is clearly the behavioral scientist. Ideally, such professionals would have a strong background in basic counseling as well as training in medical physiology, health education, and business administration. While I know of no such programs, the training of the clinical health psychologist as conducted in the psychology departments of the University of Miami in Florida and the University of Oregon Medical School are highly desirable approximations, needing only the opportunity to acquire practical business and human resource development experience.

As for the work site itself, what better place to promote health? It is generally believed that education alone is insufficient to create lasting alterations in health behavior. Rather, it appears as if behavioral technologies must be brought to bear upon the health-eroding patterns many Americans pursue. The work site may well serve as an ideal forum for the structuring and implementation of such behaviorally based programs.

Finally, preliminary data indicate that occupational health promotion efforts are positive additions to the work site. It remains to be seen if they are truly cost effective. All in all, the future looks promising. If, as some have suggested, health psychology is the psychology of the future, then occupational health psychology may well be the business of the future.

George S. Everly, Jr., PhD, is currently Director of the Psychophysiology and Health Psychology Laboratory at Loyola College in Maryland. He received his PhD in 1978 from the University of Maryland and received post-doctoral training at the University of Miami and Harvard University. His specialty area is in clinical health psychology and behavioral medicine. This contribution was prepared while Dr. Everly was a Visiting Scholar at Harvard University. Dr. Everly may be contacted at 301 Candlewood Court, Millersville, MD 21108.

RESOURCES

American Institute of Certified Public Accountants. (1981, November). Dear employees: Don't get sick. *CPA Client Bulletin, 2.*

Berry, C. (1981). *Good Health for Employees and Reduced Costs for Industry.* Washington, DC: Health Insurance Association of America.

Cohen, W. (1985). Health promotion in the workplace. *American Psychologist, 40,* 43-216.

Everly, G., & Feldman, R. (1985). *Occupational Health Promotion.* New York: Macmillan.

Goldberg, P. (1978). *Executive Health.* New York: McGraw-Hill.

Green, L. (1981, July). Emerging federal perspectives on health promotion. *Health Promotion Monographs* (Whole No. 1).

Hollander, R., Lengermann, J., & DeMuth, N. (1985). Cost-effectiveness and cost-benefit analyses of occupational health promotion. In G. Everly & R. Feldman, *Occupational Health Promotion* (pp. 298-300). New York: Macmillan.

Knowles, J. (1977). *Doing Better and Feeling Worse.* New York: Norton.

National Chamber Foundation. (1978). *How Business Can Promote Good Health for Employees and Their Families.* Washington, DC: Author.

Olive, P., & Kirkpatrick, M. (1982). *Employee Health Enhancement.* Cambridge, MA: Little.

Schein, E. (1969). *Process Consultation.* Reading, MA: Addison-Wesley.

Smith, K., Haight, G., & Everly, G. (1986). The evaluation of corporate wellness investments. *The Internal Auditor, 43,* 28-34.

Spencer, L. (1984). How to calculate the costs and benefits of an HRD program. *Training, 42,* 39-50.

Weiss, S. (1985). The case of worksite health promotion. In G. Everly & R. Feldman, *Occupational Health Promotion* (pp. ix-xviii). New York: Macmillan.

A CLINICIAN'S GUIDE TO SELECTING PARENT TRAINING PROGRAMS

Richard F. Dangel and W. Ted Blevins

With the burgeoning supply of materials devoted to parenting comes the challenge for clinicians to identify those most appropriate for specific families. Unfortunately, we know little about matching services with particular characteristics to families with particular needs. Far too often, we steer families to those that we have used before. The purpose of this contribution is to discuss several considerations in selecting parenting materials and to review representative programs.

ISSUES IN SELECTION

The task you face as a clinician is to find or provide the right service to the right client. For example, Mrs. Jones may display serious deficiencies in basic child management skills; Mr. Smith may harbor deep resentment towards his wife and children for restricting his freedom; Mrs. Williams may require support and instruction to deal effectively with her autistic toddler. Each family requires something different. As you search for parenting materials, you may wish to consider the following issues to more accurately guide your clients.

PROGRAM OBJECTIVES

It is not uncommon to find parenting programs claiming success with nearly everyone for nearly everything. Yet, those of us with experience read these claims with suspicion. One of the first dimensions for you to consider is exactly what the program is supposed to do. What are the expected outcomes? How will the participants be different when they have completed the program? Will we see changes in the parents' behaviors, attitudes, and perceptions? Will we see changes in the way their children act, feel, and think? Some programs state their objectives explicitly; others only imply certain objectives. Matching your clients' needs with the correct service can only be done if you have discerned the specific objectives of the program you are considering.

Once you have identified the program objectives, consider how they were derived. Some objectives reflect empirical findings. For example, an objective such as "Parents will employ positive reinforcement to increase the frequency of desirable child behavior" might find strong support in the literature. Other objectives might be included because they have widespread popular appeal or because they mirror the interests of the program developer. Ask yourself, "What evidence is there that these particular objectives will be worthwhile to my client?"

Do the objectives suggest the program should be used as a primary service, or ancillary to, say, ongoing psychotherapy? If additional services are required for the parenting program to be most effective, are they available? How do the program objectives fit with other treatment objectives the client may have?

Finally, identify what information about the program is available for parents. Parents often terminate before they finish a program. If we educate them regarding what to expect before they begin a program, and involve them in the selection process, they will be more likely to finish.

PARENT POPULATION

Most programs reach certain groups of parents more effectively than others. One must ask which parent population the program is designed to reach. Parent demographic characteristics may be important. For example, does this program require participation by both mother and father? Will it work with single-parent families? What educational background must participants have? Can the program involve voluntary as well as involuntary or court-ordered parents? What motivation level is required? If the program uses a group format, must parents be homogeneous along certain dimensions? If so, what dimensions, and can they be reliably assessed? Finally, are any psychological characteristics useful to screen parents in or out? For example, must parents be receptive to feedback? May they be depressed, alcoholic, abusive, or psychotic?

CHILD POPULATION

You should also determine what child population the program best serves. Are particular child characteristics, such as age, sex, handicapping conditions, and special needs important? Are the objectives of the program compatible with the characteristics of the child you are trying to reach? Are they developmentally sound? For example, does the program aim to teach early adolescents to comply with an unreasonable percentage of parent requests? How much participation is required of the child? What child motivation level is required? Specifying clearly the characteristics of the child population you are serving and the population the program is best equipped to reach will result in a more favorable outcome for your clients.

THEORETICAL BASE

All programs operate from some theoretical base, although they differ in how explicitly they describe this base and how directly the program follows the theory. For example, a program may be described as behavioral, yet it may include many components that have little to do with behavioral theory. Or, a program may claim to be Adlerian and employ Adlerian terminology, but teach behavioral principles. Select a program that operates from a theoretical base with which you are comfortable and competent.

CLINICIAN CHARACTERISTICS

Consider the skill level required to serve as the clinician using a particular program. Many programs recommend the user hold at least a bachelor's or master's degree; some suggest a doctorate. Others require specialized training and certification before the service can be delivered. Programs that serve populations with exceptional needs (e.g., parents of mentally retarded or multiply handicapped children) may work best when delivered by a clinician with specialized expertise in that area.

Your level of participation may vary across programs. Some require you to lead the group, present didactic information, supervise behavior change plans, monitor attendance, and take a very active role in general. Others simply require someone to prepare the meeting room and start the videotape machine. Make sure that you understand and can meet the requirements of your involvement. Also consider whether you are comfortable with the recommended posture; for example, if you prefer a directive approach, select programs that appear to accommodate your style.

PACKAGING CHARACTERISTICS

Though you should not select or reject a program solely because of its packaging characteristics, how a program is packaged can contribute to success or failure. How much appeal will the instructional materials have for consumers? Are handouts attractive, colorful, easy to read and understand? If the program requires special equipment, is it convenient, available, in working order? Does the program require parents to have special equipment at home, for example, a videocassette player or tape recorder? Finally, consider program cost. As with any product, cost must be weighed against likely benefits to consumers, ease of use, durability, and so on. For example, you may prefer to use videotape instructional materials which can be effective but very expensive.

GENERAL PROGRAM CHARACTERISTICS

Consider how long the program is designed to run. For example, will parents attend a meeting once per week for 6 or 8 weeks? Does this schedule fit with requirements imposed by your setting and your client population? We find that requiring parents to participate for much longer than 8 weeks can challenge even the most skillful parent trainer and the most committed parent. Can parents begin at any time or must they start only at the first week? What provisions can be made for parents who miss a meeting? Does content build sequentially? Will parents who already demonstrate competence in a particular area covered by the program find the material boring, and perhaps drop out, or is the program self-paced? Does the program require groups of parents, or can it be offered to individuals?

What teaching methods are employed - didactic instruction, role-plays, group discussions, reading, pencil and paper assignments, homework? Are the teaching methods consistent with what you know to be effective to accomplish your objectives with your client population? If not, can the format be modified to better meet the needs of your clients? Does the program provide for maintenance of the changes parents make and for booster training when needed?

PROGRAM EFFECTIVENESS

One of the most important dimensions to consider when selecting a parenting program is information regarding the program's effectiveness. You should examine data on both short and long term results. Compare results with the implicit and explicit program objectives. If the program claims to enhance parenting skills, for example, how has this outcome been demonstrated? Look for research conducted by the program developers and by others to see if the program has scientifically proven results. How well do these results agree with what you know about similar programs? For example, if a particular program suggests it can produce remarkable results with multiproblem families in two short sessions, you should be very skeptical. Are data available to show if any improvements accomplished by the parents are maintained over time? If you teach parents how to use specific skills to solve one problem, do they also learn how to apply the same skills to solve other problems? Do the benefits show up with all children in the family or only with the target child? What do past participants have to say about the program? Did they like it? Are they convinced their participation helped their children? Would they recommend the program to a friend?

Evaluating the effectiveness of a program is no easy task. Interpreting evaluations to determine if the results apply to the families you are attempting to serve is equally difficult. Nevertheless, as clinicians, we have a strong obligation to provide the best service available and to present a realistic picture of what probable outcomes a family might expect if they participate. Both of these obligations can be met only by demanding that evaluations be completed to support claims of program effectiveness.

GATHERING INFORMATION

Such practical issues as financial constraints, access to equipment, time pressures, agency theoretical orientation, a finite number of programs from which to choose, limited information available about each, and client population characteristics often force you to make a compromise decision. This does not abrogate your responsibility to make a thoughtful choice.

To make this choice, begin collecting any written materials you can about parenting programs. Professional publications typically include advertisements for parenting programs. Even though a particular program may clearly not be appropriate for you, what you learn about available programs might aid in your selection.

Once you have read distributor literature, preview the materials. Most programs are available for screening before purchase. This screening can answer many of your questions. Invite other professionals, including those with viewpoints different from yours, to assist you with your preview. Ask some of your clients to look over the materials. What do they think? Try out a lesson or two. Feedback from potential consumers can be most informative. Call the distributor and the developer if you have specific questions. Ask them for research that documents program effectiveness. Also request the names and addresses of others who have used the program and who may be able to share their experiences.

Review the scientific literature. Psychology, social work, education, nursing, and child development journals frequently include descriptions of programs and results from program evaluations. A literature review can provide you not only with information about a specific program, but also with program characteristics that seem to produce favorable results.

No single program provides all the answers for all families, or even for any one family. Your task is to select the program that meets more of the criteria you consider to be important than any other program.

SAMPLE PARENTING PROGRAMS

This section describes representative parenting materials. Because no single manuscript can even list, let alone review, all that is available, we have selected materials that share at least one of the following characteristics. They may be well-known, available to consumers, national rather than local, and illustrative of a particular type. Any review is subjective and what follows is no exception. We tried to answer as many questions as possible from the preceding section of this contribution for each program. Programs were rated against their particular aims. Each program was evaluated by two independent reviewers. The following key describes our ratings:

> ******** Excellent
> ******* Good
> ****** Acceptable
> ***** Requires substantial clinical expertise

VIDEOTAPE/AUDIOCASSETTE/PACKAGED PROGRAMS

These programs employ media as a major training component. For the most part, they are based on behavioral principles and rely on well-defined structure and sequence to present skill-oriented content. All lack thorough empirical validation.

****** Active Parenting.** Order from Active Parenting, Inc., 4669 Roswell Road, N. E., Atlanta, GA 30342 (800-235-7755). Cost: $295. Active Parenting is based on an Adlerian-Dreikurs framework and teaches such familiar topics as "I" messages, avoiding communication blocks, and listening for feelings, all within a democratic family structure. The complete kit includes advertising materials to bolster attendance and newspaper press releases. According to the authors, the program attains 97% success rate with Active Parenting principles and an 84% immediate improvement with children. The videotapes should prompt lively discussion, and they illustrate clearly the main points. For a videotape package, the cost is exceptionally reasonable. Major limitations are that many of the concepts are somewhat abstract rather than precise skills, so they may not be appropriate for lower socioeconomic families or for families whose children display high rates of aggression or noncompliance.

****** WINNING!** Order from WINNING!, P. O. Box 32, Arlington, TX 76004 (817-273-3407). Cost: Basic Program $995, Advanced Program $995. WINNING! includes a Basic Series of eight videotaped lessons, Parenting Specialist Handbook, Parent Goal Sheets, Practice Records, Graduation Certificates (Graduates become official WINNERS!), and an advanced series of 14 videotaped lessons. Each basic lesson shows 35 to 50 vignettes of families from diverse ethnic and socioeconomic backgrounds employing a single behavioral skill (e.g., praise, rewards, time out). Each advanced lesson shows parents solving a common child management problem (e.g., fighting, temper tantrums, back talk, bedwetting, etc.) by using the skills from the basic series. The program has undergone considerable evaluation and is now employed in 35 states and three countries. Limitations include cost, which many agencies find prohibitive, and the focus, which is exclusively on child management skills for parents of 3 to 12 year olds.

*** Parents and Children.** Order from Research Press, 2612 N. Mattis Avenue, Champaign, IL 61826 (217-352-3273). Cost: Purchase $240, 3-day rental $55. This videocassette or 16 mm film program aims to teach the purposeful use of behavioral principles to influence child behavior. Dr. Richard M. Foxx, the program developer, provides narration after the parent-child vignettes. The program does not include a leader's guide, which may limit its usefulness, and most of the examples appear geared towards children under 8 or 9 years old. The program is relatively expensive and requires considerable clinician support.

**** Behavioral Principles for Parents.** Order from Research Press, 2612 N. Mattis Avenue, Champaign, IL 61826 (217-352-3273). Cost: Purchase $240, 3-day rental $55. This program uses 31 vignettes to demonstrate common behavioral principles. The vignettes are more realistic and believable than those in other programs, and they invite discussion. The leader's guide is well organized and clearly written. Appropriate parent population includes a range of socioeconomic groups with children between 3 and 8 years old.

***** Nurturing Program.** Order from Family Development Associates, P. O. Box 94365, Schaumberg, IL 60194 (715-833-0904). Cost: about $600. This program employs film-strips, audiocassettes, charts, toys, and manuals for both parents and children. It attempts to teach nurturing concepts and skills, which include self-awareness, focusing on appropriate developmental capabilities of children, and some behavior management. Limited field testing suggests changes in targeted attitudes. Changes in actual parenting behaviors were not measured. The program introduces diverse and useful content. It appears likely to prompt discussion and to encourage parents and children to think about some of their behavior. Limitations are that many parents may have difficulty learning specific skills from the program and the program requires an experienced clinician.

For the most part, parenting programs have not kept up with the increasing availability of media technology as a training device. Furthermore, most existing programs show only skills based on behavioral principles as applied to young children. The materials are also limited because most show only one or two vignettes to illustrate very complex social interaction skills. While a single vignette may be useful to prompt discussion, rarely is it sufficient to teach new, difficult skills. Folklore and research support the notion that a picture is worth a thousand words, but high development costs associated with the production of multimedia materials, distribution expenses, disagreements over appropriate content, and the difficulty in translating ambiguous theory into specific parenting skills continue to limit the materials available in this category.

ORGANIZATIONAL PROGRAMS

These programs are offered by national organizations. Their availability varies across communities. Typically, organizational programs aim to reach specific populations served by the organization, such as parents whose children have birth defects. Usually the services are offered directly by the agency, although some organizations offer training for clinicians.

Red Cross. Local Red Cross chapters offer parenting services. One of their most common programs, Preparation for Parenthood, uses written materials, group participation, and lecture to present information to prospective teen or single parents, or to those providing care to young children. The format and content are tailored to the needs and interests of each group. The service is free or inexpensive. Because each chapter employs different staff, and the needs of each group of parents influence the content, no summary comments can be made except that the written materials include much useful information and are easy to read. Contact your local Red Cross chapter for specifics.

March of Dimes. Order from March of Dimes Birth Defects Foundation, 1275 Mamaroneck Avenue, White Plains, NY 10605, or contact your local chapter. Cost: Varies depending on materials ordered. The March of Dimes offers several parenting education programs, each designed to reach specific populations and to disseminate specific information. Two of their most popular programs are described here.

*** *Parenthood Education Program* is geared to low socioeconomic, school aged parents. It provides information on health care and nutrition during pregnancy. The program is to be used by teachers and is available in Spanish. The materials are well written, accurate, and should be well received by the target population.

**** *Starting a Healthy Family Series* (Four Parts) covers the significance of starting a family (Part I), the impact on a family of a child with special needs (Part II), parenting an adolescent with a birth defect (Part III), and communication with children (Part IV). Most parts include written materials for parents and children, a teacher's guide, and audiocassettes. In terms of information, the entire series is a masterpiece. The information is presented accurately, thoroughly, and sensitively. Cost is very reasonable, around $20. Evaluation data are not available, but the high quality of the materials suggests that at a minimum, most participants will think differently at the end than when they began.

YWCA. Contact the local chapter. The YWCA works under a national mandate to help prepare teen parents for the responsibilities they face. While each local charter has flexibility in terms of how it meets this priority, all share a common curriculum designed to cover such topics as child development, child discipline, life skills, nutrition, job search, and infant diet. The program uses lectures, didactic instruction, materials written at the sixth grade level, and audiovisual aids. Quality will vary across locations, but the basic materials seem sound.

SELF-HELP PARENTING GROUPS

Self-help organizations exist for virtually any concern, and parenting is no exception. Four major self-help resources are identified here.

National Information Center for Handicapped Children and Youth, P. O. Box 1492, Washington, DC 20013. Offers information and toll-free referral service to parents of children with 11 types of handicaps (deaf, deaf-blind, hard-of-hearing, mentally retarded, multiply handicapped, orthopedically impaired, other health-impaired, seriously emotionally disturbed, specific learning disabled, speech impaired, and visually handicapped).

Parent Care Headquarters, University of Utah Medical Center, 50 N. Medical Drive, Room 2A210, Salt Lake City, UT 84132 (801-581-5323). Provides information, magazines, and a newsletter to parents and professionals concerned with critically ill newborns.

Compassionate Friends, P. O. Box 3696, Oak Brook, IL 60521 (312-323-5010). Offers support, information including an outstanding book list, and friendship to parents dealing with the loss of a child.

Parents Anonymous, Inc., 7120 Franklin Avenue, Los Angeles, CA 90046 (800-421-0353). Offers a standardized program nationwide. May be associated with Mental Health-Mental Retardation or Family Services, or the independently listed. There is no fee for services.

TELEVISION

Parents can tune in to television to get practical advice and procedures for dealing with their children. Two popular shows are reviewed here.

What Every Baby Knows, with Dr. Berry Brazelton, Lifetime, 1211 Avenue of the Americas, Department A, New York, NY 10036. This series provides considerable information and reassurance to its intended audience, primarily parents of infants to preschool-age children. Role-play exercises are used to demonstrate specific procedures, and questions and answers from the audience promote a nonthreatening format. Check local stations for broadcast information.

Mother's Day, with Host Joan Lunden, Lifetime, 1211 Avenue of the Americas, Department A, New York, NY 10036. This series invites guests to share information relevant to a wide variety of parents. Topics cover everything from sex education to childhood developmental problems. Generally, the dialogue is easy to understand and useful information is disseminated. The most serious limitation is time; most guests only have time to introduce their topic and present a few key points. The interested viewer would have to follow up with independent research to learn more, although the series often identifies related resources.

MAGAZINES

Several magazines that address topics relevant to parenting are available at bookstores and supermarkets. Popular ones include *Single Parent Magazine*, *Parents*, and *Working Mother*. Each of these magazines presents a variety of articles covering much of the same material. Each relies on contributing experts to discuss such topics as the "Terrible Twos," time management, parent-child communication, dating, marital stress, and child management. Contributions range from excellent to poor, but given the spectrum of topics, there is bound to be something for everyone.

POPULAR BOOKS

A quick trip to any local bookstore will reveal over 75 popular books dealing with parenting. Topics include how to: teach your infant to read, swim, play the violin, do math and gymnastics; get tough with your troubled teen; get your child off drugs; make your child a genius; modify your toddler's behavior; solve your child's sleep problem; help your child lose weight and eat right; teach your child money management; and help your child live with the fear of nuclear war. Some of these topics may be of interest, and the proliferation of books suggests a lively market. If you are charged with helping parents to get educated, your responsibility may include helping them to select worthwhile reading materials, or at least to consume critically. Again, the answers to the questions outlined in the first part of this contribution will provide some guidelines.

Many books operate with the premise that, at least for dozens of parenting problems, parents can serve as their own therapists. For certain problems, evidence exists to support this premise. Unfortunately, most books provide more information than procedure, so readers end up with considerably more understanding than "how to" knowledge, and few texts offer any empirical support upon which to base their recommendations. Consequently, parents may select two texts, both purporting to contain solutions to the same problem, and get opposing recommendations. For example, the "experts" disagree on the appropriateness of physical punishment. Parents may select the procedure with which they feel the most comfortable, but it may be ineffective or undesirable.

POPULAR PROGRAMS

Two parenting programs are probably the most well known and durable programs in use today: STEP (Systematic Training for Effective Parenting) and PET (Parent Effectiveness Training).

***** STEP**. Order from American Guidance Service, Circle Pines, MN 55014. STEP comes complete with written notebooks for parents, colorful wall placards to illustrate key points, leader's guide, and audiocassette tapes, all packaged in a handy carrying case. Cost: Under $100. STEP aims to teach child management skills, communication skills, the role of the parent in parenting, and relationship development. The basic ideas communicated in the program are excellent. Originally designed for parents of younger children, a new version of the program is available for parents of teens. The program's greatest limitation is that it is not particularly skill oriented; some of the concepts are difficult to put into practice with the information provided. Parents with less than average education or whose children display seriously problematic behavior may find the program does not meet their needs.

**** PET**. Order from Effectiveness Training, 531 Stevens Avenue, Solana Beach, CA 92075. Cost: Variable, depending on what components are purchased. Only a few years ago, PET groups were seemingly offered by virtually every mental health and social service center in the country. Now, however, PET's popularity has waned. The program includes written materials for parents and requires a certified PET leader. The program aims to teach a specific, democratic approach to solving parent-child conflicts. The approach involves problem specification, generating alternatives, negotiation, implementation, and evaluation. One of the nicest characteristics of the program is its applicability to teens. However, in our view its methods appear to have limited use in distressed families, often those most likely to seek parenting services.

FOSTER PARENTING PROGRAMS

Though many of the materials already described may be useful for foster or house parents, specific programs to meet the unique needs of these groups exist.

***** NOVA**. Order from Center for Advancement of Education, 3301 College Avenue, Fort Lauderdale, FL 33314. Cost: Variable, depending on materials and services purchased. NOVA provides information to new or aspiring foster parents concerning virtually all aspects of foster parenting. Participants learn about communication skills, discipline, raising self-esteem, record keeping, relationship building, working with biological parents, and personal hygiene. The program's greatest strength is also its greatest limitation: so much information is provided that participants may feel overwhelmed and have difficulty translating the general content into specific day-to-day practices. Nevertheless, NOVA provides critical information quickly and can help to insure at least an entry level of awareness for foster parents.

****** PRYDE**. Request information from PRYDE, Pressley Ridge School, 530 Marshall Avenue, Pittsburgh, PA 15214. The PRYDE program offers intensive training to foster parents caring for disturbed children who otherwise might require placement in residential treatment. Participants receive training in behavior modification procedures, methods to teach social skills to adolescents, relationship development, designing individual treatment planning, and data collection systems. This is one of the few programs available designed specifically for parents working with adolescents. Its greatest limitation is that program materials and procedures are still very experimental, so dissemination is restricted.

COMPUTER SOFTWARE

New and scarce, but promising, are computer software programs for clinicians and parents. Neither of the two programs described below were available for preview.

Mind Over Minors, Human Edge, Palo Alto, CA (415-493-1593). This program claims to provide parents detailed strategies for motivating children based on each child's personality. The idea sounds good, and there is certainly an array of methods to motivate youngsters. How skillful we are at matching certain motivational methods with certain personalities is questionable. Nevertheless, even a computerized catalog of techniques could be useful to parents and clinicians.

Childpace, Computerose, Arlington, TX (817-461-1333). To use this program, parents enter information about their child's development. In response, they receive text and graphics that describe their child's development compared to normative data. Future programs will then detail specific activities for parents to use to facilitate child development in language, personal and social capabilities, and fine and major motor development.

SUMMARY

The wealth of materials available to those of us who help parents makes our job both easier and more difficult: easier because we can locate materials that aim to teach almost anything to anybody; difficult because locating and evaluating the materials takes time. If we support the notion that part of our job is not only to provide, but also to evaluate our services, then we should find ourselves constantly revising our parenting materials to better meet the needs of our clients.

Richard F. Dangel, PhD, is Associate Professor and Chairman of the Direct Practice Sequence of the Graduate School of Social Work at the University of Texas at Arlington. He is a licensed child psychologist and has authored three books and numerous articles related to parenting. Current research interests include parent training, residential care and treatment of children, and the education of emotionally disturbed children. Dr. Dangel may be contacted at the Graduate School of Social Work, The University of Texas at Arlington, Box 19129, Arlington, TX 76019-0129.

W. Ted Blevins, MA, is currently the Executive Director of Lena Pope Home, Inc., in Fort Worth, Texas. In addition, he is President-Elect of the National Association of Family-Teachers, Chairman of the Residential Contract Program Council of Texas, and on the Advisory Council of the Texas Youth Commission. His interests include working to improve child care laws on the state level. Mr. Blevins can be contacted at Lena Pope Home, 4701 W. Rosedale, Forth Worth, TX 76107.

RESOURCES

Barkley, R. A. (1981). *Hyperactive Children: A Handbook for Diagnosis and Treatment.* New York: Guilford Press.

Becker, W. C. (1971). *Parents Are Teachers: A Child Management Program.* Champaign, IL: Research Press.

Bijou, S. W., & Baer, D. M. (1978). *Behavior Analysis of Child Development.* Englewood Cliffs, NJ: Prentice-Hall.

Christophersen, E. R. (1982). *Little People: Guidelines for Common Sense Child Rearing.* Lawrence, KS: H & H Enterprises.

Clark, L. (1985). *SOS! Help for Parents.* Bowling Green, KY: Parents Press.

Dangel, R. F., & Polster, R. A. (1984). *Parent Training: Foundations of Research and Practice.* New York: Guilford Press.

Fleischman, M. J., Horne, A. M., & Arthur, J. L. (1983). *Troubled Families: A Treatment Program.* Champaign, IL: Research Press.

Hardyment, C. (1983). *Dream Babies: Three Centuries of Good Advice on Child Care.* New York: Harper & Row.

Harman, D., & Brim, O. G. (1980). *Learning to be Parents: Principles, Programs, and Methods.* Beverly Hills: Sage Publications.

Kozloff, M. A. (1979). *A Program for Families of Children with Learning and Behavior Problems.* New York: John Wiley & Sons.

Krumboltz, J. D., & Krumboltz, H. B. (1972). *Changing Children's Behavior.* Englewood Cliffs, NJ: Prentice-Hall.

Mash, E. J., Hamerlynck, L. A., & Handy, L. C. (Eds.). (1976). *Behavior Modification and Families.* New York: Brunner/Mazel.

Patterson, G. R. (1973). *Families: Applications of Social Learning to Family Life.* Champaign, IL: Research Press.

Patterson, G. R. (1982). *A Social Learning Approach: Coercive Family Process* (Vol. 3). Eugene, OR: Castalia Publishing Co.

Robinson, P. W., Newby, T. J., & Hill, R. D. (1981). *Manipulating Parents: Tactics Used by Children of All Ages and Ways Parents Can Turn the Tables.* Englewood Cliffs, NJ: Prentice-Hall.

INTRODUCTION TO SECTION V: SELECTED TOPICS

This section includes a collection of contributions that address diverse techniques and roles for clinicians in a variety of settings. In addition, there are two useful handouts which readers may copy for use with their own clients. These contributions represent a sort of potpourri of discussions which may not fit neatly into another section.

First, Raczynski provides a primer on psychological practice in medical settings. He describes the kinds of disorders frequently addressed by the psychologist working in a health care setting and discusses the more common types of interventions which would be appropriate. This is a resource article which may be viewed as a stepping stone to more specific topics in the growing field of behavioral medicine.

Wood's article describes psychological assessment and intervention in the emergency room. The psychiatric emergency room is a setting with which many clinicians do not come into contact. Wood describes basic guidelines for intervention with the acutely disturbed patient in such settings.

Knapp and his colleagues discuss the duty to protect. This is a difficult legal and clinical issue with which many clinicians are concerned. These authors discuss relevant legal precedents and suggest prudent steps for the clinician to take when dealing with a client who may act dangerously.

Kissel describes a variety of techniques which may be used to engage the "difficult" child in the playroom. How does one get the attention of a child who either appears resistant or noncompliant? His article includes a variety of practical techniques for the clinician who wishes to help such children but has a hard time getting started.

Divorce mediation is an area in which many clinicians have become involved in recent years. Cohen provides a useful perspective on mediation and offers resources for the clinician who wants to develop expertise in this process.

Finally, Anderson extensively updates a previous contribution on assessment of the mentally disabled for Social Security and SSI benefits. There have been a number of recent developments in the guidelines for evaluating the mentally disabled for such benefits. His contribution provides practical suggestions for the clinician faced with this task.

Volume 5 contains two client handouts. The first, by Yamauchi, offers 10 practical suggestions for managing stress. The second, by Salameh, provides basic guidelines for communicating more effectively. These readable handouts should be of use to clients struggling with such issues. Both may be copied for use with your clients.

SELECTED TOPICS

A PRIMER ON PSYCHOLOGICAL PRACTICE IN MEDICAL SETTINGS

James M. Raczynski

Behavioral medicine has developed dramatically in the dozen years since Birk's (1973) first use of the term in his discussion of biofeedback. In 1978, the American Psychological Association (APA) announced the addition of the Division of Health Psychology as its 38th division. Recent years have also seen the emergence of the Society of Behavioral Medicine, as well as other groups such as the Biofeedback Society of America, and at least four new specialized journals: *Journal of Behavioral Medicine*, *Behavioral Medicine*, *Behavioral Medicine Abstracts*, and *Health Psychology*.

Psychologists are presently being employed in cardiovascular settings, such as Departments of Medicine or Rehabilitation; work with pain patients, usually in Departments of Anesthesiology or Rehabilitation Medicine; Departments of Neurology and Neurosurgery, where work is being done with neuropsychology and cognitive and physical rehabilitation; work with gastrointestinal and neurogenital disorders, such as irritable bowel syndrome, incontinence, and gynecological problems; oncology settings, where psychological distress and anticipatory nausea are being dealt with; areas with visual disorders, such as myopia, blepharospasms, and even extraocular motility disorders; work with eating disorders, such as obesity, anorexia, and bulimia; pulmonary disorders; metabolic disorders, such as diabetes; and in areas of health promotion and disease prevention, such as diet, weight, smoking, alcohol and drug use, exercise, and stress reduction programs. In general, psychologists now practice in medical settings spread much farther than Departments of Psychiatry in encompassing health areas from primary to tertiary settings.

HISTORICAL DEVELOPMENTS

A variety of factors has been enumerated as contributing to the development of behavioral medicine during the 1970s, and a number of different terms have emerged to describe psychologists' roles in medical settings. While Gentry and Matarazzo (1981) trace the relationship between naturopathic medicine and philosophic psychology to the first records of civilization, it was not until the years between 1964 and 1968 that the number of psychologists in the APA who were on faculties of U.S. medical schools exceeded a thousand. Millon (1982) attributes much of this early expansion of psychologists' roles in medical settings to the inroads made by psychologists in medical and health clinical functions that resulted in fee-generating services. Psychologists were able to generate their salaries through fee-producing activities and to support their roles in medical school settings. At about the same time, Neal Miller and colleagues (Miller, 1969) began reporting the effects of biofeedback in visceral learning with animals, and the whole biofeedback movement quickly evolved. Other behavioral psychologists were concurrently making advances in treating such health-related behaviors as weight control, smoking, and alcohol and drug use problems. Importantly, two other trends also were occurring.

The first of these recent trends was an increase in health costs and a movement toward cost containment. Consequently, the stage was set for other health professionals to begin working with medical patients in improving health care services. Second, as

Doleys, Meredith, and Ciminero (1982) and others have noted, there has evolved a general recognition of the inadequacies of the "medical model" at both the lay and professional levels. Biopsychosocial models have evolved during the 1970s to replace exclusively physiologically oriented medical models. With this expansion of the roles of psychologists in medical settings, a variety of descriptive terms has emerged. To add to the old term "psychosomatic medicine," labels including "medical psychology," "behavioral medicine," "health psychology," and "behavioral health" have evolved. While much has been written concerning the definition and differentiation of these terms (see Gentry & Matarazzo, 1981 and Millon, 1982 for a discussion), conceptual distinctions between them will not be made in this contribution.

ROLE OF PSYCHOLOGISTS IN MEDICAL SETTINGS

Not surprisingly, based on their traditional roles, psychologists take part in both assessment and treatment with medical populations. Although psychologists in health care have lacked the array of mental health assessment instruments (Millon, 1982), their contributions to differential diagnoses and in assessing psychosocial factors among the physically ill is a prominent one in medical settings. Probably sparked by the efforts at cost containment of medical expenses, intervention roles cover those from primary to tertiary strategies. In addition to their roles in assessment and treatment, some psychologists in medical settings are also members of interdisciplinary teams. It is as a part of these teams that psychologists frequently relate not only with physicians but with other health professionals, such as physical therapists, occupational therapists, speech pathologists and therapists, nursing staff, nutritionists, exercise physiologists, physicians' assistants, pharmacists, and social workers.

PSYCHOLOGICAL ASSESSMENT IN MEDICAL SETTINGS

Although clearly the role of a psychologist in medical settings has grown far beyond that of clinical diagnostician, the diagnostic testing role merges well with traditional medical beliefs of systematic patient assessment. Consequently, psychologists have readily assumed roles from neuropsychology to the use of traditional psychometric instruments and, more recently, to the use of specialized diagnostic and behavioral tools developed especially for medical populations. Generally, although this review is not comprehensive, the instruments used by psychologists in medical settings can be considered within the following categories (Green, 1982): neuropsychological, personality, symptom checklist, lifestyle inventory, and single trait measures.

Neuropsychological Assessment. Neuropsychological assessment is involved in the evaluation of brain-behavior relationships. As such, the neuropsychologist is frequently called upon to differentiate brain from behavioral disorders and to determine the behavioral correlates of impaired brain structures. However, the behavioral correlates of brain impairments depend on such factors as the location, size, rate of growth, and type of lesion. The difficulty presented to the neuropsychologist is not only in integrating the above factors into determining behavior-brain relationships, but also in covering the broad range of behaviors that may be affected by brain impairment. Consequently, the neuropsychologist depends on a variety of tests to determine brain-behavior relationships whose content spans that from simple sensory and motor functions to complex functions involving attention and concentration, memory, and problem solving ability.

Neuropsychologists generally attempt to integrate test findings from both a quantitative and a qualitative basis (Boll, O'Leary, & Barth, 1981). There are fundamentally two general test batteries that neuropsychologists employ: the Halstead-Reitan Battery and allied procedures (Boll, 1981) and the Luria-Nebraska Neuropsychological Examination (Luria, 1973). Despite the utility of neurological diagnostic procedures, such as the electroencephalogram and newer neuroradiological procedures, the value of neuropsychological assessment procedures has been demonstrated in providing information concerning the location and extent of brain damage as well as the behavior and psychological functions that are impaired or left intact. Such information is very useful in making psychological and behavioral plans for neurologically impaired individuals.

Personality Assessment Measures. Personality assessment measures are frequently used by psychologists in medical settings for two reasons: (a) as a means of determining personality changes occurring with brain impairment or in reaction to physical disorders, and (b) as a way of ruling out psychopathology in medical problems. An example of the former use might be that of administering a personality inventory to a patient who has suffered a stroke; an example of the latter might be the administration of personality inventories to chronic pain patients as a way of ruling out major forms of psychopathology. All of the personality inventories developed for nonmedical populations, such as the 16 Personality Factor Inventory (16-PF) and the Minnesota Multiphasic Personality Inventory (MMPI), have probably been used with medical populations, and norms for many of these have been developed for such populations. Some inventories have also been developed expressly for medical populations, such as the Millon Behavioral Health Inventory (MBHI) (Millon, Green, & Meagher, 1982b).

Symptom Checklist. Symptom checklists have evolved as a way of quickly and accurately surveying patients' symptomatology. The two of these checklists most commonly used in medical settings are probably the Cornell Medical Index (CMI) and the Symptom Check List-90 (SCL-90). The CMI (Brodman, Erdman, & Wolff, 1949) is a 195-item true-false inventory which was developed to reflect pertinent medical and psychological data. The SCL-90 (Derogatis, 1977) is a 90-item scale with each item having a 5-point scale of distress; it was developed for use with both psychiatric and medical populations.

Lifestyle Inventories. A variety of lifestyle inventories have been developed for use with medical populations. The two most commonly encountered types of lifestyle inventories are those which have been developed to assess Type A behavior and life events. The former type is exemplified by the Jenkins Activity Survey (JAS) (Jenkins, Zyzanski, & Rosenman, 1979), which has been found to be predictive of the development of coronary heart disease in some studies (Jenkins, Rosenman, & Zyzanski, 1974). An example of the latter inventory is the Life Experiences Survey (LES) (Sarason, Johnson, & Siegel, 1978) which was developed to assess an individual's perceptions of the life stresses experienced during the preceding 12 months.

Single Trait Measures. A number of instruments have also been developed for the assessment of single traits or states. Examples of these instruments which are often used in medical settings include the Beck Depression Inventory (BDI) (Beck, 1972); the State-Trait Anxiety Inventory (STAI) (Spielberger, Gorsuch, & Lushene, 1970); the Hopelessness Scale (Beck et al., 1974); and the Multidimensional Health Locus of Control Scales (MHLC) (K. A. Wallston, B. S. Wallston, & DeVellis, 1978). These instruments, as well as many others, are commonly used in medical settings when a quick measure of a particular dimension is desired.

INTERVENTIONS

Psychologists in medical settings become involved in interventions of three basic types: primary interventions involving work with asymptomatic, healthy individuals to promote healthy lifestyles; secondary interventions involving work with individuals who have symptoms or risk factors for disease before the disorder actually develops; and tertiary interventions involving rehabilitation of individuals who are symptomatic. Thus, conducting a community program designed to increase exercise and promote a heart-healthy diet, low in saturated fats and high in fiber, would be an example of primary intervention. Interventions designed to decrease smoking, control weight, reduce Type A behaviors, lower serum lipid levels, control diabetes, and reduce blood pressure among individuals who already display these risk factors for cardiovascular diseases are examples of secondary interventions. Interventions such as those designed to lower the chances of a recurrence among individuals who have already had a myocardial infarction by reducing their Type A behaviors (e.g., Suinn, 1975) or other risk factors are considered tertiary interventions. Judging from the literature, most interventions in medical, as well as nonmedical settings are of the tertiary type, although frequent references are made to secondary interventions, and primary interventions certainly are increasing.

PSYCHOLOGISTS' ROLES ON INTERDISCIPLINARY TEAMS

Because psychologists most often work with tertiary interventions involving patients with established diseases, they frequently find themselves collaborating with other health professionals as members of an interdisciplinary team. In fact, the interdisciplinary nature of applying behavioral science knowledge to health and illness is emphasized in Schwartz and Weiss's (1978) definition of behavioral medicine and Matarazzo's (1980) definition of behavioral health. Psychologists' roles in medical settings thus frequently depart from their roles in mental health settings, where they commonly serve as independent practitioners. By contrast, medical setting psychologists typically establish the value of their contribution to the total management of the patients' health and illness, but must work with other health professionals who also make professional contributions.

SPECIALIZED INTERVENTIONS IN MEDICAL SETTINGS

Although much of the work done by psychologists in medical settings is not substantially different from that performed in a mental health milieu, certain interventions are unique to medical settings. These specialized interventions include biofeedback, stress management programs, and interventions designed to improve adherence to and compliance with medical procedures.

BIOFEEDBACK

Although many biofeedback applications can be found in nonmedical settings, the use of biofeedback techniques with psychophysiological disorders in medical settings is probably much more commonplace. Even in medical settings, however, there is much variability in the frequency with which these procedures are used. This variability can be accounted for in several ways. First, most third-party payers currently view biofeedback as experimental rather than as a clinical procedure with demonstrable efficacy; consequently, most insurors refuse to reimburse for biofeedback per se. Second, while most researchers would probably agree that biofeedback has been demonstrated as efficacious with some physical disorders, controversy still exists as to whether or not it produces better results than other behavioral procedures, such as relaxation and stress management training. Finally, biofeedback researchers have failed to present an adequate model to account for how individuals acquire control over autonomic processes (Raczynski, Thompson, & Sturgis, 1982); physicians often question the procedures based on their lack of an empirically tested theoretical base despite the appealing technological look of such procedures. This lack of specificity in biofeedback models and current third-party reimbursement policies have undoubtedly hindered biofeedback's acceptance in medical settings. Nonetheless, biofeedback is frequently used in dealing with psychophysiological disorders, particularly with headache, low back pain, Raynaud's disease, neuromuscular disorders, and temporomandibular joint pain.

STRESS MANAGEMENT

There is still a great deal of ambiguity about the proper use of the term "stress" (Leventhal & Nerenz, 1983). Generally, though, stress management programs can be broken down into three types: (a) lifestyle change programs where the goal is to produce global changes in an individual's daily response to stressors; (b) programs that are targeted at decreasing an individual's stress and increasing coping abilities with specific stressful medical procedures; and (c) programs geared toward assisting individuals to cope better with illness and death.

Lifestyle Change Stress Management Programs. Lifestyle change programs tend to be multifaceted in order to create changes in a variety of areas. Generally, components of these programs include the following: relaxation training; coping skills training, such as communication, assertion, time management, problem solving, parenting, and study skills; coping imagery training; encouragement of aerobic exercise for coping and general arousal reduction; a reduction in caffeine intake and alcohol consumption; and a cognitive-behavioral focus. These generalized stress management techniques are frequently employed with populations ranging from primary to tertiary.

Stress Management with Stressful Medical Procedures. Under this category are stress management procedures targeted toward individuals receiving painful medical procedures, such as spinal taps, bone aspirations, dental procedures, and surgery. Generally, the focus of these programs is on two areas: (a) providing information about the procedure and the after-effects of the procedure; and (b) teaching coping strategies. In conveying information about medical procedures, two types of information are discussed in the literature: procedural and sensory. Procedural information involves describing the nature of the medical event; for example, when and where it will take place, why it is being conducted, what instruments will be used, how long the procedure will last, and so on. Sensory information, on the other hand, involves giving information about the stimuli that are likely to be felt, seen, heard, smelled, and tasted during or after the procedure itself; for example, the level and duration of pain to be felt during different portions of the procedure, other somatosensory stimuli that may occur, and other visual, auditory, and olfactory stimuli that are likely to be perceived during the course of the procedure. The effectiveness of providing patients with information prior to medical procedures has been at least moderately supported.

Training in coping behaviors has also been a part of many stress management programs for medical procedures, and some data suggest that both the effects of training and procedural and sensory information are dependent on individuals' coping styles. Coping behavior training has ranged from teaching relaxation skills to cognitive coping strategies and even distraction techniques. For an example of the manner in which coping styles interact with the intervention, Andrew (1970) examined minor surgery patients, one-half of whom were given surgery-related information while the remainder received no information. Subjects were divided into three coping style groups based on a sentence completion test: (a) sensitizers who readily acknowledged negative emotions such as fear and anxiety; (b) avoiders who denied negative feelings; and (c) neutrals who did not appear to show a characteristic pattern. Neutrals who received the information spent fewer days in the hospital and required less information. Sensitizers showed no significant differences as a result of the intervention. However, negative effects were seen in medication usage among the avoiders who received the information. These results suggest the complexity of an individual's cognitive or coping style and the effects of coping and information interventions; they also highlight the need for good clinical skills in designing effective individual stress management programs.

Coping with Illness and Dying. Coping interventions, in general, will vary with the chronicity and prognosis of the particular illness. The adjustments that individuals, families, and friends must make when an acute illness or injury, such as appendicitis occurs, will differ markedly from those made for a chronic or terminal illness. In addition to the treatment implications associated with the chronicity and prognosis of the problem, data also suggest that the individuals' coping style and stage of illness may be important factors to consider. For example, Hackett, Cassem, and Wishnie (1968) report that denial during the early phase after a myocardial infarction (MI) is associated with a good prognosis; however, several weeks after having an MI, excessive denial may not be adaptive and may present compliance problems with rehabilitating coronary patients.

Hence, without going into detail, it can be seen that the issues involved in intervening with medical populations to improve coping are complex. The complexity of these issues limits their consideration here, but again emphasizes the importance of good clinical skills in working with medical populations.

ADHERENCE TO AND COMPLIANCE WITH MEDICAL PROCEDURES

Unquestionably, obtaining patient compliance with and adherence to a physician's prescriptions is an extremely important area in patient management. Statistics provide alarming data regarding this problem; for example, Cohen-Cole et al. (1982), in interviewing 150 medical outpatients immediately after their clinic visit, found that only 56% of the problems listed by patients' physicians could be named by the patients. Furthermore, patients could only describe an average of 60% of the recommendations they were supposed to be following, and 23% of the patients reported that they would not follow their doctors' recommendations. Perhaps even more alarming is the finding that despite strong evidence that antihypertensive medication reduces morbidity and mortality (Hypertension Detection and Follow-Up Program Cooperative Group, 1979), recent surveys suggest that more than 70% of hypertensive patients fail to benefit from treatment due to noncompliance with medical advice (Haynes, Sackett, & Taylor, 1979). Despite the identification of over 250 factors which have been found to be related to compliance (Haynes et al., 1979), a few practical suggestions seem effective in at least marginally improving the rates of compliance.

For short-term medical regimens, such as those administered for acute infections, careful instruction regarding the need for compliance and the medical regimen itself has been found effective (Colcher & Bass, 1972). This is not particularly surprising given that Cohen-Cole et al. (1982) found that 18% of their interviewed patients reported they did not understand what their doctors had told them. Other studies have also confirmed that both written (Linkewich, Catalano, & Flack, 1974; Sharpe & Mikeal, 1974) and verbal (Dickey, Mattar, & Chudzik, 1975) instructions have greatly improved short-term compliance. Compliance has also been improved with attention to scheduling, logistical difficulties, and other barriers (Fink, Malloy, et al., 1969; Fink, F. Martin, et al., 1969). Additional strategies have included the provision of pill calendars (Dickey et al., 1975), the provision of tablets in unit dose packages (Linkewich et al., 1974), and the use of pill containers with alarms (Azrin & J. Powell, 1969).

With long-term medical regimens, merely instructing patients about the regimens does not appear to have long-lasting effects; however, instructing physicians in compliance management does appear to result in long-term effects (Inui, Yourtee, & J. Williamson, 1976). Enlisting and encouraging family support for the patient's treatment regimen may also be effective (Levine et al., 1979). Group discussions appear effective in improving attendance and medication compliance (Nessman, Carnahan, & Nugent, 1980). Finally, when applicable, the monitoring of drug levels in bodily fluids and feedback about these levels to the patient appears to be an effective compliance procedure (e.g., Eney & Goldstein, 1976).

OVERVIEW OF PSYCHOLOGICAL INTERVENTIONS IN MEDICAL AREAS

Space limitations necessitate that the following overview be brief. Interested readers are encouraged to refer to one of the numerous edited books listed at the end of this contribution for more in-depth coverage of particular areas. In addition, this overview is limited to tertiary interventions, because the bulk of a psychologist's practice in medical settings involves tertiary rather than primary or secondary strategies.

CARDIOVASCULAR DISORDERS

Cardiovascular research has demonstrated unquestionably the prominence of behavioral factors among the risks for heart attack and stroke (Blackburn, 1980). The controllable risk factors for cardiovascular disease include eating habits, elevated blood fats (lipids), obesity, sedentary lifestyle, high blood pressure, cigarette smoking, personality type, and stress. The uncontrollable risk factors include age, sex, race and ethnic origin, and heredity. Given that all of the controllable risk factors for cardiovascular disease are behavioral, it is not surprising that psychologists assume a prominent role in tertiary interventions with this disease. Psychologists become most involved in the treatment of hypertension, in cardiac rehabilitation with post-MI patients and those with coronary artery disease (CAD), and with the peripheral vascular disease, Raynaud's Disease.

Hypertension. Hypertension is variously considered either a disease in its own right or a risk factor for other diseases, such as stroke and coronary heart disease (CHD). Because hypertension involves an elevation of systolic blood pressure (the maximum pressure which occurs in arteries as the heart beats and the pulse of blood is pushed throughout the body) and/or diastolic blood pressure (the pressure which remains within the arteries between beats of the heart and resulting pulses of blood), hemorrhagic strokes (where the arterial wall is blown open and the blood spreads into the surrounding tissue) may occur when the blood pressure exceeds the strength of the arterial wall. Coronary heart disease is almost always the result of atherosclerosis, or hardening of the arteries, and occurs as fatty deposits accumulate on the walls of coronary arteries, leading to formation of fibrous tissue in the vessel wall. This reduction in the diameter of the coronary arteries eventually leads to a narrowing of the affected vessels and reduction in the blood supply to the heart and may result in symptoms of angina pectoris (pain felt in the chest due to inadequate blood to the heart) or MI where blood is so severely occluded that a heart attack may result. While there are other risk factors for CAD, such as blood lipid levels (cholesterol), hypertension also emerges as a risk factor. Various other forms of CHD also result from hypertension and the excessive pressure put on the heart and its various components such as the heart valves.

The literature is replete with psychological treatments for hypertension. Nonpharmacological interventions range from dietary manipulations (weight reduction, sodium restriction, and potassium elevation), to aerobic exercise, and to a variety of behavioral methods, including biofeedback and relaxation techniques. It is generally accepted that dietary changes to reduce weight and alter sodium and potassium levels may substantially lower blood pressure at least in some individuals (Reisin et al., 1978); however, among some hypertensives such severe dietary regimens must be followed to effect blood pressure control that compliance is often difficult. Aerobic exercise also appears to produce a moderate blood pressure reduction effect, although additional studies are needed to determine the magnitude of this effect and the mechanism which mediates it (J. E. Martin & Dubbert, 1985).

Biofeedback techniques have been examined extensively for their utility in blood pressure reduction. Most of the early studies used some form of blood pressure measure to feed back to the individuals, and while achieving statistically significant reductions in blood pressure, the overall clinical changes in blood pressure levels were disappointing. Some of the newer studies with biofeedback, however, have focused on physiological measures other than blood pressure, such as electrodermal activity, muscle tension, and peripheral temperature. This has been done for technical reasons related to problems in obtaining a continuous measure of blood pressure, as well as theoretical reasons involving the suspected etiological mechanisms of hypertension. Some of these studies, such as those conducted by Patel and her colleagues (e.g., Patel & North, 1975), have yielded very promising results, although questions still remain regarding the generalization and maintenance of these effects.

Relaxation and broader-based stress management techniques have yielded similar promising effects among individuals with hypertension (cf. McCaffrey & Blanchard, 1985). However, as with biofeedback procedures, there still remain questions concerning generalization and maintenance of these reported treatment gains, and not all of the studies to date have consistently yielded promising results.

Cardiac Rehabilitation. Medical management of post-coronary and angina patients usually involves medication regimens to effect vascular and/or cardiac changes; dietary measures to reduce caloric, cholesterol, and triglyceride levels; and an exercise component to increase exercise tolerance to produce cardiovascular conditioning effects. The various cardiac rehabilitation activities in which psychologists may become involved range from interventions dealing with emotional reactions such as anxiety and depression, to lifestyle change issues such as modifying diet, increasing activity, reducing stress and anxiety, increasing compliance with medical regimens, and modifying Type A behaviors. In general, the interventions used with cardiac rehabilitation are similar to those used in other disorders, with the possible exception of modifying Type A behaviors.

The Type A behavior pattern is one which has been associated with increased risk of CHD even in prospective research. Generally, the behaviors that have been identified within the pattern include fast and empathic speech, interruption of others, and easily aroused irritabilities. Despite the vast number of studies examining the pattern, however, there remains a great deal of controversy over the precise behaviors that are related to CHD and the physiological mechanisms that mediate the relationship (L. H. Powell, 1984). Nonetheless, Friedman et al. (1984) have demonstrated in the Recurrent Coronary Prevention Project with post-MI subjects that a Type A intervention appears to reduce the recurrence rate of MIs by almost half. The treatment consisted of teaching subjects to identify physiologic, cognitive, and behavioral arousal, to use a variety of coping techniques to reduce arousal, and to change attitudes and beliefs that are related to Type A behaviors. These results, if replicable, suggest a fruitful area for pursuit by psychologists.

Raynaud's Disease. Raynaud's disease is a disorder of the peripheral vasculature in which vasospasms occur, usually in response to either cold or emotional stimuli (Abramson, 1974). The disorder not only produces sensations of cold in the affected part, usually the fingers or toes, but may compromise the blood supply to such an extent that pain develops, and ulcerations and even the potential for gangrene may occur. In general, relaxation-based treatments, as well as biofeedback for temperature increases in the affected body region, have both shown very promising and similar results with individuals who have this problem (e.g., Keefe, Surwit, & Pilon, 1980).

PAIN

Psychologists work in the many pain centers which have been established across the country. In these settings, which usually are housed in inpatient facilities with outpatient components, the approach to treatment is typically multidisciplinary, as advocated by the leaders in the field (e.g., Fordyce, 1976). The treatment approach is coordinated to decrease the operant reinforcers for pain behaviors, decrease the use of medications, increase activity and exercise levels in a paced manner, increase strength and range of motion, increase relaxation and stress management skills, and increase coping skills. Usually, treatment consists of an inpatient portion of the program with family involvement, followed by outpatient sessions.

Chronic pain is a relatively high frequency problem which is severely debilitating to individuals and costly to the national economy. Because pain clinics have shown very promising results by decreasing medication and health care system utilization, decreasing reported pain levels, increasing activity levels, and improving employment status, pain centers have grown to an estimated 800 programs in the United States (Turk, Meichenbaum, & Genest, 1983). The two most commonly seen types of pain problems are probably low back pain and headaches, although a variety of other pain problems also are seen commonly related to phantom limb pain, arthritis, cancer, and temporomandibular joint problems.

Headaches. The two major types of headaches are muscle contraction and vascular headaches. Muscle contraction headaches have long been conceptualized as arising from elevated muscle tension levels. The symptoms accompanying this form of headache include a nonpulsating pain which is bilateral and not accompanied by symptoms characteristic of vascular headaches. On the other hand, migraine headaches, the most common form of vascular headaches, are usually characterized by pulsating pain which may be unilateral and may be accompanied by nausea. In addition, focal sensory disturbances such as visual changes, unusual smells, and peripheral somatosensory disturbances, may accompany the headache. While relatively new data suggest that these two headache types may be more appropriately characterized as points on a continuum than as discrete diagnostic types, treatment approaches have differed somewhat depending on the diagnosis.

Individuals with muscle contraction headaches, because the disturbance involves muscular elevations, are usually administered muscle tension biofeedback for lowering muscle tension levels in the forehead. Individuals with migraine headaches, on the other hand, are usually given biofeedback for elevating their finger temperature levels, because their headaches are thought to involve a generalized vascular instability problem. By elevating finger temperature, it is thought that the individuals can be taught to stabilize their vascular systems, prevent oscillations from occurring in the system which might lead to headache, and thus prevent the occurrence of headaches. Aside from employing biofeedback, most interventions with headaches also involve a relaxation or stress management component, because both forms of headaches appear to be related to stress, even though the temporal course of stressful events and headache development may differ for the two types. In general, these interventions have demonstrated major reductions in headache activity, even among individuals for whom medical management has produced little beneficial effect.

Low Back Pain. Chronic low back pain is a major health problem in the United States, with an estimated 7 million Americans incapacitated by it (LaFreniere, 1979). Although the anatomy and physiology of the back are complex, leading to complicated treatment questions, 20% to 85% of all cases of low back pain have been described as having no discernible physical basis (White & Gordon, 1982). As with headache, muscle tension biofeedback interventions have been attempted to change muscular involvement in the pain problem, and relaxation and stress management techniques are commonly used because stress and muscular tension are thought to be related to pain levels (Dolce & Raczynski, 1985). In addition, relaxation procedures are also thought to be effective in lowering pain levels by increasing production of endorphins or endogenous opiates. More than with headaches, however, interventions with back pain usually involve attempts to affect reinforcers for pain behaviors, such as postural, facial, verbal, and nonverbal expressions of pain, by structuring the inpatient environment, working with family members, and reinforcing nonpain behaviors. Finally, the multidisciplinary interventions with low back pain patients also emphasize physical therapy, occupational therapy, and coordination with vocational counselors both to get the individual back to work and, sometimes, to assist in analyzing and modifying the work place to prevent future injury.

NEUROLOGICAL DISORDERS

Aside from the neuropsychologists who are heavily involved in the neuropsychological assessment of individuals with real or suspected brain damage, psychologists are becoming active in cognitive rehabilitation of brain-damaged individuals, with neuromuscular rehabilitation, and even with epilepsy. The role of neuropsychologists in assessment has been established for some time, but the role of neuropsychologists and other psychologists interested in rehabilitation is growing.

Cognitive Rehabilitation. Brain damage can result in both cognitive deficits and emotional changes. Efforts to intervene with cognitive deficits range from relatively simplistic interventions, such as teaching individuals to use calculators when arithmetic deficits are encountered, to rather elaborate interventions, sometimes involving the use of computerized instructional techniques to retrain skills. Emotional changes are also commonly seen among brain damaged individuals and have been the focus of some interventions. While cognitive and emotional rehabilitation efforts are relatively new, results appear promising.

Neuromuscular Rehabilitation. Neuromuscular disorders may arise out of either central or peripheral neurological problems. Although neuromuscular disorders have long been the focus of physical therapy interventions, biofeedback approaches appear effective in supplementing traditional physical therapy. In addition, relaxation and stress management interventions appear effective in intervening with some movement disorders that are affected by anxiety and muscular tension (Middaugh, 1982).

Epilepsy. Seizures are paroxysmal events in which electrical discharges occur in the brain. Depending on the locus and extent of the spread of the electrical activity, the symptoms may involve changes or interruptions in motor, sensory, cognitive, or conscious functions. Despite their physiological origin, it has been noted that seizures can be related to environmental and emotional factors. The predominant interventions that have been attempted with epileptic subjects include biofeedback, psychotherapeutic, and relaxation approaches. Most of the biofeedback with epileptic subjects has been for producing increases in sensorimotor activity in the electroencephalogram (EEG). Very systematic research has demonstrated large clinical gains even with subjects who have not benefited from conventional treatment; however, complex instrumentation and techniques are required for such approaches. Traditional psychotherapeutic procedures and relaxation-based treatment approaches (Mostofsky & Iguchi, 1982) have also been demonstrated to show striking and impressive changes in seizure activity.

ONCOLOGY

Psychologists have become involved in the assessment and treatment of cancer patients. Some of this work is with terminal patients and usually involves working in a hospice setting as part of an interdisciplinary team. However, psychologists also work with nonterminal patients who have difficulty adjusting to cancer and who develop iatrogenic effects from treatments.

For patients who are having difficulty adjusting to their disease, individual psychotherapy approaches have been utilized. These usually emphasize coping mechanisms, although the approach will vary depending on the stage of the disease (Wellisch, 1981). The most commonly seen iatrogenic effect among cancer patients is conditioned nausea. Because the drugs administered in cancer treatment may have powerful emetic effects, it is not unusual to see patients undergoing such treatment experience what may be conceptualized as classical conditioning of nausea to a variety of stimuli prior to the administration of the drug. Interventions based on relaxation and biofeedback techniques have proven effective with these sorts of cases.

EATING DISORDERS

While obesity is certainly a behavioral risk factor for a variety of disorders, anorexia and bulimia are considered health problems which require tertiary intervention. Anorexia, wherein the individual loses more and more weight through restricted caloric intake and increased caloric expenditure, may pose serious health threats and may even threaten the individual's life with continued starvation. Similarly, although probably not quite as severe, bulimia with bingeing and purging of food may lead to health problems. Intervention with both of these problems is important, but it is especially critical with those individuals who are anorectics, due to the severe health consequences of this disorder.

In general, a diverse set of physical and behavioral symptoms has been associated with anorexia, including weight loss, amenorrhea, increased activity level, severe distortion in body perception, and possibly an association with family distress. The variety of proposed etiological factors is also broad, with intervention approaches ranging from psychodynamic to behavioral, although behavioral strategies appear to be the most effective type of treatment (Bellack & D. A. Williamson, 1982). Generally, the behavioral approach to anorexia is one in which the individual is hospitalized, and complaints about food and weight are ignored while eating and weight gain are reinforced. Reinforcers may include a variety of social interactions, activities, and privileges. Additional treatment components may include such strategies as systematic desensitization for hierarchies including weight gain and food consumption, family therapy, cognitive methods of altering body image perceptions, and planned booster sessions. Although these sorts of treatment packages have not been empirically validated, they appear to be the most reasonable approach to dealing with anorectic patients.

OTHER AREAS

While the above major areas represent the majority of medical settings in which psychologists are active, there are many others in which psychologists participate in tertiary assessment and treatment. Additional areas include respiratory disorders such as asthma and even tracheostomy dependence; diabetes, in which psychologists have become active in weight control and exercise interventions, as well as interventions with needle phobics; visual disorders, such as extraocular motility disorders and blepharospasms in which spasms occur in the muscles around the eyes; gastrointestinal and urogenital disorders, such as irritable bowel syndrome, incontinence, gynecological disorders, and psychosexual problems; and even health problems in geriatric and pediatric populations. In sum, with the recognition that psychological and behavioral status affects health and disease, psychologists in medical settings are becoming active in the treatment of just about every type of health problem.

PREVENTIVE BEHAVIORAL MEDICINE

Despite the degree to which psychologists in medical settings become involved in tertiary assessment and treatment, a primer of behavioral medicine would be incomplete without at least some mention of work in primary and secondary areas. Without going into detail, psychologists, particularly those who are affiliated with preventive medicine and primary care general and internal medicine, become involved in diet, weight, smoking, alcohol and drug use, and exercise areas. With the national trends in health care towards prevention, psychologists undoubtedly will continue to find themselves in demand in the prevention of disease and promotion of healthy lifestyles.

Although approaches to all of these areas, particularly those of diet, weight, smoking, and exercise promotion, have been largely behavioral in nature, we have found that success with each of these lifestyle change efforts appears to improve with the incorporation of good clinical skills. For example, when individuals have not lost weight in our behavioral programs, we have noted often that confounding issues have emerged during individual therapy. These issues have included fears of weight loss and of the heterosexual admiration which that would bring; the inability of individuals to cope when eating occupied a substantial portion of their lives and they did not have the social skills and leisure time interests to occupy the time gained by following reasonable dietary habits; and even overt attempts by spouses to sabotage weight loss efforts due to concern about the attractiveness of their spouse with weight loss. Thus, although approaches in preventive behavioral medicine often have involved structured behavioral programs, good clinical skills are needed to maximize treatment efficacy in these areas.

SUMMARY

Psychologists have historically been a part of medical settings; until fairly recently, their roles were primarily limited to traditional mental health tasks in departments of psychiatry and in cognitive assessment roles. However, over approximately the past 15 years, psychologists' roles in some medical settings, particularly in teaching hospitals, have expanded and currently extend throughout the health system from tertiary to primary settings. As this trend continues and is facilitated by the national trends towards health cost containment and disease prevention, the demands for psychologists in medical settings should continue to filter down from teaching hospitals and increase.

James M. Raczynski, PhD, is currently an Assistant Professor in the Division of General and Preventive Medicine, Department of Psychology, and School of Public Health and an Associate Scholar in the Center for Aging, University of Alabama at Birmingham. He received his doctorate from the Pennsylvania State University in 1980 and has been involved in psychophysiological and behavioral medicine research, having published numerous articles in these areas. Dr. Raczynski may be contacted at 608 MEB, Behavioral Medicine Unit, Division of General and Preventive Medicine, University of Alabama School of Medicine, University Station, Birmingham, AL 35294.

RESOURCES

Abramson, D. (1974). *Vascular Disorders of the Extremities*. New York: Harper & Row.

Andrew, J. M. (1970). Recovery from surgery, with and without preparatory instruction, for three coping styles. *Journal of Personality and Social Psychology, 15*, 223-226.

Azrin, N. H., & Powell, J. (1969). Behavioral engineering: The use of response priming to improve prescribed self-medication. *Journal of Applied Behavioral Analysis, 2*, 39-42.

Beck, A. T. (1972). *Depression: Causes and Treatment*. Philadelphia: University of Pennsylvania Press.

Beck, A. T., Weissman, A., Lester, D., & Trexler, L. (1974). The measurement of pessimism: The hopelessness scale. *Journal of Consulting and Clinical Psychology, 42*, 861-865.

Bellack, A. S., & Williamson, D. A. (1982). Obesity and anorexia nervosa. In D. M. Doleys, R. L. Meredith, & A. R. Ciminero (Eds.), *Behavioral Medicine: Assessment and Treatment Strategies* (pp. 295-316). New York: Plenum Press.

Birk, L. (Ed.). (1973). *Biofeedback: Behavioral Medicine*. New York: Grune & Stratton.

Blackburn, H. (1980). Risk factors and cardiovascular disease. In The American Heart Association (Ed.), *The American Heart Association Heartbook: A Guide to Prevention and Treatment of Cardiovascular Disease* (pp. 1-20). New York: Dutton.

Boll, T. J. (1981). The Halstead-Reitan Neuropsychological Battery. In S. B. Filskov & T. J. Boll (Eds.), *Handbook of Clinical Neuropsychology* (577-607). New York: John Wiley.

Boll, T. J., O'Leary, D. S., & Barth, J. T. (1981). A quantitative and qualitative approach to neuropsychological evaluation. In C. K. Prokop & L. A. Bradley (Eds.), *Medical Psychology Contributions to Behavioral Medicine* (pp. 67-80). New York: Academic Press.

Brodman, K., Erdman, A. J., & Wolff, H. G. (1949). *Cornell Medical Index Health Questionnaire*. New York: Cornell University Medical College.

Cohen-Cole, S. A., Boker, J., Bird, J., & Freeman, A. M. (1982). Psychiatric education for primary care: A pilot study of needs of residents. *Journal of Medical Education, 57*, 931-936.

Colcher, I. S., & Bass, J. W. (1972). Penicillin treatment of streptococcal pharyngitis: A comparison of schedules and the role of specific counseling. *Journal of the American Medical Association, 222*, 657-569.

Derogatis, L. R. (1977). *SCL-90R (Revised) Version Manual - I*. Baltimore: Author. (Available from L. G. Derogatis, PhD, 500 Henry Phipps Clinic, Johns Hopkins Hospital, Baltimore, MD 21205.)

Dickey, F. F., Mattar, M. E., & Chudzik, G. M. (1975). Pharmacist counseling increases drug regimen compliance. *Hospitals, 49*, 85-88.

DiMatteo, M. R., & DiNicola, D. D. (1982). *Achieving Patient Compliance*. New York: Pergamon Press.

Dolce, J. J., & Raczynski, J. M. (1985). Neuromuscular activity and electromyography in painful backs: Psychological and biomechanical models in assessment and treatment. *Psychological Bulletin, 97*, 502-520.

Doleys, D. M., Meredith, R. L., & Ciminero, A. R. (Eds.). (1982). *Behavioral Medicine: Assessment and Treatment Strategies*. New York: Plenum Press.

Eney, R. D., & Goldstein, E. O. (1976). Compliance of chronic asthmatics with oral administration of theophylline as measured by serum and salivary levels. *Pediatrics, 57*, 513-517.

Fink, D., Malloy, M. J., Cohen, M., Greycloud, M. A., & Martin, F. (1969). Effective patient care in the pediatric ambulatory setting: A study of the acute care clinic. *Pediatrics, 43*, 927-935.

Fink, D., Martin, F., Cohen, M., Greycloud, M. A., & Malloy, M. J. (1969). The management specialist in effective pediatric ambulatory care. *American Journal of Public Health, 59*, 527-533.

Fordyce, W. E. (1976). *Behavioral Methods for Chronic Pain and Illness*. St. Louis: Mosby.

Friedman, M., Thoresen, C. E., Gill, J. J., Powell, L. H., Ulmer, D., Thompson, L., Price, V. A., Rabin, D. D., Breall, W. S., Dixon, T., Levy, R., & Bourg, E. (1984).

Alteration of Type A behavior and reduction in cardiac recurrences in postmyocardial infarction patients. *American Heart Journal, 108,* 237-248.

Gentry, W. D., & Matarazzo, J. D. (1981). Medical psychology: Three decades of growth and development. In C. K. Prokop & L. A. Bradley (Eds.), *Medical Psychology: Contributions to Behavioral Medicine* (pp. 5-15). New York: Academic Press.

Green, C. J. (1982). Psychological assessment in medical settings. In T. Millon, C. Green, & R. Meagher (Eds.), *Handbook of Clinical Health Psychology* (pp. 339-374). New York: Plenum Press.

Hackett, T. P., Cassem, N. H., & Wishnie, H. A. (1968). The coronary care unit: An appraisal of its psychologic hazards. *New England Journal of Medicine, 274,* 1365-1370.

Haynes, R. B., Sackett, D. L., & Taylor, D. W. (1979). Practical management of low compliance with antihypertensive therapy: A guide for the busy practitioner. *Clinical Investigative Medicine, 1,* 175-180.

Hypertension Detection and Follow-Up Program Cooperative Group. (1979). Five-year findings of the hypertension detection and follow-up program: I. Reduction in mortality of persons with high blood pressure, including mild hypertension. *Journal of the American Medical Association, 242,* 2562-2571.

Inui, T., Yourtee, E., & Williamson, J. (1976). Improved outcomes in hypertension after physician tutorials. *Annals of Internal Medicine, 84,* 646-651.

Jenkins, C. D., Rosenman, R. H., & Zyzanski, S. J. (1974). Prediction of clinical coronary heart disease by a test for the coronary-prone behavior pattern. *New England Journal of Medicine, 290,* 1271-1275.

Jenkins, C. D., Zyzanski, S. J., & Rosenman, R. H. (1979). *Jenkins Activity Survey Manual.* New York: The Psychological Corporation. (Available from The Psychological Corporation, 7500 Old Oak Boulevard, Cleveland, OH 44130.)

Keefe, F. J., & Blumenthal, J. A. (Eds.). (1982). *Assessment Strategies in Behavioral Medicine.* New York: Grune & Stratton.

Keefe, F. J., Surwit, R. S., & Pilon, R. N. (1980). Biofeedback, autogenic training and progressive relaxation in the treatment of Raynaud's disease. *Journal of Applied Behavior Analysis, 13,* 3-11.

Leventhal, H., & Nerenz, D. R. (1983). A model for stress research with some implications for the control of stress disorders. In D. Meichenbaum & M. D. Jaremko (Eds.), *Stress Reduction and Prevention* (pp. 5-38). New York: Plenum Press.

LaFreniere, J. G. (1979). *The Low Back Patient.* New York: Mason.

Levine, D. M., Green, L. W., Deeds, S. G., Chwalow, J., Russell, P., & Finlay, J. (1979). Health education for hypertensive patients. *Journal of the American Medical Association, 241,* 1700-1703.

Linkewich, J. A., Catalano, R., & Flack, H. L. (1974). The effect of packaging and instruction on outpatient compliance with medication regimens. *Drug Intelligence and Clinical Pharmacy, 8,* 10-15.

Luria, A. R. (1973). *The Working Brain.* New York: Basic Books.

Martin, J. E., & Dubbert, P. M. (1985). Exercise in hypertension. *Annals of Behavioral Medicine, 7,* 13-18.

Matarazzo, J. D. (1980). Behavioral health and behavioral medicine: Frontiers for a new health psychology. *American Psychologist, 35,* 807-817.

McCaffrey, R. J., & Blanchard, E. B. (1985). Stress management approaches to the treatment of essential hypertension. *Annals of Behavioral Medicine, 7,* 5-12.

McNamara, J. R. (Ed.). (1979). *Behavioral Approaches to Medicine: Application and Analysis.* New York: Plenum Press.

Meichenbaum, D., & Jaremko, M. E. (Eds.). (1983). *Stress Reduction and Prevention.* New York: Plenum Press.

Melzack, R., & Wall, P. D. (1983). *The Challenge of Pain.* New York: Basic Books.

Middaugh, S. J. (1982). Muscle training. In D. M. Doleys, R. L. Meredith, & A. R. Ciminero (Eds.), *Behavioral Medicine: Assessment and Treatment Strategies* (pp. 145-171). New York: Plenum Press.

Miller, N. E. (1969). Learning of visceral and glandular responses. *Science, 163,* 434-445.

Millon, T. (1982). On the nature of clinical health psychology. In T. Millon, C. Green, & R. Meagher (Eds.), *Handbook of Clinical Health Psychology* (pp. 1-27). New York: Plenum Press.

Millon, T., Green, C., & Meagher, R. (Eds.). (1982). *Handbook of Clinical Health Psychology.* New York: Plenum Press. (a)

Millon, T., Green, C., & Meagher, R. (1982). *Millon Behavioral Health Inventory Manual.* Minneapolis: National Computer Systems, Inc. (Available from National Computer Systems, Professional Assessment Services, P. O. Box 1416, Minneapolis, MN 55440.) (b)

Mostofsky, D. I., & Iguchi, M. Y. (1982). Behavior control of seizure disorders. In D. M. Doleys, R. L. Meredith, & A. R. Ciminero (Eds.), *Behavioral Medicine: Assessment and Treatment Strategies* (pp. 251-268). New York: Plenum Press.

Nessman, D. B., Carnahan, J. E., & Nugent, C. A. (1980). Improving compliance: Patient operated hypertension groups. *Archives of Internal Medicine, 140,* 1427-1430.

Patel, C. H., & North, W. R. S. (1975). Randomized controlled trial of yoga and biofeedback in management of hypertension. *Lancet, ii,* 93-95.

Powell, L. H. (1984). The Type A behavior pattern: An update on conceptual, assessment, and intervention research. *Behavioral Medicine Update, 6,* 7-10.

Prokop, C. K., & Bradley, L. A. (Eds.). (1981). *Medical Psychology: Contributions to Behavioral Medicine.* New York: Academic Press.

Raczynski, J. M., Thompson, J. K., & Sturgis, E. T. (1982). An evaluation of biofeedback assessment and training paradigms. *Clinical Psychology Review, 2,* 337-348.

Reisin, E., Abel, R., Modan, M., Silverberg, D. S., Elliahou, H. E., & Modan, B. (1978). Effect of weight loss without salt reduction on the reduction of blood pressure in overweight hypertensive patients. *New England Journal of Medicine, 298,* 1-6.

Sarason, I. G., Johnson, J. H., & Siegel, J. M. (1978). Assessing the impact of life changes. *Journal of Consulting and Clinical Psychology, 46,* 932-946.

Schwartz, G. E., & Weiss, S. M. (1978). Behavioral medicine revisited: An amended definition. *Journal of Behavioral Medicine, 1,* 249-251.

Sharpe, T. R., & Mikeal, R. L. (1974). Patients compliance with antibiotic regimens. *American Journal of Hospital Pharmacy, 31,* 479-484.

Spielberger, C. D., Gorsuch, R. L., & Lushene, R. (1970). *The State-Trait Anxiety Inventory Manual.* Palo Alto, CA: Consulting Psychologists Press.

Stone, G. C., Cohen, F., & Adler, N. E. (Eds.). (1980). *Health Psychology--A Handbook.* Washington, DC: Jossey-Bass.

Stuart, R. B. (Ed.). (1982). *Adherence, compliance and generalization in behavioral medicine.* New York: Brunner/Mazel.

Suinn, R. M. (1975). The cardiac stress management program for Type A patients. *Cardiac Rehabilitation, 5,* 13-15.

Surwit, R. S., Williams, R. B., Steptoe, A., & Biersner, R. (Eds.). (1982). *Behavioral Treatment of Disease.* New York: Plenum Press.

Turk, D. C., Meichenbaum, D., & Genest, M. (1983). *Pain and Behavioral Medicine: A Cognitive Behavioral Perspective.* New York: Guilford.

Wallston, K. A., Wallston, B. S., & DeVellis, R. (1978). Development of the Multidimensional Health Locus of Control (MHLC) scales. *Health Education Monographs, 6,* 160-170.

Wellisch, D. K. (1981). Intervention with cancer patient. In C. K. Prokop & L. A. Bradley (Eds.), *Medical Psychology: Contributions to Behavioral Medicine* (pp. 223-240). New York: Academic Press.

White, A. A., & Gordon, S. L. (1982). Synopsis: Workshop on idiographic low-back pain. *Spine, 7,* 141-149.

PSYCHOLOGICAL ASSESSMENT AND INTERVENTION IN THE EMERGENCY ROOM

Keith A. Wood

The role of psychologists in psychiatric emergency rooms has varied over recent years. In the past it has been limited primarily to a position of assistance. Psychiatrists, usually psychiatric residents, generally operated this busy but often neglected service (Gerson & Bassuk, 1980). In the past few years psychologists have expanded their positions in hospital settings and increased their activities in emergency rooms (Wood & Khuri, 1985). Such ventures into new areas, however, have been limited by their lack of medical exposure and training. Some suggest that their training and comparative salaries make them poor clinical choices for an emergency psychiatric team (psychiatric social workers and nurses would be preferred), and that their role should be primarily one of research (Barton, 1983).

In spite of the limitations, psychologists have taken on more duties and responsibilities in hospital emergency rooms. Some recent studies suggest that they do as well as their medical counterparts, and in some respects they may be even better prepared to complete certain emergency psychiatric duties (Dershowitz, 1969; Rubin, 1972; Wood & Khuri, 1985). Although their practices may be slightly different from those of their psychiatric colleagues, their assessments, diagnoses, predictions, and referrals have been accepted by the medical staff and the agencies to which their patients are referred.

The training of psychologists makes them easily adaptable to the requirements of a psychiatric emergency room for several reasons:

1. Their education in various forms of assessment is quite useful in this setting, where determining a great deal about a person in a short amount of time is essential. Psychologists are able to administer a wide range of psychological tests in a systematic, reliable manner. The mental status examination, the primary assessment tool of psychiatrists, borrows heavily from these instruments but fails to follow some of the requirements psychologists use to insure reliability. It may, indeed, be advantageous to have psychologists complete such assessments.

2. Psychologists are also trained in various statistical techniques that help to analyze present data and make reasonable predictions, two very important aspects of emergency psychiatry. In the emergency room, the clinician is asked to evaluate and often re-evaluate patients to predict whether they are likely to engage in certain dangerous behaviors. Such predictions are highly prone to error, but psychologists have the skills to make and assess predictions and have shown comparative superiority in clinical psychiatric settings. Other clinicians have recognized psychologists' scientific approach to data analysis, but have considered them best used in research positions. However, this skill is very important clinically and actually gives strong support for the use of psychologists in emergency rooms.

3. Clinical diagnosis is another area of importance in emergency room psychiatry (Khuri & Wood, 1984). Of the skills needed in this setting, *DSM-III* diagnosis probably has received the least amount of formal attention in traditional psychological training programs. In spite of this, psychologists' diagnostic patterns are very similar to those of their psychiatric colleagues (Newmark, Gentry, & Ziff,

1977). Similarities may be greater since the 1980 revision making diagnostic criteria more behavioral (American Psychiatric Association, 1980). Psychologists' expertise with behavioral analysis and objective measures has resulted in greater compatibility with present diagnostic standards.

4. The final important aspect of emergency room psychiatry involves the appropriate use of other social and treatment facilities. Psychologists' training in the importance of the social environment and its influence on behavior emphasizes the need to find nonmedical alternatives for many psychiatric patients. Preliminary data suggest that psychologists are less likely to hospitalize emergency room patients and will use other resources more often than psychiatrists (Wood & Khuri, 1985).

In summary, psychologists are able to function clinically in emergency room psychiatric settings. Some areas of their specialized training make them more appropriate in psychological assessment and treatment, but their lack of medical training imposes some limitations. The extent of such limitations appears to be a function of the psychologist's coping style, the hospital bylaws, the physicians involved, state licensure limitations, and traditional patterns. In my view, such restrictions should not prevent trained psychologists from practicing in this setting.

In this contribution I will describe several key tasks of psychologists in the emergency room. These include administration of the psychiatric interview and basic treatment decisions. Because of space limitations, several other important tasks are mentioned only briefly. These are administration of the mental status examination and specific diagnostic considerations.

THE PSYCHIATRIC INTERVIEW

The psychiatric interview is very important in emergency rooms. During the interview, the psychologist should place more emphasis on the individual's presenting behavior than on less objective causative factors. A good interview results in the patient speaking freely during early phases and the interviewer questioning more during the later phases. The interviewer must be an astute observer as well as a good listener.

There are two types of psychiatric interviews commonly used in emergency rooms: triage and general. The triage interview is a preliminary assessment of the individual's immediate functioning (Slaby, Lieb, & Tancredi, 1981). Once a consult is requested, a brief screening of the patient should be made to determine if he or she needs immediate attention. If this screening has been done by the evaluating physician, the necessary information can be determined indirectly. Even so, the psychologist may need to meet and reassure both patient and staff that the situation is under control.

The general psychiatric interview involves a thorough investigation of significant events in the patient's history and an assessment of his or her overall functioning. To accurately obtain this information, the interviewer must preface fact-gathering with a process phase. Doing this correctly is vital to the rapid, accurate assessment of the emergency room psychiatric patient.

THE PROCESS INTERVIEW

During the process phase, the interviewer focuses on gaining control of the interview (see Figure 1 on the next page). Most of the content information is gathered during this phase; omitted facts are assessed during the content portion of the psychiatric interview. As seen in Figure 1, the process interview has four basic sections: (a) general observation, (b) introduction, (c) verbalization, and (d) guided topics.

During *general observation* the interviewer unobtrusively measures the patient's present and past functioning, gathering a great deal of nonverbal information about the patient prior to formally initiating the interview (B. S. Fauman & M. A. Fauman, 1981). The goal is to look for as many revealing cues as possible. Sometimes a small, easily overlooked detail may be a critical factor in the patient's mind. Such an observation could be vital to subsequent verbalizations. It is important, therefore, to look at the way

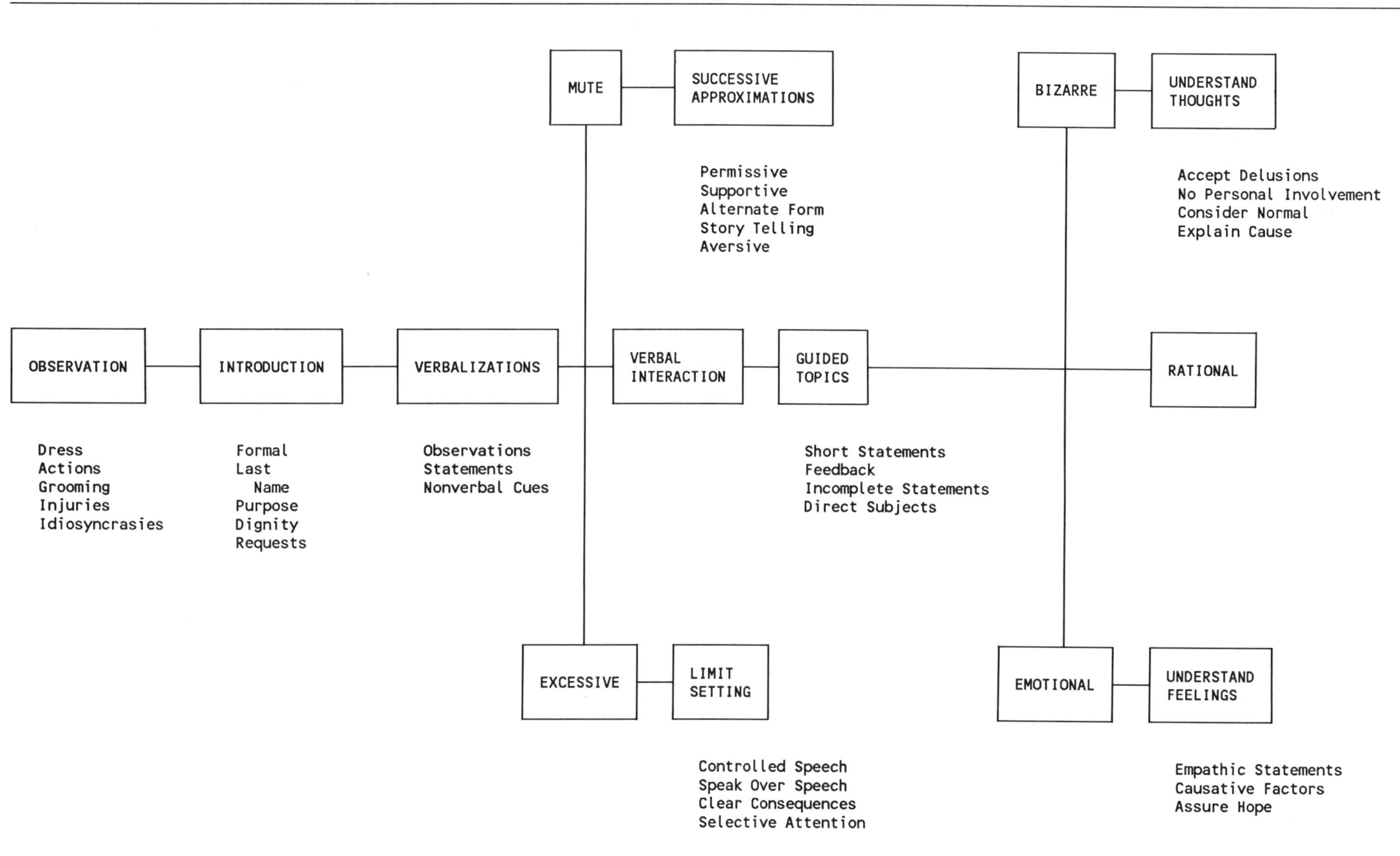

Figure 1. Emergency Room Psychiatric Process Interview

the patient is dressed. Something as simple as shoes can illustrate this point. New shoes may suggest that the patient has recently received some money, someone is taking care of him or her, or the patient is stealing. Worn shoes may imply quite a bit of walking, especially if the top portion looks new. Clean and polished shoes indicate the patient is concerned about his or her looks; dirty shoes may suggest the patient does not care about grooming matters. The wrong size shoes could mean the patient got them from a trash bin or as a "hand-me-down."

Of course, the interviewer should look at other things such as whether the socks match or are full of holes, whether the patient is wearing two or three layers of clothing, whether the clothing is appropriate, and so on. For example, patients in flamboyant clothing may be crying for attention or may be attempting to make some kind of sexual statement; patients with very revealing tops may be permissive and seductive. A torn or hole-filled shirt or blouse may suggest that the patient is wearing discards; clothes more appropriate to the opposite sex may indicate problems in identity. It is important also to look at the style and age of the clothing. Consider, for example, the collar length, the color combination, or the cut of the blouse or shirt, as well as the accessories. All these things have potential importance in the subsequent interview.

Besides dress, the interviewer should focus on the patient's general actions. A patient's lying still may suggest that he or she is tired, sleepy, or depressed. Talking to oneself is frequently associated with being disturbed about something or being unaware of one's environment. An engaging patient may reveal a desire for attention and the need to dominate, something the interviewer could use later when trying to gain more control. Repetitive, illogical actions may indicate some form of autism, retardation, or withdrawal. Pacing back and forth often indicates impending violence or anger (Wood & Khuri, 1984). Shaking may suggest extreme nervousness or trouble with alcohol or drugs.

In addition, the psychologist should notice the grooming of the patient. Matted hair or foul body odor suggest an individual who lacks interaction with others and may have used up the social resources that otherwise would see to the maintenance of his or her hygiene. An excessively dirty individual may not have had a place to sleep for some time or may have been moving about for several days. Neat but dirty clothing may indicate that the patient does not realize that time has passed. Blood on the clothing suggests that the patient has recently been injured or has inflicted injury in a physical struggle.

The observer should also notice any idiosyncrasies the patient may have. Tattoos often are associated with some special group such as a gang, some special meaning such as an old love, or some special circumstance such as being in the military. They can be quite informative and are ignored too often in emergency rooms. Scars may be associated with some significant event in the past, such as a big fight or an accident. Symbols on the patient's body may indicate membership in an organization such as a fraternity or sorority. The patient's accent could suggest a different region or country of origin. Any such information gathered prior to the influence of the interviewer's comments is a valuable asset to the subsequent interview process.

The *introduction* is the first verbal exchange the interviewer has with the patient. This is the key to the subsequent interview, and the first 15 to 20 seconds set the stage for the remainder of the interview. This is when the patient gathers his or her first impressions of the interviewer. Everything the interviewer does is important. Unlike private practitioners who have second and third chances, the emergency room evaluator must make the best of this first contact.

In the introduction, the interviewer should identify himself or herself as Dr. _________________ associated with the psychiatric department (Slaby et al., 1981). A formal but friendly climate should be set. Shaking hands should be limited to patients with whom the interviewer feels comfortable. Some patients can be physically dangerous, so caution is advised. The patient needs some personal space; staying at least one arm's length away is recommended. The patient's last name should be used unless he or she specifically suggests that the interviewer do otherwise.

During this phase the purpose of the interview should be stated. Too often interviewers approach patients and begin asking them questions with the result that patients do not know to whom they are talking or why they are being questioned. Clear but short and simple statements are best received. The interviewer should avoid talking very much or aimlessly. Setting the stage for the remainder of the interview should be the main goal at this point. The patient's dignity and privacy should be maintained. Interviewing the patient in a separate room, or at least outside the hearing range of others, is recommended. It is helpful to offer privileges such as food or drink and use of the toilet facilities before the patient has to request them. Such anticipation helps the patient feel the interviewer is sensitive, and that he or she does not have to manipulate to get such needs met. In the effort to establish oneself, the interviewer should avoid any compromising situations. If the patient starts undressing or attempts to get overly physical, the interviewer should leave or involve another professional. He or she needs to exercise caution, because emergency rooms contain a wide range of patients, many of whom are good at certain abusive games.

In an effort to establish control, it is helpful to request that the patient do something, for example, request that a prone patient sit up. This accustoms the patient to following the interviewer's lead. Such requests must be made skillfully to be effective. By gaining some control early, the interviewer may be able to go through the interview without much confrontation.

The third stage of the process interview involves initiating *verbalization*. During this phase the interviewer attempts to get the patient to talk. The patient must feel the interviewer understands and is sensitive to his or her situation (Menninger & Modlin, 1971). While accomplishing this, the interviewer must maintain some control; questions should be avoided and statements made instead. Most questions are implied statements and are thus much more threatening. A question such as "Are you hearing voices that other people are not hearing?" is more threatening than making a statement about voices.

Verbalizations are made easier by making observations. Noticing and giving feedback about changes after verbal interactions keeps the patient involved. The patient may put verbal emphasis on certain things, pause after certain statements or questions, or show softness or hardness in his or her replies. Changes in respiration rate or motor behavior, as well as factors that may be associated with such changes, should be noted. The interviewer should pay strict attention to the times at which the patient may laugh, cry, express anger, or act seductively. The patient should feel that the interviewer is aware of how he or she feels and acts without much initial interpretation.

Nonverbal cues are also important in encouraging verbalization. The interviewer should have good, nonthreatening eye contact - looking, but not getting caught in an eye-staring contest. Head nods or shakes and the use of "uh huh" and other little mumbles communicate attentive listening to the patient. The interviewer must also block out many of the extraneous noises that are often associated with busy emergency rooms. The patient should feel that his or her problem is taken seriously. At the conclusion of the verbalization phase, the patient should feel comfortable speaking to an interviewer who is in tune with him or her.

At this point in the process interview, two major problems could arise: (a) the patient could control the interview by speaking minimally or being mute, or (b) the patient could control the interview by talking too much. Either of these problems should be handled prior to continuing the interview.

Muteness. The mute patient is especially difficult because initially there is no communication. Many patients who are trying to conceal their anxieties resort to muteness. The interviewer should look for signs that suggest the patient is reacting to verbal statements, visual stimuli, or other aspects of his or her environment. Most of the patients who react to verbal or nonverbal cues should be able to speak later in the interview. The following procedures should help such patients initiate speech and speak more freely:

1. Take away the patient's control by giving permission to do something he or she is presently doing. For example, if the patient is not speaking, the interviewer might say, "I just want you to sit back, relax, and say nothing while I talk to you for a while." Thus, the interviewer takes control by giving the patient permission to continue in some resistant behavior.
2. Speak in a friendly, supportive manner, expressing empathy and understanding. Many patients do not speak much because they fear they will be misunderstood. They handle various conflicts by shutting others out. By saying something like, "I

imagine it is difficult being here surrounded by strangers asking you all types of personal questions," the interviewer may break down some of that resistance.

3. Take away the pressure to speak by giving the patient some alternative communication form. The best way to do this is to look for something the patient is already doing and force the patient to communicate by continuing or halting that behavior. For example, with a patient who is blinking quite often, a statement such as, "If you blink your eyelids, that will mean 'Yes'; if you keep them open, that will mean 'No,'" may be helpful. This allows some patients to communicate while not moving their lips. If they cooperate with this method, in all likelihood they will soon be speaking. Even if the patient decides to close his or her eyes, that is giving some control, and one can be optimistic about some subsequent verbal communication.

4. Tell an imaginary but realistic story about factors that led to the patient's being in his or her present state. This excellent technique brings together most of the information gathered during the general observation phase. Pull together as many data as possible and use reasonable hypotheses to fill in the blanks. When speaking with the patient, use pauses, allowing the patient to interject any additional information. Watch for changes in breathing, tearing, motor agitation, head nods, staring, and so on, as cues. Do not be afraid of adding to the story even if it is wrong. Frequently the patient's first statement is a correction. Here is an example: "I think I know the reason you are here. It started last night with someone you thought was quite special; you thought you could trust that person, but you were disappointed...Worse than being disappointed, you felt betrayed...You were angry and hurt at the same time, and when someone feels that way, almost anything can happen..." and so on. This is one of the best ways to get mute patients to start speaking; a correction is usually followed by an explanation of what really happened. If this technique does not work, a more adversive approach may be appropriate.

5. Place the patient in a rather uncomfortable situation which would be relieved through verbal communication. It is important to take advantage of the observations made earlier, especially of things the patient may not like, such as confrontation, engaging in repetitive acts, being touched, and so on. Some patients will obey certain commands but not speak. For example, some patients will obey commands to stand up and sit down over and over again until they finally say, "I'm tired of this. Why do I have to do this?" With a patient with whom one feels safe, putting a hand on his or her shoulder could really infringe on personal space. If the interviewer ignores the patient's stares suggesting that the interviewer remove his or her hand, the patient may be forced to give a verbal command. The interviewer should apologize when removing his or her hand. This step should be repeated if the patient fails to start speaking. Sometimes it is helpful to look away from patients who try to control by whispering or using nonverbal methods of communicating. They cannot be understood unless they speak up. Once the patient begins to talk, gradually increase his or her verbal output. Do not ask patients to tell why they were placed in the hospital. Lead them from "yes" or "no" responses, to clear content information, on to general information, and so on.

Verbosity. The excessively verbal patient presents another challenge to the interviewer. At first these patients are typically considered blessings, but when the interviewer cannot get a word in edgewise, frustration quickly ensues. Such patients need limits placed upon them, but this can be difficult. Often, as the patient talks more and louder, the interviewer has a tendency to talk more and louder. In some interviews, both the patient and the interviewer get so caught up in such verbal exchanges that it is difficult to distinguish who is the patient and who is the interviewer.

1. It is important for the interviewer to keep control of his or her voice and expression and to avoid talking faster and louder in competition with the patient. The verbosity of such patients is often contagious, and one must be careful to remain poised and talk slowly to calm the patient down.

2. The interviewer should state clear consequences to any statements made. He or she must act when statements are behaviorally violated. One might say to the patient, "If you continue to speak this way for the next 30 seconds, I will move you to a more secluded area." If the patient continues to speak the same way, then the interviewer should follow up with the consequences.

3. Selective attention can also be useful with overly verbal patients: obvious attention when the patient is talking less and obvious inattention when the patient talks more. Most patients who are hyperverbal really want to be noticed by others; therefore, the interviewer can use this device to his or her advantage. One way to accomplish this is to say, "I am going to look away from you until you stop speaking for a few seconds." If the patient stops talking, respond by saying, "Good." Then try interviewing again. Once the patient is under control, the interviewer may need to repeat some of the above-mentioned techniques to maintain the control. Though frequently mentioned, the use of chemicals to slow down such patients (or to get them to start talking) should be a last resort (Jacobs, 1984). Medication interferes with the remainder of the interviewing process. Nonchemical techniques should be tried first.

Once the patient is talking in a reasonable manner, the interviewer should begin *guiding* the patient into discussions of various *topics*. This involves directing the verbalizations into different, nonthreatening subjects and establishing the interviewer's role as "stage manager." This important phase involves close observation of the patient's verbal behavior without much emphasis on content (Puzantian, 1977).

1. The interviewer should use short statements. The less the interviewer influences the patient, the more valid the information gathered. Often patients will try to give answers they feel the interviewer wants to hear. To limit this, the interviewer should avoid asking a series of questions. Ideally, the patient should be talking approximately 75% of the time at the beginning of the interview (Rusk & Gerner, 1972). Demonstrate comprehension by using feedback statements, that is, repeating phrases the patient has made in an alternate form. By slightly exaggerating reactions, especially to very emotion-laden information presented in a very calm manner, the interviewer may disinhibit the patient and obtain a more accurate picture of his or her feelings. The interviewer may take feedback statements a step further by leaving verbal blanks to be filled in by the patient.

2. The interviewer should take advantage of the patient's statements to move the interview toward a discussion of different topics. This should occur smoothly with the interviewer in complete control. For example, the patient may say, "I've been living in Memphis for 13 years." The interviewer who wants to change the subject might respond, "Then you must be familiar with Elvis," not, "So you've been living in Memphis for some time now." The clinician's responses are significant in guiding the interview.

3. Avoid "why" questions. This asks the patient to explain away actions and events that may be important for the clinician to know about. By giving an explanation, much of the information is lost. The interviewer must remember that he or she is still gathering information, and avoid pitfalls such as emphasizing the reasons and missing the actions.

At this point in the interview, two other problems may arise. Patients may respond in either a very confusing or emotional manner so that continuing the interview may seem useless. Such problems can be reduced with the right techniques.

Bizarre Behavior. Initially the bizarre patient may seem so out of contact with reality that anything he or she says would be considered unreliable. This is especially true when interviewers go after content information prematurely. Dealing with this problem during the process stage reduces the pressure to gather specific information subsequently. The interviewer should attempt to understand how the patient is thinking, see that the thought process is somewhat stabilized, and continue with the interview. To accomplish this, the interviewer should follow four important practices:

1. Accept the patient's delusions as real. This may be difficult at times, but the interviewer needs to realize that the patient believes his or her thoughts to be real. It is not necessary for the interviewer to believe in the verity of those thoughts. The patient may say, "Since taking over as President of North America, that is United States, Canada, and Mexico, I have been under the constant watch of the Russians." It would be inappropriate to challenge such a statement at this point by saying, "But no such position exists!" A better statement might be "You must feel you have to be constantly on guard." The interviewer should be trying to understand what the patient is thinking and not trying to correct thought patterns at this point.

2. Avoid personal involvement in the patient's delusional system. The patient is likely to be even more upset upon discovery of the interviewer's true identity. The patient may have indicated that he or she thought the interviewer to be someone else by making statements such as "I know who you really are. You're the son of God, Jesus in human flesh. Speak, Master, your servant heareth. Ask and I will give you and only you from the depths of my soul." The interviewer must be cautious not to fall into the trap of getting information that might be otherwise unobtainable by accepting inclusion into the patient's delusional system. The patient can believe he or she is Jesus, Napoleon, Ronald Reagan, Joan of Arc, or whoever, but the interviewer is "Dr. ___________________." He or she must remain independent.

3. Consider the patient normal for his or her circumstances; avoid the "crazy person" stereotype. Avoid talking to patients as if their problems make them nonhuman. It is easy to consider patients with bizarre presentations as either intellectually limited or possessed with thoughts from another planet. Consequently, an interviewer might respond in a nonconstructive fashion, "If you think you own billions of dollars, then your last name must be Rockefeller." Many times these patients are much more insightful than they appear to be, at times even paranoid, and such statements can be insulting. The response of the clinician can contribute to the bizarreness of the presentation.

4. Explore the patient's bizarre thoughts even if they seem to be organically caused. Too often important information is missed if the interviewer thinks that the patient is under the influence of some chemical. It is helpful to explain the cause of the organically caused unusual experiences, but consider the chemical or condition as a disinhibitor, allowing the patient to reveal content that he or she would otherwise hide. Use this often discounted information to better understand some of the patient's less obvious feelings and perceptions. An intoxicated patient might say, "I feel so bad about how my drinking has affected my family that I really would like to kill myself." That same patient, when sober, would likely say, "I would never, never think of killing myself." The suicidal ideation during intoxication may reveal some repressed ideas and feelings that may be difficult to recognize or accept when sober. The clinician can gather this information and subsequently present it to the patient as a disinhibitor to allow greater communication about such feelings.

Emotionality. The other potential problem during this phase of the interview involves highly emotional patients. Their feelings are so intense that it is difficult for the clinician to deal with such individuals. Sometimes such patients are so excited and playful that the interviewer either gets caught up in the games or becomes frustrated and stops interviewing. Other emotional presentations seem so sad and tearful that they depress the interviewer, and for relief he or she may pull away.

It is important to understand how the patient is feeling, then attempt to stabilize the patient and continue with the interview. To accomplish this, the interviewer should:

1. Use empathic responses. The interviewer may listen carefully to the content and emotions of each statement the patient makes, then repeat them, adding a feeling statement, for example, "So you are 34 years old and never had a regular mate; you must be lonely at times." At this point the interviewer is trying to express that he or she hears what the patient is saying and feeling. To do this, it helps to

share theories concerning reasons for the patient's feelings. The goal is to agree that there are certain causes for the patient's present state.

2. Listen for possible reasons for the patient's emotionality. Specific events of which the patient is unaware may be important contributors. Many times events such as anniversaries, special events, holidays, conflicts, deaths of relatives, and so on, can significantly influence mood. The interviewer should also look for temporal patterns. With some female patients, there may be a monthly cycle (premenstrual syndrome) contributing to their feeling states.

3. Assure aid. Ideally, the interviewer should be able to communicate hope to the patient. To do this, the interviewer must believe that he or she can improve the patient's emotional state. His or her stability frequently gives the patient stability. The goal is to get the patient to a somewhat rational state so that the content portion of the interview can begin.

CONTENT INTERVIEW

The second part of the interview process involves obtaining the remaining specific information not already gathered during the process phase (see Figure 2 on the next page). Again, getting this information in response to statements rather than queries increases the reliability. Patients frequently feel pressured to answer in ways they believe the interviewer wants them to, so caution is warranted. The following is a general breakdown of areas to be covered during the content interview.

Chief Complaint. This refers to the patient's explanation of the reason for being in the psychiatric emergency room. When patients are brought by the police, their accounts may have little to do with the actual reason for admission. When patients are so psychotic that their answers make no sense, it is helpful to include under the chief complaint the description given by the police, family member, friend, caretaker, security guard, and so on. Included in the chief complaint should be behavior that led to the requirement for psychiatric attention. An example is "According to the police report, this patient was brought to the emergency room because he was walking nude in the middle of a busy street. The patient reports he was sunbathing in his shorts on his apartment deck and noticed an elderly woman trying to cross the street. He came down to help her and stopped some traffic in the process. His roommate could not be reached."

History of the Present Problem. This refers to immediate and past events leading up to the patient's being admitted to the emergency service. The emphasis here is on contributors to the present state, including significant experiences from years past.

This patient was working in a shoe factory until 2 months ago when he was dismissed after physically striking his superior. According to his family, he has been gradually more withdrawn and suspicious over the past 8 months. His wife left him 2 months ago after he badgered her with intense jealousy and suspicions. He lives alone in a low-income downtown apartment, although he receives an unemployment check.

Past Medical and Psychiatric History. This section should describe any treatment the patient has received, even that which appears unrelated to the present problem. Major illnesses, significant accidents, and unusual symptoms as well as active and past medications should be included. The amount and frequency of any medication is to be noted.

When this patient was 5, she fell off a bicycle, was unconscious, and had to be hospitalized for 2 weeks. Subsequently, she began having seizures and had to be treated with Dilantin and Phenobarbital. She has no psychiatric history but stated that her family doctor gave her some Valium for her nerves 2 years ago.

Alcohol and Drug History. The emphasis here is on the amount, timing, circumstances, and associated complications of chemical use. In regard to alcohol, the

CONTENT INTERVIEW
CLINICAL DECISIONS

INFORMATION
MENTAL STATUS EXAMINATION
DIAGNOSIS
TREATMENT
DISPOSITION

Identification
Chief Complaint
History, Present Problem
Medical/Psychiatric History
Alcohol/Drug History
Social History
Suicidal/Homicidal History
Family History

General Appearance
Motor Activity
Speech
Interview Behavior
Thought Form
Thought Content
Perception
Mood/Affect
Sensorium
Insight/Judgment

Childhood Disorders
Organic Mental Disorders
Substance Use Disorders
Schizophrenic Disorders
Paranoid Disorders
Other Psychotic Disorders
Affective Disorders
Anxiety Disorders
Somatoform Disorders
Dissociative States
Psychosexual Disorders
Facticious Disorders
Impulse Disorders
Adjustment Disorders
Personality Disorders

Chemotherapy
Crisis Intervention
Brief Psychotherapy
Family Therapy
Relationship Therapy
Grief Therapy
Education
Social Assistance

Hospitalization, Psychiatric
Crisis Stabilization Units
Emergency Housing
Medical Hospitalization
Alcohol/Drug Facilities
Jail
Nursing/Boarding Homes
Mental Health Centers
Home
Other

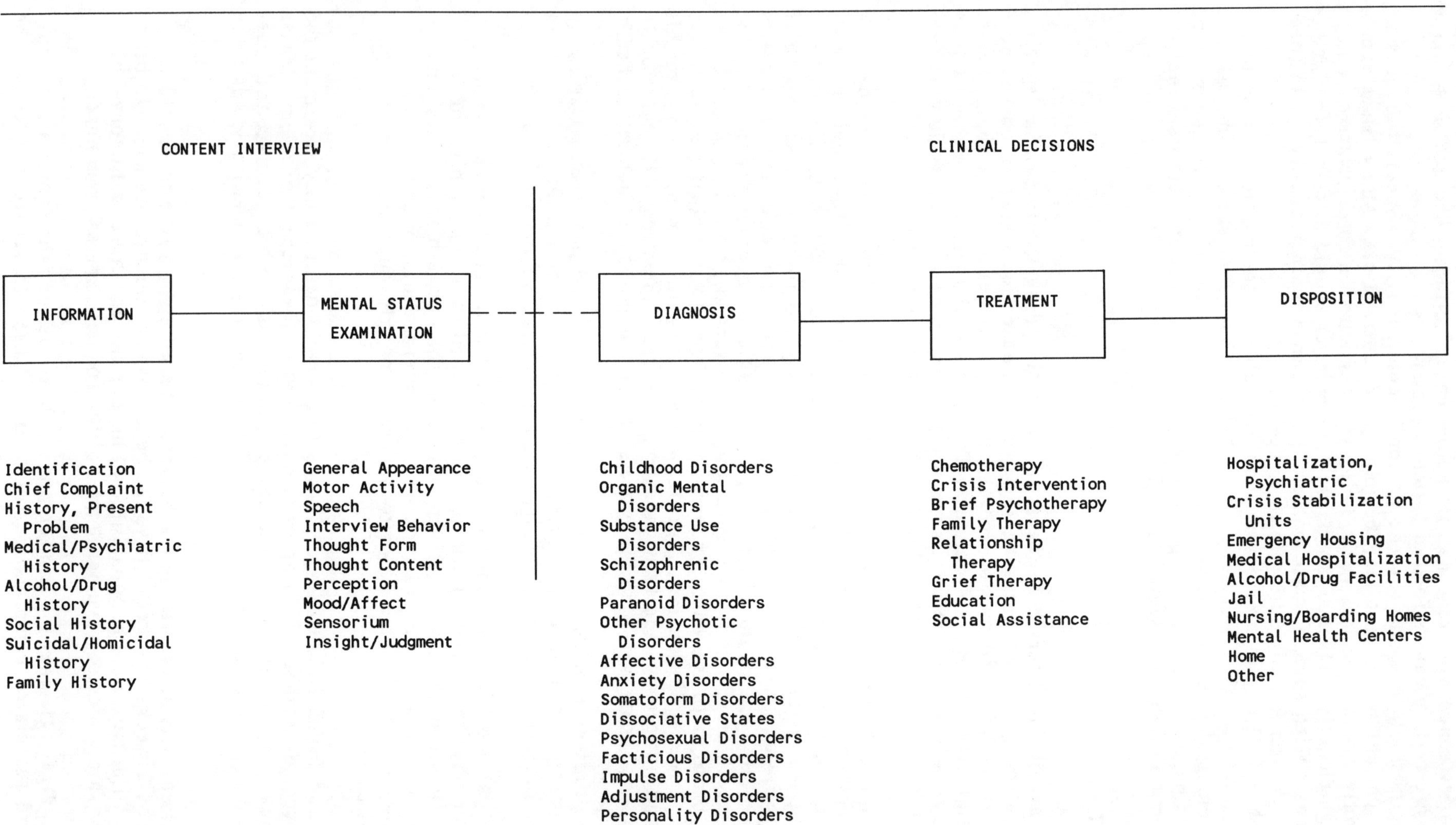

Figure 2

interviewer should determine if the patient drinks in the morning as well as evenings, with friends or alone, in good or bad situations, on weekends or weekdays, more now than in the past, and so on. A sizable number of emergency room psychiatric referrals have significant alcohol and drug histories that could have contributed to their present condition. Too often that history is never truly investigated (Knowles, 1984, provides a discussion of diagnosis of substance abusers). Many psychiatric presentations in emergency rooms are secondary to some drug effects. Getting a good history is essential for detection of such possibilities.

This patient reports drinking a glass of wine at night, on holidays, and on special occasions. He states that he uses no illegal drugs. He drinks an average of six cups of coffee per day and recently started taking some diet pills containing amphetamine. Other than the diet pills, this has been his base line behavior over the past 7 years.

Social History. Under this heading the interviewer should place the patient's social, educational, work, and criminal history, that is, his or her general lifestyle and personality traits. Has the patient had multiple intense relationships or marriages, or has he or she been able to keep a job for an extended period of time and maintain long-term friendships? Is the patient presently working and involved in a friendly relationship, or is he or she clumsy in social situations? Is there a significant criminal history, a pattern of self-destruction, or other harm?

This patient has been married seven times, the first to get away from home when she was 16. Both her academic and behavioral performance in school were poor. After a couple of suspensions she quit school in the 10th grade. She attributes many of her problems to her father's sexual molestations when she was 12 and 13. Her subsequent marriages have been with men who were either physically abusive or ran around with other women. She has no real friends and often feels bored and alone.

Suicidal and Homicidal History. This section focuses on the patient's history of self-destructive and other destructive thoughts, actions, and situations. The events and circumstances surrounding such actions should be included and considered in light of information shown to influence the probability of suicidal or homicidal behavior.

At the age of 18, she attempted to kill herself by taking a full bottle of aspirins and was subsequently hospitalized for a brief time. She states that it was secondary to several problems: her boyfriend was pressuring her, her parents didn't like him, and his parents didn't like her. She got the idea from her grandmother who died from an overdose 15 years ago. She is also having multiple conflicts with her mother.

Family Psychiatric History. This refers to treated and untreated psychiatric disorders of family members; these conditions may be either biological or environmental. Some examples are hospitalizations, mental health involvement, other psychiatric treatment, and aspects suggestive of a disorder such as alcohol use, even if it has not been treated. Some alcohol and drug abusers are self-medicators masking a psychiatric condition.

This patient was adopted at 3 months of age. He knows little about his biological parents except that his mother could not care for him because her mental condition required long-term psychiatric hospitalization. He knows nothing of his biological father. His adoptive parents have no psychiatric history, but his father is occasionally a heavy drinker. This is especially true during his depressed periods, which occur about twice a year.

OTHER ASSESSMENT FUNCTIONS

The psychiatric interview is generally followed by a mental status examination (MSE). The MSE covers the following basic sections: (a) general appearance, (b) motor activity, (c) speech, (d) interview behavior, (e) stream of thought, (f) thought content, (g) perception, (h) mood and affect, (i) sensorium, (j) intellect, and (k) insight and judgment. It is best if these are assessed on the basis of some type of structured checklist (Wood, 1981). Though this is an important part of the emergency room evaluation, further discussion is beyond the scope of this contribution.

Diagnosis represents the next logical step in the assessment process. Clinicians should make an effort to accurately diagnose the patient based on the data they have collected from the interview and MSE. A diagnosis based on *DSM-III* categories should be useful in formulating subsequent treatment decisions and a final disposition.

TREATMENT

In most psychiatric emergency rooms the emphasis has been placed on assessment and referral with little attention to actual treatment techniques. This is unfortunate because the emergency room clinician can employ a wide range of intervention strategies during this period of the patient's disequilibrium and, by doing so, reduce the likelihood of hospitalizing many patients (Feigelson et al., 1978; Kritzer & Langsley, 1967).

CHEMOTHERAPY

Psychologists are not trained or licensed to prescribe medications, but they can make recommendations in emergency room settings. To do this, the emergency room psychologist must be aware of the appropriate use of medication, including likely main and side effects.

In general, psychiatric patients do not receive psychotropic medication in emergency rooms. Several complications could arise if a patient receives chemotherapy:

1. The patient could be receiving medication from another psychiatric care source such as a mental health clinic.
2. Patients requiring a second evaluation elsewhere may not appear committable while sedated.
3. Chemotherapy may interfere with subsequent treatment attempts outside the emergency room.
4. Double dosing can result in serious side effects and increase the likelihood of extra pyramidal symptoms. This could be a problem if the patient receives two or three independent long-acting shots within a short period of time.
5. Manipulative individuals could be abusing the medication.
6. There is a lack of follow-up to assess the clinical response and adjust the medication or assess the possibility of dystonia.

Although the efficacy is limited, more medication is being prescribed to psychiatric patients than ever before (Jacobs, 1984). There are many reasons for this:

1. Patients are not able to get their medication elsewhere (i.e., they are not connected with a mental health center or private psychiatrist; they cannot afford to get it elsewhere, etc.).
2. Patients are discharged from some other program from which they obtained their medication, and they know of no other place to get a prescription.
3. Patients are referred by other agencies for crisis care (several centers having no regular physician coverage with minimal medical backup).
4. Many patients (deinstitutionalized, low income) do not know any place other than the hospital to get treatment (Menachem, Bluestone, & Steinmuller, 1983).
5. Some psychiatrists fear medical complications with selected new patients and request an emergency room evaluation prior to initiating treatment.

6. Finally, there are fewer psychiatric treatment options, resulting in more patients receiving their only care in hospital emergency rooms.

CRISIS INTERVENTION WITH POTENTIALLY DANGEROUS PATIENTS

Patients brought to the psychiatric emergency room have a high probability for potentially dangerous outbursts. The detection of impending violence and the management of explosive situations are critical skills for the emergency room clinician (Wood & Khuri, 1984).

Before beginning an interview, the clinician should evaluate the situation for danger. The position of the patient and the interviewer in reference to the door, potential weapons, and the patient's stance for potential physical aggression should be carefully assessed and modified if necessary. The clinician may want to (a) interview the patient alone, if the interviewer feels safe doing so; (b) interview the patient as privately as possible, away from the noisy part of the emergency room; (c) avoid leaving the patient alone in a room, for this could easily be interpreted as rejection; and (d) approach the patient slowly and from a distance, choosing a position for easy escape should it prove necessary.

The interviewer should not act on the natural inclination to match threats with threats; such behavior tends to further excite potentially violent patients. Rather, the clinician should acknowledge the patient's predicament and agitation. In a calm, engaging voice, the interviewer can ask "How can I help you?" showing no anxiety or fear. Sometimes it is effective to offer the patient food or drink to acknowledge sensitivity to his or her condition. During such episodes the clinician must constantly set limits. Agitated patients need authority and direction. A statement such as "Please sit down" can help relieve the patient's tension. Next the clinician should explore the patient's feelings to help him or her master the frustration. Saying "I see you are upset; do you feel dangerous to yourself or others?" could help the patient express his or her true feelings. When a patient does report dangerous impulses, it is important to find out towards whom they are directed. If the clinician believes they are serious, the potential victim may need to be warned (American Psychological Association, 1985).

If the above-mentioned verbal warnings do not work, a visual warning could be helpful. A show of force by hospital personnel frequently gives a message of not tolerating any violent action, and many patients calm down. In potentially violent situations, the interviewer should avoid (a) minimizing the chance of violence when early signs of escalating agitation are noted; (b) being isolated with such a person unless appropriate security measures have been taken; (c) engaging in behaviors which may be interpreted as aggressive, such as moving too close, touching, staring directly into the eyes, speaking loudly, using threatening expressions, or allowing several other people to interact simultaneously with the patient; (d) making promises that cannot be kept; and (e) allowing potential feelings of fear, hostility, or anger to interfere with self-control and professional understanding of the patient's circumstances.

In the event of a violent outburst, the clinician should clear the area immediately. A team of five should help control the patient, with one person holding each limb and the fifth person applying the physical restraints. While the restraints are being placed, it is advisable to explain to the patient what is being done and why. Throughout this process, it is important to reassure the patient of the clinician's concern for his or her safety and to help reduce agitation by various suggestions. If verbal, visual, and physical restraints fail to calm the patient, chemical restraint may be necessary.

Throughout all this, the clinician must be aware of his or her own feelings. Certain types of outbursts occur as a result of the way the patient is handled. In some situations, only seconds are available to deal with the situation. The interviewer's stance, attitude, affect, and verbalizations are critical if hostility is to be contained and diffused. Prejudices, emotional involvement, bias, negative attitudes, and so on, must be removed. It is important to avoid giving any message of tension.

Another role of the clinician in crisis situations is to prevent a series of crises from occurring in the emergency room. Frequently when one outburst occurs, the staff becomes increasingly tense, and this increases the likelihood of another outburst. The clinician should reassure staff members and be sensitive to their fears. If an emergency room staff person has been injured, supportive counseling may be necessary. With the increased amount of stress in emergency rooms, psychological relief is needed by both patients and staff (Menachem et al., 1983).

BRIEF PSYCHOTHERAPY

Whereas crisis intervention emphasizes the resolution of a critical period, brief psychotherapy emphasizes the removal or amelioration of specific symptoms. Using cathartic ego support or strategic intervention techniques, the clinician can effectively begin treating a range of problems (McPherson, 1984). This form of therapy should be goal-directed, with a focus on relief of symptoms and restoration of the patient's previous level of functioning. The clinician needs to understand the forces that precipitated the disruption, recognize personality factors that interfere with good functioning, look at past circumstances that resulted in similar experiences, investigate the relationship between the patient's personality traits and current problems, and understand techniques which would prevent such problems from recurring (Small, 1979).

To insure that specific changes are made in this form of psychotherapy, four steps are recommended to the clinician:

1. The interviewer should attempt to understand the patient's perception of and reactions to the problem. Some reactions are accepted as predictable for most individuals in the same situation; most responses are very individualistic and require specific attention. Once rapport has been established, the clinician should move to the next phase of the therapeutic process.
2. The interviewer should encourage insights and perceptions. This involves the mutual discovery of contributors to the problematic behavior. At this stage patients may attempt to deny major conflicts, and confrontation may be necessary to break down some of the barriers. Once the patient perceives that conflicts may lie beneath his or her overt difficulties, the clinician can move into the third phase.
3. The interviewer should develop an action plan. A specific program should be designed that allows the patient to leave the emergency room knowing just what he or she is going to do to make things better.
4. The clinician should help integrate the patient's behavioral changes and emotional state. The patient should understand why he or she is making the agreed-upon changes and how using such techniques can reduce future difficulties.

Techniques from various forms of therapy (relaxation, role playing, dream analysis, behavioral programming, etc.) are appropriate in this setting.

FAMILY THERAPY

Many emergency psychiatric patients are either brought or accompanied by family members (Perlmutter & Jones, 1985). Family members and friends are quite helpful during assessment, but they also can be beneficial in the treatment process. Because the ordinary defense mechanisms are broken down in this setting, the emergency room provides opportunity for the clinician to observe family interactions and to determine whether the patient's behavior is a function of that environment. If there are obvious communication deficits or fragmentations in the family structure, the clinician can begin improving the situation immediately (Linn, 1981). Behavioral programming often can be effective. Contingencies can be made and consequences enforced. In addition, the too-often-ignored family members of psychiatric patients should receive some support. The clinician's empathic ear can be an effective therapeutic tool in easing family tension.

RELATIONSHIP THERAPY

Frequently individuals come into the emergency room following relationship problems. Such problems are typically ignored except in crisis situations when one or both parties become explosive. Too often such altercations result in a homicide or suicide. The clinician in the emergency room has the opportunity to confront many of the couple's difficulties, aid in conflict resolution, and suggest specific behavioral changes. Such efforts may mobilize the couple to seek further professional help.

Simple, practical suggestions are best received in this setting. Finding a specific time and place for a husband and wife to discuss their marital problems may eliminate the need for outbursts that could result in another emergency room visit.

GRIEF THERAPY

There are a number of patients who appear in psychiatric emergency rooms following a significant loss. Individuals have great difficulty dealing with the loss of power (a specific position in an organization, at work, at home), possessions (source of income, house, acquisitions), relationships (death of a spouse or child, divorce), or physical function (due to aging, accident, disease). Therapeutically it is best not to prevent the patient from grieving, even though the clinician may feel uncomfortable with the process. It should be explained to the patient that feelings resulting in denial, depression, anger, and guilt are normal. It also should be emphasized that these reactions are part of the stages that lead to acceptance and reintegration. The clinician should give the patient hope by providing understanding help. Identifying stressors, explaining that time leads to improved feelings, and mobilizing family and friends are important techniques in this form of therapy (Barreira, 1984). It can be helpful to introduce the patient to various support systems that serve as coping resources.

GENERAL EDUCATION

The emergency room psychiatric clinician should explain the diagnosed disorder and prognosis to the patient and family. It is surprising how many patients and their family members are unaware of the psychiatric diagnosis, even though the patient may have been diagnosed as having schizophrenia for 20 years. Explaining the course of such disorders helps in their expectations and preparations. The clinician can give a plan of action for recurring episodes, thus reducing the chances of repeated emergencies.

SOCIAL ASSISTANCE

In addition to more direct therapeutic interventions, the psychiatric emergency room clinician can involve the patient in other social support systems (Menninger & Modlin, 1971). This can take the form of aid in getting financial assistance, transportation, religious support, food, and shelter. Specialized support groups such as Parents Without Partners or battered spouse groups could be contacted. Arrangements made while the patient is still in the emergency room increase the likelihood of subsequent involvement.

DISPOSITION

Once the assessment is complete, the diagnosis made, and treatment administered, the clinician must decide where to direct the patient from the emergency room. This decision is not always a clear one; several studies suggest that more patients are involuntarily hospitalized in psychiatric facilities than is legally warranted (American Psychological Association, 1985). If the clinician decides to hospitalize a patient against his or her will, a suit could follow for kidnapping; if the clinician releases a patient who subsequently inflicts self-harm or harms someone else, a suit could follow for inappropriate assessment and referral. The emergency room clinician must make such important disposition decisions quickly and appropriately. Patients and evaluating clinicians tend to disagree regarding patients' need for psychiatric hospitalization (Wood, Rosenthal, & Khuri, 1984). When in doubt, it is probably best to use a more conservative approach: that is, to refer the patient to the hospital.

Beyond the hospital, a variety of other dispositions exist. These include crisis stabilization units which are available in different forms, emergency housing agencies, medical hospitalization, alcohol and drug facilities, jail, nursing and boarding homes, mental health center referrals, and so on. Discussion of these various settings is beyond the scope of this contribution, but it is important that emergency room staff be both prudent and creative in their use of disposition options.

Keith A. Wood, PhD, is currently Administrative Director of Emergency Room Psychiatric Services at the Regional Medical Center, Memphis, and Assistant Professor of Psychiatry at the University of Tennessee, Memphis. Prior to his present position, he held academic and clinical positions in Huntsville, Alabama, and Memphis, Tennessee. His training is in clinical psychology and experimental analysis of behavior and he has published articles in both areas. Dr. Wood may be contacted at 66 North Pauline, Memphis, TN 38105.

RESOURCES

American Psychiatric Association. (1980). *Diagnostic and Statistical Manual of Mental Disorders* (3rd ed.). Washington, DC: Author.

American Psychological Association. (1985). *Duty to Protect* (COLI White Paper). Washington, DC: Author.

Barreira, P. J. (1984). Depression. In S. E. Hyman (Ed.), *Manual of Psychiatric Emergencies* (pp. 67-78). Boston: Little, Brown and Co.

Barton, G. M. (1983). Psychiatric staff and the emergency department: Roles, responsibilities and reciprocation. *Psychiatric Clinics of North America, 6,* 317-323.

Dershowitz, A. M. (1969, February). The psychologist's power in civil commitment: A knife that cuts both ways. *Psychology Today*, pp. 43-47.

Fauman, B. S., & Fauman, M. A. (1981). The psychiatric interview. *Emergency Psychiatry for the House Officer*. Baltimore: Williams and Wilkins.

Feigelson, E. B., Davis, E. B., MacKinnon, R., Shands, H. C., & Schwartz, C. C. (1978). The decision to hospitalize. *American Journal of Psychiatry, 135,* 354-357.

Gerson, S., & Bassuk, E. (1980). Psychiatric emergencies: An overview. *American Journal of Psychiatry, 137,* 1-11.

Jacobs, D. (1984). Psychopharmacologic management of the psychiatric emergency patient. *General Hospital Psychiatry, 6,* 203-210.

Khuri, R., & Wood, K. (1984). The role of diagnosis in a psychiatric emergency setting. *Hospital and Community Psychiatry, 35,* 715-718.

Knowles, P. L. (1984). Diagnosis and treatment decisions for alcohol and substance abusers. In P. A. Keller & L. G. Ritt (Eds.), *Innovations in Clinical Practice: A Source Book* (Vol. 3, pp. 166-178). Sarasota, FL: Professional Resource Exchange, Inc.

Kritzer, H., & Langsley, D. (1967). Training for emergency psychiatric services. *Journal of Medical Education, 42,* 1111-1115.

Linn, L. (1981). The treatment of psychiatric emergencies. In J. H. Masseurrman (Ed.), *Current Psychiatric Therapies* (pp. 177-181). New York: Grune and Stratton.

McPherson, D. E. (1984). Teaching and research in emergency psychiatry. *Canadian Journal of Psychiatry, 29,* 50-54.

Menachem, M., Bluestone, H., & Steinmuller, R. (1983). The psychiatrist as a "presence": Possible effects on emergency room staff attitudes. *General Hospital Psychiatry, 6,* 77-79.

Menninger, R. W., & Modlin, H. C. (1971). Individual violence, prevention in the violence-threatening patient. In J. Fawcett (Ed.), *Dynamics of Violence* (pp. 71-78). Chicago: American Medical Association.

Newmark, C. S., Gentry, L., & Ziff, D. R. (1977). Psychological and psychiatric opinions on schizophrenia. *Professional Psychology, 8,* 56-63.

Perimutter, R. A., & Jones, J. E. (1985). Assessment of families in psychiatric emergencies. *American Journal of Orthopsychiatry, 55,* 130-139.

Puzantian, V. (1977). *The Psychiatric Interview.* Unpublished communication, University of Tennessee Center for the Health Sciences, Memphis, TN.

Rubin, B. (1972). Prediction of dangerousness in mentally ill criminals. *Archives of General Psychiatry, 27,* 397-407.

Rusk, T., & Gerner, R. (1972). A study of the process of emergency psychotherapy. *American Journal of Psychiatry, 128,* 882-886.

Slaby, A. E., Lieb, J., & Tancredi, L. R. (1981). *Handbook of Psychiatric Emergencies.* Garden City, NY: Medical Examination Publishing.

Small, L. (1979). Models of the brief process. *The Briefer Psychotherapies* (pp. 67-83). New York: Brunner/Mazel.

Wood, K. A. (1981). *A Mental Status Evaluation Form.* Unpublished communication, University of Tennessee Center for the Health Sciences, Memphis, TN.

Wood, K. A., & Khuri, R. (1984). Violence: The emergency room patient. In J. T. Turner (Ed.), *Violence in the Medical Care Setting* (pp. 57-83). Rockville, MD: Aspen Systems.

Wood, K. A., & Khuri, R. (1985). The psychologist's role in the emergency room: A comparative study. *Professional Psychology: Research and Practice, 16,* 106-113.

Wood, K. A., & Khuri, R. (in press). *Temporal Aspects of Emergency Room Psychiatric Evaluations.* Manuscript submitted for publication.

Wood, K. A., Rosenthal, T. L., & Khuri, R. (1984). The need for hospitalization as perceived by emergency room patients and clinicians. *Hospital and Community Psychiatry, 35,* 830-832.

THE DUTY TO PROTECT: LEGAL PRINCIPLES AND THERAPEUTIC GUIDELINES

Samuel Knapp, Leon VandeCreek,
and Cindy Herzog

Psychotherapists are taught to keep client communications confidential. Clients expect that their communications will be kept secret, and psychotherapists generally believe that clients will not divulge highly personal information if they fear that their secrets will be shared. In 1976, however, the California Supreme Court ruled that a psychotherapist could be held liable for *not* breaching confidentiality to protect an innocent third party from the violence of a patient (*Tarasoff v. Regents of University of California*, 1976). The *Tarasoff* decision created anxiety and confusion among mental health professionals. Some psychotherapists misunderstood *Tarasoff* and believed that the court had promulgated regulations that unnecessarily compromised the privacy and effectiveness of psychotherapy. Others feared that subsequent court decisions might expand liability beyond that of the original *Tarasoff* decision and make psychotherapists highly vulnerable to negligence suits.

Fortunately, these fears are not justified. This contribution will explain the legal reasoning behind *Tarasoff* and the actual rulings within *Tarasoff* and subsequent cases. It will be shown that the *Tarasoff* decision is based on traditional legal principles which, if properly applied, will not interfere with sound clinical judgment. On the contrary, *Tarasoff* may actually encourage effective psychotherapy (Appelbaum, 1985; Beck, 1982; Roth & Meisel, 1977).

To understand the ruling in *Tarasoff* and subsequent cases, mental health professionals must become knowledgeable about the underlying legal principles. An understanding of these principles can guide psychotherapists in their treatment of dangerous patients.

LEGAL PRINCIPLES

The most pertinent principles are *duty to protect, foreseeability of harm*, and *identifiability of victim*. These principles have a long legal history. However, their application to the mental health field has been more recent.

According to common law, an individual has no duty to rescue or assist an injured person in an accident, although one has the duty not to harm a third party (Goldman, 1980). Courts have consistently concluded that an individual has no duty to control the behavior of another person to protect a third party until a "special relationship" has been established (Note, 1983). Special relationships may be established between clients and the custodians of psychiatric institutions, doctors, psychiatric nurses, or any mental health professional. Once this special relationship has been established, professionals must take necessary actions, which may include breaching confidentiality, to protect the public from harmful, contagious, or dangerous patients (Knapp & VandeCreek, 1982).

The duty to protect or warn typically applies only to a *foreseeable* victim of a dangerous or contagious patient. Foreseeability depends on the professional judgment of the therapist. Therapists need to use their best judgment in exercising care to protect third parties if their patients are dangerous. Professionals usually are not liable for failure to make correct judgments about foreseeability of dangerousness if they use the same knowledge and skill that other, comparable professionals utilize (Beis, 1984).

Another concept considered in several court cases related to duty to protect is *identifiability*. Therapists should be aware especially of situations in which a potential victim can be clearly identified. Then, the foreseeability of the potential dangerousness of the patient needs to be thoroughly examined (Beis, 1984).

Several courts prior to *Tarasoff* had used these principles to develop the duty to protect concept. For example, in *Skillings v. Allen* (1919), a physician was found to have a duty to warn the members of a family of the dangers of being exposed to their child's contagious disease. In another frequently cited case (*Simonsen v. Swenson*, 1920), a physician was not liable for breaking confidentiality by warning others about the contagious venereal disease of his patient. Also, in *Johnson v. State* (1968) the California Supreme Court concluded that the state had a duty to warn a foster family of the propensities for violence of a 16-year-old boy placed in their care. Finally, hospitals have been held liable for releasing dangerous mental patients when threats had been made toward identifiable victims (e.g., *Merchants National Bank and Trust Company of Fargo v. United States*, 1967).

TARASOFF AND THE DUTY TO PROTECT

The *Tarasoff* case provided little new in tort law liability. It merely took rules established for inpatients and applied them to outpatients. *Tarasoff* is important to discuss in detail because of its impact on subsequent cases and because it continues to be misunderstood (Runck, 1984). Although the entire court record is worth reading, only the necessary details are presented below.

Prosenjit Poddar, a graduate student at the University of California at Berkeley, obtained outpatient psychotherapy treatment with Dr. Lawrence Moore, a psychologist, for a severe emotional crisis after his romantic advances were rebuffed by a co-ed, Tatiana Tarasoff. During a psychotherapy session, Poddar confided his intention to kill Ms. Tarasoff when she returned from a summer vacation in Brazil. Moore took the threat seriously and consulted with two staff psychiatrists. They all agreed that the patient should be committed involuntarily to a psychiatric hospital. Moore subsequently notified the campus police that Poddar was a danger to another person and should be committed. The police officers detained Poddar for a while but did not commit him. He seemed rational, denied any intent to kill Tarasoff, and promised to avoid her. Poddar discontinued therapy with Moore, and no other attempts were made to deter him from his threatened intent to kill her. Two months later, when Ms. Tarasoff returned from Brazil, Poddar killed her.

The parents of Ms. Tarasoff initiated a wrongful death suit against the Regents of the University of California, Dr. Moore, the psychiatrists, and the police officers who released Poddar. The plaintiffs alleged that the defendants failed to commit Poddar and failed to warn their daughter of her peril.

The defendants in the case argued that dangerousness is hard to predict; hence, they should not have had to warn Tarasoff of Poddar's dangerousness. In fact, Monahan (1976) and other researchers have shown that mental health professionals have a poor track record of predicting dangerousness. Most often, they overpredict dangerousness. The court acknowledged the fact that dangerousness is hard to predict. It ruled, however, that this does not exempt therapists from their duty to protect others when such a determination of imminent danger is made. In this case, Dr. Moore had correctly predicted that Poddar was dangerous.

The defendants also argued that they should not have had to warn Ms. Tarasoff because this warning would have violated the rules of confidentiality. Psychotherapists have always viewed confidentiality as essential for effective treatment. Clients will distrust their therapists if confidentiality is breached, and therapy will be vitiated. Again, the court recognized that effective psychotherapy requires confidentiality. It stated, nevertheless, that psychotherapists have a duty to protect third parties from foreseeably dangerous patients, even if they must breach confidentiality in the process. The court ruled that "Public policy favoring protection of the confidential character of the psychotherapist-patient communications must yield to the extent to which disclosure is essential to avert danger to others. The protective privilege ends when the public peril begins" (*Tarasoff*, 1976, p. 337).

SUBSEQUENT CALIFORNIA CASES

Subsequent California cases have amplified the *Tarasoff* rules. *Mavroudis v. Superior Court for County of San Mateo* (1980) dealt with the issue of threats to unspecified persons. In this case, a hospital released a boy into the custody of his parents, whom he subsequently assaulted with a hammer. The parents wanted access to their son's psychiatric records to determine if the hospital knew they were identifiable victims of their son. The *Mavroudis* court reaffirmed the middle ground initially given in a footnote in *Tarasoff* (551 P.2d 334 at 345, footnote 11). It stated that even if the patient did not specifically state who the intended victim was, it could often be determined through a "moment's reflection." On the other hand, it recognized that the psychotherapist need not interrogate the patient or conduct a special investigation to learn the identity of the intended victim.

Another case dealt with vague and global threats against unspecified persons. In *Thompson v. County of Alameda* (1980), a juvenile had made vague threats to kill someone if he were released. Later, when released to the custody of his mother, he sexually assaulted and murdered a neighborhood child. The court ruled that the juvenile justice authorities had no obligation to warn the community. The court stated that giving a general warning for nonspecific threats made by each person paroled would be unwieldy, of little practical benefit, and would undermine the rehabilitative purposes of probation.

The *Thompson* case, however, included a strong dissent which said that warning an intended victim was not the only possible action which could have been taken. It was argued that the defendants had a duty to take reasonable steps to prevent the harm. The dissenter said that, under the circumstances of this case, the boy's mother should have been notified of the vague threats.

The assessment of dangerousness does not necessarily require that a verbal threat be made (*Jablonski v. United States*, 1983). In *Jablonski*, a federal court, applying California law, held that the psychiatrists could be held liable for failing to warn their patient's girlfriend of the danger he posed. The court noted that Jablonski had a history of violence toward his lovers. If the psychiatrists had obtained his past psychiatric records, the court argued, they would have seen that he posed an imminent threat to his girlfriend. The *Jablonski* court held the therapists liable even when they did not have actual knowledge of dangerousness because the therapists "should have known."

The duty to protect was extended in the case of *Hedlund v. Superior Court of Orange County* (1983). LaNita Wilson brought action against the psychotherapists alleging that they failed to warn her that one of their patients, Stephen Wilson (no relation), was of imminent danger to her. LaNita Wilson and Stephen were lovers, but were never married. Stephen had told a psychotherapist of his intention to seriously harm LaNita. Subsequently, Stephen shot and wounded LaNita and emotionally traumatized her infant son, who was with her at the time of the shooting.

The court concluded that the defendants had actual knowledge of Stephen's dangerousness and should have warned LaNita. Furthermore, the court agreed that the duty to protect should have extended to the infant child. The court stated:

> Nor is it unreasonable to recognize the existence of a duty to persons in close relationship to the object of a patient's threat, for the therapist must consider the existence of such persons both in evaluating the seriousness of the danger posed by the patient and in determining the appropriate steps to be taken to protect the named victim. (p. 47)

The *Hedlund* case is the only real extension of the *Tarasoff* decision. The other California cases merely amplified rules already stated in *Tarasoff*. The implications of the decision are unclear. It is not known how to identify who is in a "close relationship." Nor is it known how psychotherapists should act to protect such persons. Consider the hypothetical case in which an elementary school teacher is an identifiable victim of foreseeable danger. If warning the teacher is required, must the psychotherapist also warn the school children who are obvious bystanders? Should other teachers or school officials be warned? The *Hedlund* case suggests that if a warning is issued, the identified teacher should be alerted. The teacher may then decide how to protect those in close relationship to her.

APPLICATION OF TARASOFF TO OTHER STATES

The *Tarasoff* case is a binding precedent only in California, and courts in other states will not necessarily follow its precedent. In fact, *Tarasoff* has not been adopted by the highest court in any other state, and to date, only a few other courts have applied *Tarasoff*. A number of states have bypassed the *Tarasoff* decision because of differing circumstances in the case at trial.

In *McIntosh v. Milano* (1979), a New Jersey court accepted the *Tarasoff* doctrines. In this case, Dr. Milano, a New Jersey psychiatrist, had been treating a patient, Lee Morganstein, for 2 years before the patient murdered his next door neighbor. Morganstein had hostile feelings towards Miss McIntosh apparently because she did not reciprocate his romantic interest. He had fired a BB gun at her house and car some time prior to obtaining a pistol and murdering her.

As in the *Tarasoff* case, the court ruled that a psychiatrist must take necessary steps to protect identifiable victims of a dangerous patient. An expert witness had testified that Dr. Milano committed a "grave deviation" from accepted practice by failing to warn Miss McIntosh of Morganstein's dangerousness.

Subsequently, a federal court in Nebraska adopted the *Tarasoff* decision (*Lipari v. Sears, Roebuck, & Company*, 1980). An appellate court in New York has also indicated that it would probably accept *Tarasoff*, although the actual case addressed issues tangential to *Tarasoff* (*MacDonald v. Clinger*, 1982). As will be discussed below, numerous cases have failed to consider *Tarasoff* because the controlling facts were not identical in those cases.

REFUSAL TO EXPAND LIABILITY

In numerous cases, courts have refused to find psychotherapists liable. These have occurred when the psychotherapists followed acceptable procedures in assessing and treating their patients and reasonably could not have foreseen any harm. In addition, a court failed to find liability for failure to warn in a subsequent suicide. Finally, courts have failed to find liability when the warnings would have violated specific statutes, when the victims were already aware of the danger presented by the patient, or when the assailant-patient sought damages.

In several cases the courts have failed to find the psychotherapists liable when they followed standard procedures in assessing the degree of dangerousness and could not have reasonably foreseen the tragedy. For example, in *Leedy v. Hartnett* (1981), a patient at a Veterans Administration Hospital in Pennsylvania discharged himself and visited the plaintiffs. He got drunk during the visit and seriously injured Leedy and his wife. Leedy alleged that the hospital had a duty to warn them of Hartnett's dangerousness. The court claimed, however, that the Veterans Administration Hospital had no duty to warn the Leedys. It noted that there was no evidence "that the assailant had ever made any threats against those persons or was more likely to become violent towards people in whose presence he was comfortable" (p. 1125). Similar conclusions were reached in other cases (e.g., *Brady v. Hopper*, 1983; *Cairl v. State*, 1982; *Case v. United States*, 1981).

One court has held that the duty to protect does not extend to suicidal persons (*Bellah v. Greenson*, 1978). Tammy Bellah committed suicide while she was receiving treatment from the defendant, Dr. Greenson. Two years later, Tammy's parents brought a lawsuit against Greenson alleging that he had failed to warn them of their daughter's suicidal tendencies. Dr. Greenson was not liable because the court decided that he was not required to breach confidentiality, although the law permitted him to do so. The court stated: "Case law requires only that a therapist disclose contents of confidential communication where risk to be prevented thereby is the danger of violent assault, and not where the risk of harm is self-inflicted or mere property damage" (p. 536).

Courts refused to find liability when warnings would have violated a specific statute. In *Shaw v. Glickman* (1980), a man, his wife, and his wife's lover were being seen in group psychotherapy conducted by a psychotherapy team. Later the man entered the lover's apartment while he and the wife were in bed and shot his wife's lover five times. The assailant had never told the psychotherapy team that he planned to harm the plaintiff. The lover brought a suit against the team, however, alleging that they should have predicted the danger and warned him.

The court ruled that the psychotherapy team could not be held liable for failure to warn because the violence was not foreseeable. The Maryland court, however, went further and said that the members of the team could not lawfully disclose any information even if they had known about the imminent danger. Maryland courts do not allow breach of confidentiality even when third parties could be endangered by imminent violence. The only exception to this rule occurs when involuntary commitment of the patient is sought.

Courts have also failed to find liability when the victim is already aware of the danger. In *Matter of Estate of Votteler* (1982), a plaintiff alleged that the psychiatrist should have warned him of the threat that the patient made to him. However, the victim was already aware of the threat, while the psychiatrist was not. The court held that the doctor had used acceptable procedures in evaluating the patient's dangerousness and could not have anticipated it.

RECOMMENDATIONS FOR PSYCHOTHERAPISTS

The *Tarasoff* decision has caused confusion among many psychotherapists. Because most states have not determined if *Tarasoff* applies in their state, many psychotherapists do not know if they are bound by that doctrine. We believe it is most prudent for psychotherapists to assume they would be subject to *Tarasoff* .

The *Tarasoff* doctrine, however, does not necessarily impose an unwieldy burden on the psychotherapist. The potential for lawsuits can be greatly reduced by knowledge of the *Tarasoff* principles and by sound therapeutic judgment. The *Tarasoff* doctrine, if properly applied by the courts, does nothing to interfere with professional judgments. Specific therapeutic guidelines are provided below. Appelbaum (1985) has suggested that psychotherapists follow a three-stage procedure in analyzing their *Tarasoff* obligations. These stages are (a) identifying the procedures required to assess the degree of danger, (b) selecting the most appropriate intervention, and (c) implementing it. Liability may occur because of faulty behavior at any one of these three stages.

The first step requires that psychotherapists acquire information relevant to their evaluation of the potential for dangerousness. The *Tarasoff* court did not require psychotherapists to disclose every idle fantasy to harm others. On the contrary, the Tarasoff court stated: "A therapist should not be encouraged routinely to reveal such threats...unless such disclosures are necessary to avert danger to others" (*Tarasoff*, 1976, p. 347).

A verbal threat alone is not sufficient to make the determination of imminent dangerousness, any more than a verbal threat of suicide means that a suicide attempt is imminent. Instead, the psychotherapist must use the procedures that a reasonable clinician would use in making the assessment. This means that the psychotherapist should explore personality dynamics, background of violent behavior, access to lethal weapons, and the relationship to the intended victims. Recent articles by Finney (1982-1983) and Gutheil (1985) describe patients with histrionic and borderline personality disorders, respectively, and illustrate how the unique features of these syndromes should be considered when determining the appropriate clinical response in life-endangering situations.

Conversely, the absence of an overt threat does not necessarily rule out the possibility of imminent dangerousness. The *Jablonski* court held that the failure of the aggressor specifically to threaten the victim does not exonerate the psychotherapist from failure to assess dangerousness. Instead, the court raised the possibility that a reasonably prudent psychotherapist would have acquired previous treatment records that would have revealed a background of dangerous behavior.

The second stage delineated by Appelbaum is the selection of the appropriate intervention. It is important to note that the *Tarasoff* court did not see warning the intended victim as the only therapeutic response when danger arises. On the contrary, the court stated that the "discharge of this duty may require the psychotherapist to take one or more of various steps, depending on the nature of the case" (*Tarasoff*, 1976, p. 334), including warning the intended victim. The psychotherapist may consider one of several steps including involuntary commitment or notifying the police. Indeed, cases have been presented in which warning the intended victim was a meaningless gesture (Halleck, 1980), unnecessarily harmed the psychotherapeutic relationship (Appelbaum, 1985), or may even have precipitated violence (Adebimpe, McClung, & Gigandet, no date).

Civil commitment had been the traditional procedure for dealing with dangerous persons. With the advent of strict civil commitment laws, however, patients have often failed to qualify for a civil commitment because an overt act has not been committed or because the patients do not have the severe degree of mental illness which most states hold as a prerequisite for civil commitments.

Wexler (1980) has suggested the option of having the potential victim participate in therapy. He believes that victims sometimes unknowingly precipitate the violence against themselves. To the extent that this is true, the therapist should attend to the pathology of the relationship between the patient and the potential victim rather than to the psyche of the patient. Often the potential victim is a family member, lover, or close friend. Treatment of such a relationship should involve some contact with the potential victim as well as with the potential offender, and might take the form of family, couple, or conjoint therapy. Treatment of the pathological relationship as well as, or in lieu of, the pathological individual may be beneficial. However, the therapist must guard against unwittingly becoming a party to a criminal act.

Roth and Meisel (1977) have suggested that social or environmental manipulations may reduce the risk of danger. For example, the psychotherapist can ask patients to rid themselves of lethal weapons. They believe that psychotherapists must be frank with patients who speak seriously of harming others, and that the psychotherapist should inform the patient of the limits of confidentiality if serious threats continue. If the psychotherapist decides to warn, they suggest attempting to obtain the patient's consent first, and, if possible, making the warning in the patient's presence. Such actions allow for consideration of the future of psychotherapy with the patient.

A recent study dealt with the effects of warnings upon the psychotherapeutic relationship. Although the sample size was small and the sampling limited to psychiatrists in the Boston area, the study's conclusions supported Roth and Meisel's clinical intuition. "In every case in which a warning was warranted and discussed ahead, there was either a positive impact on therapy or no impact was apparent. However, if either the warning was not discussed ahead or was not warranted, then the impact was negative in four of five cases" (Beck, 1982, p. 194). Other anecdotal cases also support Roth and Meisel's conclusions (Appelbaum, 1985; Wulsin, Bursztajn, & Gutheil, 1983).

Appelbaum's final stage involves the appropriate implementation of the decision. This stage makes common sense because there would be no practical gain in developing an effective plan if it were not implemented. The *Tarasoff* case provides an example of failure at stage three. Dr. Moore had completed the first two stages of the three-stage procedure. He gathered enough data to make the determination of dangerousness and sought an appropriate intervention. He failed, however, in the third stage when the attempted commitment of Poddar failed. For reasons that are not clear from the case record, Moore's supervisor did not permit him to implement other strategies to prevent violence.

In any of these three stages, it is valuable to seek consultation with other mental health professionals, especially those who have expertise in dealing with potentially violent individuals. This consultation could provide insights into how to evaluate dangerousness, select the optimal intervention, or implement it effectively. In addition, psychotherapists should record management options that have been considered. These records could be invaluable if the decision were ever called into question.

Samuel Knapp, EdD, is currently a psychologist with the Rosalie G. Handler Center in Millersburg, Pennsylvania. His interests are in the legal regulation of professional psychology and the treatment of anxiety disorders. Dr. Knapp may be contacted at the Rosalie G. Handler Center, 1000 Medical Road, Millersburg, PA 17061.

Leon VandeCreek, PhD, is currently Professor of Psychology and Director of Clinical Training at Indiana University of Pennsylvania. His interests are in the areas of interface of psychology and law and professional issues. Dr. VandeCreek can be contacted at Psychology Department, Indiana University of Pennsylvania, Indiana, PA 15705.

Cindy Herzog, MA, is currently a graduate student in the Doctorate of Psychology program at Indiana University of Pennsylvania. She is interested in clinical health psychology, professional issues, and family therapy. She also works at a drug and alcohol outpatient crisis center. Ms. Herzog may be contacted at the Psychology Department, Clark Hall, Indiana University of Pennsylvania, Indiana, PA 15705.

RESOURCES

Adebimpe, V. R., McClung, J., & Gigandet, J. N. (no date). *Dangerousness in the Tarasoff Penumbra.* Unpublished manuscript.

Appelbaum, P. (1985). Tarasoff and the clinician: Problems in fulfilling the duty to protect. *American Journal of Psychiatry, 142,* 425-429.

Beck, J. (1982). When the patient threatens violence: An empirical study of clinical practice after Tarasoff. *Bulletin of the American Academy of Psychiatry and the Law, 10,* 189-201.

Beis, E. B. (1984). *Mental Health and the Law.* Rockville, MD: Aspen Systems Corporation.

Bellah v. Greenson, 73 Cal. App. 3d 892, 141 Cal. Rptr. 92 (1978).

Brady v. Hopper, 570 F. Supp. 1333 (1983).

Cairl v. State, 323 N.W.2d 20 (Minn. 1982).

Case v. United States, 523 F. Supp. 317 (1981).

Finney, J. (1982-1983). Breaking confidence: An application of the Tarasoff rule. *American Journal of Forensic Psychiatry, 3,* 135-140.

Goldman, E. B. (1980). Confidentiality and the Tarasoff case. *Ethics, Humanism, and Medicine, 38,* 237-244.

Gutheil, T. (1985). Medicolegal pitfalls in the treatment of borderline patients. *American Journal of Psychiatry, 142,* 9-13.

Halleck, S. (1980). *Law in the Practice of Psychiatry.* New York: Plenum Medical Book Company.

Hedlund v. Superior Court of Orange City, 34 Cal.3d 695, 669 P.2d 41 (Cal. 1983).

Jablonski v. United States, 712 F.2d 391 (1983).

Johnson v. State, 69 Cal.2d 782, 447 P.2d 352, 73 Cal. Rptr. 240 (1968).

Knapp, S., & VandeCreek, L. (1982). Tarasoff: Five years later. *Professional Psychology, 13,* 511-516.

Leedy v. Hartnett, 510 F. Supp. 1125 (1981).

Lipari v. Sears, Roebuck, & Company, 497 F. Supp. 185 (1980).

MacDonald v. Clinger, 446 N.Y.S.2d 801 (App. Div. 1982).

Matter of Estate of Votteler, 327 N.W.2d 759 (Iowa 1982).

Mavroudis v. Superior Court for County of San Mateo, 102 Cal. App. 3d 594, 162 Cal. Rptr. 723 (1980).

McIntosh v. Milano, 168 N.J. Super. 466, 403 A.2d 500 (1979).

Merchants National Bank and Trust Company of Fargo v. United States, 272 F. Supp. 409 (1967).

Monahan, J. (1976). The prevention of violence. In J. Monahan (Ed.), *Community Mental Health and the Criminal Justice System* (pp. 13-34). New York: Pergamon Press.

Note. (1983). Tort law: The psychiatric duty to warn. *Hamline Law Review, 6,* 513-534.

Roth, L., & Meisel, A. (1977). Dangerousness, confidentiality, and the duty to warn. *American Journal of Psychiatry, 134,* 508-511.

Runck, B. (1984). Survey shows therapists misunderstand Tarasoff rule. *Hospital and Community Psychiatry, 35,* 429-430.

Shaw v. Glickman, 45 Md. App. 718, 415 A.2d 625 (Md. App. 1980).

Simonsen v. Swenson, 177 N.W. 831 (1920).

Skillings v. Allen, 143 Minn. 323, 173 N.W. 663 (1919).

Tarasoff v. Regents of University of California, 131 Cal. Rptr. 14, 551 P.2d 334 (1976).

Thompson v. County of Alameda, 167 Cal. Rptr. 70, 614 P.2d 728 (1980).

Wexler, D. (1980). Victimology and mental health law: An agenda. *Virginia Law Review, 66,* 681-711.

Wulsin, L., Bursztajn, M., & Gutheil, T. (1983). Unexpected clinical features of the Tarasoff decision: The therapeutic alliance and the "duty to warn." *American Journal of Psychiatry, 140,* 601-603.

TECHNIQUES FOR ENGAGING "DIFFICULT" CHILDREN IN THE PLAYROOM

Stanley Kissel

A movement away from the orthodox adherence to one theory or method for understanding and alleviating childhood psychopathology to a more eclectic orientation represents one of the major changes in the realm of child psychotherapy (Halpern & Kissel, 1976; Kissel, 1977). Following the early writings of Anna Freud (1946) and Virginia Axline (1947), child clinicians would traditionally provide children materials from which they could choose and through which they could safely express themselves; therapists remained passive until invited to share in play, and would usually confine their comments to the play activity and the child's abilities. Kissel (1977) has suggested that specific methods and strategies be applied to individual children rather than forcing each child to fit a particular mold, be it Axlinian, Ginottian, or Adlerian. Schaefer and Millman (1977) and Schaefer and O'Connor (1983) have described their prescriptive approach to engaging children who are problematic. They suggest that the prescriptive approach, which emphasizes a therapist's responsibility for determining the most appropriate therapeutic technique for each particular case, will result in maximum therapeutic effectiveness in the briefest possible time period.

Each clinician enters the playroom with a conception of children as well as a particular categorization around which the child's behaviors, attitudes, feelings, and thoughts can be organized. For example, Harrington (1984) suggests understanding children from the *DSM-III* point of view and categorizes childhood disorders into five broad areas: intellectual, behavioral, emotional, physical, and developmental. Quay (1972) considers childhood psychopathology from a behavioral point of view and suggests that four patterns account for a considerable amount of the aggression, withdrawal, and immaturity often found in children showing emotional disorders. The four dimensions are: immaturity, socialized delinquency, personality disorder, and conduct disorder. Anna Freud (1965) has provided a different and highly complex psychoanalytic conceptualization of childhood pathology which is organized around the developmental tasks children experience.

The aforementioned approaches assist clinicians considerably as they attempt to understand the motivations for a child's maladaptive behavior, and also when they consider the level of pathology of their young patient. However, these approaches have not been as enlightening or helpful in suggesting specific intervention techniques.

TYPES OF CHILDREN

Throughout my years of supervising, teaching students, and providing workshops and seminars, I have utilized a straightforward categorization which has been helpful in guiding clinicians to consider specific techniques for engaging children therapeutically, whether for a diagnostic assessment with the aim of gaining information or for a more sustained therapeutic interaction with the purpose of ameliorating maladaptive behaviors and traits. For this purpose, children who are having problems can be thought of as either being *too loose* or *too tight*.

Too tight children are fearful, anxious, and have considerable difficulty expressing themselves verbally or behaviorally because they often are afraid of letting go. Children who are too loose, on the other hand, have a considerable amount of difficulty controlling their impulsive and behavioral expression of thoughts or feelings. They seem to lack concern regarding the feelings of others, have difficulty anticipating the effects or consequences of their behaviors, and have been reinforced in the past for excessive nonverbal expressions. Their ability to control themselves is poorly developed. Of course, both types of problem youngsters have difficulty with their self-esteem, as a history of maladaptive behavior often leads significant others in the environment to accentuate the negative and eliminate the positive when interacting with these children. Both types of youngsters also find it difficult to verbalize their thoughts and feelings directly. Those who are too loose cannot stand still long enough to reflect upon their performance, or they compare themselves with others negatively. The purpose of seeing a child as too loose or too tight is not suggested as an alternative to more traditional categorization or diagnostic formulizations but rather as a heuristic mediator for considering some effective and efficient techniques for engaging the child.

In general, children manifesting anxiety or depressive disorders are found to be too tight, whereas conduct and attention deficit children are found to be too loose. Before considering some specific techniques it is important to remember some of the more general considerations for engaging children therapeutically. First and foremost, adult clinicians present themselves as role models to their young patients. Clinicians convey to the child in both words and action that they are persons of authority in the playroom. That means maintaining control in the playroom by not permitting anything to occur which is harmful to either the child or the clinician. It is the therapist's responsibility to see that the room is adequately and appropriately stocked with properly functioning toys. The playroom should not be overly messy as this may confuse or inappropriately stimulate a child. Yet it cannot be a sterile operating room either. Projects which are left from session to session need to be cared for so that other children do not inadvertently destroy them or lose their parts.

When involved in board games where there is a competitive aspect, the clinician will do better to focus on the child's feelings, attitudes, and styles than on winning or losing the game. Often when playing board or competitive games, some clinicians commit a tactical error by permitting children to win because they are concerned about hurting the child's feelings. It is usually better to focus on reactions to realistic loss or developmental limitations with the aim of encouraging positive expectations for the future. Similarly, when children have such a strong need to win that they cheat or change the rules, it is important to recognize the child's needs for rule changing but to abide by the agreed upon rules. These general considerations are the background in which to apply the specific techniques that follow to successfully engage a too tight or too loose youngster.

PLAYROOM MATERIALS

The table below provides a list of materials commonly found in playrooms arranged according to the "diagnostic schema" discussed.

Loosening	Modeling	Tightening Up
Clay/Play Dough	Puppets:	Construction:
Crayons	Animals	Leather
Paints	People	Sewing
Paper	Doll house:	Models
Finger Paints	Furniture	Glue
Blocks	People	Cards
Darts, Dart Board	Doctor Kit	Board Games:
Punching Bag	Play Money	"Sorry"
Water	Blackboard	Checkers
Sandbox		Any Game with Rules
		Mirrors
		Video Recorder
		Balls

SPECIFIC TECHNIQUES FOR
ENGAGING TOO TIGHT CHILDREN

THE PICTURE-DRAWING GAME

Story telling and drawing are two well-suited techniques for engaging uptight children. Younger uptight children are made especially uncomfortable by new situations, such as the first time they meet a new doctor. Extreme inhibition, silence, or an inability to enter into play activities are some common manifestations. The picture-drawing game (Figure 1, p. 394) provides a way of quickly reducing anxiety while enlisting the child's involvement in an activity which is pleasant, nonthreatening, and consistent with both egopsychoanalytic formulations of anxiety and a Piagetian Theory of mental development. While playing this game, especially during the early encounter, the practitioner is concrete and "giving," rather than overly verbal, reflective, or "depriving."

After introducing yourself to the child, ask "Have you ever played a picture drawing game?" and immediately go to the easel or on a piece of paper draw a square. Then say, "Once upon a time there was a house," and proceed to draw in the square two smaller squares for windows and one rectangle for a door as in Drawing A. Continue by stating, "It was just like any other house with two windows, a door, a roof, and two chimneys." Add a triangle to the top and then two chimneys coming off either side as in Drawing B. "In the house there lived a little (boy/girl)." To this point you have asked nothing of the child but have given some perceptual stimulation by drawing a picture and having presented some words in a child-oriented tone. Now ask the child for a name. After a sufficient period of time if the child does not provide one, you provide the child's name and ask for his or her acknowledgment. (For purposes of our example, let the name be John.)

"Okay now, John lived in this house with his parents. One day John's parents brought him a pet doggie; what did John call his pet doggie?" As before, wait for the child to provide a name and if he or she does not, you do so. (For our example, let's call the dog Spot.) "Every day as John would go to bed he would take his pet dog Spot with him. One day when John got up, he didn't find Spot in his room. He walked out in front of the house and did not see Spot there." Upon that draw a straight line from the door of the house as in Drawing C. If the child responds "no," agree with him; if he responds "yes," say "John went to the door, and when he got close he saw the dog looked like Spot but wasn't Spot." If the child makes no response after a reasonable time, state, "He didn't find Spot." The next part of the game consists of drawing a number of lines so that they look like feet as in Drawing D. While making these lines say the following: "John began to look for his dog Spot; he went on one street and up another and then to another." You can pause and ask the child if he sees his dog; the response in all cases which you are looking to elicit is "no." Should the child say "yes," repeat as previously that he walked to the dog but it wasn't Spot. Get to the point where four legs are drawn and then tell the child, "John remembered that Spot liked to run in the park so he ran there," and draw a line which will become the tail. Ask the child if he found Spot; there the answer again should be "no." While asking him that question, draw a bushy tail and tell the child, "John kept looking and looking in the park for his dog, but could not find him," as in Drawing E.

Next, ask the child how John felt; the appropriate response is "sad." Then ask the child whether John walked home fast or slowly; regardless of what the child says, state that he felt sad and walked home slowly as in Drawing F.

Upon drawing the final line from the tail back to the house, the child should be asked, "What happened to the picture of the house?" Some children will immediately say "Spot came home," others will say "It looks like a dog," and others will seem puzzled. In any case, let the child know that the house became a picture of a dog, and ask if he or she would like to take it home. Following this you can begin to talk with the child, suggest that he or she might want to play with some toys, or, as I often do, ask the child to make a picture for me, either of a person, his or her family, an animal, or whatever.

Basically the child has been given something to take home and has been engaged in a hierarchical fashion, as you first give and then demand a little, and then demand

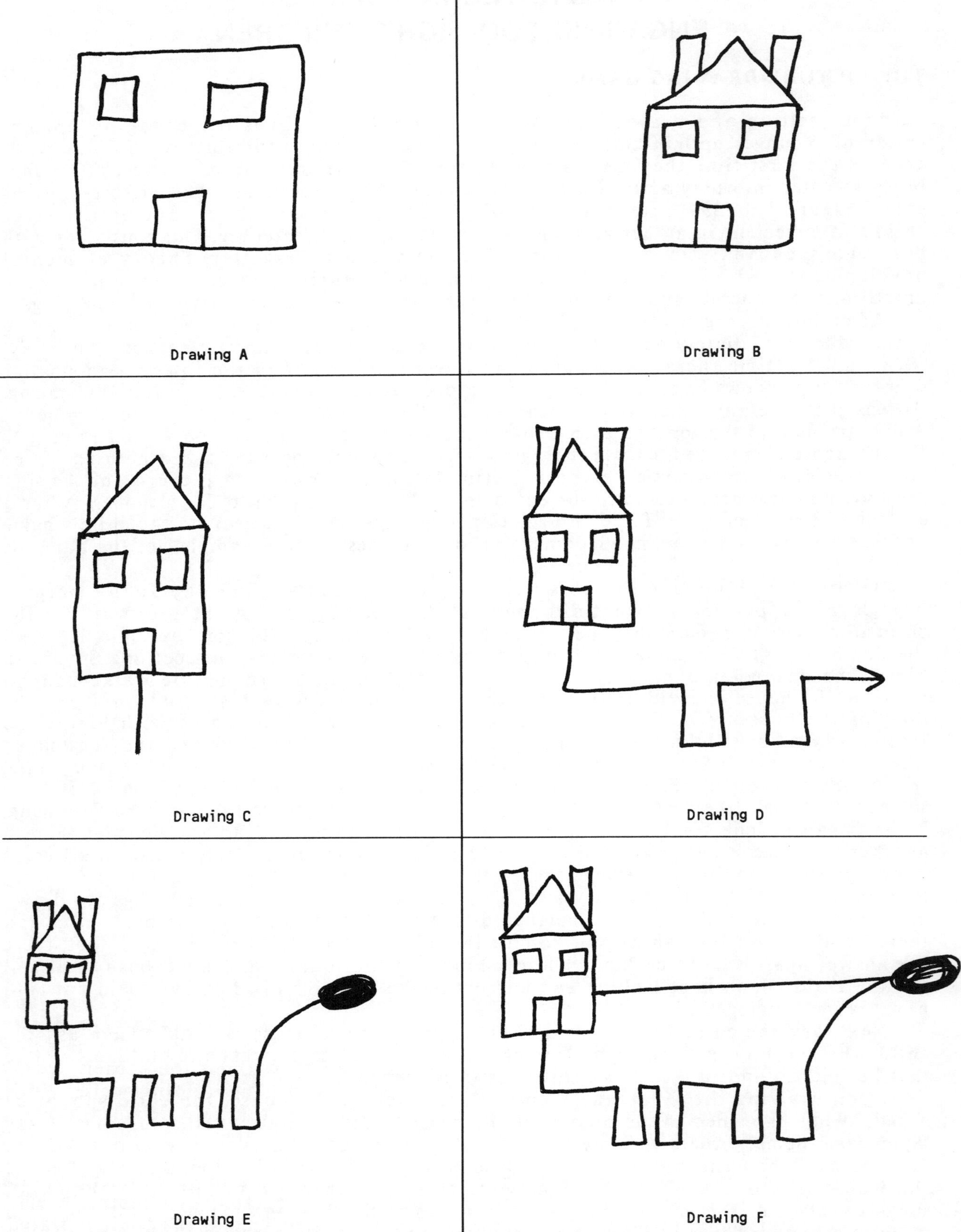

Figure 1. The Picture Drawing Game

somewhat more during the interview. Finally, the child has been asked to produce something in return which can provide diagnostic information, and also has been related to in a less threatening, anxiety reducing fashion.

TAKE A PICTURE: THE ANXIETY FADES - THE PRINT REMAINS

Anxious and frightened children often are unable to respond accurately about their worries or to perceive themselves accurately. However, many times through procedures involving active mastery, they are able to work through their uncomfortable feelings and alter their negative self-concept. Photography, and specifically the use of instant picture-taking, can be added to our graphics armamentarium which traditionally has included techniques such as spontaneous drawings, copying, and painting. The following are some examples demonstrating how instant photography can be used to engage children.

Separation Anxiety. Peggy, a 5-year-old girl who lived with her mother, father, and two younger brothers, ages 2 and 1, was referred to the clinic because her mother had accused her of being an abusing child. Peggy reportedly would hit and kick her mother until her mother began to cry. At other times, she would have extreme temper tantrums and hit and scratch herself. The mother, who was beaten many times by her husband, often witnessed by her daughter, called the clinic from a home for battered wives. Peggy was born out of wedlock when her mother was about 15. About a year later, her mother married Peggy's stepfather. We recommended time-limited foster care, counseling for the mother, and play therapy for Peggy. During the evaluation, Peggy was responsive to the diagnostician, had good eye contact, was reluctant to talk about her behavior, but did enact the hostile relationships in the family in doll play. Most significant, she was quite responsive to firm limits which were set.

At the first therapy session after foster placement, Peggy met her mother in the waiting room and easily separated. However, 20 minutes after our session ended, I was called to the waiting room because the foster worker was unable to get Peggy to separate from her mother. Peggy refused to get into the car and was crying and clinging to her mother.

I attempted some soothing comments to no avail. I then asked Peggy if she would permit me to take a picture of her mother. She stopped sobbing and permitted me to take the picture. I quickly placed myself between Peggy and her mother and offered Peggy the picture as I shooed the mother away. Somewhat stunned, the girl accepted the picture and as her mother began leaving, started to sob. I managed to get Peggy into the car and accompanied her home. She threw the picture on the floor and began sobbing. I held her, spoke comfortingly, and directed her attention to the picture of her mother, reminding her that they would see each other at the next appointment. After approximately 20 minutes, she consented to take the picture and kept looking at it. When she arrived at her foster home, she greeted the foster mother with a smile and showed the picture to her foster mother. Five sessions followed, at each of which a picture was taken. At the end of the second session, when she saw her mother outside, she asked if I might take a picture. Rather than just taking a picture of Peggy's mom, I took one of Peggy and her mother, and she took the picture and went home without a fuss.

As we began discussing the reuniting of the family, which would involve Peggy and her two brothers, I suggested that I might take a picture of all three and give this to Peggy. Six months later, I received a call from the mother, saying that all was going well. The children and mother were living in an apartment without the father. Peggy had entered kindergarten in September without incident and was doing well. While Peggy's separation fears do not necessarily indicate pathology, this case demonstrates the potential for constructively using photography with too tight children.

Limit Setting. Photography was used to reinforce limit setting in psychotherapy with a 10-year-old. The approach to limit setting followed was suggested by Ginott. Briefly, when a child attempts to break a limit, his or her wish is reflected, the limit is stated, and wherever possible substitutes are provided. Finally, further reflection on the annoyance is provided.

Frank, who was an only child, was referred to the clinic because of fire setting. When he entered fourth grade, his parents moved from another part of the state to Rochester because his father had a job change. Both parents' families lived elsewhere, and they felt out of place in Rochester, especially the mother who had been extremely close to her family. The family had one car, and thus the mother found it difficult to get away from her garden apartment. Her request for the car often led to a fight. Frank was hyperactive, although not a learning problem. After the diagnosis was made and he was put on medication in the second grade, there were no behavioral or academic problems at school. Furthermore, he was a child who had many friends, and while he was quiet around adults and thought to be a shy child by teachers, he was outgoing, playful, and at times rambunctious with his friends. His mother said much of this had changed since they moved. He had few friends and was constantly teasing and getting into fights.

When seen for an evaluation, Frank showed many of the passive-aggressive mannerisms that underachieving, latency-aged boys exhibit. He denied he was angry about coming to therapy, minimized and denied problems, had difficulty verbalizing, and was unable to choose what to do. Often he would sit silently. Following a number of minimally productive sessions, I introduced model building. After the second or third model, Frank became adventuresome and decided to move from relatively simple, snap-together models which he had completed quickly to a more complicated model. Near the end of the session, I reminded him that we had a few more minutes and suggested that he label the model so that when we met next time, we would be able to complete it. He informed me that he was quite capable of finishing it on his own at home. I acknowledged that, but reminded him of our rule that models could be taken home when they were completed but, until then, they remained the property of the clinic. I let him know I understood and reassured him that the model would be safe.

He became somewhat stronger in his request. I decided I would provide a substitute with the idea of deflecting some of his feelings. I told him that while he could not take the model home, he could take a picture of the model and show his friends what he was working on. I whipped out my One-Step, and, quick as a flash, the camera was spitting out the picture. As the print became clearer, his annoyance faded, and at our next session, he was eager to get started. As a postscript, later when he was unable to finish a model, he smiled and said he hoped he would finish it next session.

Termination Anxiety. Alice, the youngest in a family of two, wet the bed at night, was afraid to leave her mother to go to school, had frightening dreams, and often went into her mother's bed at night. Much of her anxiety and the accompanying behavioral symptoms first occurred at the time of her parents' divorce. Traditional play therapy worked well, and as we approached the termination, many of the symptoms had subsided. Alice's mother had been supported and coached so she no longer tolerated or subtly encouraged her daughter's maladaptive behaviors. The bedwetting subsided as the relationship between mother and daughter improved. However, the girl had developed a very close relationship to me, as one might expect, and as we began discussing termination, she showed indications of regressing; sleeping was interrupted by bad dreams, occasional separation anxiety, and occasional bedwetting. I asked her if I could take a picture of her to have, and so that she could remember all of the good things that occurred in therapy, I wanted her to have a picture of me. She agreed and we took pictures of each other. Her mother reported that she showed her the picture and seemed to have been helped with the worries that she had been talking about regarding not being able to see her "special friend" any longer.

MUTUAL STORY TELLING

Gardner (1971) introduced the mutual story telling technique which is based on the time-honored practice of eliciting stories from children during play therapy. After eliciting the story from the child, the therapist tells the child the story based upon his or her understanding of the psychodynamic meaning of the child's story, the child's developmental stage, and the presenting problems. The therapist's story incorporates the theme and character of the child's story but introduces healthier and more adaptive solutions and adjustments.

Kissel (1972), Kritzberg (1975), and Claman (1980) have introduced variations and elaborations of story telling techniques. Kissel (1972) has children create images and draw pictures of their stories; Kritzberg (1975) has provided a system for categorizing stories to facilitate the clinician's involvement, while Claman (1980) has children make a squiggle into a picture and then create a story about the squiggle. Kissel (1972) suggests that the child create images while listening to his or her story, and also supplies adaptive endings which are recorded and listened to by both therapist and child. Homework exercises then can be assigned to the child to provide added exposure to both conflict and active solutions. This also counteracts the child's attempt to avoid working on the conflict in the time away from therapy. Basically, these techniques help children discover better ways of adapting to anxiety-provoking situations without engendering too much anxiety in the child or the relationship. Furthermore, the novelty, structure, and active aspects of the procedure enhance a child's motivation. The following illustrates a story telling technique.

A sulky, easily angered, extremely short-statured 11-year-old was the third out-of-wedlock child in a family of five. He was referred to the clinic by the local children's department of social services because the foster parents were finding him difficult to control. The child told the following story during his fifth therapy session:

Once upon a time there was a prince and a black widow spider. The prince did not like this black widow spider so the black widow spider said, "If you marry me, I'll give you a million dollars," and so he married her and she gave him the million dollars; and she said, "If you give me a diamond ring, I'll give you a thousand dollars," and so he gave her a diamond ring and she gave him a thousand dollars. But then the black widow spider did not like him anymore, and she played a dirty trick on him. She said, "If you give me a kiss, I'll give you a billion dollars." The handsome prince kissed her and she poisoned him; then the prince died and she found another one, and she kept wandering, looking for another one because that one was no good. Then one day she met this great old goat - he was about 1 million years old - and she said, "Will you please marry me and I'll give you a thousand dollars." So the goat married her and she gave him the money, but then she did not like him anymore so she killed him too. She poisoned him just like she did the prince; and then she met a little white polar bear who was sitting in a tree and he said, "I'll marry you on one condition. If you promise not to poison me, or I'll never marry you." And so the polar bear married her, and she said, "Okay, I'll not poison you." She did not promise but she said she would not. The next day she put arsenic in his coffee, and he said, "What's in that?" She said, "Oh, just some arsenic and soon you will die - in about 10 minutes." So the polar bear began coughing and running around yelling, "I've been poisoned, let me out of here." But all the doors were locked, and he could not get out of a window because they were all locked also, and so he busted one window and climbed out and escaped and he went home. The moral of the story was never marry a poisoned lady.

I chose to focus on the child's conflict of not being able to adequately express his true wishes. The bear was interpreted as the figure who best represented the child because he was the third child and the bear, the third victim of the spider.

The story that I created duplicated the child's, except that in response to her offer of marriage, the old goat said, "I don't think so, because I am old and I don't want to get married." When the spider approached the polar bear and said, "Polar bear, marry me," the polar bear said, "I don't think I want to marry you," and the black widow spider said, "Polar bear, if you marry me, I will make you rich and give you lots of money," and the polar bear said to the black widow spider, "That's very nice of you, you must be a kind black widow spider, but I think I'd rather wait and find somebody that I really like and then get married, even though I think you're nice. Thank you for your offer and good-bye." The moral of this story was telling how you feel is better than holding it in.

When applying story-telling techniques to engage children, clinicians are faced with choosing from the number of possible choices that usually come to mind. When developing the plot, create an action story which has a beginning, middle, and especially an ending which, whenever possible, conveys an active mastery message.

Kritzberg (1975) suggests that most stories clinicians create can be categorized as mirror stories, suggestive-directive stories, or indirect-interpretive stories. Claman (1980) has found this approach helpful while using the squiggle-drawing game.

1. *Mirror stories* - In this type of story, the clinician repeats the child's story with only minor changes in plot, characters, action, outcome, and meaning (i.e., a cat can be changed to a dog, a lake to a sea). Mirror stories are effective ways of informing children that you are listening and paying attention to them as well as encouraging their self-expression. This type of story is a "safe" one to tell and can be likened to reflections or repetitions in talk therapy. The mirror story is the type of story to create when you are unable to decide upon a dynamically oriented mastery story.
2. *Suggestive-directive stories* - These stories relate to conflicts concerning general developmental-psychosocial tasks and encourage active mastery. Themes which express trust (don't be afraid of people), self-expression (talking is helpful; see example), peer relations (friends are fun, stand up to bullies), and persistence (don't be discouraged by failure) are some of the usual ones which these stories encompass. The clinician's message or parts of it are incorporated in the child's subsequent stories. If the child relates reality incidents which were handled more adaptively than in the past, then the clinician's message is being understood and assimilated.
3. *Indirect-interpretive stories* - These stories focus on a specific, current problem of a child (i.e., fear of swimming, fear of the dark, being shy, and fear of dogs). The clinician emphasizes the child's worry and uses a desensitization model with the addition of supportive elements to reduce anxiety and fear as the story unfolds.

SPECIFIC TECHNIQUES FOR
ENGAGING TOO LOOSE CHILDREN

Children who are too loose also have problems with accurately perceiving themselves and their self-worth. However, these children often hide their negative and inadequate feelings from others as well as from themselves. The belief that only providing a troubled child unconditional positive regard, genuineness, and congruence in a relationship would stimulate growth and self-enhancement is often challenged by the clinical results of work with children who are too loose. Behavior-disordered children often do not stay still long enough to experience these positive communications; children who are too loose have problems focusing their attention, have extremely low frustration and anxiety tolerance, are action rather than word oriented, and find it difficult to delay gratification. Such children's low self-esteem is often the result of chronic failure, both in school and with authority figures. Their interpersonal style is characterized by blends of (a) denial ("I didn't do it"), (b) avoidance ("I can't do it"), (d) acting out ("I won't do it"), and (d) repression ("I don't know").

MODEL BUILDING

Model building is a task well-suited for engaging children who are too loose. A 9-year-old third grader of average intelligence, with poor coordination, impulsivity, and perceptual impairment, was referred to a mental health center because of disruptive classroom behavior and poor school achievement. Initially, he was quite belligerent, often refusing to talk. He showed little awareness of the presence of different games and models in the playroom. During the third session, it was suggested that he might be interested in working on a model. The boy was provided with a few models (with a probability of completion in one session). Pieces were few, of medium size, and the instructions were mostly pictures to choose from.

His approach was characteristic of many learning-disabled and impulsively oriented children. He glued the two biggest pieces together. For the simple models, this procedure is adaptive; once "hooked," the child goes on to more difficult models. Lacking good organization skills and with limited ability to attend to details and poor frustration tolerance, the child had to repeatedly return to the beginning to insert pieces which had been left out. The first lesson learned was that working slower is faster. While his need for speed, finishing quickly, and immediate reward was recognized, he was forced by his experience to consider that things done more slowly ultimately get done more quickly. Through action rather than words, he began to learn the adaptive importance of attention to details and orderliness. Additionally, he developed a sense of accomplishment. The more difficult models also helped develop better frustration tolerance, as he had to wait 2 to 3 weeks before he could take home his completed model. Of course, the model was always found with the previous work undamaged, thus building trust in the relationship. As proficiency developed, he was required to become even more involved in the process by reading some of the instructions, relating words to numbers, and keeping a record of the sequence of completed parts. The major share of the work was done by the child, but the therapist assisted whenever necessary so that the project was a cooperative venture, and the child learned another lesson: Two heads are better than one.

Although model building may appear to place greater emphasis on *play* than *therapeutic engagement*, it requires specific knowledge, sensitivity, and flexibility on the part of the practitioner. The role of the therapist involves several key tasks:

1. *Provide materials* - models, glue, scissors, tweezers, most of the necessary materials which must be made available to the child.
2. *Establish rules* - it is better to permit the playroom rules to emerge while working on the model, than to list them at the inception of the project. For example, children may want to take their model home even if incompleted; the rule *models cannot leave until completed* should be introduced at the end of the initial model building session by emphasizing that the child can keep the model and take it home *when completed*. The need to complete one model before starting another and completing only one model per session are other usual rule-oriented encounters.
3. *Protect incompleted models* - it is extremely important that the child find his or her model intact from session to session. The therapist must protect the model from being broken by other children who visit the playroom. This can become a problem if one is sharing the playroom with a number of other practitioners.
4. *Focus the child* - guiding questions which direct children to figure out answers for themselves lead to active mastery. When children flounder or become unduly frustrated, asking them if there is anything in the model box which can help, or how they usually find out how to play new games, can lead them to discover the instructions. Helping the child to match his or her model part to the picture of it in the instructions is often enough to get a stuck child back on the track.
5. *Cooperate with the child* - although the child should do the majority of assembling the model, the therapist should help so that the project becomes a cooperative venture and not a "Walt Disney experience." Hold pieces for the child, especially when fine motor coordination may be causing problems; do some parts, if the child asks and the task is repetitive; for example, putting four wheels together in a car model. Make suggestions which can facilitate the assembly, especially as frustration mounts. It is very important to verbalize the different emotions the child might be experiencing while working on the models, such as pride, happiness, frustrations. Also, talk about experiences the child might be having outside the playroom, at home, school, or with friends.
6. *Manage resistance* - some children become so engrossed in their model that they will hardly engage in any talk with the therapist. At such times the therapist needs to secure feedback from the significant adult about what progress is being made in order to gauge modifications that need to be introduced. Confrontation regarding the avoidance of talk and limiting the time spent during each session working on the model (e.g., half session model building, half session talk; or shifting to a different activity) can be helpful.

The introduction of models requires careful planning by the clinician. Several tips may aid the process:

1. *Display some models* - the therapist can have a few models displayed in his or her office to stimulate the child's interest. Some practitioners provide some verbal structure to children explaining how they can use their time together. Model building can be included in the orientation, or a direct suggestion can be made to the child about the model.
2. *Choose appropriate models* - it is important that the first model building experience be successful. The model should be easy (see table) and able to be completed in one or, at the most, two sessions.
3. *Help children get started* - managing frustration, focusing the child's attention on the instructions, emphasizing sequencing and the importance of attending to details, and managing the experience by setting appropriate rules are the primary tasks from the therapist's point of view. Completing the model so that it looks good is the primary task from the child's point of view.

Some children will choose a model that is too difficult even though you try to persuade them otherwise. Permit this to happen! When they get discouraged, encourage; when they give up and request another model, as theirs is in shambles, permit them to change and then introduce the rule: You have to finish your model before you can start another one, and once again guide them to a model within their reach.

The table below illustrates the availability of model building kits of various degrees of difficulty.

MODEL BUILDING KITS

Complexity	Manufacturer
<u>Difficult</u>	
Large boats (hull length 20")	Revell
Large cars (1/25 scale)	Monogram
Large planes (1/48 scale)	Monogram
<u>Medium</u>	
Small cars (7 and older)	Lindberg
Snap together planes, helicopters	Revell
Intermediate size boats and planes (1/720 scale)	Revell
Glue togethers - Super Heroes	
<u>Easy</u>	
Snap together cars	Revell
Snap together animals	Aurora
Snap together boats and planes (7 and older)	Lindberg

Criteria for more complexity:

    a. Multiple pieces
    b. Much reading
    c. Long directions (# of steps)
    d. Gluing
    e. Number of sessions to complete

COLOR-YOUR-LIFE-TECHNIQUE

The Color-Your-Life Technique (O'Connor, 1983) can be used with children individually or in groups. It can be used as a tool to teach children about feelings or as a method to encourage reticent children to express their feelings. When used by those professionally trained to work with problematic children, the Color-Your-Life Technique can assist in eliciting intense feelings on the part of children, and lead to detailed explorations and discussions about their affects and associated life events.

The technique can be used with a wide variety of too loose children, but in my experience it seems to be most productive with children between the ages of 6 and 12 who are of average intelligence. A basic prerequisite is that the child have sufficient cognitive abilities to recognize and name colors as well as different states. O'Connor suggests that the technique not be used with psychotic children because of the level of concrete and associative thinking required.

The only materials required for the Color-Your-Life Technique are plain paper and any type of coloring instruments such as paints, markers, or crayons. Yellow, red, green, blue, and black, as well as other colors, should be made available to the child. The technique consists of two parts: First the child is trained in pairing feelings and colors and then the child is asked to represent his or her feelings using colors.

Therapeutically, the primary purpose of the technique is to encourage children to verbally express their feelings. Active discussion between child and therapist is encouraged. O'Connor suggests that the therapist begin by asking children if they can pair an affect with a particular color:

Therapist: "Can you tell me what feeling might go with the color red?"
Child: "Uhm, I don't know."
Therapist: "Can you think of a time when people get very red in the face? Think about cartoons you have seen. When do the characters scrunch up their faces and get red?"
Child: "When they are mad!"
Therapist: "That's right. Most people think that the color red goes along with being angry." (O'Connor, 1983, p. 254)

The child and therapist continue this type of discussion until each color is related to a specific affect. The following are some suggested pairings which are consistent with art therapy interpretations:

> Black - Sadness
> Red - Anger
> Yellow - Happiness
> Brown - Boredom
> Green - Jealousy, Envy

In the color-affect association segment of the technique, colors can be used to help children distinguish intensity of feelings. For example: being unhappy or a little sad can be differentiated from being very sad or depressed by suggesting that black goes with feelings people have when a pet or a person they care about dies, while blue is a color which goes with feelings people have when they cannot find a toy, or break something, or a friend moves away. The younger the child, the more important it is to relate affects to concrete examples in the experiences of children for purposes of maximizing differentiation between each of the color-feeling pairs.

When working with children showing specific conflicts, or when a particular issue is to be explored, other pairings can be added - for example, the use of pink and blue to represent traditional sex role stereotypes. The number and variety of color-feeling pairs is limited only by the material available and the creativity of the therapist. However, O'Connor (1983) suggests, "It is generally wise to limit the number of pairs presented at any one time to eight or nine, as this seems to be a number most children can manage successfully" (p. 254). It is also important for the therapist to remember that children may describe how they feel during subsequent treatment sessions in terms of earlier agreed upon color terms.

The second segment of the Color-Your-Life Technique is instituted after the color-feeling pairs are established. The child is given a piece of blank paper and asked to fill it up with colors to show the feelings in his or her life. Some explanation is generally necessary at this point to help the child get started. O'Connor (1983) suggests saying, "If you have been happy about half the time in your life then half the paper should be yellow. If you have been happy your whole life with no other feelings, then you should color the whole paper yellow. You may complete the coloring in whatever way you choose, using squares, circles, designs, and so forth" (p. 255). These instructions or similar ones should be continued until it is clear that the child is aware of what is desired.

It is permissible for the therapist to engage the child in verbalizations; indeed, verbalizations are encouraged while the child is drawing. Such discussions may focus on events occurring in the child's life or feelings related to the different colors.

CONCLUSION

Children who are too tight, that is extremely anxious, depressed, or fearful; or too loose, that is overactive, impulsive, or aggressive, are extremely difficult to engage in either assessment or treatment. Five specific techniques have been presented to assist the clinician in engaging such children rapidly, with the aim of making the encounter as rewarding, productive, and helpful as possible. These techniques are based upon child centered principles that involve the introduction of more structure and direction into the playroom. These approaches recognize and respect the influence of external behavior on internal adjustment and place an emphasis on active mastery. As they use these techniques, I encourage clinicians to flexibly recognize the needs of individual children, rather than rigidly force each child into a particular therapeutic mold. Successful therapy requires creative application of techniques that meet each child's needs.

Stanley Kissel, PhD, is currently Chief Psychologist of the Children and Youth Division at the Rochester Mental Health Center, and also maintains an independent clinical practice. In addition to working with children and families, he is interested in writing and lecturing. He has made numerous contributions to the professional literature including the authorhsip of four books. Dr. Kissel may be contacted at 1425 Portland Avenue, Rochester, NY 14621.

RESOURCES

Axline, V. M. (1947). *Play Therapy*. New York: Ballantine.

Claman, L. (1980). The squiggle-drawing game in child psychotherapy. *American Journal of Psychotherapy, 34,* 414-421.

Freud, A. (1946). *The Psychoanalytic Treatment of Children*. London: Imago.

Freud, A. (1965). *Normality and Pathology in Childhood*. New York: International Universities Press.

Gardner, R. H. (1971). *Therapeutic Communications with Children: The Mutual Storytelling Technique*. New York: Aronson.

Halpern, W. I., & Kissel, S. (1976). *Human Resources for Troubled Children*. New York: Wiley-Interscience.

Harrington, R. G. (1984). Assessing childhood anxiety and depressive disorders. In S. J. Weaver (Ed.), *Testing Children* (Ch. 11, pp. 161-185). Kansas City, MO: Test Corporation America.

Kissel, S. (1972). Systematic desensitization therapy with children: A case study and some suggested modifications. *Professional Psychology, 3,* 153-168.

Kissel, S. (1977). Children's services - past, present, future. *Child Psychiatry and Human Development, 7,* 197-204.

Kritzberg, N. I. (1975). *The Structured Therapeutic Game Method of Child Analytic Psychotherapy*. Hickville, NY: Exposition Press.

O'Connor, K. J. (1983). The Color-Your-Life Technique. In C. E. Schaefer & K. J. O'Connor (Eds.), *Handbook of Play Therapy* (Ch. 13, pp. 251-259). New York: Wiley-Interscience.

Quay, H. C. (1972). Patterns of aggression, withdrawal, and immaturity. In H. C. Quay & J. S. Werry (Eds.), *Psychopathological Disorders of Childhood* (pp. 1-30). New York: Wiley.

Schaefer, C. E., & Millman, H. (Eds.). (1977). *Therapies for Children - A Handbook of Effective Treatments for Problem Behaviors* (pp. 1-12). San Francisco: Jossey-Bass.

Schaefer, C. E., & O'Connor, K. (Eds.). (1983). *Handbook of Play Therapy*. New York: Wiley-Interscience.

AN INTRODUCTION TO DIVORCE MEDIATION

Stanley N. Cohen

Most marriage and family practitioners readily acknowledge that divorce, or marital dissolution as it is now commonly called, has become a fact of life. It is as much a part of the contemporary American scene as marriage itself.

The rise in divorce over the past 20 years has been dramatic to say the least. There were 413,000 divorces recorded in 1962. The figure doubled 10 years later, and annually since 1975, over 1 million couples have instituted divorce proceedings (National Center for Health Statistics, 1981). While the number of dissolutions has stabilized since 1983, annual divorce filings are expected to hover around the million mark for the next several years.

Not unexpectedly, the number of children whose parents get divorced has risen sharply. It has been estimated that of those minor children born in the 1970s, between 20% and 30% will experience the dissolution of their parents' marriage. This estimate increases to 25% and 30% if annulments and legal separations are considered (Bane, 1976).

The reality of high divorce rates, along with the profound adjustments in marital and parental relationships that must be made in the transition from an intact family situation to one of separation and divorce, has resulted in an expansion of services offered by marriage and family therapists. Practitioners now are as apt to be asked to help couples deal with divorce related economic, personal, and social issues as they are to provide couples assistance in solving their marriage and family problems.

Recently, mediation has emerged as an intervention geared specifically to assist couples in conflict over custody, visitation, spousal and child support, and other economic issues. The focus of such conflicts may be over one or a combination of these issues. Mediation can be useful to deal with these disputes at any stage of the divorce process. For example, it can help to minimize ongoing conflicts so that couples can make informed, cooperative decisions before becoming enmeshed in the divorce process. Mediation also may be a constructive alternative for those couples in the midst of divorce who are at an impasse that could result in judicial intervention. Finally, mediation can address post-divorce child related and economic problems due to changes in social and personal circumstances (e.g., remarriage) and lingering resentments over the divorce (e.g., visitation and child support defaults).

Folberg (1983) has defined mediation as:

> a process by which disputants attempt to reach a consensual settlement of issues in dispute with the assistance and facilitation of a neutral resource person or persons. At the very least, the process consists of systematically isolating points of agreement and disagreement, developing options, and considering accommodations. (p. 8)

Ricci (1980) addresses differences between counseling, mediation, and arbitration in the following manner:

> Counseling, mediation, and arbitration differ from one another in crucial ways. Counseling offers advice, alternatives, and perhaps, some therapeutic intervention. Mediation differs from arbitration in that the mediator does not take sides and aids the parties in reaching their own agreement. But arbitration means that both sides present their case to a person who is hired and empowered to judge the case and make a decision. Arbitration hearings work like courts. (p. 157)

The mediation process should be viewed as an alternative to self-help and litigation. It enables the participants to work cooperatively with each other and to assume responsibility in making decisions that can have a profound impact on the well-being of themselves and their children during and after divorce. Mediation, then, is viewed by its advocates as being a more constructive alternative to resolving divorce disputes than the adversarial arena of the courtroom.

This contribution offers an introduction to the development and implementation of mediation services to resolve disputes between couples during and after divorce. The following aspects of mediation are addressed: (a) its history as a means to resolve disputes; (b) its differences from marriage and family therapy; (c) how divorce mediation services are offered; (d) evaluation; (e) its promise, limitations, and future directions; and (f) various practical considerations.

DIVORCE MEDIATION: BRIEF HISTORICAL NOTES

The current enthusiasm and advocacy for mediation belies its long history as a method used to resolve personal disputes. In their historical reviews, both Brown (1982) and Folberg and Taylor (1984) point out that mediation as a dispute resolution technique has been used by all types of societies for thousands of years. In ancient China, for example, mediation was the principal means by which conflict between disputing parties was resolved. It continues to be practiced in the People's Republic of China, and enjoys an important place in the Chinese legal system. Similarly, a rich history of conciliation and mediation also is found in the customs of Japan.

In parts of Africa, a respected community leader traditionally has served as a mediator to assist disputing parties in cooperatively resolving their grievances. Generally, the focus has been on getting disputants to settle their differences without resorting to the use of an arbitrator or judge.

In the United States, the early Quakers used mediation and arbitration to resolve disputes. Ethnic and religious groups culturally attuned to mediation established similar systems after immigrating to the United States. One example is the Chinese Benevolent Society, which was created to resolve disputes between community members and disagreements within families. Another is the Jewish Conciliation Board, established in New York City in 1920. This community-based system, which continues to function, is a derivation of the Jewish Religious Court - a system used by ancient Hebrews for conciliation and mediation between community and family disputants.

More recently, the Federal Mediation and Conciliation Services, established in 1947, have provided assistance in resolving labor and industrial disputes. The Dispute Resolution Act was passed by Congress in 1980 and offers support for establishing alternative approaches to settling community disputes without resorting to judicial intervention. Strides also have been made by state and local governments to develop and implement programs that focus on domestic violence, consumer complaints, landlord-tenant disputes, and neighborhood disagreements.

While the mediation of family disputes has been practiced historically, specific application of mediation in response to divorce disputes has a very short history. As pointed out by Brown (1982),

> practically none of the books on divorce, children of divorce, or child custody that were published prior to 1981 even mention the word "mediation." (p. 3)

How does one account for the long delay and apparent resistance in applying mediation principles to the resolution of divorce disputes? The question is a complex one and cannot be answered fully here. However, part of the answer may involve two factors related to a long-standing perception about the negative impact of divorce on family life, and particularly on children. The first factor has been addressed by the author and a colleague (Cohen & Jones, 1983) in the following manner:

A belief commonly held by most Americans is that the family requires unconditional and permanent bonds between its members for its survival. Historically,...marriage has been defined as a lifelong commitment between two adults that typically involves maintaining a household and raising children. In other words, marital and parental relationships are thought to be one and the same. Simply stated, if your marriage dissolves or ends, so does your family.

The fact is that parenting relationships are not intended to be terminated by divorce. Indeed the laws explicitly emphasize a reordering of parental and parent-child relations, the intent being to secure access to the child by the out-of-home parent. At the same time, the manner in which parenting responsibilities are to be shared during and after divorce have been clouded by the way family law has categorized the role of divorced parents in custodial and noncustodial terms. What is of particular concern to many noncustodial parents is that they have no legal basis to be involved in the lives of their children except on a limited basis. Recent changes in family law -- for example, joint custody -- have clarified and provided a legal basis by which both parents have the opportunity to participate in decisions related to the rearing of their children.

In summary, the ideal American family is one that is intact, nuclear, and child-centered. This idea is deeply embedded in the cultural fabric of our society going back to the colonial days. Family life also has been romanticized as a life-long commitment between two adults with no distinction having been made regarding the functional difference between marital and parental relationships and the implications of disruption to family members when a divorce occurs. (pp. 468-469)

Given such deeply rooted notions about the lifelong nature and importance of family relationships to the well-being of children, any attempts to provide alternatives that promote routes out of a dysfunctional marriage are bound to be resisted strongly. Indeed, such a procedure could be viewed as breaking up families - the antithesis of a constructive intervention.

Reviewing the history of divorce also may be helpful in understanding why mediation of divorce disputes only recently has established a foothold in the United States. In ancient times, marriage and divorce were considered private matters and not subject to state control. The rise and influence of Christianity, however, conceptualized marriage as inviolate. Therefore, it was not subject to dissolution. Consequently, both marriage and divorce were controlled exclusively by the church for centuries. Eventually, government assumed control over marriage and divorce, but divorce remained very difficult to obtain. Domestic relations law came to require grounds to be established before the court could grant a divorce. One had to "prove" the other party was unfit to continue the marriage. The system was structured on an adversarial basis, which pitted party against party. Divorce was viewed as a contentious and competitive process that exacerbated and sustained bitterness even among couples who had held minimal animosity towards each other, except for the desire to terminate their marriage.

Making divorce difficult to obtain also has functioned to control divorce rates and sustain marriage. I believe that social and legal resistance to mediation have prevailed so long because of the adversarial legal procedures used to process divorce.

Coincident with sharply rising divorce rates, the reality of divorce was gradually being accepted as an aspect of contemporary life. These events coupled with break-throughs in divorce reform, as exemplified by California passing the first no-fault legislation in 1970, opened the door for mediation to be considered as a viable alternative to traditional adversarial procedures. As no-fault divorce has become accepted in this country, so has divorce mediation achieved respectability as a constructive and effective intervention in resolving divorce-related disputes.

CONTRASTING DIVORCE MEDIATION
WITH MARRIAGE AND FAMILY THERAPY

An emerging discipline commonly seeks out and clarifies its uniqueness from other similar professions. The discussion that follows is the author's understanding of Kelly's (1983) attempt to delineate basic differences between divorce mediation and psychotherapy or counseling. Additional comments put the mediation versus therapy analysis into perspective.

Kelly differentiates between mediation and counseling by examining several aspects of mediation and comparing the two approaches. These aspects include:

> the goal of mediation, the nature of the mediation process, the role of the mediator, the role of diagnosis, the place of emotional expression in the mediation process, and the mediator's techniques and interventions. (p. 35)

GOALS OF MEDIATION

The principal goal of mediating a divorce is the negotiation of those issues identified by the parties and mediator that will result in a written settlement agreement. The specificity of the goal (a settlement) contrasts with counseling goals, which generally are broad based, such as improving marital relationships, enhancing one's personal life, and the like.

While there is general agreement about the primary goal of divorce or post-divorce mediation, there is less consensus regarding subgoals germane to specific settlements. These include restructuring of parental and parent-child relationships, developing a means by which the parties can deal with each other when the need arises after their divorce, and enhancing a constructive adjustment to the divorce. In these areas, the boundaries between mediation and counseling are not clear-cut.

MEDIATION PROCESS

Mediation is viewed as goal-focused, task-oriented, and time-limited. It emphasizes the present and future considerations of the couple and their children. While short-term and crisis counseling may share some of these characteristics, there are differences in the goals, tasks, and issues of therapy.

Both clients and mediator have to deal with concrete tasks if a settlement is to be reached. Thus the focus is on external information and issues rather than on internal psychological material. In divorce mediation, clients have to be specific in identifying and valuing assets, liabilities, and other property. Workable plans must be made for custody, visitation, and child support. Mediation, therefore, is geared to focused problem solving. By contrast, therapy usually deals with internal or interpersonal material, emotions, and the quality of a person's relationship with his or her spouse. Although the business of mediation may evoke emotional reactions, these need to be contained so that the goals of mediation can be attained. Therapy often seeks to expand rather than contain the exploration of psychological material with the goal of changing behavior. The mediation experience may elicit psychological change, but the mediator, unlike the therapist, is not in a position to interpret or explore any such issues.

The mediation format is seen as being quite different from the counseling experience. Early on, client and mediator expectations, an explanation of the structure of the process, and "rules of the game" are outlined explicitly so that the mediator and the clients can move as quickly as possible toward an agreement on the issues in dispute. By contrast, counseling or therapy moves more slowly, placing an emphasis on what is troubling an individual or couple. The therapist may use several sessions establishing rapport and gathering personal and marital histories in order to develop a treatment plan for resolving a couple's problems.

ROLE OF THE MEDIATOR

A divorce mediator functions in an active manner. In many respects, the mediator serves as an educator to the couple, providing them with information that is needed for an equitable negotiated settlement. At the same time, he or she remains task-oriented, keeping the clients on target with regard to the aims, procedures, and scope of the mediation. The mediator does not make decisions, but facilitates the couple's decision making, while remaining impartial and maintaining a balance between both parties.

While helping the clients, the mediator may function like an active family therapist who is working on a specific family problem. However, there are some critical differences between the two approaches. The mediator must have skills different from those offered by a therapist if he or she is to mediate a divorce settlement. The competent mediator must have a working knowledge of domestic relations law, common monetary practices, budgetary needs, areas of divorce law that provide for the division of assets and liabilities, and income tax considerations. This specialized knowledge, in addition to specific information about the impact of divorce on parents and their children, makes the mediator's role considerably broader than that of the traditional marital therapist.

DIAGNOSIS

Diagnostic activity is limited to the purposes of mediation, and primarily is used to build strategy. Generally speaking, a mediator's concern is with the clients' reaction to the divorce, the power relationship between the couple, and present and future needs of the parties and their children. By contrast, the therapist is interested in the past history of a couple; for example, courtship, sex, developmental aspects of the family, and marital and familial role expectations. While such material is important for the therapist, it is not considered necessary to reach a successful divorce agreement.

THE PLACE OF EMOTIONS IN MEDIATION

The experienced mediator is aware of the strong emotions that may surface as a couple works toward reaching a divorce settlement. He or she also is aware that clients respond differently insofar as emotional expressions are concerned. Because of these variations, the mediator must be clear with regard to the role that emotions play in the negotiation of an agreement. The extent to which emotional expression facilitates or impedes the mediation process dictates how much of these feelings the mediator will allow to surface in the sessions. By contrast, emotional expression and a sharing of feelings about important aspects of themselves and their marriage often are desirable in counseling with couples. The expression of emotions in the counseling sessions does not necessarily interfere with the treatment process.

CONFLICT MANAGEMENT

The mediator assumes an active role in managing conflict when it emerges in the mediation sessions. This is done to provide safeguards that allow for the process to move on in a rational, task-oriented manner. Obviously, sustained conflict between clients impedes any progress being made in mediation and may result in one or both parties abandoning their efforts at reaching a negotiated settlement.

Therapy intervention, on the other hand, may welcome the expression of conflict by clients. It is considered useful in understanding important aspects of the problems which brought an individual or couple to counseling. In fact, the conflict management techniques used by mediators could be seen as counterproductive in therapy that seeks to understand the dynamics of a couple's conflict to work towards its resolution.

NEGOTIATION STRATEGIES

Clients who elect to mediate their divorce vary in their readiness to reach an agreement. The process is straightforward and relatively quick when the clients are open and flexible. However, if they are locked into a fixed position with little to trade, the mediator needs negotiating skills to avoid an impasse and ultimate termination of the process. Because therapists traditionally have no training in bargaining techniques, their approach relies heavily on exploration, interpretation, and subsequent emotional and behavioral change in helping couples resolve their difficulties.

TRANSITION FROM THERAPIST TO MEDIATOR

The preceding discussion has underscored key differences in the techniques mediators and therapists use in helping their clients resolve interpersonal problems and conflicts. In a sense, the above material clouds the fact that the majority of persons who currently practice mediation come from professional mental health backgrounds. The transition for many therapists to mediator clearly has been made without a great deal of difficulty.

How can this occur when the goals of mediation and marriage and family therapy seem relatively disparate? First, the theoretical orientation of a therapist bears some relationship to the ease with which they can function as mediators. For example, it may be difficult, without considerable training, for a psychodynamically oriented therapist who primarily works with individuals on a long-term basis to feel comfortable with mediation. On the other hand, therapists who have a behavioral orientation, work conjointly with couples, use a crisis or short-term counseling model, and are familiar with conflict resolution techniques, probably will make an effective transition to mediator. If you conceptualize the two examples as opposite ends of a continuum, you may informally assess your orientation's compatibility with mediation. Beyond the transition issue, almost all therapists will need to enhance their skills and knowledge about divorce law and procedures, bargaining and dispute resolution strategies, state and federal tax considerations, the divorcing process and its impact on parents and children, and the economics of divorce.

MEDIATION AS PRACTICED IN COURT-RELATED AND NONCOURT-RELATED SETTINGS

There are two settings where divorce mediation services are offered: court-related and noncourt-related. The focus of what is mediated varies both across and within these settings.

COURT-CONNECTED SERVICES

Mediation services typically have developed as an extension of marital interventions provided by professionally staffed counseling units which are part of a judicial jurisdiction. These units are called conciliation courts, and they originally provided marriage counseling focused on the reconciliation of couples who had either filed for divorce or were considering such an action. The oldest conciliation court was established in Los Angeles in 1955; it served as a model system for other such services in California and other jurisdictions in the country. The focus of service was reconciliation in the Los Angeles Conciliation Court, but the counseling approach was similar to divorce media-tion; short-term counseling in a confidential conjoint setting helped couples to negotiate a formal reconciliation agreement.

As divorce rates increased, conciliation courts expanded their services to include divorce counseling and custody evaluations. Again in response to a growing awareness of the value of mediation as an alternative to court litigation, the state of California in 1982 mandated mediation services for any couple in dispute over custody or visitation issues. Although mandated mediation services have not been totally accepted by all judicial systems, court-connected mediation programs have proliferated.

Typically, court-connected mediation services are limited to the resolution of custody and visitation disputes. Response to this type of divorce mediation has been mixed. As is pointed out by Milne (1983):

Separating the mediation of parent child-issues from financial and property issues allows children to be treated as an issue in their own right, and it lessens the potential for using them as pawns in the negotiation process. However, separation of issues can segment a divorce agreement artificially when property, finances, and children are indeed related and when decisions made in one area affect decisions made in the other area. (p. 19)

There has also been criticism of court-connected mediation programs that allow information obtained during the mediation process to be given to the judge and the parties' attorneys. Implicit in this situation is the covert ability of the mediator to influence an agreement made by the parties. Those who support this practice point to the fact that court-connected mediators often work with highly conflicted couples who are not likely to reach an agreement through less aggressive means.

THE PRIVATE SECTOR

One type of divorce mediator is the sole practitioner. Most typical is the mental health professional who provides divorce mediation in addition to other therapeutic services (Pearson, Ring, & Milne, 1983). To a lesser degree, lawyers also provide divorce mediation. Usually, they continue to practice law while offering mediation to selected clients.

Often, sole practitioners team up with each other and work together as co-mediators. The team often is composed of an attorney and a counselor. These practitioners usually maintain their legal and counseling services and co-mediate on a part-time basis.

Private mediation service operates on a fee for service, and independently establishes policy and procedures. The type of services offered by these practitioners is varied insofar as the issues mediated, the model of mediation used, and the professional orientation of the mediator. This wide variation occasions criticism of these providers, and makes them susceptible to calls for the development of mediation standards and practices.

The agency or clinic that offers divorce mediation is also found in the private sector. This type of organization typically is patterned along the lines of a mental health agency and offers a wide range of services. Within this type of system, certain individuals are advocates of divorce mediation. These persons may have participated in mediation training, and they offer the service as part of their professional practice. Other agencies specify divorce mediation as one of the services provided; many of these agencies are advocates for children, and therefore are motivated to provide mediation dealing with custody and visitation.

EVALUATION OF DIVORCE MEDIATION

This section summarizes selected research findings that recently have been reported about divorce mediation. The discussion is framed around two projects. One project, the Denver Custody Mediation Project, evaluated the effectiveness of private-based mediation in resolving custody and visitation disputes out of court. The second project focused on the effectiveness of three court-connected mediation services located in Los Angeles, Minneapolis, and Connecticut, in resolving custody and visitation issues. These projects, under the direction of Jessica Pearson, offer a relatively reliable assessment of mediation because of their scale and longitudinal design (Pearson & Thoennes, 1984a).

THE FINDINGS

Mandated court-connected services, not unexpectedly, attract the highest participation rates. In Los Angeles County (where mediation is mandatory), there were close to 4500 mediation cases involving custody and visitation in 1982. Typically, however, mediation services that are voluntary do not draw large numbers of participants. The Denver Project offered free mediation, and half of the referred parties chose not to use the service (Pearson, Thoennes, & Vanderkooi, 1982a). A 1981 survey of public and private mediation programs (Pearson et al., 1983) found that over 93% of those services identified as private-based conducted less than 50 mediations annually, and slightly over half saw fewer than 10 cases.

Pearson, Thoennes, and Vanderkooi (1982b) suggest that differences in those who mediate and those who do not may explain some of the resistance. The pro-mediation group scores higher on traditional socioeconomic indicators, and seems to communicate better with their spouses. Women who try mediation find it less distant and impersonal than the court system. Men apparently opt for mediation because they see their chance of winning custody as being low in the courtroom. Further, men who are ambivalent about the divorce or who are reconciliation prone seem eager to try mediation.

Attorneys play an important part in their client's choice about using mediation. Among those who tried mediation, 72% of the women and 69% of the men indicated they were encouraged by their attorneys. Among those couples that chose not to use mediation, only 18% of the women and 32% of the men indicated that their attorneys suggested mediation (Pearson et al., 1982b).

The preceding data suggest that low participation in mediation may be associated with low public awareness of the service and with attitudes of lawyers. As long as mediation maintains a low community profile, it may only be used by higher income, better-educated divorcing couples or by those who are required to mediate their disputes by court jurisdiction, as in California.

Although some advocates voice concern about making mediation of divorce issues compulsory, there is not much evidence to support such concern (Pearson & Thoennes, 1984b). First, mandatory mediation seems to enjoy a healthy public support, with between 60% and 70% of those using court-connected mediation services in Los Angeles, Minneapolis, and Connecticut favoring such programs. The pro-position is very high, of course, among those who reached agreement (85%). More interesting is the fact that between 62% and 68% of those couples who failed in their mediation attempts also support a mandated approach to the resolution of divorce disputes.

Mediation agreements vary and are difficult to interpret, primarily because there are different definitions as to what constitutes agreement. In addition, it is hard to ascertain the extent to which "unsuccessful" couples who use mediation reached a settlement after they used the service. Some programs dealing with domestic relations disputes report agreement rates of 70% (Irving et al., 1981) and 80% (Wixted, 1982). Included in these figures are agreements to continue further sessions of mediation as well as temporary agreements.

More frequently, however, mediation services report agreement reached between disputant couples ranging from 40% to 65%. In the three court-connected mediation services studied by Pearson (Pearson & Thoennes, 1984a), the resolution of child custody and visitation disputes approximated 40%. An additional 20% to 30% of couples using mediation reported partial or temporary agreements.

Most civil complaints terminate either by dismissal, default, or a negotiated settlement. To find out whether mediation is as effective as pending litigation, Pearson, Thoennes, and Vanderkooi (1982a, 1982b) compared disputing parties who used mediation with another group who went to court to resolve the issues. Sixty percent of the mediating couples reached agreement, and a majority of those who tried but could not reach a mediated agreement stipulated an agreement prior to appearing in court. In contrast, only half of the nonmediating group stipulated before going to court, while the remaining disputants relied on a judicial resolution of their disagreements.

Thoennes and Pearson (1985) found no set of case and client variables highly predictive of success in mediation. However, there were patterns suggestive of successful outcomes. Higher-income clients were able or willing to mediate more often than lower-income clients. Those couples who mediated successfully also appeared more willing to communicate or cooperate with each other. There is a lower incidence of pathology, such as substance abuse or spouse abuse, among successful clients.

There also appears to be a relationship between mediation success and the scope and duration of the disagreement(s). Successful mediations are more likely to occur if cases are mediated early in the divorcing process and if there are not multiple ongoing disputes. This is particularly true if the cases do not involve serious disputes about child and spousal support and the division of property. This information points to the need for diverting divorce disputants to mediation as soon as possible.

Finally, mediator experience appears to be related to a successful outcome in mediation, as found by Pearson and Thoennes (1984b) in their study of mediators. For example, 30% of cases seen by new mediators resulted in resolution of the disputes; successful mediation increased to over 60% of all cases when the mediator was more experienced.

Agreements also are more likely when couples perceive their mediator to be neutral, thus underscoring the importance of impartiality in the sessions. Further, successful mediation is tied to a client's perception that the mediator should be task-oriented and focus on solutions to the disputes. Clients who reached full agreement in mediation reported (Pearson & Thoennes, 1984b):

> the mediator understood the...problems..., gave the respondent a chance to express...views, reduced...tension..., focused...on the children, did not spend...time on the past, provided information about child development and adjustment, and helped to identify...custody and visitation alternatives. (p. 18)

Mediation appears to foster accommodation and compromise in custody and visitation matters. For example, couples who reached agreement in mediation seemed to choose joint custody more often than nonmediating couples. Also, in those cases where sole custody was agreed upon, more visitation time was provided than in nonmediated agreements (Pearson & Thoennes, 1984b). The mediation process seems to allow for more give and take by couples than in situations where disputes are adjudicated.

Three factors have been cited by those clients supportive of mediation (Pearson & Thoennes, 1984a). First, mediation was viewed as beneficial in helping couples focus on their children's needs. Second, the mediation process was viewed as providing an opportunity to air grievances - a chance to express one's point of view about the dispute. Third, mediating couples felt the process helped keep the discussion on target and prevented arguing, which allowed for a focus on the issues to be resolved, namely custody and visitation. In addition, successful mediation clients were somewhat more satisfied with the outcomes than those using adversarial means to resolve custody and visitation issues.

Despite high levels of satisfaction with mediation, there also were dissatisfactions voiced by its users. Half of the sample in the Pearson study of the three court-connected mediation services reported tension and unpleasantness in the sessions. A slightly smaller percentage of clients reported feeling defensive. Considering the emotionality around issues of custody and visitation, these comments are not totally unexpected. Other dissatisfactions revolved around misconceptions about mediation. For example, many parties thought that the process might save the marriage, and began the sessions angry and upset. Others thought the mediators would make the final custody decision.

Finally, mediation seems to have little impact on the relationship between the couple. About 20% of the parties reported that mediation helped them understand their ex-spouse's point of view, and only a third felt it had helped them understand themselves (Pearson & Thoennes, 1984a). Mediation, then, seems limited in affecting long-term relationship patterns; thus, it should not be viewed as a substitute for counseling and support services.

THE PROMISE, LIMITATIONS, AND FUTURE DIRECTIONS

A reluctant acceptance of the reality of divorce in contemporary life has necessitated the creation of a humane and fair way to resolve divorce disputes that provides couples with a voice in life decisions affecting themselves and their children during and after divorce. Mediation is now viewed as one such means, and such services have proliferated in both the public and private sector.

Although the practice of mediation has just emerged over the past few years, public support for it has grown. In addition, increased research attention has focused on its effectiveness. Preliminary reports by researchers point to its efficacy while acknowledging that it is not a panacea. Yet, it appears to be at least as effective as adjudication, and couples are far more satisfied using mediation than having to go to court to solve their problems. Data from the research done thus far support the use of mediation services whenever possible as an alternative to resolving issues in the adversarial atmosphere of the courtroom.

Although mediation enjoys an increasing acceptance among clients, mental health professionals, judges, and attorneys, some perspective should be maintained about its appeal and effectiveness. For example, mediation should not be viewed as a mechanism by which all divorce related disputes can be settled, notwithstanding assertions to the contrary by some of its ardent advocates. Judicial adjudication will still be needed for some individuals or couples who either are not amenable to mediation or who want their day in court. Indeed, couples have a legal right to use the court system if they so desire.

As with any emerging discipline, it is appropriate to examine the development and practice of mediation critically in order to enhance its professional growth. It is important to address issues that can mold the practice of divorce mediation into an identifiable service that can be responsibly offered to the public. Issues that seem pertinent center on (a) continuing to clarify and develop a generic framework for all forms of public and private based divorce mediation without limiting the ways in which it is currently practiced; (b) educating the public about the thrust and focus of mediation and its value as a dispute resolution technique; (c) working with legal, judicial, and mental health professionals to provide an understanding of the interdisciplinary nature of mediation; (d) developing realistic standards and practices of mediation that reflect and distinguish its legitimacy as a discipline; (e) continuing to support research related to the effectiveness of mediation and the qualities important in training competent mediators; and (f) advocating training programs that reflect the combined legal and behavioral science perspective that distinguishes the practice of mediation.

PRACTICAL CONSIDERATIONS

The following information is intended to assist mental health practitioners who are interested in expanding their clinical services to include divorce mediation. It is important that such individuals assess their skills and obtain mediation training, particularly if they are not experienced in working with attorneys, knowledgeable about domestic relations law, or familiar with the financial aspects of family life. With the recent emergence of clinical mediation as a discipline, there has been a proliferation of training seminars and workshops offered throughout the United States and Canada. As with any new profession, the quality of mediation training varies and should be assessed carefully. Increasingly, universities and colleges are offering courses in mediation. Such courses generally are offered by education and counseling departments, and taught by adjunct or primary faculty who have training in mediation or are practicing mediators. Regional educational institutions can provide information on the availability of local mediation training programs.

Another source of training are institutes or workshops offered or sponsored by associations with a particular focus on mediation and other dispute resolution techniques. The administrative offices of the following associations generally have information about training opportunities:

Association of Family and Conciliation Courts (AFCC), OHSU - Department of Psychiatry, GH 149, 3181 Sam Jackson Road, Portland, OR 97201, Phone: (503) 220-5651.

Academy of Family Mediators (AFM), c/o Nancy Thode, Executive Director, 80 Perkins Road, Greenwich, CT 06830, Phone: (203) 629-1131.

Society of Professionals in Dispute Resolution (SPIDR), 1730 Rhode Island Avenue, N.W., Suite 509, Washington, DC 20036, Phone: (202) 833-2188.

These associations provide a variety of educational materials and information that is helpful to practitioners providing services to families. They also hold annual conferences that bring together many interdisciplinary professionals who have been instrumental in the development of mediation training and services. In addition, AFCC and AFM publish the *Conciliation Courts Review* and the *Mediation Quarterly*, respectively. These professional journals primarily publish articles related to family and divorce mediation. Anyone interested in mediation may wish to consider membership in one or more of these associations.

Liability coverage should also be reviewed carefully to ascertain whether mediation is covered under the terms of your insurance plan. Generally, mediation is not specified as part of services covered by a typical policy written for mental health professionals. It now is possible to obtain mediation liability insurance; information is available from the previously mentioned associations.

In summary, the future of mediation appears promising. It has achieved a high degree of public support considering its recent arrival as an alternative means to resolve divorce related disputes. Private and public services have proliferated and further growth seems assured as mediation becomes more well-known.

Notwithstanding the emergence of mediation as a viable service, most couples complete their divorce without using the services of mental health professionals. Consequently, a limited clientele seeks out services, and it is difficult to maintain a full-time mediation practice. Practitioners trained in mediation, therefore, typically provide broad based mental health services to individuals, couples, and families, of which mediation is an integral part.

Stanley N. Cohen, PhD, currently serves as Executive Director of the Association of Family and Conciliation Courts, and is a faculty member of the Department of Psychiatry at the Oregon State Health Sciences University, Portland, Oregon. He is a Fellow and Approved Training Supervisor of the American Association of Marriage and Family Therapists. His interest areas are clinical and research aspects of marriage, family, and divorce and he has published articles in these areas. He serves on the editorial boards of *The Journal of Divorce, Journal of Psychotherapy and the Family,* and *The Conciliation Courts Review.* Dr. Cohen may be contacted c/o OHSU, Psychiatry, 3181 Sam Jackson Road, Portland, OR 97201.

RESOURCES

Bane, M. J. (1976). *Here to Stay: American Families in the Twentieth Century.* New York: Basic Books.

Brown, D. G. (1982). Divorce and family mediation: History, review, future directions. *Conciliation Courts Review, 20*(2), 1-37.

Cohen, S. N., & Jones, F. N. (1983). Issues of divorce in family therapy. In B. Wolman & G. Stricker, *Handbook of Family and Marital Therapy* (pp. 465-478). New York and London: Plenum Press.

Coogler, O. J. (1978). *Structured Mediation in Divorce Settlements: A Handbook for Marital Mediators.* Lexington, MA: Lexington Books.

Folberg, J. (1983). Mediation overview: History and practice. *Mediation Quarterly, 1,* 3-13.

Folberg, J., & Taylor, A. (1984). *Mediation: A Comprehensive Guide to Resolving Conflicts Without Litigation.* San Francisco: Jossey-Bass.

Haynes, J. M. (1981). *Divorce Mediation: A Practical Guide for Therapists and Counselors.* New York: Springer.

Irving, H., Benjamin, M., Bohm, P., & MacDonald, G. (1981). *Final Research Report of the Conciliation Project: Provincial Court (Family Division).* Toronto: Ministry of Attorney General.

Kelly, J. B. (1983). Mediation and psychotherapy: Distinguishing the differences. *Mediation Quarterly, 1,* 33-44.

Kressel, K. (1985). *The Process of Divorce: How Professionals and Couples Negotiate Settlements.* New York: Basic Books.

Lemmon, J. A. (1985). *Family Mediation Practice.* New York: Free Press.

Milne, A. (1983). Divorce mediation: The state of the art. *Mediation Quarterly, 1,* 15-31.

National Center for Health Statistics. (1981). *Annual Summary of Births, Deaths, Marriages, and Divorces* (Monthly Vital Statistics Report, 29:13). Washington, DC: U.S. Government Printing Office.

Pearson, J., Ring, M., & Milne, A. (1983). A portrait of divorce mediation services in the public and private sector. *Conciliation Courts Review, 21*(1), 1-24.

Pearson, J., & Thoennes, N. (1984). A preliminary portrait of client reactions to three court programs. *Mediation Quarterly, 5,* 21-40. (a)

Pearson, J., & Thoennes, N. (1984). *Research on Divorce Mediation: A Review of Major Findings* (13th Quarterly Report, Grant #90-CW-634). Divorce Mediation Research Project from the Department of Health and Human Services, Children's Bureau. (b)

Pearson, J., Thoennes, N., & Vanderkooi, L. (1982). Mediation of contested child custody disputes. *The Colorado Lawyer, 2,* 337-355. (a)

Pearson, J., Thoennes, N., & Vanderkooi, L. (1982). The decision to mediate: Profiles of individuals who accept and reject the opportunity to mediate contested child custody and visitation issues. *The Journal of Divorce, 6,* 17-35. (b)

Ricci, I. (1980). *Mom's House/Dad's House: Making Shared Custody Work.* New York: MacMillan Publishing Co.

Saposnek, D. J. (1983). *Mediating Child Custody Disputes: A Systematic Guide for Family Therapists, Court Counselors, Attorneys, and Judges.* San Francisco: Jossey-Bass.

Thoennes, N., & Pearson, J. (1985). Predicting outcomes in divorce mediation: The influence of people and process. *Journal of Social Issues, 41,* 115-126.

Weitzman, L. J. (1985). *The Divorce Revolution: The Unexpected Social and Economic Consequences for Women and Men in America.* New York: The Free Press.

Wixted, S. (1982). *The Children's Hearing Project: A Mediation Program for Children and Families, Alternative Means of Family Dispute Resolution.* Washington, DC: American Bar Association Special Committee on Alternative Means of Dispute Resolution.

RECENT DEVELOPMENTS IN ASSESSMENT OF THE MENTALLY DISABLED FOR SOCIAL SECURITY AND SSI BENEFITS

Jack R. Anderson

During the past 3 years the adjudication of mental disability claims for Social Security and SSI benefits has been significantly modified. Previous assessment processes and procedures were successfully challenged by class-action suits, resulting in benefits being restored to tens of thousands of claimants because their cessations were determined to have violated the law. New legislation was enacted requiring changes in federal regulations. As a consequence, mental listings were doubled in number from four to eight; the Psychiatric Review Technique (PRT), Form SSA-2506 BK, used in the assessment process, was revised; and the Mental Residual Functional Capacity (RFC) Assessment, Form SSA-4734-F4-SUP, was expanded from the consideration of seven basic mental activities to twenty. These two SSA forms should be in the possession of every mental health professional involved in the adjudication process at any level. They may be obtained from your state agencies' professional relations divisions by calling them on their WATS lines.

During the past 15 years that I have been active in this program, I have examined several thousand claimants and prepared consultative reports for state agencies and administrative law judges. As director of Nebraska Public Institutions, I coordinated with the Director of Welfare the conversion of benefits from state and county programs to SSI. As medical director of a disability determination unit, I have consulted with state agency examiners on more than 5000 claims. In this contribution, I will explain my approach to interviewing claimants and preparing consultative reports.

OBTAINING DOCUMENTATION

As soon as I receive a request to perform a consultative examination, whether it comes from the state agency or the claimant, I look for documentation. If there is none I immediately telephone the state agency and ask the examiner assigned to the claim for all relevant documents: hospital records, clinical records, court proceedings, vocational history, the original claim application - anything and everything that is available. I request that these be sent to me before my appointment with the claimant. I also ask that, if at all possible, the claimant be accompanied by a relative, friend, or neighbor who can furnish an objective account of the claimant's current activities and history.

ASSESSMENT AND REPORT PREPARATION

DAILY ACTIVITIES

When the claimant is interviewed, I begin by asking about daily activities. I want to know exactly how the claimant spends every hour of the day, every day of the week. All of the rhythms and living activities of the day and night are explored in detail:

sleeping, eating, drinking, dressing, bathing, grooming, communicating. With whom does the claimant live? Who does the cooking? Who pays the rent? How about transportation? How did the claimant get to the interview? How does the claimant survive on a day-to-day basis with no income? Does the claimant participate in household work, yard work, babysitting, or recreational activities? Does he or she use drugs or alcohol? Is the claimant in treatment? Is he or she receiving medication?

One purpose of the intensive development of specific daily activity details is to focus attention on the goal of the examination, which is to determine eligibility for disability benefits, not to formulate a diagnosis or treatment plan.

In the recent modifications of the adjudication process, with input from the various organizations of mental health professionals, 20 separate mental abilities necessary to get and hold a job were developed and classified into four categories as follows (from mental RFC):

A. Understanding and Memory

1. The ability to remember locations and work-like procedures
2. The ability to understand and remember short and simple instructions
3. The ability to understand and remember detailed instructions

B. Sustained Concentration and Persistence

4. The ability to carry out very short and simple instructions
5. The ability to carry out detailed instructions
6. The ability to maintain attention and concentration for extended periods
7. The ability to perform activities within a schedule, maintain regular attendance, and be punctual within customary tolerance
8. The ability to sustain an ordinary routine without special supervision
9. The ability to work in coordination with or proximity to others without being distracted by them
10. The ability to make simple work-related decisions
11. The ability to complete a normal workday and workweek without interruptions from psychologically based symptoms and to perform at a consistent pace without an unreasonable number and length of rest periods

C. Social Interaction

12. The ability to interact appropriately with the general public
13. The ability to ask simple questions or request assistance
14. The ability to accept instructions and respond appropriately to criticism from supervisors
15. The ability to get along with co-workers or peers without distracting them or exhibiting behavioral extremes
16. The ability to maintain socially appropriate behavior and to adhere to basic standards of neatness and cleanliness

D. Adaptation

17. The ability to respond appropriately to changes in the work setting
18. The ability to be aware of normal hazards and take appropriate precautions
19. The ability to travel in unfamiliar places or use public transportation
20. The ability to set realistic goals or make plans independently of others

As I develop daily activities material from the claimant and whomever else is available, I refer to this list frequently. By the time this portion of the interview is completed, I have usually formulated an opinion about whether the claimant's mental impairment would preclude his or her sustained employment within the constraints and stresses of the normal work environment.

PRESENT ILLNESS

The next portion of the interview is spent in developing the history of the claimant's mental impairment. The hospital, clinical, and other records furnished by the state agency, the claimant, or other sources are used to assist the claimant in completing this anamnesis. It is important to develop adequate information about the effects of the impairment on the claimant's activities from the beginning. If the claimant is able to function currently but was unable to work for 12 consecutive months or more in the past, this may establish eligibility for a closed period of benefits. If the claimant worked effectively for sustained periods of time prior to the development of the impairment, it is important to estimate as closely as possible when the impairment became so severe that it precluded employment. Developing symptoms have often resulted in termination of the claimant's employment even before the impairment was recognized and diagnosed. This date, the "onset date" of severe impairment, is necessary for determining the duration of severity. If the severity has lasted, or is expected to last, for 12 months from onset, eligibility will probably be established.

For cyclic conditions, the length of time of each exacerbation and remission should be carefully noted. Under current, liberalized adjudication policies, documented impairments that occur so frequently as to preclude sustained employment may be grounds for benefit allowance even though the claimant currently appears able to work.

PERSONAL HISTORY

The amount of time spent on this part of the interview depends on the nature of the impairment. If the condition is a chronic brain syndrome resulting from a head injury, stroke, or CNS disease, and the claimant had no prior psychiatric history, in my opinion, that is enough information for this section. For other diagnoses it is often appropriate to develop more detailed histories of the claimant's early development and subsequent family, community, school, work, social, sexual, and marital adjustments. For claimants with personality disorders, substance addiction disorders, and conditions with confusing or unclear diagnostic features, I ask specifically and in detail about disciplinary problems in school, police records (even traffic violations), and adjustment in any military service.

Again, it is important to remember the purpose of the examination when completing this part of the interview. Only enough information to facilitate adjudication should be included. Details about familial dynamics and interpersonal relationships that are necessary for therapeutic planning are out of place in the disability consultative examination and report.

DIAGNOSIS

By the time I have reviewed the record and interviewed the claimant long enough to gather information for the above three sections, I have usually arrived at a diagnosis. I use *DSM-III* terminology and coding. I also decide within which of the official listing categories the diagnosis is properly classified. These categories are (a) organic mental disorders; (b) schizophrenic, paranoid, and other psychotic disorders; (c) affective disorders; (d) mental retardation and autism; (e) anxiety related disorders; (f) somatoform disorders; (g) personality disorders; and (h) substance addiction disorders.

MENTAL STATUS

A complete mental status examination should be accomplished and reported, using any of the professionally accepted outlines or formats. In addition, while the claimant is still in the office, I review the signs and symptoms included in the PRT as evidence of each of the listings to be sure that I have inquired about mental status findings associated with the diagnosis and listing I have selected for this claimant. These diagnostic "clusters" or "syndromes" are as follows:

1. Organic mental disorders (at least one of the following):

   (a) disorientation to time and place; (b) memory impairment; (c) perceptual or thinking disturbances; (d) change in personality; (e) disturbance in mood; (f) emotional lability and impairment in impulse control; (g) loss of measured intellectual ability of at least 15 IQ points from pre-morbid levels, or overall impairment clearly within the severely impaired range of neuropsychological testing (e.g., the Luria-Nebraska, Halstead-Reitan, etc.).

2. Schizophrenic, paranoid, and other psychotic disorders (at least one of the following):

   (a) delusions or hallucinations; (b) catatonic or other grossly disorganized behavior; (c) incoherence, loosening of associations, illogical thinking, or poverty of content of speech associated with one of the following: blunt affect, flat affect, or inappropriate affect; (d) emotional withdrawal or isolation.

3. Affective disorders:

   Depressive (at least four of the following): (a) anhedonia or pervasive loss of interest in almost all activities; (b) appetite disturbance with change in weight; (c) sleep disturbance; (d) psychomotor agitation or retardation; (e) decreased energy; (f) feelings of guilt or worthlessness; (g) difficulty concentrating or thinking; (h) thoughts of suicide; or (i) hallucinations, delusions, or paranoid thinking.

   Manic syndrome (at least three of the following): (a) hyperactivity; (b) pressure of speech; (c) flight of ideas; (d) inflated self-esteem (grandiosity); (e) decreased need for sleep; (f) easy distractibility; (g) involvement in activities that have a high probability of painful consequences which are not recognized; or (h) hallucinations, delusions, or paranoid thinking.

4. Mental retardation and autism (at least one of the following):

   (a) mental incapacity evidenced by dependence upon others for personal needs (e.g., toileting, eating, bathing, or dressing) and inability to follow directions, such that the use of standardized tests of intellectual functioning is precluded; (b) a valid verbal, performance, or full scale IQ of 59 or less; (c) a valid verbal, performance, or full scale IQ of 60 to 69 inclusive and a physical or other mental impairment imposing additional and significant work-related limitation of function; or (d) a valid verbal, performance, or full scale IQ of 60 to 69 inclusive or, in the case of autism, gross deficits of social and communicative skills.

5. Anxiety related disorders (at least one of the following):

   (a) generalized persistent anxiety accompanied by at least three of the following: motor tension, autonomic hyperactivity, apprehensive expectation, or vigilance and scanning; (b) a persistent irrational fear of a specific object, activity, or situation which results in a compelling desire to avoid it; (c) recurrent severe panic attacks manifested by a sudden, unpredictable onset of intense apprehension, fear, terror, and sense of impending doom occurring on the average of at least once a week; (d) recurrent obsessions or compulsions which are a source of marked distress; or (e) recurrent and intrusive recollections of a traumatic experience (flashbacks) which are a source of marked distress.

6. Somatoform disorders (at least one of the following):

   (a) a history of multiple physical symptoms of several years' duration beginning before age 30 that have caused the individual to take medicine frequently, see a physician often, and alter life patterns significantly; (b) persistent nonorganic disturbance of vision, speech, hearing, use of a limb, sensation, or control of movement (e.g., akinesia, dyskinesia, coordination disturbances, or psychogenic seizures); or (c) unrealistic interpretation of physical signs or sensations associated with the pre-occupation or belief that one has a serious disease or injury.

7. Personality disorders (at least one of the following):

   (a) seclusiveness or autistic thinking; (b) pathologically inappropriate suspiciousness or hostility; (c) oddities of thought, perception, speech, and behavior; (d) persistent disturbances of mood or affect; (e) pathologic dependence, passivity, or aggressivity; (f) intense and unstable interpersonal relationships and impulsive and damaging behavior.

8. Substance addiction disorders:

   Behavioral or physical changes associated with the regular use of substances that affect the central nervous system; for example, organic mental disorders, affective disorders, anxiety disorders, personality disorders, peripheral neuropathies, liver damage, gastritis, pancreatitis, or seizures.

These symptom clusters and syndromes are taken almost word for word from the PRT. Because of their length and detail, they may appear formidable to a busy practicing clinician; however, only one of the eight diagnostic syndromes needs to be reviewed for each claimant. I have found that it takes less than a minute to check my mental status findings against the appropriate symptom cluster for each claimant, and I believe the practice has sharpened my diagnostic and interviewing skills in addition to improving my reports.

At every level of adjudication, the above lists of mental activities, diagnostic categories, and symptom clusters constitute the assessment vocabulary. State agency examiners, psychologists, and psychiatrists, hearing officers, and administrative law judges all use this frame of reference and terminology which is mandated by law and regulation. Mental health professionals, the only ones who communicate directly with the claimants, can expedite the adjudicative process and increase its validity and reliability if they follow the same guidelines and terminology in their examinations and reports.

ABILITY TO MANAGE FUNDS

The examining clinician is expected to express his or her opinion as to the claimant's ability to manage his or her own money. One format for this purpose is included in Volume 4 of the *Innovations in Clinical Practice* series. The state agency and the Social Security Administration are not bound to accept the examiner's opinion, but they usually do unless there is contradictory evidence in the claimant's records. If I feel that the claimant's impairment significantly effects his or her judgment, even sporadically, I give the opinion that the claimant is not capable of managing funds so that a custodian or guardian can be appointed to protect the claimant's financial well-being. Many state agency examiners and mental health professionals believe that an examining consultant's opinion that a claimant is capable of managing funds is inconsistent with a finding of mental disability. I, therefore, include a detailed explanation in the rare instances that I say a mentally disabled claimant is financially competent.

IMPACT OF MENTAL IMPAIRMENT ON ABILITY TO WORK

There are three general kinds of opinions to be expressed in this section:

1. "No clinical or historical evidence of a medically determinable mental impairment was found."
2. "There is evidence of a mental impairment, but it is not considered to be so severe as to preclude work activity."
3. "The mental impairment is documented, has lasted or is expected to last for 12 consecutive months from onset, and the symptoms (from the PRT) affect some of the work-related mental activities (from the RFC) to the degree that the claimant

would not be expected to meet the mental demands of even simple, unskilled work on a sustained basis in a competitive work environment."

Any one of these three opinions, to carry any probative weight, has to be consistent with the preceding sections. The first two need no further elaboration. The third is an opinion that the claimant is eligible for disability benefits and should summarize the relevant clinical and historical findings upon which the opinion is based. For example:

The hospital records indicate the claimant incurred a closed head injury 10 months prior to this examination. Since then, clinical records show memory impairment and emotional lability (items 1, b. and 1, f., Mental Status checklist above - from PRT). The claimant frequently laughed and cried during the interview and was unable to remember any of four unrelated words after 3 minutes. In fact, the claimant was unable to recall being given the test words. These symptoms are considered to limit the claimant's ability to remember locations, work-like procedures, and instructions (items 2 and 3 from RFC) so severely as to preclude even simple, unskilled work.

In addition, the emotional lability would prevent the claimant from getting along with co-workers or peers without distracting them or exhibiting behavioral extremes (item 15 from RFC).

State agencies, of course, are not bound by the consultative examiner's opinion about the claimant's eligibility for benefits. Nonetheless, I believe this paragraph should be included in every report. The adjudicative set tends to keep the examination and report appropriate to disability assessment rather than diagnosis and treatment. The examining mental health professional, because he or she has a direct sample of the claimant's behavior, is probably better able to assess ability to work than the state agency staff who have nothing to base their opinions on but records.

Over the years I have found that the opinions I gave in my consultative reports were generally upheld in the adjudicative process, either in the initial claim determination, the reconsideration, or at the administrative law judge hearing. Now that the expanded PRT and RFC are being used, I believe examining mental health professionals stand an even better chance than before of having their opinions upheld, if they follow the above guidelines.

ADVOCACY

I always explain to the claimants and their friends and relatives that the decision concerning their eligibility for disability benefits is made by the state agency and SSA, not by me. Some of them are referred by well-meaning county welfare workers who do not understand the disability criteria, or by insurance agencies that require SSA disability adjudication prior to establishing other insurance benefits. When these claimants are obviously not eligible for Social Security or SSI benefits, I attempt to interpret the disability criteria to them without specifically giving them my opinion. I believe that careful interpretation of reality is nearly always therapeutic, and hope a claimant will be encouraged to seek employment rather than waiting for a ship that will never come in.

If it is obvious to me that a claimant does meet mental disability eligibility criteria, I carefully explain to the claimant (and, whenever possible, to a competent relative or friend) that the best course of action is to engage an attorney who specializes in disability claims. Claimants are protected by law from excessive legal fees; their charts are clearly marked "attorney representation," which assures careful consideration of their claims at every level of adjudication; and they will have legal representation at the administrative law judge hearing, if it goes that far.

The mentally disabled are doubly disadvantaged. The same symptoms that keep them from working often prevent them from successfully pursuing their disability claims. We mental health professionals have a social obligation to provide advocacy for these individuals. We can do a great deal to improve the quality of their lives if we will only devote the necessary time and energy to provide disability reports that will result in their receiving the financial benefits to which they are legally entitled.

Jack R. Anderson, MD, is currently a graduate student in economics at the University of Alabama at Tuscaloosa. He is a retired U.S. Army psychiatrist and former Director of Public Institutions for the state of Nebraska, as well as a Professor of Clinical Psychiatry at the University of Alabama Medical Center. His primary interest in the advocacy of the disabled led him to his present graduate work. In addition to work in the graduate program, he examines and prepares reports for mental disability claimants at Bryce Hospital in Tuscaloosa. Dr. Anderson may be contacted at 3536 Wynwood Drive, Birmingham, AL 35210.

RESOURCES

Anderson, J. R. (1983). How to evaluate claimants for Social Security and SSI benefits. In P. A. Keller & L. G. Ritt (Eds.), *Innovations in Clinical Practice: A Source Book* (Vol. 2, pp. 436-441). Sarasota, FL: Professional Resource Exchange, Inc.
U.S. Department of Health and Human Services. (1985, February 4). *Federal Old-Age, Survivors, and Disability Insurance; Listing of Impairments--Mental Disorders* (FEDERAL REGISTER, 20 CFR Part 404). Washington, DC: U.S. Government Printing Office.

INTRODUCTION TO THE HANDOUTS

Many clinicians have discovered that informational handouts and brochures are helpful in their work with clients. Well designed materials can provide clients with important information, prevent misunderstandings, and facilitate treatment. As in our previous volumes, we have included some carefully selected handouts which may be copied for use with your clients.

"Stress Management: Ten Self-Care Techniques" is designed as a handout for clients trying to cope more effectively with their reactions to stressful circumstances. Following a brief discussion of stress, the author provides 10 practical suggestions for reducing distress. The handout was prepared by Kent T. Yamauchi who is currently a clinical psychologist and Assistant Professor at the Psychological Services of Pasadena City College. His interests include cognitive-behavioral self-management, health promotion, and brief psychotherapy. Dr. Yamauchi may be contacted at Psychological Services, C-232, Pasadena City College, 1570 East Colorado Boulevard, Pasadena, CA 91106-2003.

The second handout, "Communicating More Effectively," offers suggestions about how to increase the effectiveness of communications. Elements of good communication and practical examples are provided to illustrate the discussion. The author, Waleed A. Salameh, feels that providing his patients with handouts such as the one included here can be helpful in reducing their anxiety, providing objective cognitive information, and creating an openness to the psychotherapeutic process. Dr. Salameh is a licensed clinical and consulting psychologist in private practice in San Diego, California. His other contribution to this volume, "The Effective Use of Humor in Psychotherapy" can be found on page 157. Dr. Salameh can be contacted at 1335 Hotel Circle South, Suite 316-17, San Diego, CA 92108-3487.

STRESS MANAGEMENT: TEN SELF-CARE TECHNIQUES

Many people don't realize it, but stress is a very natural and important part of life. Without stress there would be no life at all!

We need stress (eustress), but not too much stress for too long (distress). Our body is designed to react to both types of stress. Eustress helps keep us alert, motivates us to face challenges, and drives us to solve problems. These low levels of stress are manageable and can be thought of as necessary and normal stimulation.

Distress, on the other hand, results when our bodies over-react to events. It leads to what has been called a "fight or flight" reaction. Such reactions may have been useful in times long ago when our ancestors were frequently faced with life or death matters. Nowadays, such occurrences are not usual. Yet, we react to many daily situations as if they were life or death issues. Our bodies really don't know the difference between a saber-toothed tiger and an employer correcting our work. It is how we perceive and interpret the events of life that dictates how our bodies react. If we think something is very scary or worrisome, our bodies react accordingly.

When we view something as manageable, though, our body doesn't go haywire; it remains alert, but not alarmed. The activation of our sympathetic nervous system (a very important part of our general nervous system) mobilizes us for quick action. The more we sense danger (social or physical), the more our body reacts. Have you ever been called upon to give an extemporaneous talk and found that your heart pounded so loudly and your mouth was so dry that you thought you just couldn't do it? That's over-reaction.

Problems can occur when overactivation of the sympathetic system is unnecessary. If we react too strongly or let the small over-reactions (the daily hassles) pile up, we may run into physical, as well as psychological, problems. Gastrointestinal problems (e.g., diarrhea or nausea), depression, or severe headaches can come about from acute distress. Insomnia, heart disease, and distress habits (e.g., drinking, overeating, smoking, and using drugs) can result from the accumulation of the small distresses.

What we all need is to learn to approach matters in more realistic and reasonable ways. Strong reactions are better reserved for serious situations. Manageable reactions are better for the everyday issues that we all have to face.

ARE YOU A REACTOR OR AN OVER-REACTOR?

Below are situations that cause stress in some and distress in others. Imagine yourself in each one right now. How are you reacting?

- Driving your car in rush hour
- Misplacing something in the house
- Waiting in a long line at the grocery store or bank
- Being blamed for something

- Getting a last minute work assignment
- Having something break while using it
- Dealing with incompetence at work
- Planning your budget

SOME HEALTHFUL HINTS

Basically, we need to modify our over-reactions to situations. Rather than seeing situations as psychologically or physically threatening and thereby activating our sympathetic nervous system, our *para*sympathetic nervous system (that part which helps lower physiological arousal) needs to be called into play. The following suggestions are designed to reduce distress. Try them. They work!

1. *Learn to Relax.* Throughout the day, take "minibreaks." Sit down and get comfortable, slowly take a deep breath in, hold it, and then exhale *very* slowly. At the same time, let your shoulder muscles droop, smile, and say something positive like, "I am r-e-l-a-x-e-d." Be sure to get sufficient rest at night.

2. *Practice Acceptance.* Many people get distressed over things they won't let themselves accept. Often these are things that can't be changed, like someone else's feelings or beliefs. If something unjust bothers you, that is different. If you act in a responsible way, the chances are you will manage stress effectively.

3. *Talk Rationally to Yourself.* Ask yourself what real impact the stressful situation will have on you in a day or a week and see if you can let the negative thoughts go. Think through whether the situation is your problem or the other's. If it is yours, approach it calmly and firmly; if it is the other's, there is not much you can do about it. Rather than condemn yourself with hindsight thinking like, "I should have...," think about what you can learn from the error and plan for the future. Watch out for perfectionism - set realistic and attainable goals. Remember, everyone makes errors. Be careful of procrastination - breaking tasks into smaller units will help and prioritizing will help get things done.

4. *Get Organized.* Develop a realistic schedule of daily activities that includes time for work, sleep, relationships, and recreation. Use a daily "things to do" list. Improve your physical surroundings by cleaning your house and straightening up your office. Use your time and energy as efficiently as possible.

5. *Exercise.* Physical activity has always provided relief from stress. In the past, daily work was largely physical. Now that physical exertion is no longer a requirement for earning a living, we don't get rid of stress so easily while working. It accumulates very quickly. We need to develop a regular exercise program to help reduce the effects of stress before it becomes distress. Try aerobics, walking, jogging, dancing, swimming, and the like.

6. *Reduce Time Urgency.* If you frequently check your watch or worry about what you do with your time, learn to take things a bit slower. Allow plenty of time to get things done. Plan your schedule ahead of time. Recognize that you can only do so much in a given period. Practice the notion of "pace, not race."

7. *Disarm Yourself.* Every situation in life does not require you to be competitive. Adjust your approach to an event according to its demands. You don't have to raise your voice in a simple discussion. Playing tennis with a friend doesn't have to be an Olympic trial. Leave behind your "weapons" of shouting, having the last word, putting someone else down, and blaming.

8. *Quiet Time.* Balance your family, social, and work demands with special private times. Hobbies are good antidotes for daily pressures. Unwind by taking a quiet stroll, soaking in a hot bath, watching a sunset, or listening to calming music.

9. *Watch Your Habits.* Eat sensibly - a balanced diet will provide all the necessary energy you will need during the day. Avoid nonprescription drugs and minimize your alcohol use - you need to be mentally and physically alert to deal with stress. Be mindful of the effects of excessive caffeine and sugar on nervousness. Put out the cigarettes - they restrict blood circulation and affect the stress response.

10. *Talk to Friends.* Friends can be good medicine. Daily doses of conversation, regular social engagements, and occasional sharing of deep feelings and thoughts can reduce stress quite nicely.

FOR MORE INFORMATION

You can learn more about managing stress through books and audio cassette tapes available at public libraries and bookstores. Among the more popular books are *Stress Without Distress* by Dr. Hans Selye, *Mind As Healer, Mind As Slayer* by Dr. Kenneth Pelletier, and *Relaxation Response* by Dr. Herbert Benson. A useful cassette tape is *A Six Second Technique to Control Stress* by Dr. Charles Stroebel.

For an individualized stress management program, you may wish to consult a health care professional specializing in health promotion. For a referral, contact the local office of your state's psychological association, or the department of psychology at a nearby college or university.

This handout was prepared by Kent T. Yamauchi, PhD.

COMMUNICATING MORE EFFECTIVELY

Effective communication is a key ingredient in professional success and personal fulfillment. We all need to effectively communicate our thoughts and emotional reactions to co-workers, friends, or others. Because our educational system does not provide any direct guidelines for teaching communication, we usually end up with hit-or-miss communication; sometimes we get our point across but many times we don't. We also tend to forget that communication is a two-way street: A complete communication cycle includes both the ability to clearly express a message and to accurately understand the messages of others. Communication researcher Dr. Paul Waltzawick says in his book, *The Language of Change*, that human communication has three major characteristics: (a) We cannot not communicate - even silent persons are communicating something about themselves through the silence. (b) Human communication is multileveled - your words could be saying one thing but your body language or clothing could be communicating another message. (c) The message sent is not necessarily the message received - because of the different angles each person uses to interpret information, you cannot assume that what you meant has been understood by the other person.

Psychological research and clinical experience have enabled us to determine 11 important qualities of effective communication:

1. *Respect.* Communication usually improves in situations where people show consideration for each other's choices and viewpoints, even when they may personally disagree with a given viewpoint. For example, your teenage son will be more receptive to your comments about his low school grades if you express your feelings about the situation without blaming or accusing him ("I am sad because I want to help you succeed, but I don't know how"), thus making it possible for him to respond positively.

2. *Empathy.* By actively listening to what is going on with the other person and feeding back to him or her your understanding about what you just heard, you are recognizing that person's feelings and experiences. For example, in response to his daughter's excited comments about her recent job promotion a father might empathically say, "This promotion means a lot to you, doesn't it! It makes you really happy to be recognized for the good work you do."

3. *Concreteness.* Communication cannot be productive unless it goes beyond vagueness and zeros in on specifics. Feeling bored during an interaction is usually a sign that the communication is too general and, therefore, cannot hold one's attention. For example, a manager cannot expect "higher productivity" from his employees unless he concretely defines what he wants, such as (a) showing up to work at exactly 7:30 a.m.; (b) turning out 10% more of a specific product within a period of 6 months; (c) giving X shares of company stock to those employees who achieve and maintain (a) and (b) within the next 6 months.

4. *Immediacy.* Communication is more relevant when it focuses on present reality. For example, instead of reciting all the past hurts or anticipated fears relating to her relationship with her boyfriend, a woman might choose to limit the expression of her hurt to the present instance: "I feel sad and undermined right now because you're telling me that you're cancelling our weekend plans so you can go watch the game at your friend's house."

5. *Warmth.* This includes all verbal and nonverbal cues by which we can show positive concern in our relationship with others. A person can express warmth by maintaining direct eye contact and sitting face-to-face during communication, being mentally available to what the other is expressing, noting positive things about the other person ("I like the colors of your dress," "I appreciate your courteous ways in dealing with other people," etc.), and making encouraging remarks about plans and projects which are important to others ("Did you obtain approval for the loan to buy your new house?" "Your good grades in college should help you gain admission to law school," etc.). Along the same lines, sending a "thank you" note to a gracious host or to a supportive co-worker would also represent an appropriately welcome expression of warmth.

6. *Genuineness.* This means a person truly believes what he or she is communicating, and that the person's actions are generally consistent with what he or she says. The genuine communicator is open and candid but gentle and compassionate; there are no hidden meanings behind what is being said. For example, parents are not very convincing when they preach to their children about the benefits of physical exercise if they refuse to make time for exercise in their own lives.

7. *Self-Disclosure.* Communication is facilitated when a person is able to share with others the relevant incidents from his or her own life. Because we all share similar fears and needs and a common core of biological, developmental, and social experiences, it is inevitable that disclosing personal information would bring two people a little closer. For example, a father would be much closer to his adolescent son if he shared some of his own adolescent experiences related to finding his identity, discovering sexuality, rebelling against rules, and so on. Using the "I" format in conversation, instead of the impersonal or accusatory "you," is another aspect of self-disclosure which shows that you are "owning" your feelings. "You always ignore my opinions" might become "I fear that my opinions are not that important to you."

8. *Interpersonal Patience.* It requires time and effort to really listen to another person. Because different individuals have different levels of expressiveness, it is important for communicators to pace themselves with each other's expression, instead of imposing their own style upon others. In conversation, it is helpful to decrease signs of impatience ("Ya, ya, I know what you mean," tapping on a desk while talking, fingering with objects), increase signs of active listening (a nod of the head combined with an "um hmm," "Yes," "I follow you," "I see your point"), and check to see if the other person is still listening ("Are you with me?" "Am I making any sense to you?" "Is this clear to you?").

9. *Confrontation.* The content of communication is not always emotionally neutral or necessarily pleasant to another person's ears. There are times when we need to confront or question differences between what someone says and actually does, or what is fantasized and what really happens. Confrontation is also used to express disagreement or to let others know where you stand on important issues. It is often difficult to confront because most of us react defensively when we feel criticized. Consequently, confrontation is practically ineffective without affirmation. It is useful to associate affirmation (the expression of constructive aspects in others) with confrontation so that the confrontation can be digested, leading to a productive outcome. Care should also be taken to assure the person you are confronting that you are not questioning his or her personal worth, but rather a specific action or behavior - confrontation should not be confused with rudeness, explosiveness, or the expression of dogmatic views. For example, if a husband puts his wife down in front of guests, she might confront his behavior by saying, "You know, I really appreciated your tenderness and support 2 weeks ago when mother passed away. But I feel you are being callous and distant when you put me down in front of our guests. I am hurt by the rise and fall of your caring about me."

10. *Social Assertiveness.* This behavior is an alternative to passivity and aggression in social interactions. You are not being socially assertive if you sulk, swallow your reactions, act like a persecuted martyr, expect others to read your mind and then feel disappointed when they don't fulfill your needs, or *always* place other people's priorities before your own. Neither are you being assertive when you demand instead of request, violate the rights of others, act like you own the planet, blurt out your feelings without regard for how they might affect others, and constantly force other people's hand to get what you want. Both approaches lead to broken or disappointing relationships and avoidance. On the other hand, you *are* being assertive when you can request and refuse, stand up for your rights, not feel guilty when you say "No" (to what you don't want) or embarrassed when you say "Yes" (to what you really want), deal with problems when they come up instead of ignoring them, take risks in expressing yourself honestly, and make your needs known in a social context. For example, when a nonsmoking employee is asked to share an office with another employee who smokes, he can assertively tell his associate, "I am bothered by cigarette smoke because it makes my eyes red and gives me a sore throat. Since this office has no windows, would you mind taking your smoking break at the employees lounge?" If the employee does not obtain satisfaction with his associate, he could then approach the supervisor about sharing an office with another nonsmoker.

11. *Humor.* Humor, according to Victor Borge, is "the shortest distance between two people"; it is the spice of communication, a powerful way of breaking defensive barriers, and a refreshing means of conveying information. Getting your point across with humor can be much more effective than using a solemn or scathing approach. It often works to introduce humor to interactions by using self-directed or situational humor - humorous aspects about your life or about the circumstances under which an interaction is taking place. Later, unobtrusive other-directed humor (humorous aspects of others' lives) can be used when the ambience becomes more relaxed. For example, an excellent teacher I once had began his classes by saying, "I have a lot of things to teach you! I'm a garbage can of knowledge!" Once everyone was relaxed and laughing, he would then go to the heart of his lecture, using humor along the way to convey material in a stimulating format.

All the above characteristics, when understood and applied, lead to effective communication. The rewards of effective communication are a sense of personal fulfillment and a substantial enrichment of interpersonal relationships. I now encourage you to step back, take a good look at your communication patterns, and see where you need to make changes. Then you can start integrating the above suggestions with your own style in a personally relevant manner.

This handout was prepared by Waleed A. Salameh, PhD.

INFORMATION FOR CONTRIBUTORS

The editors of *Innovations in Clinical Practice* welcome the opportunity to review manuscripts which are consistent with the goals of the series. Manuscripts will be reviewed only if they are not simultaneously under consideration elsewhere. While we will attempt to handle all manuscripts with care, it is important to note that we assume no responsibility for unsolicited manuscripts. Any obligations we make to contributors are specified by written agreement after manuscript acceptance, and we reserve the right to accept or reject manuscripts at our discretion. All submissions should be accompanied by the author's current vita or a brief letter outlining the author's professional experience and training relevant to the topic. Manuscripts which are accepted are subject to editing.

MANUSCRIPT SUBMISSION

Interested contributors should submit an original and two copies of double-spaced manuscripts with a vita or letter describing their relevant experience to: Senior Editor, *Innovations in Clinical Practice*, Professional Resource Exchange, Inc., P. O. Box 15560, Sarasota, FL 34277-1560. Receipt of all manuscripts will be acknowledged and authors will be contacted again and notified of our editorial decision following review. Contributions not accepted for publication can be returned only if authors include a large, self-addressed envelope with sufficient postage.

MANUSCRIPT PREPARATION

Brief contributions are preferred, and unsolicited manuscripts should not exceed 25 double-spaced typed pages. Each manuscript should begin with a title page which includes the name(s), address(es), and telephone number(s) of the author(s). The second page should have the title of the paper centered at the top, but should not contain the names of the author(s). No abstract is required. Manuscripts should generally follow the style specified by the current *Publication Manual of the American Psychological Association* (1983). There is, however, an exception in that each article should include a "resource" instead of a "reference" section and "reference notes." The use of footnotes is discouraged. Contributors may refer to the contents of the present volume for a general sense of the style which should be followed. Three levels of headings may be used to facilitate the organization of contributions: (a) a centered main heading, (b) a flush side heading, and (c) an indented side heading. Manuscripts should be written in a concise, professional, but readable manner. Writing in the first person, for example, is quite acceptable. Sexist language should be avoided.

ASSESSMENT INSTRUMENTS AND FORMS

The *Innovations* volumes contain informal clinical assessment instruments and checklists. We do not usually publish formal psychological tests. Assessment instruments are designed to help the clinician be more thorough in collecting information. Contributors of assessment instruments should write for the special instructions which pertain to this type of material.

INDEX

Volumes 1, 2, 3, 4, and 5

(Volume numbers are noted in **bold** print)

A

Addison's disease, **3**: 45-46, **5**: 92
Adolescent Sentence Completion Test (see Sentence Completion Test for...)
Adrenal gland dysfunction, **3**: 45-46
Acute porphyria, **3**: 50
Affective disorders (also see Depression), **3**: 5-25
    bipolar disorder, **3**: 11-12, 112
    cyclothymic disorder, **3**: 12
    depression in older adults,
        assessment of, **3**: 100-116
        treatment of, **3**: 117-131
    dexamethasone suppression test, **3**: 7-8
    diagnosis, **3**: 5-19
    dysthymic disorder, **3**: 12-13
    major depression, **3**: 9-11,
        in older adults, **3**: 100-102
    medical disorders associated with, **3**: 16-17
    treatment, **3**: 19-22
Agoraphobia, **4**: 5-20
    defined, **4**: 5-7
    demographics of, **4**: 8
    differential diagnosis of, **4**: 7-8
    drug therapy for, **4**: 19-20
    etiology of, **4**: 8-13
        agoraphobic spiral, **4**: 12
        biological factors, **4**: 11-12
        existential aspects, **4**: 10-11
        secondary gain, **4**: 10
        sensitization, **4**: 8-9
        social conditioning, **4**: 12
    treatment of, **4**: 13-20
        comprehensive treatment chart, **4**: 14
        exposure therapy, **4**: 13-17
        sequence, **4**: 17-19
AIDS (Acquired Immune Deficiency Syndrome), **3**: 79-80, **5**: 221-230
    basic information, **5**: 221-222
    social and psychological impact, **5**: 223-227

AIDS (Continued)
    treatment of clients with, **5:** 221-230
        managing clinical symptoms, **5:** 227-229
        therapist issues, **5:** 229
Alcohol abuse,
    Alcohol History Form, **3:** 169
    Alcoholics Anonymous and treatment, **5:** 83-90
    associated with other drug abuse, **3:** 173-174
        aftercare, **3:** 176-177
        Drug History Form, **3:** 175
        treatment for, **3:** 174-176
    diagnosis and treatment decisions, **3:** 166-178
    marital treatment of, **5:** 152-154
    patient risk and prognosis, **3:** 170
    referral and treatment, **3:** 171-173
        inpatient treatment, **3:** 172
        outpatient treatment, **3:** 172-173
    screening indicators, **5:** 78-79
    symptoms, **3:** 166-170
        alcohol history, **3:** 168-170
    treatment issues, **5:** 71-82
Alcoholics Anonymous, **5:** 83-90
Anger,
    assessment of, **2:** 185-187
    cognitive model of, **2:** 182-185
    determinants of, **2:** 187-189
    stress inoculation therapy for, **2:** 181-201
    treatment procedure for, **2:** 193-199
Anorexia nervosa, **5:** 5-28
    appropriate body weight determination, **5:** 36-37
    assessment, **5:** 5-28
        assessment framework, **5:** 6-11
        psychometric, **5:** 19-23
        symptoms, **5:** 7-15
        techniques, **5:** 15-21
    attitudes toward weight and shape, **5:** 8-9, 40
    defined, **5:** 6
    diagnostic issues, **5:** 11-15
    dieting and extreme weight control, **5:** 9-10
    medical consultation, **5:** 31
    monitoring body weight, **5:** 37
    predisposing factors, **5:** 6-8
    starvation consequences, **5:** 33
    symptoms, **5:** 7-15
    treatment, **5:** 29-44
        cognitive behavioral methods, **5:** 38-39
        initial interviews, **5:** 32-33
        meal planning, **5:** 34-35
        normalization of eating and weight, **5:** 33-37
        psychological issues, **5:** 39-42
        resistance, **5:** 31-32
        therapeutic relationship, **5:** 32
        two-track approach, **5:** 30-31
Answering machines, **5:** 271-276
Antianxiety medications, **1:** 400-439
    brand name index, **1:** 402
Antidepressant medications, **1:** 400-439, **2:** 174-180, **3:** 20
    brand name index, **1:** 402
    lithium carbonate, **2:** 178, **3:** 430-432
    monoamine oxidase inhibitors, **2:** 178

Antidepressant medications (Continued)
    table of common antidepressants, **2:** 177
    tricyclics, **2:** 177
Antipsychotic medications, **3:** 419-454
    brand name index, **3:** 421
Assertiveness training in marital therapy, **5:** 146-150
Autoimmune disorders, **3:** 52

B

Balance sheet (form for client problem solving), **2:** 80
Battered clients, **1:** 8-9
Behavioral medicine (also see specific topics, e.g., Pain),
    assessment, **5:** 352-353
    history, **5:** 351-352
    interventions, **5:** 353-361
    psychologist's roles, **5:** 352-354
Bereavement,
    interviewing the bereaved, **1:** 89-111
Binge eating and vomiting, **5:** 10 ,17, 37-38
Biofeedback,
    certification and training, **2:** 157-158
    electrodermal feedback, **2:** 148-149
    electroencephalographic feedback, **2:** 149-151
    electromyographic feedback, **2:** 145-147
    insurance reimbursement for, **2:** 153-157
    major instruments reviewed, **2:** 145-151
    and microcomputers, **1:** 199
    with Myofacial Pain Dysfunction Syndrome, **2:** 339, **5:** 195
    overview of, **2:** 142-160
    professional issues, **2:** 153-160, **5:** 354
    professional societies, **2:** 160
    for tension headache (EMG), **1:** 146-148
    thermal feedback, **2:** 147-148
    treatment programs, **2:** 151-153
Body image disturbances in eating disorders, **5:** 18
Borderline personality disorder, **5:** 103-135
    assessment, **5:** 103-112
        diagnostic issues, **5:** 105-107
        differential diagnosis, **5:** 108-110
        structured interviews, **5:** 110-111
    defined, **5:** 103-104
    morbidity, **5:** 105
    prevalence, **5:** 104-105
    treatment considerations, **5:** 113-135
       · aggression, **5:** 125-126
        cognitive-behavioral approaches, **5:** 124
        countertransference, **5:** 126-127
        exploratory versus supportive approaches, **5:** 113-114
        families, **5:** 123-124
        group psychotherapies, **5:** 124-125
        hospitalization, **5:** 128
        Kernberg's approach, **5:** 115-118
        psychopharmacology, **5:** 125
        self-destructive behaviors, **5:** 127-128
        traditional psychotherapeutic approaches, **5:** 114-123
        Winnicott's approach, **5:** 118-120
        work skills, **5:** 124

Boyd Developmental Progress Scale, 3: 306-309
    administration and scoring, 3: 307-308
    construction, 3: 306
    scale, 3: 309
Brain electrical activity mapping, 5: 98-99
Brain function and psychological assessment of children, 3: 154-157
Brief Psychiatric Rating Scale (for adults), 2: 307-315
    history form, 2: 315
    instrument, 2: 314
    introduction, 2: 307-313
Brief Psychiatric Rating Scale for Children, 3: 257-266
    history form, 3: 265
    instrument, 3: 264
    introduction, 3: 257-263
Bruxism, 2: 338
Bulimia nervosa,
    appropriate body weight determination, 5: 36-37
    assessment, 5: 5-28
        assessment framework, 5: 6-11
        psychometric, 5: 19-23
        symptoms, 5: 7-15
        techniques, 5: 15-21
    attitudes toward weight and shape, 5: 8-9, 40
    binge eating and vomiting, 5: 10, 17, 37-38
    defined, 5: 6
    diagnostic issues, 5: 11-15
    dieting and extreme weight control, 5: 9-10
    medical consultation, 5: 31
    monitoring body weight, 5: 37
    predisposing factors, 5: 6-8
    starvation consequences, 5: 33
    symptoms, 5: 7-15
    treatment, 5: 29-44
        cognitive-behavioral methods, 5: 38-39
        initial interviews, 5: 32-33
        issues, 5: 37-38
        meal planning, 5: 34-35
        normalization of eating and weight, 5: 33-37
        psychological issues, 5: 39-42
        resistance, 5: 31-32
        therapeutic relationship, 5: 32
        two-track approach, 5: 30-31
Burnout, clinician, 3: 221-228
    contributing factors, 3: 222-226
    recognition of, 3: 221-222
    prevention strategies, 3: 226-227
    treatment issues, 3: 224-226

C

Cardiopulmonary disorders and anxiety, 5: 92-93
Cardiovascular disorders, 5: 356-358
    cardiac rehabilitation, 5: 357-358
    hypertension, 5: 357
    Raynaud's disease, 5: 358

Cancer patients, **4:** 153-171, **5:** 360
    assessment of, **4:** 156-159
        expectations, **4:** 158
        will to live, **4:** 157-158
    caregiver support networks, **4:** 166
    mobilizing the inner healer, **4:** 162-166
    therapeutic posture with, **4:** 154-155
    treatment plan for, **4:** 159-162
Career and life planning tools for practitioners, **4:** 435-444
    planning needs, **4:** 435-436
    planning process, **4:** 436
    planning resources and instruments, **4:** 436-441
        ability, **4:** 440-441
        general, **4:** 437
        interests, **4:** 439-440
        personality, **4:** 441
        skills, **4:** 438
        values, **4:** 437-438
Catharsis in psychotherapy, **4:** 35-49
    emotions, **4:** 37-39
    history of, **4:** 35-37
    role of, **4:** 39-41
Cathartic techniques, **4:** 41-46
Chaisson's technique, **1:** 33
Child abusing clients, **1:** 9-10
Child custody (see Custody)
Children,
    techniques for, **5:** 391-403
        color-your-life-technique, **5:** 400-402
        model building, **5:** 398-400
        mutual story telling, **5:** 396-398
        picture drawing game, **5:** 393-395
        picture taking, **5:** 395-396
        playroom materials, **5:** 392
        too tight children, **5:** 393-398
        too loose children, **5:** 398-402
        types of children, **5:** 391-397
    theraplay technique for, **5:** 177-187
        case illustration, **5:** 183-185
        diagnosis, **5:** 179-180
        intervention techniques, **5:** 180-181
        parent-child activities, **5:** 177-179
        phases of therapy, **5:** 183
Children's chronic illnesses (see Chronic illness in children)
Children's Current Symptom Checklist, **2:** 256-271
Chromatography, **5:** 95
Chronic illness in children, **4:** 173-186
    helping the child cope, **4:** 177-180
    impact on the family, **4:** 180-182
    managing the illness, **4:** 174-177
        communicating with the physician, **4:** 175-176
        defining patient and parent responsibilities, **4:** 176
        learning about the illness, **4:** 175
        motivating the patient, **4:** 176-177
Chronic pain,
    activity and, **1:** 128
    anxiety and, **1:** 129
    conditioning of, **1:** 128-129
    depression and, **1:** 130
    diagnosis of, **1:** 130-132

Chronic pain (Continued)
    distraction and, **1:** 127-128
    Hendler Screening Test for Chronic Back Pain Patients, **2:** 272-277
    management of, **1:** 126-140
    meaning of, **1:** 127
    Myofacial Pain Dysfunction Syndrome (MPDS), **5:** 189-201
    neurophysiology of, **1:** 126-127
    patient characteristics and, **1:** 129-130
    treatment, **1:** 132-137, **5:** 189-201, 358-359
        with drugs, **1:** 132-134
        with biofeedback, **1:** 134
        with hypnosis, **1:** 135
        with medical-surgical techniques, **1:** 136
        with physical therapy, **1:** 135
        with psychotherapies, **1:** 134-135
        success, **1:** 136-137
Client advisory boards, **3:** 217-219
Client materials, **1:** 376-399, **2:** 442-450, **3:** 455-467
    About Your Appointment for Psychological Testing, **2:** 450
    Communicating More Effectively, **5:** 431-433
    Confidentiality, **1:** 379-380
    Coping with Loss and Grief, **2:** 447-449
    Differences in Sexual Desire, **3:** 464-467
    Fee Information, **1:** 381
    A Guide to Psychotherapy, **2:** 443-446
    How to Communicate Effectively, **1:** 377-378
    Me? Go for Psychotherapy? Not a Chance!, **3:** 459-463
    Office Policy Statement, **4:** 348-349
    Parents Are Forever, **4:** 469-479
    Plain Talk about Dealing with the Angry Child, **4:** 481-483
    Stress Management: Ten Self-Care Techniques, **5:** 427-429
    Talking with Children About Separation and Divorce, **1:** 382-383
    The Therapy Process and First Session Evaluation, **4:** 352-353
    Understanding Family Therapy, **3:** 456-458
    Understanding and Managing Stress, **1:** 391-399
    Visitation Guidelines for Noncustodial Children, **4:** 110-113
Client snatching, **5:** 257-259
Cognitive therapy,
    basic concepts, **1:** 38-41
    for Borderline personality disorder, **5:** 124
    for depressed older adults, **3:** 119-123
    for depression, **1:** 37-52
    for eating disorders, **5:** 38-39
    for martial problems, **5:** 137-156
    for offenders, **4:** 115-125
    procedures, **1:** 41-48
Collection (fees),
    form letter, **1:** 225
    use of small claims court, **5:** 245-255
Color-your-life-technique for children, **5:** 400-402
Communicating More Effectively (client handout), **5:** 431-433
Communication skills for clinicians, **2:** 135-143
    indirect techniques, **2:** 139-142
    law of requisite variety, **2:** 136-137
    utilization of behavior, **2:** 137-139
Community interventions, **3:** 319-335
Community mental health ideology, **3:** 327
Community psychology competencies, **3:** 326
Competency assessment, civil, **3:** 310-315
    Competency Assessment Inventory, **3:** 311-315

Competency to Stand Trial Assessment Instrument, **2**: 278-284
    instrument, **2**: 283
    introduction, **2**: 278-282
Complaints, handling client, **2**: 206-207
Compliance to medical procedures, **5**: 356
Computer testing program design using BASIC, **3**: 229-242
    advanced techniques, **3**: 237-241
    five-factor inventory, **3**: 231-237
Computerized axial tomography, **5**: 96
Computerized literature searches (Online database searches for information), **4**: 229-242
Computerizing the clinical office, **4**: 215-227
    applications and software, **4**: 215-219
    database access software, **4**: 239-240, 242
    hardware, **4**: 219-226
Confidential communications (also see Privileged communication), **1**: 357, **2**: 209-210, 399-401, **3**: 391-405
    duty to protect, **5**: 383-390
    in group therapy, **3**: 410-412
Confidentiality (client handout), **1**: 379-380
Conflicts of interest in psychotherapy, **2**: 213-214, 404-407
Consent for Release of Professional Information (form), **1**: 218
Consultation (also see specific consultees), **1**: 320-333, **3**: 319-335, 336-342
    assessing requests for, **3**: 336-342
    context, **1**: 327-330
    contracts, **1**: 329-330, **3**: 334
        with police agencies, **2**: 373-375
    defined, **1**: 321-322, **3**: 337
    with dentists (see Dentists), **2**: 331-347
    with emergency medical technicians, **4**: 377-390
    ethical issues in, **2**: 319-330
        informed consent, **2**: 324-325
    examples, **3**: 320-335
    fees (also see Fees), **2**: 250-262
    for helping skills training, **4**: 391-411
    history of, **1**: 320-321
    in hospitals (see this heading), **3**: 379-390
    legal issues in, **2**: 327-328
    model of, **1**: 322-323
    organization development (see this heading), **2**: 348-360
    with police (see this heading), **2**: 371-387
    with schools (see this heading), **3**: 343-352
    sequential contracts in, **1**: 322-327
Consumer approach to clinical practice, **3**: 213-220
    client right safeguards, **3**: 214-219
Contracts,
    for consultation, **1**: 329-330
        with police, **2**: 373-375
    for therapy, **3**: 214-216
Contributor information, **4**: 485
Coping statements (in stress inoculation), **1**: 119-121
Coping Strategies Scales for Depressed Patients, **5**: 287-297
    introduction, **5**: 287-290
    scale (COSTS), **5**: 291-297
Couples groups, in divorce therapy, **2**: 8-9
Court testimony (see Expert witness roles)
Covert conditioning, **1**: 68-70
Covert modeling, **1**: 70
Criminal offenders (see Offenders)
Crises, repeating, **1**: 11-13

Crisis intervention (also see specific types of crises, e.g., Suicide), 1: 1-15
    crisis assessment checklist, 4: 267-284
    emergency room assessment and intervention, 5: 365-381
        disposition, 5: 379-380
        psychiatric interview, 5: 366-375
            content interview, 5: 373-376
            process interview, 5: 366-373
        training of psychologists for, 5: 365-366
        treatment, 5: 376-379
            chemotherapy, 5: 376-377
            dangerous patients, 5: 377-378
            therapies, 5: 378-379
    with families, 2: 126-128
    with police personnel, 2: 381-383
    with sexual assault victims, 4: 71-74
    with suicidal crises, 2: 167-171
Cushing's disease, 5: 92
Custody, mediating child, 3: 26-40
    case studies, 3: 32-37
    child and family issues, 3: 27-29
    clinician roles in, 3: 31-32
    guidelines for deciding disputed custody, 3: 29-30
    Permission to Release Custody Evaluation (form), 4: 358
    specific recommendations, 3: 37-39
    visitation guidelines for noncustodial children, 4: 110-113

D

Dangerous clients, 1: 7-8
    duty to protect others, 5: 383-390
    in the emergency room, 5: 377-378
Database searching (see Online database searches for information)
Death (also see Bereavement),
    leading causes of, 5: 332
Decision Making Grid (form), 2: 78
Delirium, 3: 47-48, 5: 92
Dementia, 3: 46-47, 110-111, 5: 92
Dental Anxiety Scale, 2: 333
Dentists, consultation with, 2: 331-347
    dental fear, 2: 332-335
    oral habit problems, 2: 337-339
    patient compliance, 2: 339
    pediatric dentistry, 2: 335-337
        Maternal Questionnaire (regarding children's dental fears), 2: 336
Depression (also see Affective disorders)
    anorexia nervosa and, 5: 14-15
    assessment in older adults, 3: 100-116
        clinical interview for, 3: 102-108
        Dexamethasone suppression test, 5: 94-95
        major depressive episodes, 3: 100-102
        screening measures for, 3: 113-114
        treatment planning issues in, 3: 108-112
    cognitive therapy for, 1: 37-52
    Coping Strategies Scales (COSTS), 5: 287-297
    diagnosis, 3: 5-19
    educational approaches for older adults, 3: 126-127
    endogenous, in older adults, 3: 106-107
    evaluating the depressed patient, 2: 174-176, 3: 5-19
    major, 3: 9-11

Depression (Continued)
    medical disorders associated with, **3:** 16-17, 108-109
    medication for (also see Antidepressant medications), **2:** 174-180, **3:** 20
    structured enrichment program for, **1:** 304-307
    symptoms in older adults, **3:** 104-108
    treatment, **3:** 19-22
    treatment in older adults, **3:** 117-131
        behavioral therapy, **3:** 120-123
        cognitive therapy, **3:** 119-123
        electroconvulsive therapy, **3:** 125-126
        family therapy, **3:** 123-124
        group therapy, **3:** 124
        psychodynamic therapy, **3:** 123
        somatic therapies, **3:** 124-125
    treatment planning for older adults, **3:** 108-112
Dexamethasone suppression test, **3:** 7-8, **5:** 94-95
Diagnostic system, use of a, **2:** 210-211
Diagnostic technology (see Psychiatric diagnostic technology), **5:** 91-102
Disability evaluations for Social Security and SSI, **2:** 436-441, **5:** 417-423
    advocacy, **5:** 422-423
    assessment and report preparation, **5:** 417-422
        ability to manage funds, **5:** 421
        ability to work, **5:** 421-422
        daily activities, **5:** 417-418
        diagnosis, **5:** 419
        mental status, **5:** 419
        personal history, **5:** 419
        present illness, **5:** 419
    documentation, **5:** 417
Disclosure of patient records (also see Privilege and Confidentiality), **1:** 355-357, **2:** 209-210, 399-401
Divorce mediation, **5:** 405-416
    contrasted with therapy, **5:** 408-410
    court settings, **5:** 410-411
    defined, **5:** 405-406
    evaluation of, **5:** 411-413
    future directions, **5:** 413-414
    goals and processes, **5:** 408-410
    history, **5:** 406-407
    private practice of, **5:** 411
    training resources, **5:** 414-415
Divorce, Suggestions for Talking with Children About Divorce (client handout), **1:** 384-385
Divorce Therapy, **2:** 5-16
    dialectic model of defined, **2:** 6-7, 12-13
    during divorce, **2:** 9-11
    post-divorce issues, **2:** 11-14
    predivorce stages, **2:** 7-9
DSM-III Classification and Codes, **1:** 443-450
Duty to protect, **5:** 383-390
    legal principles, **5:** 383-384
    recommendations for therapists, **5:** 387-389
    Tarasoff implications, **5:** 384-386
Dying patients (also see Grief, Hospices), **1:** 344-345

E

Eating Attitudes Test (EAT-26), **5:** 22
Eating Record, Daily, **5:** 23

Electroconvulsive therapy, **3:** 21-22
    for depressed older adults, **3:** 125-126
Electrodermal biofeedback, **2:** 148-149
Electroencephalographic biofeedback, **2:** 149-151
Electromyographic biofeedback, **2:** 145-147
Emergency medical technicians, training psychological skills, **4:** 377-390
Emergency room assessment and intervention, **5:** 365-381
    disposition, **5:** 379-380
    psychiatric interview, **5:** 366-375
        content interview, **5:** 373-376
        process interview, **5:** 366-373
    training of psychologists for, **5:** 365-366
    treatment, **5:** 376-379
        chemotherapy, **5:** 376-377
        dangerous patients, **5:** 377-378
        therapies, **5:** 378-379
Emotional expression,
    in cancer patients, **4:** 157
    in psychotherapy (also see Catharsis), **4:** 35-49
Employee assistance program (EAP), **1:** 334-342, **3:** 353-364, **5:** 264-265
    components, **1:** 336
    costs, **1:** 340-341, **3:** 361-363
    defined, **3:** 353-354
    implementation, **1:** 336-341
    marketing, **3:** 356-361
    models, **1:** 334-335, **5:** 264-265
    planning considerations, **1:** 335-336
    in private practice settings, **3:** 355-356
Endocrine disorders, **3:** 43-46, **5:** 92
Enuresis, **2:** 86-100
    associated characteristics, **2:** 87-90
    theoretical formulations, **2:** 86-87
    treatment, **2:** 90-97
        with conditioning, **2:** 92-96
            urine alarm instructions, **2:** 94
        with dry bed training, **2:** 96-97
        with medication, **2:** 91
        with retention control, **2:** 96
Epilepsy, **5:** 92, 98, 359-360
Ericksonian approaches to strategic hypnotherapy, **5:** 45-58
    case study, **5:** 54-57
    hypnosis defined, **5:** 46-47
    indirection, **5:** 47-49
        indirect suggestions and binds, **5:** 48
        metaphors and anecdotes, **5:** 48-49
    induction steps, **5:** 53-54
    process, **5:** 52-54
    strategic applications, **5:** 50-52
    utilization, **5:** 49-50
    versus traditional approaches, **5:** 47-50
Ethics (also see specific topics, e.g., Confidentiality)
    in clinical practice, **2:** 399-410
    colleague relationships, **5:** 257-259
    conflicts of interest in psychotherapy, **2:** 213-214, 404-407
    in consultation, **2:** 319-330
    in group therapy, **3:** 406-418
    for insurance procedures, **1:** 440-442
    interprofessional relations, **2:** 407-409
    malpractice, **2:** 205-216
    in the media, **2:** 365-367

Evaluation of service questionnaires, **2:** 285-291
    Assessment of Therapy Progress, **2:** 287-288
    Client Satisfaction Survey **2:** 288-289
    Introduction to questionnaires, **2:** 285-286
    Referring Professional Satisfaction Survey, **2:** 290-291
    Therapist Evaluation Questionnaire, **4:** 354-357
Evaluation of therapy, **2:** 285-286, **3:** 217
Excessive somnolence, disorders of (DOES), **2:** 64-66
Executive assessment, **4:** 445-458
    areas to assess, **4:** 449-451
    assessment process, **4:** 451-453
    preliminary considerations, **4:** 445-448
    report, **4:** 453-454
Experiential psychotherapy sessions, **5:** 59-68
    being the deeper experiencing, **5:** 64-65
    carrying experiences forward, **5:** 61-62
    experiencing new ways of being and behaving, **5:** 65-68
    getting into the experiential state, **5:** 59-61
    integrating relationships with deeper experiences, **5:** 62-64
Expert witness roles, **1:** 355-361, **3:** 367-378
    cross-examination, **3:** 368-370
    initial forensic interview, **4:** 467-474
    legal terms glossary, **4:** 459-466
    post-trial, **1:** 359
    pre-trial, **1:** 356-357, **3:** 374-378
    and privileged communication, **3:** 399-402
    subpoenas, **1:** 355-357, **3:** 399
    trial, **1:** 357-359
    vocational assessments, **3:** 373-375
    witness fees, **1:** 357,359
    witness stand suggestions, **1:** 358-359, **3:** 368-373
Extramarital affairs, **3:** 179-198
    described, **3:** 179-180
    discovery, **3:** 190-195
    therapy model, **3:** 180-190
    triad interview approach, **3:** 195-197

F

Family,
    genogram construction and interpretation, **5:** 203-208
    the healthy, **2:** 118-119
Family life cycle stages, **2:** 130-132
Family Therapist Rating Scale, **3:** 243-256
    applications, **3:** 245-246
    development, **3:** 243-245
    rater guidelines, **3:** 249-250
    scale, **3:** 251-253
Family therapy, **2:** 113-134
    with family crises, **2:** 126-128
    holistic approach in, **2:** 113-114
    indications for, **2:** 119-120
    individual focus in, **2:** 117-118
    interview goals and procedures in, **2:** 122-123
    practical considerations in, **2:** 119-129
    resistance in, **2:** 121-122

Family therapy (Continued)
    with substance abusing adolescents, **3:** 132-142
        assessment and treatment, **3:** 138-141
        family styles, **3:** 132-138
    structural, **2:** 101-112
    systems/interpersonal focus in, **2:** 114-117
    therapist's role in, **2:** 120-121
    for transitional problems (e.g., divorce, stepfamilies), **2:** 124-126
    Understanding Family Therapy (client handout), **3:** 456-458
    who to include or exclude in, **2:** 120-121
Fee Information (client handout), **1:** 381
Fees (also see Insurance reimbursement),
    consulting, **2:** 250-262
        collection, **2:** 259-262
        fee arrangements, **2:** 256-259
        how to establish, **2:** 250-256
    late, **2:** 214, 260-261
Feminist psychotherapy, **3:** 143-152
    history, **3:** 143-145
    therapy program, **3:** 147-151
    treatment philosophy, **3:** 146-147
    women's studies, **3:** 145-146
Filial therapy, **2:** 26-39
    evaluation and planning phase, **2:** 34-36
    generalization phase, **2:** 32-34
    home play sessions, **2:** 30-32
    parents' practice sessions, **2:** 30
    teaching of play sessions, **2:** 28-30
Flooding with agoraphobia, **4:** 13
Forensic consultation (also see Expert witness roles), **3:** 374-378
Forensic interview, conducting the initial, **4:** 467-474
Forms and instruments,
    Alcohol History Form, **3:** 169
    Application for Psychological Services, **4:** 350-351
    Assessment of Therapy Progress, **2:** 287-288
    Balance Sheet (for personal problem solving), **2:** 80
    Boyd Developmental Progress Scale, **3:** 309
    Brief Psychiatric Rating Scale (for Adults), **2:** 314
        History form, **2:** 315
    Brief Psychiatric Rating Scale for Children, **3:** 264
        History form, **3:** 265
    Case Summary and Treatment plan, **1:** 45
    Client Satisfaction Survey **2:** 288-289
    Collection form letter, **1:** 225
    Competency Assessment Inventory, **3:** 311-315
    Competency to Stand Trial Assessment Instrument, **2:** 283
    Consent for Release of Professional Information, **1:** 218
    Consent to Record Sessions, **4:** 359
    Contract for participant in residential workshop group, **1:** 83
    Coping Strategies Scales (COSTS), for depressed patients, **5:** 291-296
    Crisis Assessment Summary, **4:** 273-283
    Current Symptom Checklist for Children, **2:** 267-270
    Daily Eating Record, **5:** 23
    Daily Record of Dysfunctional Thoughts, **1:** 48
    Decision Making Grid, **2:** 78
    Dental Anxiety Scale, **2:** 333
    Diet Diary Record of Food Intake and Related Behavior, **4:** 135
    Drug History Form, **3:** 175
    Eating Attitudes Test (EAT-26), **5:** 22

Forms and instruments (Continued)
    Family Therapist Rating Scale, **3:** 251-253
    Global Assessment Scale, **2:** 301
    Group Therapy Contract, **3:** 216
    Group Therapy Contract for Participants, **1:** 83
    Hendler Screening Test for Chronic Back Pain Patients, **2:** 274-277
    Humorous Sentence Completion Blank, **5:** 170-171
    Individual Client Information Questionnaire, **1:** 215-217
    Individual Psychotherapy Contract, **3:** 215
    Insurance Claim Form, **1:** 224
    Insurance Information for Patients, **1:** 186
    Jackson Incest Blame Scale, **4:** 66-68
    Level of Functioning Scale, **2:** 302
    Marital Information Form, **2:** 293-296
    Marriage Problems, Scale of, **1:** 250-255
    Maternal Questionnaire (regarding children's dental fears), **2:** 336
    Mental Status Examination form, **1:** 229-230
    Mental Status Examination-Revised, **5:** 281-284
    Mini-Mental State Examination, **4:** 309
    Obstacles Analysis Worksheet (for personal problem solving), **2:** 82
    Office Policy Statement, **4:** 348-349
    Parenting Skills Inventory, **3:** 284-287
    Parent's Questionnaire (for assessment of hyperkinesis), **1:** 261-262
    Patient's Health Questionnaire, **5:** 198-199
    Payment Agreement Form, **1:** 222-223
    Permission to Release Information, **1:** 219
    Permission to Release Custody Evaluation, **4:** 358
    Physical Stress Location Chart, **1:** 295
    Police officer selection background information form, **5:** 327-328
    Problem Analysis Grid, **2:** 75
    Problem Solving Inventory, **1:** 235-238
    Problem Solving Worksheet, **2:** 81
    Psychotherapy Problem Checklist, **3:** 218
    Reasons for Living Inventory, **4:** 326-329
    Referral acknowledgment form letters, **1:** 226
    Referring Professional Satisfaction Survey, **2:** 290-291
    Release form cover letters, **1:** 220-221
    Scale of Marriage Problems, **1:** 250-255
    Sentence Completion Test for Adolescents, **3:** 303-304
    Sexual History Inventory, **4:** 334-343
    Social Adjustment Self-Report Questionnaire, **5:** 302-306
    Spouse Abuse Scale, **1:** 25
    Strain Questionnaire, **5:** 309-312
    Substance Abuse Screening Check List, **1:** 291-292
    Suicidal Death Prediction Scales, **1:** 272-288
        older females, **1:** 284-286
        older males, **1:** 281-283
        younger females, **1:** 286-287
        younger males, **1:** 283-284
    Summary/Profile Sheet for Reporting Test Scores, **3:** 289-293
    Teacher's Questionnaire (for assessment of hyperkinesis), **1:** 263
    Therapist Evaluation Questionnaire, **4:** 354-357
    Therapy notes, **1:** 44
    Treatment Record Form, **3:** 294-299
    View Sharing Inventory for Couples, **4:** 289-303
    Vocational Performance Assessment, **3:** 375-376
    Vocational Screening Profile (planning worksheet), **4:** 311-319
Foster parenting programs, **5:** 346
Freud family genogram, **5:** 208
Fuller Psychophysiologic Profile, **2:** 152

G

Gay clients, psychotherapeutic issues with, **3:** 69-84
    AIDS victims, **3:** 79-80, **5:** 221-230
        basic information, **5:** 221-222
        social and psychological impact, **5:** 223-227
        treatment of clients, **5:** 221-230
            managing clinical symptoms, **5:** 227-229
            therapist issues, **5:** 229
    coming out process, **3:** 73-74
    differential diagnosis, **3:** 74-75
    gay and lesbian social relationships, **3:** 77-79
    illness model of homosexuality, **3:** 69-70
    therapeutic goals, **3:** 70-77
Genograms, **5:** 203-220
    construction, **5:** 204-211
    Freud's family genogram, **5:** 208
    future of, **5:** 218
    interpretation, **5:** 211-218
Global Assessment Scale, **2:** 301
Goal attainment scaling in marital therapy, **4:** 95-100
Grief,
    Coping with Loss and Grief (client handout), **2:** 447-449
    crisis intervention with, **1:** 10-11
    Guide to Interviewing the Bereaved, **1:** 89-111
        interview components, **1:** 93-97
        Long form interview schedule, **1:** 104-106
        Short form interview schedule, **1:** 106-108
    uncomplicated bereavement, **3:** 112
    unresolved in cancer patients, **4:** 156-157
Group therapy,
    confidentiality, **3:** 410-412
    contracts for participants, **1:** 83, **3:** 216
    designing, **1:** 78-79
    early stages, **1:** 84-87
    ethical guidelines, **1:** 79, **3:** 415-417
    ethical issues, **3:** 406-418
    informed consent in, **3:** 407-408
    leader values in, **3:** 413-414
    practical strategies for planning, **1:** 78-88
    pregroup sessions, **1:** 78-84
    recruiting members, **1:** 79
    rights of participants, **3:** 408-409, 412-413
    risks, **3:** 409-410
    screening members, **1:** 79-81, **3:** 406-407
    structured exercises, **2:** 411-435
    termination and follow-up, **3:** 414-415
Guided affective imagery, **1:** 70-71

H

Health care delivery systems (also see Practice and specific issues), **5:** 261-269
Health Maintenance Organizations (HMOs), **4:** 205-207, **5:** 262, 266
Health psychology,
    in medical settings, **5:** 351-364
        assessment, **5:** 352-353
        history, **5:** 351-352

Health psychology (Continued)
        interventions, **5:** 353-361
        psychologist's roles, **5:** 352-354
     in occupational settings, **5:** 331-338
       case example, **5:** 335-336
       current status, **5:** 333-334
       rationale, **5:** 331-333
       systems consultation approach, **5:** 334-335
     training the occupational health psychologist, **5:** 337
Health questionnaire, **5:** 198-199
Helping skills training, consultant's guide, **4:** 391-411
Hendler Screening Test for Chronic Back Pain Patients, **2:** 272-277
    instrument, **2:** 274-277
    introduction, **2:** 272-273
Homosexuality, illness model of (also see Gay clients), **3:** 69-70
Hospices, **1:** 343-352
    consultation with, **3:** 330
    functions, **1:** 343-344
    mental health clinician roles, **1:** 349-350
    needs of dying patients, **1:** 344-345
    preparation for hospice work, **1:** 347-348
    staff, **1:** 345-347
Hospital consultation (also see Medical settings), **3:** 379-390
    hospital privileges, **3:** 380-382
    patient assessment, **3:** 384-387
      relevant instruments, **3:** 386-387
    physician referrals, **3:** 382-383
    professional issues, **3:** 388-389
Hostage negotiation training for police, **2:** 380-381
Humor Immersion Training, **5:** 164-171
Humor in psychotherapy, **5:** 157-175
    indirect suggestions, **5:** 160-164
    limitations and ethical considerations, **5:** 172-173
    rationale, **5:** 157-158
    therapeutic techniques, **5:** 167-168
    therapist traits, **5:** 158-160
Humor Rating Scale, **5:** 159-160
Humorous Sentence Completion Blank, **5:** 170-171
Hyperkinesis,
    Parent and teacher rating forms for assessment of, **1:** 257-264
      application, **1:** 259-260
      hyperkinesis index, **1:** 259-260
      normative data, **1:** 257-259
Hypnosis,
    applications, **1:** 34-35
    chronic pain and, **1:** 135
    defined, **1:** 31-32, **5:** 46-47
    Ericksonian approaches to hypnotherapy, **5:** 45-58
    induction procedures, **1:** 32-33
    primer, **1:** 30-36

I

Imagery,
    communication and, **1:** 71
    coping, **1:** 121
    countertransference and, **1:** 72
    in stress inoculation, **1:** 118-119

Imagery (Continued)
    therapeutic techniques, **1:** 67-77
    therapist's checklist for using, **1:** 73-75
Impaired clinicians (see Burnout)
Incest (also see Sexual assault victims), **3:** 55-68, **4:** 53-54
    assessment of victims, **4:** 54-58
    cues, **3:** 59
    dynamics, **3:** 56-58
    Jackson Incest Blame Scale, **4:** 66-68
    prevention programs for children, **3:** 67-68
    problem checklist, **3:** 61
    treating adult victims, **3:** 63-66, **4:** 58-65
    treating incestuous families, **3:** 59-67
Independent practice (see Practice)
Independent practitioner association (IPA), **5:** 266-277
Individual Client Information Questionnaire, **1:** 215-217
Informed consent to treatment, **2:** 401-404
Insomnias (DIMS), **2:** 61-64
Insulin production dysfunction, **3:** 46
Insurance, malpractice, **2:** 214, **4:** 246-250
Insurance reimbursement, **1:** 184-193
    accepting assignment, **1:** 191-192
    basic steps, **1:** 184-185
    for biofeedback, **2:** 153-157
    charges, **1:** 189-191
    claim form instructions, **1:** 185-191
    claim rejections, **1:** 192
    coinsurance, **1:** 191
    diagnosis, **1:** 185-187
    insurance claim form, **1:** 224
    Insurance Information for Patients form, **1:** 186
    peer review, **1:** 192
    procedure codes, **1:** 187-189
    Usual, customary, and reasonable charges (UCR), **1:** 189-191

L

Law enforcement candidate screening (see Police selection)
Lawsuits against mental health professionals (also see Malpractice), **4:** 244-245
Legal terms glossary, **4:** 459-466
Lesbian clients, psychotherapeutic issues with (also see Gay clients), **3:** 69-84
Level of functioning scales, **2:** 287-306
    sample scales, **2:** 301-302
    scale characteristics, **2:** 289-303
    selection and use, **2:** 303-306

M

Magnetic resonance imaging, **5:** 96-98
Malpractice,
    in consultation, **2:** 319-330
    insurance, **4:** 248-250
    prevention, **4:** 243-251
    in psychotherapy, **2:** 205-216
Management consultation (also see Organization development),
    with police, **2:** 383-384

Marital communication, **4**: 82-92, **5**: 137-142
    (also see View Sharing Inventory for couples)
Marital Information Form, **2**: 292-296
Marital therapy,
    cognitive-behavioral techniques, **5**: 137-156
        assessment, **5**: 142-145
        cognitive restructuring techniques, **5**: 150-151
        communication and assertiveness training, **5**: 146-150
        discrimination training, **5**: 145-146
        theory and model, **5**: 137-142
        treatment, **5**: 145-154
    goal attainment scaling in, **4**: 95-100
Marketing psychotherapy services, **2**: 233-241
Marriage and family structured enrichment programs, **1**: 299-308
    depression enrichment program, **1**: 304-307
    prevention philosophy, **1**: 299-300
    relationship enhancement therapy, **2**: 40-53
    social skills training, **1**: 301-303
Marriage problems,
    midlife marital crises, **4**: 79-93
        healthy couples, **4**: 81-87
        midrange and dysfunctional couples, **4**: 87-91
    scale of, **1**: 240-256
        administration and scoring, **1**: 247-249
        construction, **1**: 240-247
        forms, **1**: 250-255
Media, and mental health professions, **2**: 361-370
    achieving behavior change, **2**: 362
    Association for Media Psychology, **2**: 367-368
    ethics, **2**: 364-367
    interactive cable television, **2**: 364-365
    motion pictures, **2**: 365
    preparation, **2**: 368-369
    print media, **2**: 362-363
    radio, **2**: 365-367
    television, **2**: 363-364
Mediation (see specific types, e.g., Divorce)
Medical considerations in psychiatric syndromes, **3**: 41-54, **5**: 91-102
    anxiety, **5**: 93
    depression, **5**: 92
    eating disorders, **5**: 31
    endocrine disorders, **3**: 43-46
    hysteria, **5**: 93
    metabolic disorders, **3**: 50-51
    neurological disorders, **3**: 46-50
    psychosis, **5**: 93
    tumors and malignancy, **3**: 51
Medical settings, practice in
        assessment, **5**: 352-353
        history, **5**: 351-352
        interventions, **5**: 353-361
        psychologist's roles, **5**: 352-354
Medications (see listings for major types of psychiatric medications (e.g., Antidepressant
        medications)
    causing emotional symptoms, **5**: 93
Mental Status Examinations, **1**: 227-230, **4**: 305-310, **5**: 279-285
    in the disability evaluation, **5**: 419-420
    in the emergency room, **5**: 373-374
Metabolic disorders, **3**: 50, **5**: 92

Microcomputers,
    biofeedback and, **1**: 199
    in clinical practice, **1**: 199-210, **4**: 215-227
        applications and software, **4**: 215-219
    database access software, **4**: 239-240, 242
    functioning of, **1**: 200-203
    printers for, **1**: 196-197
    selection of, **1**: 204-205, **4**: 219-226
    test administration and scoring with, **1**: 200, 205-208
    word processing, **1**: 194-198, 203, **4**: 215-219
Midlife marital issues, **4**: 79-93
Migraine headache, **1**: 141
Mini-Mental State Examination,
    development and administration, **4**: 305-308
    examination, **4**: 309
Mother's support groups, **3**: 321-322
Muscle contraction headaches,
    assessment, **1**: 143-145
    EMG (electromyographic feedback) use with, **1**: 141-143
    etiology, **1**: 141-143
    medication of, **1**: 143
    psychophysiological stress profile for, **1**: 145
    treatment, **1**: 141-150
    Myofacial Pain Dysfunction Syndrome (MPDS), **1**: 141, **2**: 338-339, **5**: 189-201
Mutual story telling technique for children, **5**: 396-398
Myofacial Pain Dysfunction Syndrome (MPDS), **5**: 189-201
    assessment, **5**: 190-192
    case history, **5**: 190
    treatment, **5**: 192-197
        biteplates, **5**: 194
        education and self-management, **5**: 192-193
        physical therapy, **5**: 194
        psychological approaches, **5**: 194-196
        psychopharmacology, **5**: 193
        secondary treatment, **5**: 193
        transcutaneous stimulation, **5**: 194
        treatment failures, **5**: 196-197

N

Neoplastic disorders, **5**: 92
Neurological disorders, **3**: 46-50, **5**: 92, 359-360
Neuropsychological assessment procedures, **3**: 157-159
    Halstead-Reitan Battery, **3**: 158
    Luria-Nebraska Battery, **3**: 158-159
Neuropsychological screening, **2**: 17-25
    assessment process, **2**: 18-19
        for intellectual functioning, **2**: 19
        for language related skills, **2**: 20
        for new learning and problem solving, **2**: 19-20
        for sensory-perceptual functions, **2**: 20
        for visual-spatial abilities, **2**: 20
    case illustrations, **2**: 21-23
    of children, **3**: 153-165
        age considerations in, **3**: 160-161
        special considerations in, **3**: 161-162
        use of common instruments for, **3**: 159-161
        referral questions in, **3**: 162-163

Neuropsychological screening (Continued)
    tests, **2:** 20-21, 23-24, **3:** 159-161
    for traumatic injury, **2:** 391-394
Nursing homes, inservice training for, **3:** 323

O

Obesity, **4:** 127-152
    abnormal attitudes toward weight and shape, **5:** 8-9
    appropriate body weight determination, **5:** 36-37
    assessment of, **4:** 130-132
    classification of, **4:** 129-130
    definition of, **4:** 127
    diet diary record, **4:** 135
    dieting and extreme weight control, **5:** 9-10
    epidemiology of, **4:** 127-128
    medical complications of, **4:** 128-129
    treatment, **4:** 132-147
        for mild obesity, **4:** 133-141
        for moderate obesity, **4:** 141-144
        for severe obesity, **4:** 141-147
Occupational health psychology (see Health psychology)
Offenders,
    cognitive-behavioral interventions with, **4:** 115-125
    interventions, **4:** 119-123
    offense formula, **4:** 115-116
    treatment tasks, **4:** 116-119
Office design and selection, **3:** 201-212, **5:** 233-244
    design considerations, **3:** 204-206
    furniture and accessories, **3:** 206-212
    institutional offices, **3:** 202
    residential offices, **3:** 203
    space sharing, **3:** 202
Office leases, **3:** 203-204
Online database searches for information, **4:** 229-242
    advantages and limitations, **4:** 230-231
    database access software, **4:** 239-240, 242
    database vendors, **4:** 231-232
    databases, **4:** 232-234
    sample searches, **4:** 234-237
    who should search, **4:** 238-240
Organization development, **2:** 348-360
    assessment, **2:** 353-354
    consultant roles, **2:** 357-359, **3:** 330-331
    defined, **2:** 348-351
    interventions, **2:** 354-357
    models, **2:** 351-353
Overweight (see Obesity)

P

Pain (see Chronic pain or specific form of pain, e.g., MPDS)
Parathyroid gland dysfunction, **3:** 44-45
Parent rating forms for assessment of hyperkinesis, **1:** 257-264
Parent training as child therapists (see Filial therapy), **2:** 26-39

Parent training programs, **5:** 339-348
    computer programs, **5:** 346-347
    foster parenting programs, **5:** 346
    issues in selection, **5:** 339-341
    organizational programs, **5:** 343-344
    sample programs, **5:** 342-348
        Active Parenting, **5:** 342
        Behavioral Principles for Parents, **5:** 343
        Nurturing Program, **5:** 343
        Parent Effectiveness Training, **5:** 346
        Parents and Children, **5:** 343
        STEP, **5:** 346
        WINNING, **5:** 342-343
    self-help parenting groups, **5:** 344
Parenting skills, assessment of, **3:** 276-288
    Parenting Skills Inventory, **3:** 284-287
Patient's Health Questionnaire, **5:** 198-199
Payment agreement form, **1:** 222-223
Pediatric psychology, **4:** 415-434
    case examples, **4:** 427-431
    chronic illness of children, **4:** 183-186
    history of, **4:** 416
    referrals to pediatric psychologists, **4:** 417-420
    roles of the pediatric psychologist, **4:** 420-427
Peer review for insurance claims, **1:** 192
Permission to Release Information (form), **1:** 219
Personal Problem Solving Inventory, **1:** 231-239
    administration, **1:** 232-233
    development, **1:** 231-232
    interpretation, **1:** 233-234
    inventory, **1:** 235-238
Physical causes for psychiatric syndromes (also see Medical considerations), **3:** 41-54
Physical Stress Location Chart, **1:** 293-295
    chart, **1:** 295
    directions, **1:** 293-294
Picture drawing game for children, **5:** 393-395
Play therapy,
    with difficult children, **5:** 391-403
        color-your-life-technique, **5:** 400-402
        model building, **5:** 398-400
        mutual story telling, **5:** 396-398
        picture drawing game, **5:** 393-395
        picture taking, **5:** 395-396
        playroom materials, **5:** 392
        techniques for too tight children, **5:** 393-398
        techniques for too loose children, **5:** 398-402
        types of children, **5:** 391-397
    theraplay technique for children, **5:** 177-187
        case illustration, **5:** 183-185
        diagnosis, **5:** 179-180
        intervention techniques, **5:** 180-181
        parent-child activities, **5:** 177-179
        phases of therapy, **5:** 183
Police, consultation with, **2:** 371-387
    areas of intervention, **2:** 377-385
        counseling and crisis intervention, **2:** 381-382
        hostage negotiation, **2:** 380-381
        inservice training, **2:** 380-381
        management consultation, **2:** 383-384

Police, consultation with (Continued)
      post traumatic situations, **2:** 382-383
      recruit training, **2:** 378-379, **3:** 332,
      selection, **2:** 377-378, **5:** 317-330
   contractual considerations, **2:** 373-376
   cultural considerations, **2:** 371-372
   entry issues, **2:** 373
Police selection, **5:** 317-330
   background information form, **5:** 327-328
   ethical and legal issues, **5:** 317-319
   history, **5:** 317
   instruments and techniques, **5:** 321-323
   purposes of evaluation, **5:** 319-321
   recommended procedures, **5:** 324
   research on, **5:** 323-324
   screening battery components, **5:** 324-325
Positron emission tomography, **5:** 100
Post accident anxiety syndrome (see Traumatic injury cases), **2:** 393
Post traumatic situations with police, **2:** 382-383
Post-traumatic stress disorder in veterans, **4:** 23-34
   diagnosis, **4:** 24-26
   historical background, **4:** 23-24
   symptoms, **4:** 24-26
   treatment, **4:** 26-32
      family therapy, **4:** 28-29
      group therapy, **4:** 27-28
      individual therapy, **4:** 29-32
      inpatient vs. outpatient therapy, **4:** 32
Practice,
   answering machines in, **5:** 271-276
   California experiences, **5:** 262-263
   checklist and resources guide, **2:** 242-249
   contracts,
      capitated, **5:** 264
      fee for service, **5:** 264
   descriptions of four types, **5:** 233-244
   rural setting for, **4:** 253-263
   sales and purchase, **2:** 217-222
      sample contract, **2:** 220
   types of professional, **5:** 261-269
      EAPs, **5:** 264-265
      HMOs, **5:** 264, 266
      PPOs, **4:** 203-213, **5:** 266-269
Preferred Provider Organizations (PPOs), **4:** 203-213
   considerations in joining, **5:** 267-269
   defined, **4:** 203-204, **5:** 266-279
   development and management, **4:** 206-212
   future of, **4:** 212
   history of, **4:** 204-206
   The Psychological Health Plan (TPHP), **4:** 207-213
Preventive activities, **3:** 319-335
Private practice (see Practice or specific topic, e.g., Office design)
Privileged communication, **3:** 391-405
   and confidentiality, **2:** 401
   in consultation, **2:** 328
   defined, **1:** 357, **3:** 392-393
   exceptions, **3:** 400-402, **5:** 383-390
   in legal proceedings, **3:** 399-400
   persons and data covered, **3:** 394-396

Problem solving strategies for clients, **2:** 73-85
    Balance Sheet (form), **2:** 80
    brainstorming plus, **2:** 76-77
    decision making, **2:** 78-80
    generating alternatives, **2:** 74-77
    Obstacles Analysis Worksheet, **2:** 82
    Personal Problem Solving Inventory (also see main heading), **1:** 231-239
    Problem Analysis Grid (form), **2:** 75
    problem definition, **2:** 73-74
    problem solving worksheet, **2:** 81
Progressive muscle relaxation (see Relaxation)
PsycAlert, **4:** 232-233
Psychiatric diagnostic technology (also see specific tests), **5:** 91-102
The Psychological Health Plan (TPHP), **4:** 207-213
Psychological Testing, About Your Appointment for, (client handout), **2:** 450
Psychophysiological Stress Profile (PSP) (in muscle contraction headaches), **1:** 145
Psychotherapy,
    A Guide to Psychotherapy (client handout), **2:** 443-446
    Me? Go for Psychotherapy? Not a Chance! (client handout), **3:** 459-463
Psychotherapy Problem Checklist, **3:** 218
PsycInfo, **4:** 232

R

Radio and mental health professionals (see Media)
Radioimmunoassay, **5:** 95-96
Reasons for Living Inventory, **4:** 321-330
Recording of sessions, consent form, **4:** 359
Re-Evaluation Counseling, **4:** 36
Referral acknowledgment form letters, **1:** 226
Regional cerebral blood flow, **5:** 99-100
Rehabilitation (also see Medical settings or specific problem), **5:** 359
Relationship enhancement therapy (for marital and family relations), **2:** 40-53
    applications, **2:** 42
    formats, **2:** 43
    goals, **2:** 41
    paradigms, **2:** 49-50
    research, **2:** 42
    skills for clients, **2:** 46-47
    theory, **2:** 43-46
    therapist considerations in, **2:** 47-49
Relaxation,
    progressive muscle relaxation, **1:** 151-170
        antianxiety medication and, **1:** 164-165
        general tension and, **1:** 152-154
        headache and, **1:** 156-157
        historical development of, **1:** 151-152
        hypertension and, **1:** 157-159
        insomnia and, **1:** 154-156
        overcontrolled clients and, **1:** 162-164
        physical disabilities and, **1:** 165-166
        physical setting, **1:** 159-160
        taped relaxation, **1:** 161-162
        therapist preparation for administration of, **1:** 160-161
    instruction script, **1:** 172-174
    in stress inoculation, **1:** 117
Release forms and cover letters, **1:** 219-221

Remarried families, **4:** 101-114
    assessment of, **4:** 103-104
        genogram, **4:** 103-104
    structural differences in, **4:** 101-102
    treatment of, **4:** 102-110
        goals, **4:** 104-105
        groups, **4:** 108
        multiple impact therapy, **4:** 108
        therapist, **4:** 108-110
    visitation guidelines, **4:** 110-112
Report writing via a word processor, **2:** 223-232
    developing interpretive statements, **2:** 229-231
    sample report, **2:** 225-228
Right to know, client's, **2:** 403-404
Risk management for malpractice (also see Malpractice), **4:** 246-250
Rural professional practice, **4:** 253-263

S

School consultation,
    consultant as conceptualizer, **3:** 348-350
    consultant as participant, **3:** 344-348
    early secondary intervention program, **3:** 324
    preschool, **3:** 322-325
    organizational perspectives, **3:** 343-352
Seizure disorders, **3:** 48
Selection assessment for police, **2:** 377-378
Self-help groups in treatment of substance abusers, **5:** 83-90
Sentence Completion Test for Adolescents, **3:** 300-305
    introduction, **3:** 300-302
    test, **3:** 303-304
Serum drug levels, **5:** 95
Sex therapy, **4:** 187-200
    assessment for, **1:** 54-58, **3:** 267-275, **4:** 190-192
        conjoint interviews, **1:** 54-56,
        individual interviews, **1:** 56-57, **4:** 190-191
        questionnaire use, **1:** 57
        referral for specialized consultation, **1:** 58
    assumptions of, **1:** 53-54
    for:
        common dissatisfactions, **1:** 58-64
        erectile dysfunction, **4:** 196
        female primary orgasmic problems, **4:** 194
        female secondary inorgasmic dysfunction, **4:** 194-195
        inhibited ejaculation, **4:** 195
        lack of arousal, **4:** 196
        low sexual desire, **4:** 197
        premature ejaculation, **4:** 195
        vaginismus and dyspareunia, **4:** 197
Sexism in psychotherapy (also see Feminist therapy), **1:** 363-375
Sexual assault, **4:** 51-78
    attribution of blame, **4:** 53
        Jackson Incest Blame Scale, **4:** 66-69
    definitional issues, **4:** 51-52
    incidence and prevalence, **4:** 52
Sexual assault syndrome, **4:** 53-54
    assessment of sexual assault victims, **4:** 54-58

Sexual assault syndrome (Continued)
    treatment of, **4:** 58-65
        behavioral, **4:** 62-64
        client issues, **4:** 59-60
        crisis intervention, **4:** 61-62, 71-74
        group treatment, **4:** 64-65
        therapist issues, **4:** 58-59
    victim interview guide, **4:** 69-70
Sexual disorders, **4:** 187-200
    arousal phase dysfunctions, **4:** 189
    assessment of, **4:** 190-192
        interview, **4:** 190-191
        medical, **4:** 191-192
        Sexual History Inventory, **4:** 331-344
    definitions, **4:** 188-190
    desire phase dysfunctions, **4:** 189-190
    orgasm phase dysfunctions, **4:** 188-189
Sexual dissatisfaction,
    assessment of, **1:** 54-58
    Differences in Sexual Desire (client handout), **3:** 464-467
    treatment for, **1:** 58-64
Sexual dysfunction, structured assessment outline for, **3:** 267-275
Sexual History Inventory, **4:** 331-344
Sleep,
    characteristics, **2:** 54-57
    disorders primer, **2:** 54-72
    rules for better habits, **2:** 59-60
    stages and cycles, **2:** 55-57
Sleep disorders, **2:** 54-72
    assessment, **2:** 57-58
    classification and treatment, **2:** 61-69
    excessive somnolence (DOES), **2:** 64-66
    insomnias (DIMS), **2:** 61-64
    narcolepsy, **2:** 65
    parasomnias, **2:** 67-69
    pharmacological treatment of, **2:** 60
    sleep apnea, **2:** 65-66
    sleep terrors, **2:** 69-69
    of sleep-wake schedule, **2:** 67
    sleepwalking (somnambulism), **2:** 68
Small claims court for fee collection, **5:** 245-255
    claim preparation, **5:** 247
    counterclaims, **5:** 250-251
    judgment, **5:** 253-255
    overview, **5:** 245-247
    trial, **5:** 252-253
    trial preparation, **5:** 249-251
Smoking,
    impact, **5:** 332
    treatment and prevention, **3:** 85-99
        coping skills, **3:** 90-91
        maintenance after quitting, **3:** 91-93
        preparation for quitting, **3:** 86-90
        nicotine fading, **3:** 88-89
        oversmoking, **3:** 87-88
        prevention, **3:** 94-95
Social Adjustment Self-Report Questionnaire,
    introduction, **5:** 299-301
    questionnaire, **5:** 302-306

Social Security and SSI evaluations, **2:** 436-441, **5:** 417-423
   advocacy, **5:** 422-423
   assessment and report preparation, **5:** 417-422
      ability to manage funds, **5:** 421
      ability to work, **5:** 421-422
      daily activities, **5:** 417-418
      diagnosis, **5:** 419
      mental status, **5:** 419
      personal history, **5:** 419
      present illness, **5:** 419
   documentation, **5:** 417
Sociotropy and depression, **1:** 49
Sport psychology, **4:** 363-376
   clinical issues, **4:** 364-367
   defined, **4:** 363-364
   enhancing sport performance, **4:** 368-370
   professional issues, **4:** 370-371
   therapeutic applications of sport, **4:** 367-368
Spouse Abuse, **1:** 16-29
   assessment, **1:** 16-21
   immediate intervention for, **1:** 8-9, 22
   scale, **1:** 25
   treatment, **1:** 22-24
Standard of care, **2:** 207-209
   in medical settings, **3:** 388-389
Strain Questionnaire,
   introduction, **5:** 309-312
   questionnaire, **5:** 313
Stress,
   and anger, **2:** 182-185
   assessment of, **1:** 314-315
   in cancer patients, **4:** 156
   developing a workshop for management of, **1:** 309-319
   and health, **1:** 311-312
   management strategies, **1:** 312-314, **5:** 354-355
      with police personnel, **2:** 378-380
   psychophysiology, **1:** 310-311
   reduction training at the YMCA, **3:** 329
   Strain Questionnaire for measurement of, **5:** 309-312
   Stress Management: Ten Self-Care Techniques (client handout), **5:** 427-429
   Understanding and Managing Stress (client handout), **1:** 391-399
Stress inoculation, **1:** 112-125
   for anger control (also see Anger), **2:** 181-201
   application phase, **1:** 121-122
   conceptual basis, **1:** 112-113
   educational phase, **1:** 114-117
   rehearsal phase, **1:** 117-121
Structural family therapy, **2:** 101-112
   defined, **2:** 101-103
   initial session, **2:** 108-111
   techniques, **2:** 103-108
Structured group exercises, **2:** 411-435
Subpoenas (also see Expert witness roles), **1:** 356-357, **3:** 399
Substance abuse (also see Alcohol abuse),
   in adolescents, **3:** 132-142
   Alcoholics Anonymous and treatment, **5:** 83-90
   associated with alcohol abuse, **3:** 173-174
      aftercare, **3:** 176-177
      Drug History Form, **3:** 175
      treatment for, **3:** 174-176

Substance abuse (Continued)
    controlled ingestion issue, **5**: 75
    denial and rationalization of, **5**: 75-78
    indicators of, **5**: 78-79
    medication in treatment for, **5**: 73-75
    practical issues in treating, **5**: 71-82
    psychological testing for, **5**: 72-73
    self-help groups for, **5**: 83-90
    treatment considerations, **5**: 79-81
Substance Abuse Screening Check List, **1**: 289-292
    check list, **1**: 291
    instructions and interpretation, **1**: 289-290
Suicide,
    behaviors, **2**: 164-165
    borderline personality disorders, **5**: 127-128
    crisis intervention in, **2**: 167-171
    death prediction scales, **1**: 256-289
        instructions, **1**: 272-280
        predictive efficiency, **1**: 269-271
        older females, **1**: 284-286
        older males, **1**: 281-283
        younger females, **1**: 286-287
        younger males, **1**: 283-284
    factors, **2**: 161-163
    intervention, **1**: 5-7, **2**: 161-173
    legal considerations, **2**: 172
    in older adults, **3**: 102
    plan, **2**: 162
    prevention procedures, **2**: 161-173
    research issues, **1**: 265-266
    traditional signs, **2**: 165-166
    typical patterns, **2**: 163-164
Supervision, need for, **2**: 209

T

Tarasoff ruling (also see Duty to protect), **5**: 384-386
Teacher rating forms for assessment of hyperkinesis, **1**: 257-264
Television and mental health professionals (see Media)
Temporomandibular joint (TMJ) pain (also see Myofacial Pain Dysfunction Syndrome), **1**:
    141, **2**: 338-339, **5**: 189-201
Tension headaches (see Muscle contraction headaches)
Test administration and scoring by microcomputer, **3**: 229-242
Test Score Summary/Profile Sheet, **3**: 289-293
Theraplay technique for children, **5**: 177-187
    case illustration, **5**: 183-185
    diagnosis, **5**: 179-180
    intervention techniques, **5**: 180-181
    parent-child activities, **5**: 177-179
    phases of therapy, **5**: 183
Therapy groups (see Groups)
Thermal biofeedback, **2**: 147-148
Thumbsucking, **2**: 337-338
Thyroid dysfunction, **3**: 44
Thyrotropin releasing hormone test, **5**: 95
Time management techniques for clinicians, **1**: 177-183
Tranquilizers (see Antianxiety or Antipsychotic medications)

Traumatic injury cases, **2:** 391-398
    assessment, **2:** 393-394
    post accident anxiety syndrome, **2:** 393
    post concussive syndrome, **2:** 392
    treatment, **2:** 394-396
Treatment Record Form, **3:** 294-299
Tumors,
    brain, **3:** 48-49, **5:** 92
    other, **3:** 51, **5:** 92

V

View Sharing Inventory for couples,
    introduction, **4:** 285-288
    inventory, **4:** 289-304
Violence, (also see Anger)
    client, **1:** 7-8
    marital, **1:** 8-9, 16-29
Vitamin deficiencies, **3:** 50
Vocational Performance Assessment, **3:** 375-376
Vocational Screening Profile (planning worksheet), **4:** 311-319
Volunteer citizen boards, **3:** 331-332

W

Weight (see Obesity)
Wilson's disease, **3:** 50-51, **5:** 92
Word processing for the clinical office, **1:** 194-198, **4:** 215-218
    automated report writing, **2:** 223-232
        developing interpretive statements, **2:** 229-231
        sample report, **2:** 225-228
    creating documents, **1:** 195-196
    defined, **1:** 194-195
    printers, **1:** 196-197

CONTINUING EDUCATION AVAILABLE FOR HOME STUDY

Innovations in Clinical Practice: A Source Book is now available for continuing education study in your home or office. This best-selling, comprehensive source of practical clinical information is complemented by examination modules which may be used to earn continuing education credits.

Credits may be obtained by successfully completing examinations based on those contributions in each volume which have been selected by the editorial advisory board. Each of these contributions explores a timely topic designed to enhance your clinical skills and provide the knowledge necessary for effective practice. After studying these selections, a multiple-choice examination is completed and returned to the Professional Resource Exchange for scoring. Upon passing the examination (80% of test items answered correctly), your credits will be recorded and you will receive a copy of your official transcript.

The continuing education modules for Volumes 3 and 4 of *Innovations in Clinical Practice* are currently available and each module contains examination materials for 20 credits (equivalent to 20 hours of continuing education activity). The Volume 5 module will be available in October 1986 and will earn approximately 20 credits. The cost of each module is only $45.

The *Innovations in Clinical Practice* Continuing Education Program is one of the most efficient ways to stay current on new clinical techniques and obtain formal credit for your study. If your professional associations and state boards do not currently require formal CE activities, you may still wish to consider this program as an excellent means of receiving feedback on your professional development. This self-study program is...

Relevant - selections are packed with information pertinent to your practice.

Inexpensive - typically less than half the cost of obtaining credits through workshops and these expenses are still tax deductible as a professional expense.

Convenient - study at your own pace in the comfort of your home or office.

Useful - the volume will always be available as a practical reference and resource for day-to-day use in your professional practice.

Effective - as a means of staying up to date and obtaining feedback on your knowledge acquisition and professional development. In many states with continuing education requirements, credits earned from APA approved sponsors are automatically approved for licensure renewal. Consult your profession's state board for their policies regarding the status of programs offered by APA approved sponsors.

The Professional Resource Exchange is approved by the American Psychological Association to offer Category I continuing education for psychologists. The APA approved sponsor maintains responsibility for the program.

ORDER FORM

I want to order *Innovations in Clinical Practice: A Source Book*. Please send me:

Deluxe Binder Editions ($44.95 per copy + shipping**)...Vol 1___2___3__ 4__ 5___ $_______

Hardbound Editions ($39.95 per copy + shipping**)............................Vol 3___4___5___ $______

CE Modules ($45 per module + shipping**)..Vol 3___4___5___ $______
        (See NOTE* at bottom of this form regarding the CE Program)

        Florida Residents: please add sales tax (5%)...........................$______
   **Shipping & Handling (Books = $2.50 per copy in US, $4.00 foreign,
      CE Modules = no charge in US, $2.00 foreign).........................$______

Total Order (Orders from Individuals & Private Institutions Must Be Prepaid) $______

Check or money order enclosed (USA currency) ______
Please charge my: MasterCard ______ Visa ______

Credit Card Number:_______________________________ Expiration Date:_________________

Telephone: (_____)_____-_______ Profession:_______________ Highest Degree:____________

Have you previously ordered from the Professional Resource Exchange? Yes_____No______

Do you currently receive our catalogs?   Yes____No_____

SHIP TO: ____

(please print)   ____

                 ____

                 ____

Please make check payable to the Professional Resource Exchange and mail your order to:

Professional Resource Exchange / Post Office Box 15560 / Sarasota, FL 34277-1560

Phone Orders (MasterCard & Visa only), call (813) 366-7913 (weekdays: 9:30-4:30 EST)

We usually ship in-stock items within 48 hours. Items ordered prior to publication will be shipped within 15 days after publication. If shipment will be delayed 30 days over normal shipping time, you will be notified and a refund will be made if desired. Fifteen day return privilege if not satisfied. Availability and prices on all products are subject to change without notice.

*Note: Volume 3 and 4 Modules each earn 20 CE Credits and are currently available. The Volume 1 and 2 Modules have been discontinued. The Volume 5 Module will earn approximately 20 CE Credits and will be available in October 1986. In order to participate in the CE programs, you must purchase a Module and either purchase or have access to the corresponding *Innovations* volume.

Revised: May, 1986

TABLES OF CONTENTS
FOR OTHER VOLUMES
IN THE INNOVATIONS SERIES

VOLUME 1

CLINICAL ISSUES AND APPLICATIONS
Crisis Intervention: Helping Clients in Turmoil
    Charles P. Ewing
Counseling the Violent Husband
    Daniel G. Saunders
A Primer on Clinical Hypnosis
    Harold H. Smith, Jr.
Cognitive Therapy for Depression: History, Concepts and Procedures
    Raymond P. Harrison and Aaron T. Beck
Enhancing Sexual Intimacy
    Leslie R. Schover
Primer on Therapeutic Imagery Techniques
    Kenneth S. Pope
Practical Strategies for Therapy Groups
    Gerald Corey
Interviewing the Bereaved
    Regina Flesch
Primer on Stress Inoculation
    Robert A. Martin
Management of Chronic Pain
    Edward C. Covington
Techniques for Treatment of Muscle Contraction Headaches
    Thomas S. Budzynski
Progressive Muscle Relaxation: Appropriate and Inappropriate Applications
    Richard K. Russell and Michael W. Gribble
How to Use Relaxation Training with Clients
    Richard N. Feil
PRACTICE MANAGEMENT AND PROFESSIONAL DEVELOPMENT
Time Management Techniques for Clinicians
    William E. Cooper
How to Collect Insurance Reimbursement
    Stanley E. Jones
Word Processing for the Clinical Office
    Peter A. Keller
Microcomputers in Clinical Practice
    Richard M. Samuels and Kenneth Herman
INSTRUMENTS AND OFFICE FORMS
Introduction to Office Forms
    Peter A. Keller and Lawrence G. Ritt
Structured Mental Status Examination
    William G. Crary and C. Warner Johnson

Utilizing a Personal Problem Solving Inventory
    P. Paul Heppner
A Scale of Marriage Problems
    Clifford H. Swensen and Anthony Fiore
Parent and Teacher Rating Forms for the Assessment of Hyperkinesis in Children
    C. Keith Conners
Suicidal Death Prediction Scales
    Dan J. Lettieri
Substance Abuse Screening Check List
    Bruce D. Forman
Physical Stress Location Chart
    James B. Blakley
COMMUNITY INTERVENTIONS
Skill Training and Structured Enrichment Programs for Marriage and Family Life
    Luciano L'Abate
How to Develop a Stress Management Workshop
    J. Dennis Murray and Joel E. Grace
Consultation: A Practical Approach
    Francis T. Miller
Developing Employee Assistance Programs
    Charles M. Vehlow and Carroll L. Kropp
The Hospice Concept and Roles for the Clinician
    Martin D. Schaefer and J. Dennis Murray
SELECTED TOPICS
The Mental Health Professional as Expert Witness
    John F. Nichols
Some of My Best Friends Are Sexist: An Essay in Therapist Self-Exploration
    Judith F. D'Augelli
Introduction to Materials for Clients
    *Peter A. Keller, Lawrence G. Ritt, Arthur M. Bodin, The Association of Family and
        Conciliation Courts, Joel E. Grace, and Stephen H. Davis*
Comprehensive Guide to Antidepressants and Mild Antianxiety Medications
    James W. Long
Codes of Ethics for Insurance Procedures
    Oklahoma Psychological Association
DSM-III Classification and Codes
    American Psychiatric Association

VOLUME 2

CLINICAL ISSUES AND APPLICATIONS
Stages and Techniques of Divorce Therapy
    Florence W. Kaslow
Neuropsychological Screening
    Susan B. Filskov
Introduction to Filial Therapy: Training Parents as Therapists
    Louise F. Guerney
Marital and Family Relationship Enhancement Therapy
    Bernard Guerney, Jr.
A Sleep Disorders Primer
    Peter J. Hauri and Terry S. Proeger
Strategies for Facilitating Client's Personal Problem Solving
    P. Paul Heppner
The Treatment of Enuresis
    Suzanne Bennett Johnson
Techniques of Structural Family Therapy
    William Silver
Practical Issues and Applications in Family Therapy
    Terry M. Levy

Creative Communication for Clinicians
    Charles M. Citrenbaum, William I. Cohen, and Mark E. King
Advances in Biofeedback: A Behavioral Medicine Approach to Treatment of Stress
    Related Disorders
    George Fuller-von Bozzay
Suicide Prevention Procedures
    Calvin J. Frederick
Antidepressant Medication in the Outpatient Treatment of Depression: Guide for Non-
    medical Psychotherapists
    Kenneth Byrne and Stephen L. Stern
Stress Inoculation Therapy for Anger Control
    Raymond W. Novaco

PRACTICE MANAGEMENT AND PROFESSIONAL DEVELOPMENT
Avoiding Malpractice in Psychotherapy
    Robert Henley Woody
I Sold My Private Practice
    Robert D. Weitz
Psychological Test Analysis and Report Writing Via a Word Processor
    Ken R. Vincent
How to Improve the Marketing of Therapy Services
    Herbert E. Klein
Independent Practice: Checklist and Resources Guide
    Peter A. Keller and Lawrence G. Ritt
How to Establish and Collect Consulting Fees
    Robert E. Kelley

INSTRUMENTS AND OFFICE FORMS
Current Symptom Checklist for Children
    C. Eugene Walker
Hendler Screening Test for Chronic Back Pain Patients
    Nelson Hendler
Competency to Stand Trial Assessment Instrument
    Paul D. Lipsitt and David Lelos
Evaluation of Service Questionnaires
    Peter A. Keller and J. Dennis Murray
Marital Intake Form
    Rhonda S. Keller
Level of Functioning Scales: Their Use in Clinical Practice
    Frederick L. Newman
Brief Psychiatric Rating Scale and Brief Psychiatric History Form
    John E. Overall

COMMUNITY INTERVENTIONS
Ethical Issues in Consultation
    Leonard J. Haas
Consultation with Dentists: Innovative Roles for the Clinician
    Barbara D. Ingersoll and Michael J. Geboy
The Concepts and Techniques of Organization Development: An Introduction
    Leonard D. Goodstein and Phyliss Cooke
The Mental Health Professions and the Media
    Jacqueline C. Bouhoutsos
New Roles in Consultation with Police
    W. Parke Fitzhugh

SELECTED TOPICS
Roles for Clinicians in Assessment and Treatment of Traumatic Injury Cases
    Harold H. Smith, Jr.
Ethical Issues in Clinical Practice
    Charles P. Ewing
155 Exercises: A Starting Point for Leading Structured Groups
    John M. Russell
How to Evaluate Claimants for Social Security and SSI Benefits
    Jack R. Anderson

CLIENT HANDOUTS
A Guide to Psychotherapy
   Patricia Lacks, Jennifer Stolz, and Jeffrey Levine
Coping with Loss and Grief
   J. Dennis Murray
About your Appointment for Psychological Testing
   Peter A. Keller

VOLUME 3

CLINICAL ISSUES AND APPLICATIONS
Advances in Identification and Management of Affective Disorders
   Janyce D. Tarell and A. John Rush
Evaluating and Mediating Child Custody Cases
   Andrew P. Musetto
Psychiatric Syndromes with Physical Causes
   Earl L. Loschen
Treating Incestuous Families and Victims
   Blair Justice and Rita Justice
Psychotherapeutic Issues with Gay and Lesbian Clients
   John C. Gonsiorek
Treatment and Prevention of Smoking
   Harry A. Lando
Assessing Depression in Older Adults
   Ruth Czirr and Dolores Gallagher
Treating Depression in Older Adults
   Dolores Gallagher and Ruth Czirr
Family Therapy and the Substance Abusing Adolescent
   W. Robert Nay
Feminist Psychotherapy: Theory and Implementation
   Lili Sikorski-Smith
Neuropsychological Screening of Children
   Lawrence C. Hartlage
Diagnosis and Treatment Decisions for Alcohol and Substance Abusers
   Philip L. Knowles
An Innovative Strategy for Treating Extramarital Affairs
   Tom McGinnis
PRACTICE MANAGEMENT AND PROFESSIONAL DEVELOPMENT
Selecting and Designing Office Space
   Stanley Kissel
Using a Consumer Approach in Clinical Practice
   James K. Morrison
Impaired Clinicians: Coping with "Burnout"
   Herbert J. Freudenberger
Designing a Testing Program for Your Personal Computer
   Richard N. Feil
Rating Family Therapy Skills
   Fred P. Piercy, Roger A. Laird, and Mary Jo Zygmond
INSTRUMENTS AND OFFICE FORMS
A Brief Scale for Rating Psychopathology in Children
   John E. Overall and Betty Pfefferbaum
Structured Assessment of Sexual Dysfunction
   Gwen K. Weber Burch
A Systematic Approach to Assessing Parenting Skills
   Mark H. Lewin and Richard L. Wolfe
A Summary/Profile Sheet for Reporting Test Scores
   John K. McHenry
Treatment Record Form
   Ruth B. Schumacher

A Sentence Completion Test for Adolescents
  H. Marie Boultinghouse
Boyd Developmental Progress Scale
  Robert D. Boyd
A Form for Assessing Civil Competency
COMMUNITY INTERVENTIONS
Introduction to Community and Prevention Activities
  Judith A. Kramer and Brenna H. Bry
Understanding and Responding to Consultation Requests
  Thomas E. Backer
Organizational Perspectives on School Consultation
  Christopher B. Keys
Developing an Employee Assistance Program within a Clinical Practice
  Jack D. McInroy and Scott G. Howard
SELECTED TOPICS
Testifying as an Expert Witness
  Kenneth N. Anchor
Hospital Consultation
  C. Wayne Winkle
Privileged Communication
  Suanna J. Wilson
Ethical Issues in Group Therapy
  Gerald Corey
A Guide to Antipsychotic Medications
  James W. Long
CLIENT HANDOUTS
Understanding Family Therapy
  Terry Levy
Me? Go for Psychotherapy? Not a Chance!
  Val Farmer
Differences in Sexual Desire
  Jerry M. Friedman
INDEX OF VOLUMES 1, 2, & 3

VOLUME 4

CLINICAL ISSUES AND APPLICATIONS:
Treating Agoraphobia: A Multidimensional View
  Andrew P. Musetto
Post-Traumatic Stress Disorders in Veterans
  Steven M. Silver
Catharsis in Psychotherapy
  Michael P. Nichols and Robert A. Pierce
Assessment and Treatment of Sexual Assault Victims
  Thomas L. Jackson, Randal P. Quevillon, and Patricia A. Petretic-Jackson
Strategies for Coping with Midlife Marital Crises
  Florence W. Kaslow
Goal Attainment Scaling in Marital Assessment and Therapy
  David S. Hargrove
A Therapeutic Approach to the Remarried Family
  Helen Crohn, Clifford J. Sager, and Hollis Steer Brown
Cognitive-Behavioral Intervention with Offenders
  Seth R. Krieger
Treatment of Obesity in Adults: A Clinical Perspective
  Thomas A. Wadden
Psychotherapy with Cancer Patients
  A. David Feinstein
Helping Children and Families Cope with Chronic Illness
  Suzanne Bennett Johnson

Advances in Sex Therapy Techniques
   Jerry Friedman and Joseph Czekala
PRACTICE MANAGEMENT AND PROFESSIONAL DEVELOPMENT
Preferred Provider Organizations
   Arthur J. Bindman and Thomas J. Hefele
Computerizing the Clinical Office
   Seth R. Krieger
Using Online Database Searches for Information
   Fred Batt
Malpractice Prevention and Risk Management for Clinicians
   Edward T. Negley
Establishing and Maintaining an Independent Rural Practice
   Donald W. Tiffany, Richard P. Schellenberg, and Phyllis G. Tiffany
INSTRUMENTS AND FORMS:
An Assessment Checklist for Crisis Therapy
   Karl A. Slaikeu
The View Sharing Inventory for Couples
   Jan Cavanaugh and Bernard Guerney, Jr.
The Mini-Mental State Examination
   Miriam P. Spencer and Marshal F. Folstein
The Vocational Screening Profile
   Richard Shick
The Reasons for Living Inventory
   Marsha M. Linehan
The Sexual History Inventory
   Stephen D. Fabick
A Collection of Office Forms
   Carroll L. Meek; Editors
COMMUNITY INTERVENTIONS:
Sport Psychology: Developing Clinical Possibilities
   Steven R. Heyman
Psychological Skills for Emergency Medical Technicians: A Training Guide
   Michael A. Hoge and Richard Hirschman
Interpersonal Helping Skills Training: A Consultant's Guide
   Eldon K. Marshall and P. David Kurtz
SELECTED TOPICS:
An Introduction to Pediatric Psychology
   C. Eugene Walker, Michael D. Miller, and Rebecca Smith
Career and Life Planning: Tools for Practitioners
   Mary J. Heppner and P. Paul Heppner
The Clinician and Executive Assessment
   John H. Bone
An Annotated Glossary of Legal Terms for Mental Health Clinicians
   Samuel Knapp and Leon VandeCreek
Conducting the Initial Forensic Interview
   Kenneth Byrne
CLIENT HANDOUTS
Parents Are Forever: A Message about Divorce
   Association of Family Conciliation Courts
Plain Talk about Dealing with the Angry Child
   Luleen S. Anderson
INDEX OF VOLUMES 1, 2, 3, & 4